Fluid, Electrolyte, and Acid-Base Physiology

FOURTH EDITION

Fluid, Electrolyte, and Acid-Base Physiology

A Problem-Based Approach

Mitchell L. Halperin, MD, FRCPC
St. Michael's Hospital
University of Toronto
Toronto, Canada

Kamel S. Kamel, MD, FRCPC
St. Michael's Hospital
University of Toronto
Toronto, Canada

Marc B. Goldstein, MD, FRCPC
St. Michael's Hospital
University of Toronto
Toronto, Canada

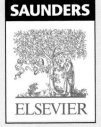

SAUNDERS

ELSEVIER

SAUNDERS
ELSEVIER

1600 John F. Kennedy Boulevard
Suite 1800
Philadelphia, PA 19103-2899

FLUID, ELECTROLYTE, AND ACID-BASE PHYSIOLOGY:
A PROBLEM-BASED APPROACH   ISBN: 978-1-4160-2442-2

Notice

Knowledge and best practice in this field are constantly changing. As new research
and experience broaden our knowledge, changes in practice, treatment, and drug
therapy may become necessary or appropriate. Readers are advised to check the
most current information provided (i) on procedures featured or (ii) by the man-
ufacturer of each product to be administered, to verify the recommended dose
or formula, the method and duration of administration, and contraindications.
It is the responsibility of the practitioners, relying on their own experience and
knowledge of the patient, to make diagnoses, to determine dosages and the best
treatment for each individual patient, and to take all appropriate safety precautions. To the fullest extent of the law, neither the Publisher nor the Authors assume
any liability for any injury and/or damage to persons or property arising out of or
related to any use of the material contained in this book.

The Publisher

Library of Congress Cataloging-in-Publication Data

Halperin, M. L. (Mitchell L.)
    Fluid, electrolyte, and acid-base physiology : a problem-based
approach / Mitchell L. Halperin, Kamel S. Kamel, Marc B. Goldstein. —4th ed.
        p. ; cm.
    Includes bibliographical references and index.
    ISBN 978-1-4160-2442-2
    1. Water-electrolyte imbalances. 2. Acid-base imbalances.
3. Water-electrolyte imbalances—Case studies. 4. Acid-base
imbalances—Case studies. I. Kamel, Kamel S. II. Goldstein, Marc B.
III. Title.
    [DNLM: 1. Acid-Base Imbalance—physiopathology. 2. Water-Electrolyte
Imbalance—physiopathology. 3. Acid-Base Imbalance—diagnosis.
4. Potassium—metabolism. 5. Water-Electrolyte Imbalance—diagnosis. WD
220 H195f 2009]
    RC630.H34 2009
    616.3′992—dc22

                                                    2008020019

Acquisitions Editor: Adrianne Brigido
Developmental Editor: Angela Norton
Project Manager: Bryan Hayward
Design Direction: Steven Stave

Printed in the United States of America

Last digit is the print number: 9 8 7 6 5 4 3 2 1

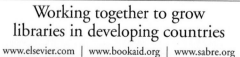

To Brenda, Marylin, and Ellen:
We are indeed extremely
grateful for your patience;
your strong,
unwavering support;
and your understanding.

Preface

There has been a long interval between this, the fourth edition of *Fluid, Electrolyte, and Acid-Base Physiology,* and the third edition of the book. This delay was caused, in part, by our decision to virtually rewrite the text, which resulted from our collaboration with Professor Kamel S. Kamel, whose input has had a major impact on the content of the current edition. A creative and critical individual who is highly motivated to understand "why things happen in biology," Dr. Kamel encouraged us to intensify our traditionally bold challenge of some of the classical thinking on physiologic processes. This iconoclastic emphasis we applied, for example, to our clinical approach to disorders that include abnormalities in acid-base, salt and water, and/or potassium homeostasis.

In each section of the book, we begin with a chapter in which we highlight principles of physiology and biochemistry. The greater part of each chapter describes more classical aspects, but with a focus that is often distinct from that of other textbooks. In the last part of each chapter, we turn our attention to integrative physiology, providing new insights that rely on a deductive analysis rather than on available experimental evidence (which has been known to impose certain constraints). Our goals here are to raise questions and to reject mere repetition of currently accepted dogma in favor of demonstrating a different way of thinking. Thus, although not every reader will agree with our explanations, they serve the essential function of indicating where controversies and uncertainties exist.

In Chapter 1, Principles of Acid-Base Physiology, for example, we encourage the reader to take a critical look at how we describe "good" and "bad" buffering of hydrogen ions. Because base balance is largely ignored in classical descriptions of acid-base balance in favor of a primary focus on acid balance, we have included a strong emphasis on base balance. We also stress that the renal contribution to acid-base balance must occur *without* sacrificing the need to minimize the risk of forming kidney stones (i.e., it is essential to maintain a urine pH close to 6 and to have a concentration of citrate that is close to that of calcium in the urine). In the final part of Chapter 1, we encourage the reader to think broadly by asking a question with far-reaching implications: *Why is the normal blood pH 7.40?* The analysis begins with issues that concern survival; moves to respiratory physiology, mitochondrial metabolism, and bone physiology that helps maintain an "ideal" concentration of ionized calcium in plasma; and then returns to the acid-base physiology during a sprint.

In the section on integrative physiology in Chapter 9, Sodium and Water Physiology, we emphasize regulation and also question many of the accepted dogmas about the urine concentrating mechanisms. We begin with a function/control analysis of regulation, aided by a new discovery of great importance: the absence of aquaporin 1 water channels in the thin descending limbs of the loop of Henle. The focus of regulation is on inhibitory control mechanisms that act on the medullary thick ascending limb of the loop of Henle, which leads us to propose a system of regulation that begins paradoxically with dilution of the medullary interstitial compartment (rather than with the so-called single effect in the loop of Henle). In this way, not only is the reader spared the discomfort of wrestling with the elusive (and incomplete or incorrect) countercurrent multiplier hypothesis. We present an alternative way to examine events that is consistent with the facts and allows for the regulation of the reabsorption of Na^+ and Cl^- in the medullary thick ascending limbs of the loop of Henle.

An emphasis on biochemistry contributes to the most important feature of this book: improvement of the reader's understanding by providing the rationale for the regulation of each major component of physiology. In Chapter 5, Ketoacidosis, we highlight principles of metabolic regulation. In this context, we look at the possible role for the uncoupling of oxidative phosphorylation in diabetic ketoacidosis, a discussion that leads us to consider the generation of reactive oxygen species and how the body reacts to this threat. Similarly, Chapter 6, Metabolic Acidosis, contains a strong biochemical component in its discussion of lactic acidosis and pyroglutamic acidosis.

By providing increased detail about regulation, we provide the background for the reader to deduce how a metabolic process is likely to be controlled, by asking the question *What is the primary function of this process?* An examination of the principal types of regulation, control by the quantity of enzyme, the concentration of substrate, and/or the concentration of its key product follows. Because changing the quantity of enzyme usually occurs after a considerable delay and because controls exerted by the concentration of substrate are designed primarily to remove a dangerous substrate, acute control is most often initiated by inhibitory influences, which commence when the concentration of the key product rises or falls sufficiently (see, e.g., the discussion of concentration of the urine in Chapter 9).

The final emphasis in this area is the examination of control mechanisms from a Paleolithic perspective, since control mechanisms to ensure survival were most likely to have developed during this period. Parenthetically, the pressures of modern times are unlikely to have a sufficiently large *control strength* to overcome these primitive inhibitory control mechanisms. In this regard, it is tempting to speculate, for example, that genes for obesity were "good" in Paleolithic times, when food could not be stored for prolonged periods. In contrast, because these genes decrease the human lifespan by predisposing individuals to disorders such as diabetes mellitus and cardiovascular disease, they are considered "bad" today. Admittedly, in various parts of the book, we allowed our excitement with respect to interesting ideas in biology to take us beyond a basic description of the topics.

Also featured prominently throughout the book is integrative physiology, and we encourage readers to take the time to examine the pathophysiology far beyond the area of discussion. For example, in the management of diabetic ketoacidosis, readers are challenged to think deeply about cerebral edema and to consider how the incidence of this serious complication can be minimized. Similarly, in the course of discussing the renal role in maintaining acid-base homeostasis, we integrate into the physiology the importance of minimizing the likelihood of renal stone formation (i.e., the importance of maintaining a urine pH close to 6 and a concentration of citrate that is close to that of calcium in the urine).

The clinical areas in the chapters also have a unique focus. We begin consistently with emergencies on first contact, with "Patient, please do not die!" as our theme. The anticipation of dangers that might be induced by our therapy and the strategies needed to prevent them from occurring ensue, followed by a diagnostic workup in which principles of physiology are applied to the bedside.

How to Use This Book

Although the fourth edition of *Fluid, Electrolyte, and Acid-Base Physiology* has been extensively rewritten, we remain committed to our basic philosophy of *learning by understanding*. An introduction and a series of objectives emphasize the focus of each chapter, and key points are highlighted in shaded boxes. To accommodate a diverse readership, we include margin notes, a series of questions with answers (in the form of discussions) at the end of each chapter, and for those who are interested in more in-depth information, there are sections on integrative physiology. The placement of these features is designed to minimize disruption of the flow of the text for the general reader. Each major group of disorders is preceded by a chapter on the relevant basic science, which readers can peruse before or after they turn to the clinical chapters. Those who want quick answers to vexing clinical challenges can consult the list of diagnostic flow charts (illustrations that provide the diagnostic approach for given disorders, which are indexed in their own table of contents, to permit easier access to them).

Retaining our commitment to the Socratic process of learning, we challenge readers with case studies followed by questions. By returning to the case study questions after they complete a chapter, readers can ensure that they have succeeded in learning the key points. Additional questions posed throughout the chapters should keep readers engaged and challenged.

Interconversion of Units

Because some readers will be more familiar with the International System of Units (SI units) and others will prefer the conventional units used in the United States, we provide the following conversion table. To convert units, multiply the reported value by the appropriate conversion factor.

PARAMETER	CONVENTIONAL TO SI UNITS	SI TO CONVENTIONAL UNITS
Na, K, Cl, HCO3	× 1 = mmol/L	× 1 = mEq/L
Ca	× 0.25 = mmol/L	× 4.0 = mg/dL
Urea	× 0.36 = mmol/L	× 2.8 = mg/dL
Creatinine	× 88.4 = µmol/L	× 0.0113 = mg/dL
Glucose	× 0.055 = mmol/L	× 18 = mg/dL
Albumin	× 10 = g/L	× 0.1 = mg/dL

List of Abbreviations

We have used a common form of abbreviation for the concentrations of electrolytes and metabolites in this book. This system is as follows:

P = Concentration of a substance in plasma; the subscript is the substance in question. Examples of the common ions follow:

P_{Na} = Concentration of sodium (Na^+) in plasma
P_K = Concentration of potassium (K^+) in plasma
P_{Cl} = Concentration of chloride (Cl^-) in plasma
P_{HCO3} = Concentration of bicarbonate (HCO_3^-) in plasma

Examples of the common metabolites follow:

$P_{Glucose}$ = Concentration of glucose in plasma
$P_{Ketoacid\ anions}$ = Concentration of ketoacid anions in plasma
P_{Urea} = Concentration of urea in plasma
$P_{Creatinine}$ = Concentration of creatinine in plasma
$P_{Albumin}$ = Concentration of albumin in plasma

U = Concentration of a substance in urine; the subscript is the substance in question. Examples of the common ions follow:

U_{Na} = Concentration of sodium (Na^+) in urine
U_K = Concentration of potassium (K^+) in urine
U_{Cl} = Concentration of chloride (Cl^-) in urine
U_{HCO3} = Concentration of bicarbonate (HCO_3^-) in urine

Examples of the common metabolites follow:

$U_{Glucose}$ = Concentration of glucose in urine
$U_{Ketoacid\ anions}$ = Concentration of ketoacid anions in urine
U_{Urea} = Concentration of urea in urine
$U_{Creatinine}$ = Concentration of creatinine in urine
$U_{Albumin}$ = Concentration of albumin in urine

FE = Fractional excretion, which is the ratio of their rate of excretion divided by the quantity filtered in a given time period. Examples of the common ions follow:

FE_{Na} = Concentration of sodium (Na^+) in urine
FE_K = Concentration of potassium (K^+) in urine
FE_{Cl} = Concentration of chloride (Cl^-) in urine
FE_{HCO3} = Concentration of bicarbonate (HCO_3^-) in urine

Additional abbreviations are defined at their first occurrence in each chapter.

Contents

List of Cases

List of Flow Charts

section one
Acid-Base

chapter 1

Principles of Acid-Base Physiology

Introduction

Our goal in this chapter is to describe the physiology of hydrogen ions (H^+). It quickly becomes apparent that many issues are difficult to understand unless one stops frequently to examine the "big picture." For example, based on the chemistry, H^+ are the smallest ions (atomic weight 1) and their concentration in body fluids is tiny (a millionfold lower than that of HCO_3^-, their major partner). On the other hand, H^+ are extremely powerful in that they are intimately involved in the capture of energy from fuel oxidation in a form that permits humans to survive by driving the production of adenosine triphosphate (ATP). In this context, the electrical charge on the proton is far more important than its chemical concentration.

DEFINITIONS

ACIDEMIA VERSUS ACIDOSIS
- Acidemia describes an increased concentration of H^+ in plasma.
- Acidosis is a process in which there is an addition of H^+ to the body; this may or may not cause acidemia.

ACIDS AND BASES
Acids are compounds that are capable of donating H^+; bases are compounds that are capable of accepting H^+. When an acid (HA) dissociates, it yields H^+ and its conjugate base or anions (A^-).

$$HA \rightleftharpoons H^+ + A^-$$

VALENCE
Valence is the net electrical charge on a compound or an element.

The concentration of H^+ in body fluids must be maintained in a very narrow range. If this concentration rises, H^+ will bind to very important compounds (proteins), and this changes their charge, shape, and possibly their function, with potentially dire consequences. Accordingly, it is not surprising that there is a H^+ removal process (the bicarbonate buffer system) that reacts with H^+ even if the concentration of H^+ is not elevated. The strategy that permits this H^+ removal system to function is that a low P_{CO_2} obliges H^+ to react with HCO_3^- (see equation at the end of this paragraph). Therefore, a high H^+ concentration stimulates breathing and thereby ensures that there is a lower concentration of CO_2 in each liter of alveolar air and hence in the arterial blood. As we stress throughout this chapter, the P_{CO_2} that is directly related to the majority of the bicarbonate buffer system is the P_{CO_2} in capillaries of skeletal muscle rather than the arterial P_{CO_2}; the former is revealed by measuring the brachial or femoral venous P_{CO_2}.

$$H^+ + HCO_3^- \rightleftharpoons CO_2 + H_2O$$

As shown in the preceding equation, this *safe* way to remove H^+ leads to a deficit of HCO_3^-. Accordingly, one must have another system that adds new HCO_3^- to the body as long as acidemia persists; this is the task of the kidney. The most important component is the excretion of ammonium ions (NH_4^+) because the kidney makes $NH_4^+ + HCO_3^-$ in the same metabolic process (see equation).

$$Glutamine \rightarrow 2\,NH_4^+ + 2\,HCO_3^-$$

The diet also produces an alkali load, which the kidneys eliminate. The chemical form to excrete this alkali must be such that it does not lead to the formation of precipitates in the urine. This is achieved by excreting alkali as a family of organic anions rather than as HCO_3^-, because the latter raises the urine pH, which may lead to the precipitation of calcium and phosphate. Hence, another theme in this chapter is that the H^+ concentration in the urine is regulated in a safe range to minimize the risk of forming kidney stones. Maintaining a urine pH of about 6 will permit a high rate of excretion of NH_4^+, and this diminishes the risk of precipitation or uric acid.

ABBREVIATIONS
ATP, adenosine triphosphate
ADP, adenosine diphosphate

ACID-BASE TERMS
Concentration of H^+: The normal value in plasma is 40 ± 2-nmol/L.
pH: This is the negative logarithm of the [H^+]; its normal value in plasma is 7.40 ± 0.02.
HCO_3^-: HCO_3^-, the conjugate base of carbonic acid, is the "H^+ remover" of the bicarbonate buffer system; its concentration in plasma is close to 25 mmol/L, but there are large fluctuations throughout the day (22 to 31 mmol/L).
P_{CO_2}: The major carbon waste product of fuel oxidation is carbon dioxide. Its concentration (or P_{CO_2}, which is its partial pressure) must be low in *venous* blood to ensure that the bicarbonate buffer system can minimize changes in the concentration of H^+. The normal arterial P_{CO_2} is 40 ± 2 mm Hg. The P_{CO_2} in blood draining skeletal muscles is ~6 mm Hg > the arterial P_{CO_2} at rest.

OBJECTIVES

■ To describe the major processes that lead to acid and to base balance.

ACHIEVE ACID BALANCE

1. *Production of acids:* This is revealed when *new* anions are found in the body and/or in excreted fluids.
2. *Buffering of H^+:* This should minimize H^+ binding to proteins in vital organs (i.e., the brain and the heart). To do so, H^+ must react with HCO_3^-. The vast majority of HCO_3^- in the body is in the interstitial and intracellular compartments of skeletal muscle. The key to achieving this function is to have a low P_{CO_2} in the arterial blood and in the capillaries of skeletal muscle.
3. *Kidneys add new HCO_3^- to the body:* This occurs primarily when NH_4^+ are excreted in the urine.

ACHIEVE BASE BALANCE

1. *Input of alkali:* This occurs primarily when fruit and vegetables are ingested because they contain the K^+ salts of organic acids that are metabolized to yield HCO_3^-.

2. *Elimination of alkali:* This occurs when a family of organic anions is excreted; it is a two-step process: (1) The alkali load stimulates the production of endogenous organic acids, the H^+ of which eliminate HCO_3^-, and (2) the kidneys excrete these organic anions with K^+ in the urine.

CREATE AN IDEAL URINE COMPOSITION
1. The kidneys maintain acid and base balance without increasing the risk of forming kidney stones because the urine pH is maintained close to 6.0.
2. Eliminating alkali via the excretion of organic anions (e.g., citrate) lowers the concentration of ionized calcium in the urine.

PART A
CHEMISTRY OF H⁺

H⁺ AND THE REGENERATION OF ATP

Two important properties allow H^+ to lead to the synthesis of ATP. First, H^+ can cross cell membranes only if there is a special H^+ hole (pore, channel) or transporter. Second, there is a special H^+ channel in the inner mitochondrial membrane that is coupled to ATP regeneration (Fig. 1-1). In more detail, H^+ are first actively pumped out of mitochondria using energy derived from the oxidation of fuels—this creates a very large electrical and a small chemical driving force for H^+ to enter mitochondria via a special H^+ channel. This couples the entry of H^+ and the system for the formation of ATP. It has two components, the H^+ channel and a H^+-ATP synthase, which converts ADP plus inorganic phosphate to ATP (this process is called *oxidative phosphorylation; see margin note*).

Uncoupling of oxidative phosphorylation

At times, when it is advantageous to have a faster rate of fuel oxidation, the body permits H^+ to enter mitochondria by a different H^+ route, one that is not linked to the conversion of ADP to ATP (see Chapter 5, page 145, for a possible role for uncoupler proteins in ketoacid formation).

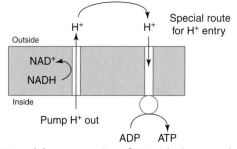

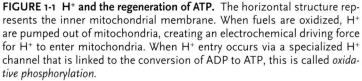

FIGURE 1-1 H⁺ and the regeneration of ATP. The horizontal structure represents the inner mitochondrial membrane. When fuels are oxidized, H^+ are pumped out of mitochondria, creating an electrochemical driving force for H^+ to enter mitochondria. When H^+ entry occurs via a specialized H^+ channel that is linked to the conversion of ADP to ATP, this is called *oxidative phosphorylation.*

H⁺-ATPase
- The H^+-ATPase catalyzes the reverse reaction of the synthesis of ATP; it pumps H^+ across membranes using the energy from the hydrolysis of ATP.
- This pump carries out an important function (i.e., removing hormones from their receptors in special compartments of the cell). It is also important for the renal excretion of NH_4^+.

ATP AND ADP
When work is performed, the energy is provided when the terminal high-energy phosphate bond in ATP is hydrolyzed; this results in the production of ADP (see equations).

$$Work + ATP \rightarrow ADP + Pi$$

$$ADP + Pi + O_2 \rightarrow ATP$$

(Pi, inorganic phosphate.)

ATP/ADP TURNOVER
- It is crucial to appreciate that the actual concentration of ATP is small (~5 mmol/L) and that of ADP is extremely tiny (~0.02 mmol/L), but their rate of *turnover* can be enormous.
- The weight of ATP in the brain is just a few grams (0.005 mol/L × molecular weight ~700 g/mol).
- The brain consumes close to 3 mmol of O_2 per minute or 4.5 moles of O_2 per day. Because 6 moles of ATP are formed per mole of O_2 consumed, the brain regenerates 27 moles of ATP per day (4.5 moles/day of O_2 × 6 ATP/O_2). Hence, the turnover of ATP in the brain is almost 20 kg (27 moles × mol wt ~700 g/1000 = 18.9 kg).

CONCENTRATION OF H⁺

Think of the concentration of H^+ from the following three perspectives.

1. In relation to the concentration of other ions in the extracellular fluid (ECF) compartment, the normal concentration of H^+ is extremely small (0.000040 mmol/L, or 40 ± 2 nmol/L). In fact, the concentration of its partner, HCO_3^- (~25 mmol/L), is almost one millionfold higher than that of H^+.

2. The concentration of H^+ should be examined relative to the affinity of H^+ for chemical groups on organic or inorganic compounds in the body. This comparison provides insights as to whether H^+ will be bound or remain free.

3. A quantitative perspective is obtained by examining the rates of production and removal of H^+. An enormous number of H^+ are formed and removed each day (>70,000,000 nmol versus the amount of free H^+ in the body at any one time [~3000 nmol]; *see margin note*); small discrepancies between the rate of formation versus the rate of removal of H^+ can result in major changes in concentration of H^+ if this is sustained.

AMOUNT OF H⁺ IN THE BODY
Extracellular fluid (ECF): 15 L × 40 nmol/L = 600 nmol
Intracellular fluid (ICF): 30 L × 80 nmol/L = 2400 nmol

BENEFIT OF H⁺ BINDING TO HEMOGLOBIN
When H^+ bind to hemoglobin in systemic capillaries, hemoglobin can off-load oxygen (O_2) at a higher P_{O_2} to improve the diffusion of O_2 to cells. In contrast, when H^+ dissociate from hemoglobin in the capillaries in the lungs (driven by a higher P_{O_2}), this leads to a greater uptake of O_2 from alveolar air for a given alveolar P_{O_2} (see Chapter 8, page 235 for more discussion of this topic).

RISKS ASSOCIATED WITH H⁺

Proteins have an "ideal" shape that maintains their structural integrity and permits them to carry out essential functions (enzymes, transporters, contractile elements). H^+ have a high affinity to bind to the amino acid histidine in proteins at the pH in cells. When the concentration of H^+ rises, these bound H^+ change the charge, shape, and possibly the function of these proteins. Accordingly, there must be a mechanism to keep the concentration of H^+ very low. Moreover, this mechanism must be very efficient because of the enormous daily turnover of H^+. Nevertheless, there are examples when this binding of H^+ to proteins has important biologic functions (*see margin note*).

QUESTIONS

(Discussions on page 34)

1-1 *In certain locations in the body, H^+ remain free and are not bound. What is the advantage in having such a high concentration of H^+?*

1-2 *What is the rationale for the statement, "In biology only weak acids kill"?*

PART B
DAILY BALANCE OF H⁺

PRODUCTION AND REMOVAL OF H⁺

- *H^+ production:* H^+ are generated when neutral compounds are converted to anions.
- *H^+ removal:* H^+ are removed when anions are converted to neutral products.

METABOLIC PROCESS
- A metabolic process analysis is a way of examining the overall impact of metabolism by considering only the substrates and the products while ignoring all intermediates (see Chapter 5, page 113 for more details).
- A metabolic process is made up of a series of metabolic pathways that carry out a specific function. They are usually located in more than one organ.
- Examples:

1. Diet fuel → ATP + CO_2 + H_2O

2. Diet fuel → storage compounds

3. Storage compounds → ATP + CO_2 + H_2O

To determine whether H^+ are produced or removed during metabolism, we use a "metabolic process" analysis (*see margin note*).

To establish the balance for H^+ in a metabolic process, one need only examine the valences of all of its substrates and products. If the sum of all of these valences is equal, there is no net production or removal of H^+. When the products of a metabolic process have a greater anionic charge than its substrates, H^+ are produced (e.g., incomplete oxidation of the major energy fuels, carbohydrates, and fats). Conversely, when the products of a metabolic process have a lesser anionic charge than its substrates, H^+ are removed.

In a typical Western diet, 85% of kilocalories are in the form of carbohydrates and fat. Although their metabolism produces a large amount of H^+, this is not a *net* H^+ load because subsequent metabolic steps remove these H^+ as fast as they are formed (see following equations for the oxidation of carbohydrates {glucose} and fat [triglycerides]). The only time there is a *net* H^+ load is when the complete oxidation of these fuels does not occur. Faster production of H^+ from oxidation of glucose occurs during hypoxia (see Chapter 6, page 165 for more discussion), whereas faster production of H^+ from neutral fat (triglycerides) occurs during states with a net lack of insulin (see Chapter 5, page 117 for more discussion).

$$\text{Glucose} \rightarrow \text{L-lactate}^- + H^+ \rightarrow CO_2 + H_2O$$
$$\text{Triglycerides} \rightarrow \text{ketoacid anions}^- + H^+ \rightarrow CO_2 + H_2O$$

The metabolism of certain dietary constituents leads to the addition of H^+ (e.g., proteins) or HCO_3^- (fruits and vegetables) to the body. A general overview of the components of the daily turnover of H^+ is illustrated in Figure 1-2. Notwithstanding, one must examine balances for *both* acids and bases to have a true assessment of H^+ balance.

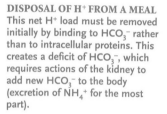

DISPOSAL OF H^+ FROM A MEAL
This net H^+ load must be removed initially by binding to HCO_3^- rather than to intracellular proteins. This creates a deficit of HCO_3^-, which requires actions of the kidney to add new HCO_3^- to the body (excretion of NH_4^+ for the most part).

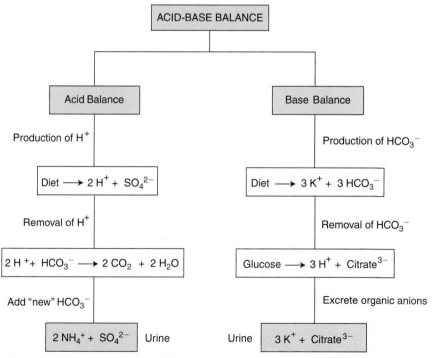

FIGURE 1-2 Overview of the daily turnover of H^+. Acid balance is shown on the *left*, and base balance is shown on the *right*. There are three components to acid balance: (1) There is the production of H^+, (2) HCO_3^- removes this H^+ load, and (3) the kidneys add new HCO_3^- to the body when NH_4^+ is excreted in the urine. There are also three components to base balance: (1) The alkali load of the diet is converted to HCO_3^- in the liver, (2) organic acids are formed in the liver and their H^+ remove HCO_3^-, and (3) the HCO_3^- load drives the excretion of these new organic anions along with the K^+ from the diet in the urine.

Acid balance

> - H^+ are produced when the valence of the products of a metabolic process have a net negative charge as compared to its substrates.

Oxidation of two classes of amino acids (cationic amino acids [e.g., lysine, arginine] and sulfur-containing amino acids [e.g., cysteine, methionine]) yields an H^+ load (Table 1-1). In contrast, H^+ are removed during the oxidation of anionic amino acids (e.g., glutamate, aspartate) because all of their products are electroneutral (urea, glucose, or $CO_2 + H_2O$). Because the number of cationic and anionic amino acids is close to equal in the amino acid mixture in beefsteak, the H^+ load that causes a deficit of HCO_3^- is mainly from the metabolism of sulfur-containing amino acids that yield H_2SO_4.

H_2SO_4

H^+ cannot be eliminated by metabolism of SO_4^{2-} to neutral end products (because no such pathway exists) or by being excreted bound to SO_4^{2-} in the urine (because of the low affinity of SO_4^{2-} for H^+). Hence, these H^+ must be titrated initially with HCO_3^- and, as a result, CO_2 is formed. Acid balance is restored when these SO_4^{2-} are excreted in the urine with an equivalent amount of NH_4^+ because new HCO_3^- is generated in this process (Fig. 1-3).

$H_2PO_4^-$

The diet consists primarily of intracellular organic phosphates in nucleic acids (RNA, DNA) and phospholipids, which are monovalent; hence, their accompanying cation is K^+. On metabolism to inorganic phosphate ($H_2PO_4^-$), which has a pK of 6.8, close to one bound H^+ is released at pH values in the body per $H_2PO_4^-$ formed (Fig. 1-4). These H^+ react with HCO_3^-, creating a deficit of HCO_3^- in the body. To achieve H^+ balance, new HCO_3^- must be regenerated. This occurs in two steps: (1) The kidney converts $CO_2 + H_2O$ to H^+ and HCO_3^-, and (2) these H^+ are secreted and bind to filtered HPO_4^{2-} anions. Thus $H_2PO_4^-$ is excreted when the urine pH is in the usual range (i.e., ~6) while HCO_3^- is added to the body. Hence, elimination of H^+ produced during the metabolism of organic phosphates does not require the excretion of NH_4^+.

TABLE 1-1 **H^+ FORMATION OR REMOVAL IN METABOLIC REACTIONS**

Reactions that yield H^+ (more net negative charge in products than in substrates)
Glucose $\rightarrow$ L-lactate$^-$ + H^+ (new L-lactate anions)
C_{16} fatty acid $\rightarrow$ 4 ketoacid anions$^-$ + 4 H^+ (new ketoacid anions)
Cysteine $\rightarrow$ urea + CO_2 + H_2O + 2 H^+ + SO_4^{2-} (new SO_4^{2-} anions)
Lysine$^+$ $\rightarrow$ urea + CO_2 + H_2O + H^+ (loss of cationic charge in lysine)
Reactions that remove H^+ (more net positive charge in products than in substrates)
L-Lactate$^-$ + H^+ $\rightarrow$ glucose (L-lactate anion removed)
Glutamate$^-$ $\rightarrow$ urea + CO_2 + H_2O
Citrate^{3-} + 3 H^+ $\rightarrow$ CO_2 + H_2O (citrate anion removed)
H^+ are neither produced nor removed in the following reactions
Glucose $\rightarrow$ glycogen or CO_2 + H_2O (neutrals to neutrals)
Triglyceride $\rightarrow$ CO_2 + H_2O (neutrals to neutrals)
Alanine $\rightarrow$ urea + glucose or CO_2 + H_2O (neutrals to neutrals)

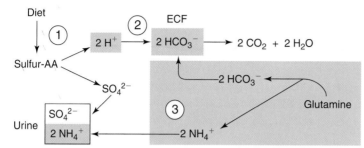

FIGURE 1-3 H⁺ balance during the metabolism of sulfur-containing amino acids. Renal events are represented in the *large shaded area*. When sulfur-containing amino acids are converted to SO_4^{2-} anions, H^+ are produced (*site 1*). H^+ react with HCO_3^-, and this produces a deficit of HCO_3^- in the body (*site 2*). To achieve H^+ balance, new HCO_3^- must be regenerated. Metabolism of the amino acid glutamine in cells of proximal tubules produces NH_4^+ and a dicarboxylate anion. HCO_3^- are added to the body when the anion is metabolized to a neutral end product and NH_4^+ is excreted in the urine with SO_4^{2-} anions (*site 3*).

Base balance

All the emphasis so far has been on the production and removal of H^+. The diet, however, also provides an alkali load that is produced during the metabolism of a variety of organic anions in fruit and vegetables (Fig. 1-5). Although it would have been very "nice" from a bookkeeping point of view to have these HCO_3^- titrate the H^+ load from H_2SO_4 produced during the metabolism of sulfur-containing amino acids, this occurs only to a minor extent. The advantage of not having the dietary alkali load titrate dietary acid becomes evident when the composition of the urine is examined in the context of minimizing the risk of kidney stone formation.

The site where dietary organic anions are first converted to HCO_3^- is the liver. This avoids having a potentially toxic anion enter the systemic circulation (e.g., citrate anions chelate ionized calcium in plasma; see Case 6-1, page 186). In response to the alkali load, endogenous acids are produced. Although many different organic acids are produced in the liver, the fate of their H^+ is similar—removal by HCO_3^-. To prevent the synthesis of HCO_3^- at a later time, these conjugate bases (e.g., citrate anions) are made into end products of metabolism by being excreted with K^+ in the urine (*see margin note*). As discussed later, the pH of cells of the proximal convoluted tubule

QUANTITIES
- Each day, 360 mEq of organic anions are filtered (glomerular filtration rate [GFR] of 180 L/day; [OA⁻] ~2 mEq/L). Of these anions, 90% are reabsorbed and ~10% are excreted.
- An alkali load diminishes the renal reabsorption of organic anions such as citrate and increases their excretion in the urine.

ABBREVIATION
OA, organic anions

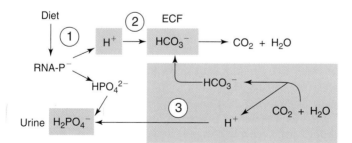

FIGURE 1-4 H⁺ balance during the metabolism of organic phosphates. Because dietary phosphate is an organic phosphate, it has a valence of −1 (derived mainly from phosphate in muscle cells). The product of its metabolism is divalent inorganic phosphate (HPO_4^{2-}) plus 1 H^+ (*site 1*). These H^+ remove HCO_3^- from the body (*site 2*). New HCO_3^- are regenerated when the kidney secretes H^+, which bind to filtered HPO_4^{2-} in the lumen of the nephron (*site 3; see large shaded area*).

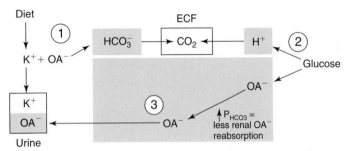

FIGURE 1-5 Overview of base balance. Base balance is achieved in three steps. The first is the production of HCO_3^- from dietary K^+ salts of organic anions in the liver (*site 1*). This is followed by the production of organic acids in the liver; their H^+ titrate these HCO_3^- (*site 2*). The renal component of the process is shown in the *large shaded area* (*site 3*). The organic anions are filtered and only partially reabsorbed by the kidney; hence, they are made into end products of metabolism by being excreted in the urine.

URINE CITRATE AS A WINDOW ON pH OF THE PROXIMAL TUBULE CELL
- When there is a low pH in cells of the proximal convoluted tubule, citrate is avidly reabsorbed and the urine is virtually citrate-free.
- A high intracellular pH in proximal convoluted tubule cells diminishes the reabsorption of citrate and thereby increases its excretion rate.

plays an important role in determining the rate of excretion of citrate (*see margin note*).

From an integrative physiology point of view, the elimination of dietary alkali in the form of organic anions has a number of advantages in terms of minimizing the risk of kidney stone formation. In more detail, it avoids the excretion of HCO_3^-; hence, the likelihood of kidney stones that form when the urine pH is too high (e.g., $CaHPO_4$). In addition, the elimination of this dietary alkali in the form of citrate anions lessens the likelihood of forming calcium-containing kidney stones because citrate anions chelate ionized calcium in the urine.

QUESTION

(Discussion on page 35)

1-3 *Does consumption of citrus fruit, which contains a large quantity of citric acid and its K^+ salt, cause a net acid and/or a net alkali load?*

BUFFERING OF H^+

- The most important goal of buffering is to minimize the binding of H^+ to intracellular proteins.

Binding of H^+ to proteins

The traditional view of the buffering of H^+ is "*proton*-centered" (i.e., it focuses solely on the concentration of H^+). It is based on the premise that H^+ are very dangerous; therefore, anything that minimizes a rise in their concentration is beneficial. Its weakness is that this view of buffering does not consider the price to pay to achieve this goal (e.g., a possible change in protein function). An argument to support this view is that a high concentration of H^+ may depress myocardial function. Notwithstanding, because a very high cardiac output is present during a sprint when the blood pH may be below 7.0, this conclusion should be questioned.

We emphasize a different interpretation and suggest that a "*brain protein*–centered" view of buffering of H^+ in the patient with metabolic acidosis may offer a better way to understand the pathophysiology, and it has important implications for therapy. The major tenet of this view is that the role of buffering is not simply to lower the concentration of H⁺ but, of even greater importance, to minimize the binding of H⁺ to proteins in cells of vital organs (e.g., the brain and the heart; see following equation). If H⁺ do not bind to proteins, these macromolecules maintain the normal charge and shape so that they can function in an optimal fashion as enzymes, transporters, contractile elements, and structural compounds.

$$H^+ + Protein^0 \rightleftharpoons H \bullet Protein^+$$

Bicarbonate buffer system

- This buffer system removes H⁺ without requiring a high concentration of H⁺.

Because the bicarbonate buffer system at pH 7.4 is very far displaced from its pK′ (pH ~ 6.1), it is not a typical chemical buffer. Rather, it becomes an effective way to remove H⁺ when there is a *low* P_{CO_2}, which "pulls" the bicarbonate buffer system equation to the right (see following equation). As a result, the concentration of H⁺ falls, which decreases the binding of H⁺ to proteins. In addition, the bicarbonate buffer system is capable of removing a large quantity of H⁺ because there is a large amount of HCO_3^- in the body (*see margin note*).

$$H^+ + HCO_3^- \rightleftharpoons H_2CO_3 \rightleftharpoons H_2O + CO_2 \rightarrow loss\ via\ lungs$$

QUANTITY OF BICARBONATE
IN THE BODY
ECF compartment: 25 mmol/L ×
15 L = 375 mmol
ICF compartment: 12.5 mmol/L ×
30 L = 375 mmol

What ensures that the bicarbonate buffer system and not the protein system will remove the bulk of the added H⁺?

- A low P_{CO_2} is a prerequisite for optimal function of the bicarbonate buffer system.

The bicarbonate buffer system can "outcompete" proteins for H⁺ removal because when ventilation is stimulated by acidemia, the arterial P_{CO_2} will be lower (Fig. 1-6). As a result, H⁺ reacts with HCO_3^- and the concentration of both reactants decreases in a 1:1 ratio (see earlier equation). Notwithstanding, the percentage of decline in the concentration of H⁺ is much larger than the fall in the P_{HCO3} as the former is close to a millionfold lower than the latter (*see margin note*).

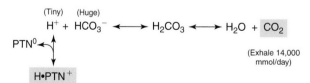

FIGURE 1-6 **Buffer systems.** Proteins in cells have an "ideal charge" (depicted as PTN⁰). Binding of H⁺ to these proteins increases their net positive charge (H•PTN⁺) and may compromise their function. Hence, the key principle is that new H⁺ must be removed by binding to HCO_3^- so that very few H⁺ can bind to proteins (PTN⁰) in cells. To force H⁺ to bind to HCO_3^-, the P_{CO_2} must fall in cells despite the fact that cells produce an enormous quantity of CO_2.

PHYSIOLOGY OF THE
BICARBONATE BUFFER SYSTEM
- Regulation of the bicarbonate buffer system (BBS) is by the capillary P_{CO_2}. This highlights the need to measure the brachial or femoral venous P_{CO_2} in patients with metabolic acidosis both to understand if the BBS removed H⁺ and to design therapy for that patient to improve the function of the BBS in skeletal muscle (i.e., lower the venous P_{CO_2} if the effective arterial blood volume is low).
- There is an important setting where it is advantageous not to remove H⁺ by the BBS because there will soon be a large and late H⁺ load: the metabolic buffering of H⁺ when L-lactic acid is produced in a sprint (see page 31 in this chapter).

Which P_{CO_2} is important for the bicarbonate buffer system to function optimally?

Arterial P_{CO_2}

> • The arterial P_{CO_2} reflects, but is not equal to, the P_{CO_2} in brain cells; it sets a minimum possible value for the P_{CO_2} in capillaries of all other organs in the body.

The only cells in the body that have the *same* P_{CO_2} as in arterial blood are the red blood cells that are located in the arterial blood volume. Therefore, the arterial P_{CO_2} does not reveal whether the bicarbonate buffer system has operated efficiently in the vast majority of the ICF and ECF compartments. Notwithstanding, the arterial P_{CO_2} sets the lower limit for the P_{CO_2} in capillaries. Furthermore, the arterial P_{CO_2} is important because it reflects the P_{CO_2} in brain cells but in an indirect fashion. In more detail, the rate of production of CO_2 in the brain is relatively constant because cerebral oxygen consumption does not vary appreciably. The brain produces 1 mmol CO_2 per mmol O_2 it consumes, as the brain oxidizes glucose as its primary fuel. In addition, the rate of blood flow to the brain undergoes only minimal variation throughout the day owing to autoregulation. Accordingly, the arterial P_{CO_2} reflects the P_{CO_2} in brain cells in the absence of a marked degree of contraction of the effective arterial blood volume during which the brain fails to autoregulate its rate of blood flow.

The process to lower the arterial P_{CO_2} begins with stimulation of the respiratory center in the brain. It is an ideal response because it ensures that the brain will always have an "ideal" P_{CO_2} in its ECF and ICF compartments so that there is only a minimal binding of H^+ to intracellular proteins during metabolic acidosis, which decreases possible detrimental effects on neuronal function (*see margin note*).

Capillary P_{CO_2}

The capillary P_{CO_2} is higher than the arterial P_{CO_2} because cells in the body consume O_2 and add CO_2 to their capillary blood. CO_2 diffuses rapidly because distances are short and time is not a limiting factor; thus, the P_{CO_2} in capillaries is virtually identical to the P_{CO_2} in cells *and* in the interstitial compartment of the ECF in a given region. Therefore, the capillary P_{CO_2} reveals whether the bicarbonate buffer system has operated efficiently in the vast majority of the ICF and ECF compartments in the body (Table 1-2). The capillary P_{CO_2} is influenced by arterial P_{CO_2} and the rate of addition of CO_2 to capillary blood in individual organs of the body. In more detail, if most of the oxygen in each liter of blood delivered to a certain area is consumed, the P_{CO_2} in its capillary blood rises appreciably (*see margin note*). There are two conditions is which most of the O_2 delivered in a liter of blood is consumed: (1) a rise in the rate of metabolism without a change in the rate of blood flow, or (2) a decrease in the rate of blood flow with no change in the rate of O_2 consumption.

Venous P_{CO_2}

Although the capillary P_{CO_2} reveals whether the bicarbonate buffer system has operated efficiently in the vast majority of the ICF and ECF compartments in the area drained by this capillary bed, one cannot measure it directly. The venous P_{CO_2}, however, closely reflects the

---

CONCENTRATION OF H^+ IN BRAIN CELLS
In response to acidemia, alveolar ventilation is stimulated and the arterial P_{CO_2} falls. Nevertheless, this cannot bring the pH in brain cells back to normal—otherwise there would not be a persisting stimulus to alveolar ventilation. Hence, there will always be a minimal degree of H^+ binding to proteins in brain cells during acidemia.

CO_2 ADDED PER LITER OF BLOOD FLOW
• Close to 3 mmol/min of O_2 are extracted in skeletal muscle, which receives close to 1 L/min of blood flow. This results in an average capillary P_{CO_2} that is 6 mm Hg higher than the arterial P_{CO_2}.
• When skeletal muscle cells extract more than 3 mmol O_2 per liter of blood flow, more CO_2 is added to each liter of capillary blood and its P_{CO_2} is higher. This compromises the effectiveness of the bicarbonate buffer system.

TABLE 1-2 **THE BLOOD P_{CO_2} AND ITS IMPLICATIONS FOR "BRAIN PROTEIN–CENTERED" BUFFERING OF H^+**

SITE OF SAMPLING	BBS BUFFERING	FUNCTIONAL IMPLICATIONS
• Arterial P_{CO_2}	• Reflects the P_{CO_2} in brain if the blood flow rate is autoregulated	• Assess alveolar ventilation • Sets the lower limit for the capillary P_{CO_2}
• Mixed venous P_{CO_2}	• Not really able to define site of H^+ buffering	• Cannot tell if H^+ are bound to brain proteins
• Brachial vein P_{CO_2}	• Reflects the P_{CO_2} in skeletal muscle cells and their interstitial compartment	• A low venous P_{CO_2} is needed to force H^+ to be buffered by HCO_3^- in muscle cells • Assess if H^+ are bound to proteins in the brain

BBS, bicarbonate buffer system.

capillary P_{CO_2} in its drainage bed. There is, however, one caveat—if an appreciable quantity of blood shunts from the arterial to the venous circulation and bypasses cells, this venous P_{CO_2} does not reflect the P_{CO_2} in the interstitial space and in cells in its drainage bed.

Which venous P_{CO_2} should be measured in clinical medicine to assess the effectiveness of the bicarbonate buffer system?

The focus should be on skeletal muscle because of its size—it is the organ with the largest content of HCO_3^- (Fig. 1-7). If this organ fails to remove the bulk of the H^+ load during metabolic acidosis, acidemia becomes more severe and the brain is forced to bind more H^+ to its intracellular proteins. Therefore, the P_{CO_2} should be measured in brachial or femoral venous blood to assess the effectiveness of the bicarbonate buffer system.

Failure of the bicarbonate buffer system

• The P_{CO_2} in venous blood is much higher than the arterial P_{CO_2} when more O_2 is extracted and thereby more CO_2 is added *per liter of blood flow*.

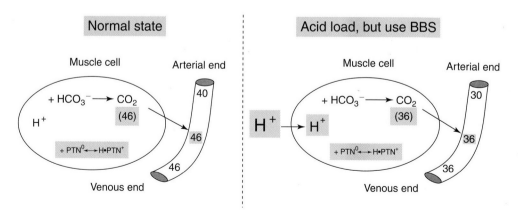

FIGURE 1-7 Effectiveness of the bicarbonate buffer system (BBS) in skeletal muscle. The *large oval* represents a skeletal muscle cell, and the *curved cylindrical structure* to its *right* represents its capillary. The normal state is shown on the *left*, and buffering of a H^+ load is shown on the *right*. Notice that a lower arterial P_{CO_2} favors the diffusion of CO_2 from cells into the capillary and that the venous P_{CO_2} is virtually equal to the P_{CO_2} in cells. Hence, new H^+ are forced to react with HCO_3^- in cells because the P_{CO_2} in cells has declined; of even greater importance, the concentration of H^+ in cells does not rise appreciably, and very few H^+ bind to proteins in cells.

AUTOREGULATION OF BLOOD FLOW TO THE BRAIN
When the effective arterial blood volume is very low, autoregulation of brain blood flow fails, and the P_{CO_2} in the jugular vein rises abruptly. As a result, the brain is not able to remove H^+ by its bicarbonate buffer system and more H^+ binds to its proteins, with potentially dire consequences.

The P_{CO_2} in venous blood draining skeletal muscle is much higher than the arterial P_{CO_2} in two circumstances. First, if more oxygen is consumed and the rate of blood flow does not rise by a commensurate amount (e.g., during vigorous exercise); second, if the rate of blood flow has decreased and there is no major decline in the rate of consumption of oxygen (Fig. 1-8). The main cause of failure of the bicarbonate buffer system in skeletal muscle is a very marked decline in its blood supply—this is present when metabolic acidosis is accompanied by a contracted effective arterial blood volume. As a result, the circulating H^+ concentration rises, which increases the H^+ burden for brain cells. As long as the blood flow to the brain is maintained by autoregulation, its venous P_{CO_2} does not rise and it can still use its bicarbonate buffer system (*see margin note*); nevertheless, this is not sufficient to prevent more H^+ from binding to its intracellular proteins with potential untoward effects.

In summary, patients with metabolic acidosis *and* a contracted ECF volume have a high P_{CO_2} in venous blood draining skeletal muscle, and therefore they fail to titrate a H^+ load with their bicarbonate buffer system in skeletal muscle. Hence, there is a much higher H^+ burden in their brain cells, with possible detrimental effects (e.g., mental status deterioration in patients with diabetic ketoacidosis and a contracted ECF volume). This high venous P_{CO_2} falls appreciably when sufficient saline is infused to improve hemodynamics. Hence, enough saline should be given to these patients to ensure that the P_{CO_2} in the brachial or femoral venous blood is not more than 10 mm Hg higher than the arterial P_{CO_2}.

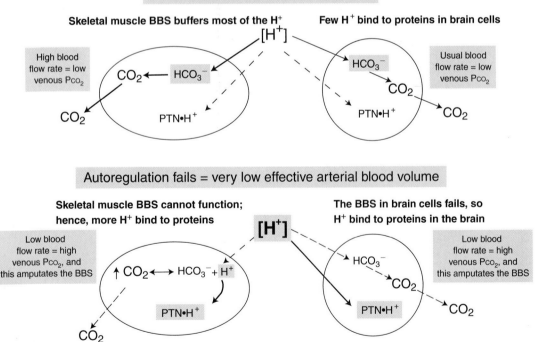

FIGURE 1-8 Buffering of H^+ in the brain in a patient with a contracted effective arterial blood volume. Buffering of H^+ in a patient with a normal effective arterial blood volume and thereby a low venous P_{CO_2} is depicted in the *top portion of the figure*. The vast majority of H^+ removal occurs by bicarbonate buffer system (BBS) in the interstitial space and in cells of skeletal muscles. Buffering of a H^+ load in a patient with a contracted effective arterial blood volume and thereby a high venous P_{CO_2} is depicted in the *bottom portion of the figure*. A high P_{CO_2} prevents H^+ removal by the bicarbonate buffer system in muscles. As a result, the circulating H^+ concentration rises, which increases the H^+ burden for brain cells.

Buffering of H+ during a sprint

Buffering of H^+ produced during a sprint requires a new H^+ acceptor that binds a large quantity of H^+ *without* causing the formation of CO_2. Although the bicarbonate buffer system cannot operate in this setting because the venous P_{CO_2} is very high, it does become very important just after exercise ceases (see the discussion of metabolic buffering in Part C, page 31).

QUESTIONS

(Discussions on page 35)

1-4 *Why is the L-lactic acidosis observed during cardiogenic shock so much more devastating than the L-lactic acidosis observed during a sprint if the $P_{L\text{-}lactate}$, arterial pH, and P_{HCO3} are identical?*

1-5 *The heart extracts close to 70% of the oxygen from each liter of coronary artery blood. What conclusions can you draw about buffering of H^+ in the heart? Might there be advantages owing to this high extraction of O_2 per liter of blood flow?*

ROLE OF THE KIDNEY IN ACID-BASE BALANCE

The kidneys must perform two tasks to maintain acid balance (for base balance, see page 9). First, the kidney must reabsorb virtually 100% of the filtered HCO_3^-; this is achieved primarily by H^+ secretion in the proximal convoluted tubule. Second, the kidneys must add new HCO_3^- to the body when there is an acid load; this is achieved principally by excreting more NH_4^+.

BASE BALANCE
This is described in more detail on page 9.

Reabsorption of filtered HCO_3^-

- The kidneys must prevent the excretion of the very large quantity of filtered HCO_3^-.
- This is primarily the task of the proximal convoluted tubule.
- Performing this function does not raise the quantity of HCO_3^- in the body.

It is important at the outset to recognize that a huge amount of HCO_3^- is filtered and reabsorbed each day (GFR of 180 L/day × P_{HCO3} 25 mmol/L = 4500 mmol). Approximately 90% of this HCO_3^- (~4000 mmol/day) is reabsorbed in an indirect fashion by the proximal convoluted tubule (Table 1-3).

Reabsorption of $NaHCO_3$ in the proximal convoluted tubule

The bulk of filtered HCO_3^- is reabsorbed in an indirect fashion in the proximal convoluted tubule as a result of H^+ secretion, which causes HCO_3^- to disappear from the tubular lumen and reappear in the blood (Fig. 1-9). There is no direct acid-base impact of this reabsorption of HCO_3^- because it does not result in a positive balance of HCO_3^-. Nevertheless, should this process fail, there is an initial loss of $NaHCO_3$ in the urine and the development of metabolic acidosis (this disorder is called *proximal renal tubular acidosis;* it is discussed on page 85 in Chapter 4).

CAUTION
The numbers are minimum estimates, as the last site of micropuncture in the proximal convoluted tubule is not the end of this nephron segment.

TABLE 1-3   QUANTITY OF HCO₃⁻ REABSORBED IN THE NEPHRON

The numbers are estimates for a 70-kg adult based on micropuncture data in rats (*see margin note*). We used a GFR of 180 L/day and a P_{HCO_3} of 25 mmol/L in the normal state and we used 10 mmol/L in the patient with metabolic acidosis. In the normal state, virtually 100% of filtered HCO_3^- is reabsorbed and about 90% of this occurs in the proximal convoluted tubule. In this example, we assumed that the filtered load of HCO_3^- during chronic metabolic acidosis was reduced to 1800 mmol/day. Although H^+ secretion in the proximal convoluted tubule is stimulated, there are too few H^+ acceptors in its lumen due to the low filtered load of HCO_3^- to permit high rates of proximal H^+ secretion.

EVENT	HCO_3^- (mmol/day)	
	NORMAL STATE	*METABOLIC ACIDOSIS*
Filtration	4500	1800
Reabsorption (total)	4495	1800
Proximal	4000	1620
Distal	495	180

The events in the proximal convoluted tubule result in conservation of both Na^+ and HCO_3^- and can be viewed as two parallel stories—one dealing with the reabsorption of Na^+ and the other dealing with the secretion of H^+.

The Na⁺ story

- This story has three components: (1) at the luminal membrane, (2) in the cell, and (3) at the basolateral membrane.
- In general, this process is regulated by signals related to the need to reabsorb Na^+ (higher when the effective arterial blood volume is low).

In the luminal membrane, Na^+ are transported on a special transporter that causes H^+ to move in the opposite direction (the Na^+/H^+ exchanger-3 [NHE-3]). This is an electroneutral event because for every Na^+ reabsorbed, one H^+ is secreted into the lumen. The intracellular component is the very low concentration of Na^+ inside proximal convoluted tubule cells, which provides the driving force to reabsorb Na^+ by NHE-3. The basolateral story focuses on the Na-K-ATPase in

ABBREVIATION
NBC, Na-bicarbonate cotransporter

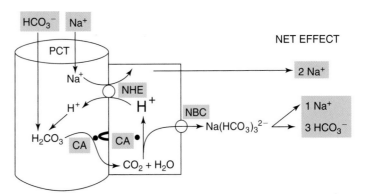

FIGURE 1-9   Reabsorption of NaHCO₃ in the proximal convoluted tubule. The components of the process of indirect reabsorption of $NaHCO_3$ are shown in the figure. H^+ secretion is largely via a renal-specific Na^+/H^+ exchanger (NHE). HCO_3^- exits the cell via Na-bicarbonate cotransporter (NBC). This process requires a luminal CA_{IV} and intracellular CA_{II}. CA, carbonic anhydrase.

the basolateral membrane. This ion transporter provides the driving force for the overall process—maintaining the low concentration of Na^+ in these cells; it transports three Na^+ out of the cell in conjunction with the entry of two K^+ (*see margin note*).

The H+ story

- This story has components in three locations: (1) at the luminal membrane, (2) in the cell, and (3) at the basolateral membrane.
- This process is limited by the filtered load of HCO_3^- and stimulated by a high concentration of H^+ in proximal convoluted tubular cells.

On the luminal membrane, there are two unique features: the NHE-3 and the luminal carbonic anhydrase (CA_{IV}). The latter enzyme hydrolyzes carbonic acid that is formed in the lumen to CO_2 and H_2O. The enzyme-catalyzed rate of hydrolysis of H_2CO_3 is virtually as fast as the rate of generation of H_2CO_3. If rapid catalysis did not occur, indirect reabsorption of HCO_3^- would be retarded and urinary excretion of HCO_3^- would ensue.

Inside the cell, there are two important components of the H^+ story. First, there is a different carbonic anhydrase enzyme (CA_{II}), which prevents the accumulation of OH^- (in other words, it makes HCO_3^- available inside cells). Second, there is a modifier site on NHE-3 to which H^+ bind, and this activates this ion exchanger.

On the basolateral membrane, there is a unique transport system for the exit of HCO_3^- from these cells, which permits an ion complex of one Na^+ and the equivalent of three HCO_3^- to exit as a divalent anion, $Na(HCO_3^-)_3^{2-}$—this is called the *Na-bicarbonate cotransporter*.

Regulation of proximal H+ secretion

- NHE-3 has a high capacity, but the "leaky" tight junctions in the proximal convoluted tubule prevent the generation of steep concentration gradients for H^+.
- Regulators of $NaHCO_3$ reabsorption in the proximal convoluted tubule include the filtered load of HCO_3^-, the luminal concentration of H^+; the intracellular concentration of H^+; stimuli for Na^+ reabsorption; and, importantly, the hormone angiotensin II.

The filtered load of HCO_3^-. The proximal convoluted tubule reabsorbs close to 90% of the 4500 mmol of HCO_3^- that are filtered each day (see Table 1-3). In this quantitative example, lowering the P_{HCO3} to 10 mmol/L during metabolic acidosis reduces the filtered load of HCO_3^- to 1800 mmol/day. Even though H^+ secretion in the proximal convoluted tubule will be stimulated by the high concentration of H^+ in proximal convoluted tubule cells, the reabsorption of $NaHCO_3$ must be reduced by more than 50% because there are no other luminal H^+ acceptors of quantitative importance (*see margin note*).

Luminal [H^+]. A higher concentration of H^+ in the lumen of the proximal convoluted tubule inhibits H^+ secretion in patients with metabolic acidosis (see Table 1-3). This same scenario occurs when a patient is given acetazolamide, a drug that inhibits luminal carbonic anhydrase. In this case, H^+ secretion is diminished because of the rise in the concentration of carbonic acid (H_2CO_3) and thereby H^+ in the lumen; hence, less of the filtered HCO_3^- is reclaimed.

NBC AND Na^+ TRANSPORT

- Close to 5% of Na^+ exits proximal convoluted tubule cells as a $Na(HCO_3^-)_3^{2-}$ ion complex, which moves passively down its electrochemical gradient. This Na^+ is reabsorbed without requiring the hydrolysis of ATP (it bypasses the Na-K-ATPase in proximal convoluted tubule cells).
- This process accounts for the reabsorption of 1260 mmol of Na^+ per day with a stoichiometry of 1 Na^+ per 3 HCO_3^- on the NBC exit step and a GFR of 180 L/day (i.e., 21 mmol of HCO_3^- per liter of GFR are reabsorbed in the proximal convoluted tubule).

NHE AND SECRETION OF NH_4^+ IN THE PROXIMAL CONVOLUTED TUBULE

- In a patient with chronic metabolic acidosis, there is less filtered HCO_3^-; hence this transporter has a diminished role in the reabsorption of $NaHCO_3$.
- NH_4^+ excretion is important in this setting. Activation of NHE-3 by intracellular acidosis should allow for the entry of more NH_4^+ into the lumen of the proximal convoluted tubule on this transporter.

Concentration of H^+ in proximal convoluted tubule cells. A rise in the concentration of H^+ in proximal convoluted tubule cells stimulates the secretion of H^+ for two reasons. First, the higher concentration of H^+ may cause more H^+ secretion by NHE-3. Second, and of greater importance, the binding of H^+ to a modifier site on NHE-3 activates this cation exchanger. As shown in Table 1-3, this activation is not very important during metabolic acidosis because of the small filtered load of HCO_3^-. Intracellular acidosis can help explain why the P_{HCO3} is elevated in patients with hypokalemia or chronic respiratory acidosis.

Avidity for the reabsorption of Na^+

- The most important regulator of the reabsorption of NaHCO$_3$ in the proximal convoluted tubule is angiotensin II.

When the effective arterial blood volume is contracted, proximal Na^+ reabsorption (and thereby H^+ secretion) rises because of the higher concentration of angiotensin II. In contrast, there is inhibition of the reabsorption of NaHCO$_3$ in the proximal convoluted tubule when NaHCO$_3$ is given. Part of the mechanism involves a fall in the concentration of H^+ in the ICF, which diminishes flux through the NHE-3 despite an increase in the number of H^+ acceptors in the lumen. In addition, the Na^+ load expands the effective arterial blood volume, leading to lower levels of angiotensin II and thereby inhibition of the reabsorption of NaHCO$_3$ in the proximal convoluted tubule. This seems to negate the direct effect of the increased filtered load of HCO_3^- to stimulate the reabsorption of HCO_3^- in the proximal convoluted tubule; thus, there is a prompt excretion of the excess HCO_3^-.

Minor factors. Hypercalcemia and/or a low parathyroid hormone level stimulate proximal H^+ secretion by NHE-3.

Renal threshold for reabsorption of HCO_3^-

- There is no renal threshold for the reabsorption of NaHCO$_3$ in the proximal convoluted tubule as long as the effective arterial blood volume is not expanded, which prevents a fall in the level of angiotensin II.

If there were a renal threshold for the reabsorption of NaHCO$_3$ in the kidney, it would represent the highest P_{HCO3} at which H^+ secretion is sufficient to "reclaim" virtually all of the filtered HCO_3^- (Fig. 1-10). Although this has been demonstrated experimentally, one must ask, "What were the conditions in these experiments?" The demonstration of this renal threshold for the reabsorption of NaHCO$_3$ occurs only when experimental animals or humans were given an infusion of NaHCO$_3$. This, however, expands the effective arterial blood volume owing to the load of Na^+, which lowers angiotensin II levels and thereby depresses the reabsorption of the extra NaHCO$_3$. In addition, the alkali load lowers the concentration of H^+ in proximal convoluted tubule cells and thereby removes this stimulator for NHE-3. In conclusion, because this does not represent a physiologic setting where the P_{HCO3} is increased, it may not be the correct experimental setting to define normal physiology.

In fact, there is no renal threshold for the reabsorption of NaHCO$_3$ when the P_{HCO3} is raised *without* expanding the effective arterial blood volume (see Fig. 1-10). The best example of this in normal

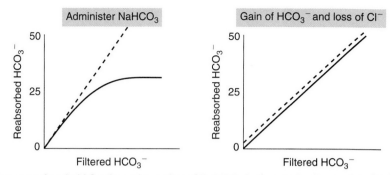

FIGURE 1-10 Apparent threshold for the reabsorption of NaHCO$_3$ in the proximal convoluted tubule. The quantity of HCO$_3^-$ filtered (GFR × P$_{HCO_3}$) is depicted on the x-axis, and the quantity of HCO$_3^-$ reabsorbed at this same GFR is depicted on the y-axis. The *dashed line* represents equality between filtered and reabsorbed HCO$_3^-$. When the P$_{HCO_3}$ is below the normal value, all the filtered HCO$_3^-$ are reabsorbed and there is no bicarbonaturia. As shown in the *left portion of the figure*, when the P$_{HCO_3}$ is increased *and* the effective arterial blood volume is expanded (administer NaHCO$_3$), virtually all of the extra filtered HCO$_3^-$ escape reabsorption in the proximal convoluted tubule (i.e., when the P$_{HCO_3}$ exceeds 25 to 30 mmol/L) and is excreted in the urine. In contrast, as shown in the *right portion of the figure*, when the P$_{HCO_3}$ is increased *without* expanding the effective arterial blood volume (e.g., deficit of HCl), virtually all of the extra filtered HCO$_3^-$ are reabsorbed in the proximal convoluted tubule and there is no bicarbonaturia despite a very high P$_{HCO_3}$. Hence, there is an apparent threshold for the reabsorption of NaHCO$_3$ in the proximal convoluted tubule only when the effective arterial blood volume is expanded.

physiology is the alkaline tide owing to secretion of HCl into the lumen of the stomach (see Fig. 7-2, page 198). Electroneutrality is maintained because there is an exchange of Cl$^-$ for HCO$_3^-$ in the ECF compartment with a 1:1 stoichiometry. After this occurs, the P$_{HCO3}$ rises toward 30 mmol/L, but the urine contains very little HCO$_3^-$. Hence, subjects on a typical Western diet have an effective arterial blood volume that leads to angiotensin II levels that are sufficient to stimulate proximal H$^+$ secretion despite the presence of alkalemia.

Reabsorption of NaHCO$_3$ in the loop of Henle

It is not clear how much filtered HCO$_3^-$ leaves the proximal convoluted tubule, but approximately 100 mmol enters the distal convoluted tubule. Hence close to 300 mmol of HCO$_3^-$ are removed either in the pars recta of the proximal tubule or in the thick ascending limb of the loop of Henle, where H$^+$ secretion is via an NHE-3 (*see margin note*).

Reabsorption of NaHCO$_3$ in the distal nephron

A small quantity of HCO$_3^-$ is delivered to the distal nephron in normal physiology, and this is reabsorbed when H$^+$ are secreted by an H$^+$-ATPase in the α-intercalated cells. When the H$^+$—derived from the dissociation of H$_2$O—are secreted, intracellular OH$^-$ are formed; OH$^-$ are removed instantaneously by combining with CO$_2$ to form HCO$_3^-$, and the process is catalyzed by carbonic anhydrase II. HCO$_3^-$ exit via a Cl$^-$/HCO$_3^-$ anion exchanger in the basolateral membrane.

Net acid excretion

- The net acid excretion formula ignores the major form of elimination of alkali (excretion of urinary organic anions or "potential HCO$_3^-$"); hence, it measures only the excretion of acid.

LIMITATION IN MICROPUNCTURE DATA
It is likely that greater than 90% of filtered HCO$_3^-$ is reabsorbed in the proximal convoluted tubule, as the last micropuncture site in the proximal convoluted tubule is on the cortical surface and there is a considerable length of this nephron segment before it reaches the renal medulla.

ABBREVIATION
NAE, net acid excretion

When faced with an acid or alkali load, the kidney must eliminate the resulting H^+ and/or the HCO_3^-. There is no bicarbonaturia, because the urine pH is usually close to 6 for most of the 24-hour period; thus, the NAE formula fails to consider the renal component of base balance (see Fig. 1-5). Therefore, this formula must be revised as described in the following equations:

$$\text{Old version: NAE} = U_{H2PO4} + U_{NH4} - U_{HCO3}$$

$$\text{Revised version: NAE} = U_{H2PO4} + U_{NH4} - U_{HCO3} - U_{OA}$$

Excretion of ammonium

- For every NH_4^+ excreted in the urine, one new HCO_3^- is added to the body.

The metabolic process that leads to acid balance is described in Figure 1-11. Oxidation of sulfur-containing amino acids in proteins results in a H^+ load. These H^+ are eliminated after reacting with HCO_3^- in the body. The kidneys must replace this deficit of HCO_3^- in the body by forming new HCO_3^- and NH_4^+ in a 1:1 stoichiometry and excreting the NH_4^+ in the urine to make it an end product of metabolism (*see margin note*; Fig. 1-12).

Quantities: The usual rate of excretion of NH_4^+ is 20 to 40 mmol/day. In chronic acidosis, the kidney can excrete close to 3 mmol NH_4^+/kg body weight/day in children and close to 200 mmol/day in adults.

Biochemistry of NH_4^+ production

The first segment of this pathway has three steps (glutamine entry into mitochondria of the proximal convoluted tubule, its hydrolysis by glutaminase to form glutamate, and the conversion of glutamate

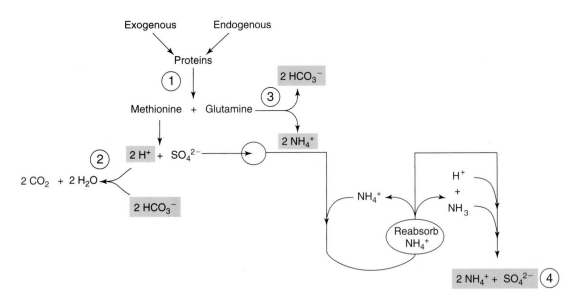

FIGURE 1-11 Overview of acid balance: Focus on NH_4^+. Sulfur-containing amino acids (e.g., methionine) are converted to H^+ and SO_4^{2-} anions (*site 1*). A deficit of HCO_3^- is created when these new H^+ react with HCO_3^- (*site 2*). Glutamine (*see margin note*) is converted to NH_4^+ and HCO_3^- in cells of the proximal convoluted tubule; the new HCO_3^- are added to the body to replace the deficit of HCO_3^- (*site 3*). NH_4^+ is made into an end product of this metabolic process by being excreted in the urine in equivalent amounts to SO_4^{2-} anions (*site 4*).

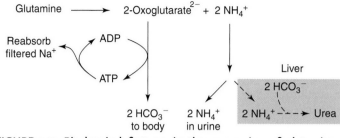

FIGURE 1-12 Biochemical features in the conversion of glutamine to HCO_3^- and NH_4^+. The metabolism of glutamine occurs in mitochondria of proximal convoluted tubule cells. Initially, glutamine is converted to 2-oxoglutarate^{2-} plus 2 NH_4^+. Two new HCO_3^- are generated and added to the body after the 2-oxoglutarate^{2-} is converted to neutral end products. To complete the process of HCO_3^- gain, NH_4^+ must be excreted in the urine; this prevents the conversion of NH_4^+ and HCO_3^- to urea in the liver (*shaded rectangle*).

to 2-oxoglutarate^{2-}). The final products are two NH_4^+ and the anion 2-oxoglutarate^{2-}. The next segment is the conversion of 2-oxoglutarate^{2-} to the neutral end products CO_2 and glucose, which results in the formation of the new HCO_3^-. All of these products plus the new HCO_3^- are added to the renal venous blood. The function of the last segment of the process is to maintain this gain of new HCO_3^-; it is accomplished when NH_4^+ is excreted in the urine (see Fig. 1-12).

Signals to augment the oxidation of glutamine in the proximal convoluted tubule

- Because the overall function of this metabolic process is to add *new* HCO_3^- to the body when there is a deficit of HCO_3^-, it is not surprising that it is activated when there is a chronic H^+ load.

The signal to synthesize more NH_4^+ (a sustained high concentration of H^+) has to be recognized in a location that is central to the overall process, in cells of the proximal convoluted tubule. Just how intracellular acidosis in the proximal convoluted tubule stimulates the production of NH_4^+ and HCO_3^- is not known with certainty. Possible mechanisms are listed in the margin (*see margin note*). Because a high H^+ concentration in proximal convoluted tubule cells is also present during chronic hypokalemia, renal ammoniagenesis is augmented in this setting (*see margin note*). The converse is also true; hyperkalemia is the most common cause of metabolic acidosis owing to a diminished rate of production of NH_4^+ because it causes a lower H^+ concentration (higher pH) in cells of the proximal convoluted tubule.

Selection of fuels for oxidation in the proximal convoluted tubule

- There is a lag period before glutamine is "selected" as the fuel for oxidation so that NH_4^+ production does not rise appreciably during acute and transient acidosis.

When there is a large H^+ load owing to the overproduction of L-lactic acid, there is no need to augment the oxidation of glutamine to eliminate this H^+ load because the L-lactate anion is metabolized

GLUTAMINE
- Glutamine is the most abundant amino acid in proteins; it can also be made in the liver and skeletal muscle; hence, its availability is not likely to limit renal ammoniagenesis except in severely malnourished patients.
- Glutamine is an important fuel for the intestinal tract, and it is also a precursor of reduced glutathione, an important mitochondrial antioxidant (see Chapter 6, page 183).

MECHANISMS THAT MAY STIMULATE NH_4^+ + HCO_3^- PRODUCTION DURING CHRONIC METABOLIC ACIDOSIS
- Enhanced entry of glutamine into mitochondria of proximal convoluted tubule cells
- Induction of the enzyme catalyzing the first step in glutamine metabolism (phosphate-dependent glutaminase)
- Activation of a key enzyme step (e.g., 2-oxoglutarate dehydrogenase)

HYPOKALEMIA AND NH_4^+ PRODUCTION IN THE KIDNEY
Electroneutrality must be present; you must consider the effects of the anion as well.
- *Low intake of K^+ and potential HCO_3^-:* This will increase the net input of H^+, and this stimulates NH_4^+ production.
- *Low intake of K^+ and $H_2PO_4^-$:* This will decrease the net input of H^+ and inhibit NH_4^+ production.
- *Deficit of KCl (e.g., chronic vomiting):* This leads to extracellular alkalemia (inhibits NH_4^+ production) and a high ICF [H^+] in the PCT (stimulates NH_4^+ production).

and new HCO_3^- are produced in a relatively short period of time. An obvious example of this scenario is the acute and severe L-lactic acidosis during a sprint. Hence, it is not surprising that the proximal convoluted tubule cells continue to oxidize fuels of carbohydrate (L-lactate$^-$) or fat origin (fatty acids) in this setting. This lag period offers a biologic advantage because the excretion of NH_4^+ would cause the catabolism of lean body mass to provide the substrate, glutamine, for NH_4^+ production during the first days of fasting.

Diminished availability of ADP decreases the conversion of glutamine to NH_4^+

• ADP is generated when renal work is performed.

Close to 80% of filtered Na^+ (~22,500 mmol/day) is reabsorbed in the entire proximal convoluted tubule, the site where NH_4^+ is formed. ADP is produced because this work requires the hydrolysis of the terminal high-energy phosphate bond in ATP (Fig. 1-13). Although several fuels may be oxidized to convert ADP back to ATP, glutamine is "selected" when a sustained acid load has caused a deficit in HCO_3^- and a higher concentration of H^+. In this context, the oxidation of glutamine occurs almost exclusively in mitochondria in proximal convoluted tubule cells because this nephron segment reabsorbs close to four fifths of filtered Na^+ and thereby generates enough ADP to permit a high rate of production of $NH_4^+ + HCO_3^-$ when needed. Hence, it is not surprising that there is limited amount of ADP when the GFR falls (see Fig. 1-13). This accounts for the low rate of excretion of NH_4^+ in patients with renal insufficiency, even in the presence of metabolic acidosis. If there were a high availability of alternate fuels

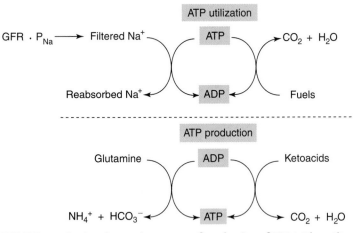

FIGURE 1-13 Setting the maximum rate of production of NH_4^+. The utilization of ATP in the proximal convoluted tubule is depicted in the *top portion of the figure*; ATP is used primarily to reabsorb filtered Na^+. This generates the ADP needed to permit the oxidation of glutamine to form NH_4^+ and new HCO_3^-, which is depicted in the *bottom portion of the figure*. Fuels compete for the available ADP; glutamine is selected in the presence of chronic metabolic acidosis and NH_4^+ production is increased, providing that there is enough filtered Na^+ to have high rates of ADP generation. In contrast, in the presence of high filtered loads of ketoacids, less glutamine can be oxidized as ketoacids compete for ADP. GFR, glomerular filtration rate.

competing with glutamine for this limited amount of ADP, there could be a lower than expected rate of production of NH_4^+. One example is the ketoacidosis of chronic starvation where the goal is to have equal excretion rates of NH_4^+ and ketoacid anions. This requires a lower rate of excretion of NH_4^+ in this setting of metabolic acidosis owing to the oxidation of some of the reabsorbed ketoacids (oxidation of β-hydroxybutyrate and glutamine require almost identical amounts of ADP; see Fig. 1-13).

Transport of NH_4^+ into the lumen of the proximal convoluted tubule

- In quantitative terms, virtually 100% of the NH_4^+ to be excreted is added to the luminal fluid that exits from the proximal convoluted tubule in the rat with chronic metabolic acidosis.

The major mechanism for the entry of NH_4^+ into the lumen of proximal convoluted tubule is by NH_4^+ replacing H^+ on NHE-3, thus making it a Na^+/NH_4^+ cation exchanger. The remainder of the NH_4^+ exits the kidney via the renal vein.

Medullary transfer of NH_4^+

This process has two components:
- The generation of a high concentration of NH_4^+/NH_3 in the renal medullary interstitium.
- The entry of NH_3 into the lumen of the medullary collecting duct.

This segment of the process to excrete NH_4^+ begins with the reabsorption of NH_4^+ in the medullary thick ascending limb (mTAL) of the loop of Henle. This is achieved by having NH_4^+ replace K^+ on the luminal Na^+, K^+, $2Cl^-$ cotransporter (NKCC-2). There is a second step for this segment of the process, the medullary recycling of NH_4^+. It begins with the movement of NH_4^+ from the interstitial compartment where the concentration of NH_4^+ is high into the thin descending limb of the loop of Henle, where the concentration of NH_4^+ is low. The net effect of this countercurrent exchange is to raise the concentrations of NH_4^+ and NH_3 deep in the medullary interstitial compartment (Fig. 1-14). The mechanism for the entry of NH_3 into the lumen of the medullary collecting duct is discussed later in this chapter.

Function of the shunt of NH_4^+ from the loop of Henle into the lumen of the medullary collecting duct

- The main function of this shunt process may *not* be to increase the excretion of NH_4^+.

There are two possible functions of this medullary shunt for NH_4^+/NH_3. First, it could enable the kidney to have a higher and possibly more precisely controlled rate of excretion of NH_4^+. Second, because the net effect of adding NH_3 into the lumen of the medullary collecting duct is a higher luminal pH as NH_3 is a H^+ acceptor, the function of this segment of the process may be to raise the pH in the luminal fluid in this nephron segment when H^+ secretion is stimulated. Each of these possible functions is discussed in more detail in the following paragraphs.

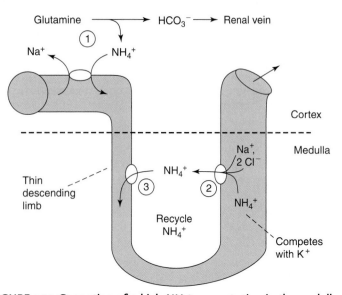

FIGURE 1-14 Generation of a high NH$_4^+$ concentration in the medullary interstitial compartment. The *U-shaped structure* is the loop of Henle. The first step in the process that raises the concentration of NH$_4^+$ in the medullary interstitial compartment is NH$_4^+$ production in the proximal convoluted tubule; NH$_4^+$ enter the lumen on the Na$^+$/H$^+$ exchanger (*site 1*). The second step is the reabsorption of NH$_4^+$ via the Na$^+$, K$^+$, 2 Cl$^-$ cotransporter (NKCC-2) in the medullary thick ascending limb (*site 2*). The third step is the entry of NH$_4^+$ ultimately into the descending limb of the loop of Henle, completing a countercurrent exchange of NH$_4^+$ (*site 3*).

The medullary shunt of NH$_4^+$/NH$_3$ allows for a higher rate of excretion of NH$_4^+$. The only data that speak to this issue are from experiments carried out in rats given a chronic acid load to augment the rate of excretion of NH$_4^+$. The data from these studies indicate that close to 75% of NH$_4^+$ excreted was added between the earliest and terminal segments of the cortical distal nephron. Therefore, the medullary shunt pathway for NH$_4^+$/NH$_3$ accounts for only a *small* proportion of the quantity of NH$_4^+$ excretion in the rat with metabolic acidosis (Fig. 1-15; *see margin note*).

APPLYING DATA FROM RATS TO HUMANS
- There is a danger in assuming that a human is a 70-kg rat. The major difference for the excretion of NH$_4^+$ is that the diet of the rat supplies 10-fold more alkali than acid. Therefore, the most important acid-base function in the rat is to excrete organic anions rather than to excrete NH$_4^+$.
- Humans with damage to their medullary interstitial compartment have a low rate of excretion of NH$_4^+$ and develop metabolic acidosis on this basis. Hence the medullary shunt for NH$_4^+$ may be important for NH$_4^+$ excretion in humans (see the discussion of Question 4-1, page 108).

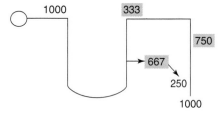

FIGURE 1-15 Quantitative analysis of NH$_4^+$ excretion: Role of the medullary shunt. The *stylized structure* represents a nephron. The data were derived from studies in rats with chronic metabolic acidosis. Of note, the amount of NH$_4^+$ added to the proximal convoluted tubule is similar to the amount of NH$_4^+$ excreted in the final urine (1000 nmol/min); two thirds of this NH$_4^+$ is reabsorbed in the medullary thick ascending limb. There is a large addition of NH$_4^+$ into luminal fluid in the cortical distal nephron so that most of the NH$_4^+$ to be excreted are present in fluid entering the medullary collecting duct (*see margin note*). Hence, the addition of NH$_4^+$ via the medullary shunt accounts for perhaps 20% to 25% of the NH$_4^+$ excreted in these rats.

The medullary shunt of NH₄⁺/NH₃ adjusts the urine pH to close to 6.0

> • The renal medullary shunt pathway for NH_3 is part of a system that maintains the urine pH close to 6.0, without compromising the ability of the kidney to achieve acid-base balance.

One way to evaluate the function of the medullary NH_4^+/NH_3 shunt pathway is to observe what happens to the rate of excretion of NH_4^+ and the urine pH when this NH_4^+ shunt pathway is inhibited. Blocking the reabsorption of NH_4^+ in the loop of Henle in *rats* with chronic metabolic acidosis and a high rate of excretion of NH_4^+ did decrease the medullary interstitial concentration of NH_4^+, but it did *not* decrease the rate of excretion of NH_4^+. Hence, this shunt process does not appear to be critical for excreting NH_4^+ in rats. On the other hand, when this shunt was inhibited, the urine pH declined significantly; this suggests that this medullary shunt pathway may be important to raise the urine pH toward 6.0 by adding NH_3 into the inner medullary collecting duct when distal H^+ secretion is stimulated by the metabolic acidosis. The secondary effect is to have a small increase in the net addition of NH_4^+ to the urine. Therefore, the renal medullary shunt pathway is part of a system that maintains the urine pH close to 6.0, without compromising the role of the kidney in achieving acid-base balance. In fact, the highest rates of NH_4^+ excretion in a person with *chronic* metabolic acidosis occur while the urine pH is close to 6.0 (Fig. 1-16).

Diffusion of NH₃ in the renal medulla: A more detailed examination

Historical note. The main process for transport of NH_3 into the lumen of the medullary collecting duct has been described as "diffusion trapping." In essence, distal H^+ secretion lowers the urine pH below 6.0, which decreases the NH_3 concentration in the lumen of the medullary collecting duct to permit more NH_3 to diffuse from the medullary interstitial compartment to the lumen of the medullary collecting duct. The question, however, is, "Does the decline in the NH_3 concentration

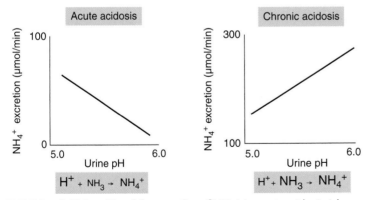

FIGURE 1-16 Urine pH and the excretion of NH₄⁺. In acute acidosis (shown on the *left*), distal H^+ secretion is stimulated, but there is a lag period before a high rate of ammoniagenesis is achieved. The urine pH is low (temporarily), and there is only a *modest* rise in the rate of NH_4^+ excretion. In chronic metabolic acidosis (shown on the *right*), both the H^+ secretory rate and the NH_3 availability are greatly increased. The increase in NH_3 availability is relatively larger than the increment in H^+ secretion. The medullary shunt of NH_4^+/NH_3 adjusts the urine pH to a value of close to 6.0.

Note the difference in scale for NH_4^+ on the y-axis of each panel.

TABLE 1-4 **CONCENTRATION DIFFERENCE OF NH$_3$ IN THE RENAL MEDULLARY INTERSTITIAL COMPARTMENT**

In this calculation, we assumed that the interstitial fluid pH is 7.3. The concentration of NH$_3$ in the interstitial compartment is set at 20 in arbitrary units. Lowering the urine pH toward 6.3 is the only pH range where there is a quantitatively important effect on the concentration difference for NH$_3$ between the interstitial compartment and the lumen of the medullary collecting duct. Said another way, only a large defect in distal H$^+$ secretion (a very high urine pH) would have a large negative impact on the rate of diffusion of NH$_3$ into the medullary collecting duct.

INTERSTITIAL [NH$_3$]	LUMEN		DIFFERENCE IN [NH$_3$]
	pH	*[NH$_3$]*	
20	7.0	10	10
20	6.7	5.0	15
20	6.3	2.0	18
20	6.0	1.0	19
20	5.0	0.1	19.9

ENTRY OF NH$_4^+$ INTO THE DISTAL NEPHRON

- The concentration of NH$_3$ in the renal medullary interstitial compartment is too low to support rapid rates of diffusion of NH$_3$.
- There are two proposed mechanisms for the entry of NH$_3$ into the lumen of the collecting duct, an NH$_4^+$/H$^+$ antiporter and an NH$_3$ channel. Notwithstanding, they achieve the same net result: the entry of NH$_3$ into the luminal compartment.
- There are two types of Rh glycoproteins, one on the basolateral and another on the luminal membrane of these cells that permit this function to occur. Cell membranes provide a barrier for the diffusion of NH$_3$. Perhaps a high luminal concentration of H$^+$ facilitates the opening of NH$_3$ channels.

DIFFUSION

The concentration difference for NH$_3$ depends for the most part on the concentration of NH$_3$ in the compartment from which its diffusion is initiated (the medullary interstitium) rather than where it ends up (the lumen of the medullary collecting duct) because only the former has a high concentration of NH$_3$. In fact, lowering the luminal NH$_3$ concentration from a *tiny* to a *very tiny* value does *not* have an important influence on the rate of diffusion of NH$_3$.

in the lumen of the medullary collecting duct aid the diffusion of NH$_3$ appreciably in the physiologic range of urine pH values (~6.0)?"

Synopsis of diffusion. Diffusion is a passive process. To be efficient, a large *concentration difference* is required for a substance to diffuse, the distance for diffusion must be short enough, and barriers for diffusion must be absent or bypassed. We examine the diffusion of NH$_3$ from the medullary interstitial compartment into the lumen of the medullary collecting duct in this context.

1. *Concentration difference for NH$_3$:* To understand whether distal H$^+$ secretion influences this *concentration difference* for NH$_3$ in the medullary collecting duct in a major way, one must examine this process in quantitative terms (*see margin note*). As shown in Table 1-4, lowering the luminal H$^+$ concentration by distal H$^+$ secretion is potentially important in this context if the urine pH is greater than 6.3. In contrast, lowering the urine pH below 6.3 has a progressively minor additional effect to raise the concentration difference for NH$_3$; hence, it cannot augment the driving force for NH$_3$ diffusion by an appreciable amount. Nevertheless, ongoing H$^+$ secretion must match the addition of NH$_3$ into the lumen of the medullary collecting duct to prevent a rise in the urine pH to a range that could compromise additional diffusion of NH$_3$.

2. *Remove the barrier for diffusion of NH$_3$:* There are two competing theories concerning the mechanism for the transfer NH$_3$ from the loop of Henle to the lumen of the medullary collecting duct (Fig. 1-17). The important physiologic fact is that the net effect is identical—the entry of NH$_3$ into the luminal fluid of the medullary collecting duct (*see margin note*).

QUESTION

(Discussion on page 36)

1-6 *What changes would you expect to find in the urine if the transport system that adds NH$_3$ to the lumen of the inner medullary collecting duct were to "disappear" (be knocked out) in a rodent?*

Secretion of H$^+$ in the distal nephron

H$^+$ pumps. H$^+$ pumps are located primarily in the luminal membranes of the mitochondria-rich α-intercalated cells (Fig. 1-18). There are two major H$^+$ pumps in this segment, an H$^+$-ATPase (in contrast to the NHE-3 of the proximal nephron) and an H$^+$/K$^+$-ATPase, but only

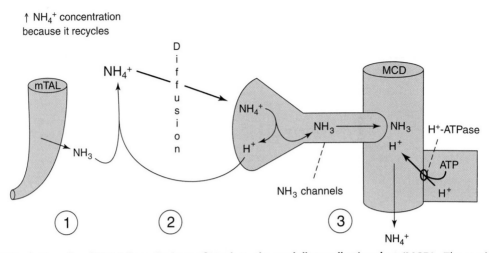

FIGURE 1-17 **Transfer of NH$_4^+$ from the loop of Henle to the medullary collecting duct (MCD).** The medullary thick ascending limb (mTAL) of the loop of Henle is shown to the *far left* and the MCD is shown to the *far right* The *funnel-shaped structure* in the MCD represents a NH$_3$ channel. The added NH$_3$ from the mTAL is converted to NH$_4^+$ by H$^+$ arriving from *site 3*. Recycling of NH$_4^+$ in the loop of Henle raises the concentration of NH$_4^+$ in the medullary interstitium (*site 1*) to aid its diffusion (*site 2*). NH$_4^+$ enters the hydrophobic mouth of the NH$_3$ channel, where it is converted to H$^+$ and NH$_3$ (*site 3*). This raises the local concentration of NH$_3$ close to 1000-fold and permits NH$_3$ to diffuse into the lumen of the MCD if this channel is open.

the former is particularly important from an acid-base perspective (*see margin note*). The H$^+$-ATPase helps reabsorb any remaining filtered HCO$_3^-$ and also excrete more NH$_4^+$ while the urine pH is 6.0. Secretion of H$^+$ is an electrogenic process that creates a lumen-positive voltage. Because the lumen of the medullary collecting duct can maintain only a very small positive voltage, either an anion (such as Cl$^-$) must be secreted along with H$^+$ or a cation (such as Na$^+$ or K$^+$) must be reabsorbed in the medullary collecting duct for H$^+$ secretion to continue.

Quantities. Distal nephron H$^+$ secretion is required to reabsorb close to 100 mmol of filtered HCO$_3^-$, and it may promote the net addition of close to 20 mmol/day of NH$_4^+$ (extrapolating data from the rat).

Urine pH and the excretion of NH$_4^+$

The urine pH is not useful to know how much NH$_4^+$ is being excreted when its value is less than 6.5. Notwithstanding, the urine pH is very useful to determine why the rate of excretion of NH$_4^+$

H$^+$/K$^+$-ATPase
The main function of the H$^+$/K$^+$-ATPase is to reabsorb K$^+$. This reabsorption of K$^+$ and secretion of H$^+$ requires that there be H$^+$ acceptors available in the lumen of the distal nephron. These luminal H$^+$ acceptors are HCO$_3^-$ and NH$_3$ because virtually all the HPO$_4^{2-}$ has already been converted to H$_2$PO$_4^-$ in upstream nephron segments.

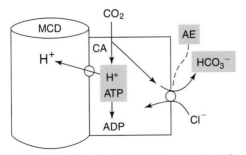

FIGURE 1-18 **Secretion of H$^+$ by the H$^+$-ATPase in the distal nephron.** The H$^+$-ATPase is located in the luminal membrane and in secretory vesicles (precursors or stores of H$^+$ pumps) inside α-intercalated cells. H$^+$ secretion generates a steep H$^+$ concentration gradient because the luminal membrane is relatively impermeable to H$^+$. The resulting HCO$_3^-$ exits the cell via a basolateral HCO$_3^-$/Cl$^-$ anion exchanger (AE).

is low. A low urine pH (~ 5.0) suggests that there is a limited availability of NH_3 in the medullary interstitial compartment (usually low production of NH_4^+ in the proximal convoluted tubule) or possibly a low NH_3 channel open probability in the medullary collecting duct. On the other hand, if the urine pH is unduly high (>6.5), the defect is in distal H^+ secretion or is one of an abnormally high secretion of HCO_3^-.

URINE pH AND KIDNEY STONE FORMATION

> • The elimination of an acid load via the excretion of NH_4^+ and of an alkali load via the excretion of alkali in the form of organic anions ensures that the urine pH can be maintained close to 6.0.

Acid and base balances must be achieved while maintaining an ideal composition of the urine to prevent the precipitation of solutes and minimize the risk of forming kidney stones. The central factors are the pH of the urine (Fig. 1-19) and the concentration of poorly soluble constituents in the urine. The safe range for the urine pH is close to 6.0 for most of the day.

Low urine pH and uric acid stones

A low urine pH increases the risk of forming uric acid kidney stones because uric acid is poorly soluble in water and its pK is close to 5.3 (see Fig. 1-19; *see margin note*). The medullary shunt for NH_3 minimizes the likelihood of having a urine pH of close to 5 because it provides the H^+ acceptor, NH_3, to adjust the urine pH to a value close to 6.0 when H^+ secretion in the distal nephron is stimulated by acidemia.

High urine pH and $CaHPO_4$ kidney stones

The excretion of dietary alkali in the form of organic anions minimizes the likelihood of having a urine pH that is in the high 6 range. Of greater importance, one of these urinary organic anions (i.e., citrate)

URINE pH AND NH_4^+ EXCRETION
A low urine pH is not a critical determinant of the rate of excretion of NH_4^+ in chronic metabolic acidosis. In fact, one can have the highest rate of excretion of NH_4^+ while the urine pH is close to 6.0.

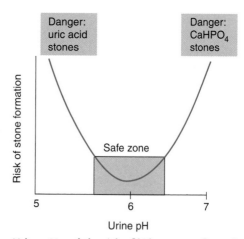

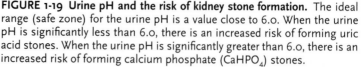

FIGURE 1-19 Urine pH and the risk of kidney stone formation. The ideal range (safe zone) for the urine pH is a value close to 6.0. When the urine pH is significantly less than 6.0, there is an increased risk of forming uric acid stones. When the urine pH is significantly greater than 6.0, there is an increased risk of forming calcium phosphate ($CaHPO_4$) stones.

chelates ionized calcium in the urine. Therefore, the combination of avoiding bicarbonaturia and the resulting high urine pH (which lowers the concentration of HPO_4^{2-}) as well as chelating ionized calcium with citrate helps minimize the risk of precipitation of $CaHPO_4$ in the renal papilla at the orifices of the inner medullary collecting duct.

PART C
INTEGRATIVE PHYSIOLOGY

WHY IS THE NORMAL BLOOD pH 7.40?

- We wondered why the blood pH in humans is 7.40 and not some other value.

Because there are three parameters in the bicarbonate buffer equation—the arterial pH, P_{CO_2}, and P_{HCO3}—once two have been set, the third must follow. To select the first one to examine, we decided to turn to the most important element for survival—the continued regeneration of ATP—and consider this process in Paleolithic times, when our control systems developed. To improve our analysis, we examined this process under maximum stress. ATP must be regenerated at extremely high rates during the "fight or flight" response; thus, our focus was on the need to supply O_2 at maximum rates. Because CO_2 is formed when O_2 is consumed, it seemed logical to start with the arterial P_{CO_2}. To deduce what would be the most appropriate value for the arterial P_{CO_2}, we ask the following questions.

What is needed to deliver the largest quantity of O_2 in blood?

- Ensure that hemoglobin in blood is fully saturated with O_2.

O_2 is poorly soluble in water, so it is transported in a bound form in blood (i.e., bound to hemoglobin in red blood cells). Hemoglobin is fully saturated with O_2 when the P_{O_2} in blood is 100 mm Hg. Therefore, the P_{O_2} in alveolar air should be very close to 100 mm Hg at *all* times.

What is needed to have a P_{O_2} of 100 mm Hg in alveolar air?

- Do not extract *more than* one third of the O_2 from each liter of inspired air.

The content of O_2 in air is directly proportional to its P_{O_2} because there are no bound forms of O_2 in air (Fig. 1-20). The P_{O_2} of humidified air is 150 mm Hg (*see margin note*). Therefore, after extracting one third of the oxygen in inspired air, the P_{O_2} in alveolar air is 100 mm Hg (*see margin note*).

What is the relationship between O_2 consumption and CO_2 production?

- To maintain an alveolar P_{O_2} of 100 mm Hg, the P_{CO_2} must be 40 mm Hg in alveolar air and thus in the arterial blood.

CONCENTRATION OF O_2 IN AIR
Air is 21% O_2, and the water vapor pressure at 37° C is 47 mm Hg. Because the atmospheric pressure is about 760 mm Hg, the P_{O_2} is about 150 mm Hg (0.21 × [760 – 47 mm Hg]).

P_{O_2} OF ALVEOLAR AIR DURING VIGOROUS EXERCISE
- When the rate of consumption of O_2 rises, many more liters of air must be inspired per minute to ensure that the P_{O_2} in alveoli *continues* to be close to 100 mm Hg (extract only one third of the O_2 from each liter of inspired air). In fact, the capacity to breathe must greatly exceed the maximum cardiac output.
- If more than one third of the O_2 is extracted in the lungs, the P_{O_2} falls in alveolar air and thus each liter of arterial blood carries less O_2 because its P_{O_2} is lower.

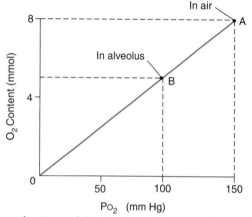

FIGURE 1-20 The Po$_2$ and the content of O$_2$ in one liter of air. The *top dashed line* represents inspired air with its Po$_2$ of 150 mm Hg and its O$_2$ concentration of 8 mmol/L (*point A*). In the alveolus, the Po$_2$ of air is 100 mm Hg if one third of the content of O$_2$ in air is extracted in the lungs (*point B*).

RESPIRATORY QUOTIENT
The ratio of CO$_2$ produced to O$_2$ consumed is called the *RQ*.
- When carbohydrates are oxidized, the RQ is 1.0.
  $C_6H_{12}O_6 + 6 O_2 \rightarrow 6 CO_2 + 6 H_2O$
- When fatty acids are oxidized, the RQ is 0.7.
  $C_{16}H_{32}O_2 + 23 O_2 \rightarrow 16 CO_2 + 16 H_2O$
- When a typical Western diet is consumed, the RQ is close to 0.8 because of the mixture of fat and carbohydrate in the diet.
- Because the brain oxidizes glucose as its primary fuel, its RQ is 1.0.

The ratio of oxygen consumption and CO$_2$ production is called the *respiratory quotient* (RQ). When a typical Western diet is consumed, the RQ is close to 0.8 (*see margin note*). Thus, the rise in the Pco$_2$ in the alveolar air is 0.8 times the fall in its Po$_2$. When one third of the content of oxygen in alveolar air is extracted, the Pco$_2$ in alveolar air rises by 40 mm Hg (RQ of 0.8 × 50 mm Hg). *This means that the Pco$_2$ in arterial blood is 40 mm Hg.*

What is the consequence of having an arterial Pco$_2$ at 40 mm Hg?

- Regulation of alveolar ventilation is required to maintain a Pco$_2$ of 40 mm Hg in arterial blood.

One can anticipate that it is necessary to have control mechanisms to ensure that the Pco$_2$ in arterial blood remains very close to 40 mm Hg—this is achieved because the arterial Pco$_2$ is a regulator of alveolar ventilation. Nevertheless, the controls described so far do not indicate how to regulate the blood pH. To understand the possibilities, recognize that there are two variables remaining. Hence, either the pH or the P$_{HCO3}$ must be regulated to determine the value of the third parameter in the bicarbonate buffer system (see following equation). We cannot determine with certainty which one it is, but we explore this issue further by asking the following question.

$$H^+ + HCO_3^- \rightleftharpoons H_2CO_3 \rightleftharpoons CO_2 + H_2O$$

What is an ideal P$_{HCO3}$?

- If function is known, controls can be deduced.
- An obvious role of HCO$_3^-$ is in the buffering of H$^+$; a less obvious role is to ensure that the concentration of ionized calcium in the ECF equals that of divalent inorganic phosphate.

The following issues are important to select the ideal P_{HCO3}. First, the P_{HCO3} should be as high as possible to remove the H^+ load during the recovery period of vigorous exercise. Second, the P_{HCO3} cannot be too high because this will increase the concentration of carbonate (CO_3^{2-}) and lead to a lower concentration of ionized Ca^{2+}, owing to precipitation of calcium carbonate ($CaCO_3$) in the ECF compartment. Thus, when the P_{HCO3} is 25 mmol/L, the concentration of ionized Ca^{2+} will be 1.2 mmol/L (*see margin note*).

For optimal bone turnover, it is advantageous to have near-equal concentrations of ionized Ca^{2+} and HPO_4^{2-}. Since the pH is 7.4 in the ECF compartment and four fifths of total inorganic phosphate is in the form of HPO_4^{2-}, the total inorganic phosphate should be close to 1.5 mmol/L to achieve this stoichiometry (1.2 mmol/L/0.8).

What conclusions can be drawn?

The normal values for the concentrations of H^+ (pH), P_{CO_2}, and P_{HCO3} are 40 nmol/L (7.40), 40 mm Hg, and 25 mmol/L, respectively, and this has several advantages. The P_{CO_2} is likely to be dictated by considerations related to O_2 transport. To have a high concentration of HCO_3^-, but also one that produces the ideal ionized Ca^{2+} concentration in the ECF compartment, the P_{HCO3} should be close to 25 mmol/L. Accordingly, this leads to a concentration of H^+ of 40 nmol/L (pH 7.40). This concentration of H^+ allows a certain number of H^+ to bind to the receptors for hormones on the exterior surface of cells. If the concentration of H^+ is significantly higher, hormones such as adrenaline and insulin, which have very important functions, will bind less well to their specific receptors.

METABOLIC BUFFERING OF H⁺ DURING A SPRINT

There are four phases of ATP regeneration during a sprint, and each is associated with a very large flux of H^+. In a broader perspective, skeletal muscle cells must deal with these large inputs and outputs of H^+ without compromising the functions of other organs in the body, especially those that are essential for survival (e.g., the brain and the heart).

Acid-base changes in a sprint

A synopsis of these events is provided in the box that follows:

> **Alkaline phase**
> - *Production of alkali*: When phosphocreatine is converted to creatine and HPO_4^{2-}, and half of the HPO_4^{2-} is converted to $H_2PO_4^-$, there is a net removal H^+ (i.e., a gain of alkali; *see margin note*).
> - *Removal of this alkali load*: The source of H^+ to remove this alkali is mainly nonbicarbonate buffers (e.g., carnosine). In addition, some HCO_3^- is exported from muscle cells (along with K^+).
>
> **Acid phase**
> - *Production of H^+*: When work is performed, the energy is supplied when ATP^{4-} is converted to $ADP^{3-} + HPO_4^{2-}$. Accumulation of ADP^{3-} drives anaerobic glycolysis (i.e., conversion of

glucose to two L-lactate anions plus ATP^{4-}). Nevertheless, the quantity of these adenine nucleotides is very small relative to the turnover of ATP^{4-}. The sum of these events is the net addition of one H^+ per L-lactate anion, but the protons come from the hydrolysis of ATP^{4-}.

- *Removal of the H^+ load*: The bicarbonate buffer system in skeletal muscle cannot remove H^+ during vigorous exercise because the P_{CO_2} in its capillary blood is high (owing to extraction of the vast majority of O_2 in each liter of blood flow and its subsequent conversion to CO_2). Hence, muscle cells must have abundant nonbicarbonate buffers to remove these H^+ in the acidosis phase of a sprint; the H^+ acceptors are HPO_4^{2-} and proton-free histidines in carnosine and in proteins.
- When the H^+ load is very high, the concentration of H^+ rises, and this forces additional H^+ to bind to proteins, which forces cessation of exercise.

Recovery phase

- During the recovery from vigorous exercise, there is a sudden, large H^+ load produced during the regeneration of phosphocreatine^{2-}. At this time, the bicarbonate buffer system must be recruited to remove H^+, and it does so when there is a fall in the P_{CO_2} in the capillary blood of muscle.

The alkaline phase of ischemic exercise

Hydrolysis of phosphocreatine (P-Cr^{2-})

The alkaline phase is initiated by muscular work in which ATP^{4-} is converted to ADP^{3-} plus HPO_4^{2-} (equation 1). Although H^+ are generated in this reaction, the important biologic consequence is the accumulation of ADP^{3-}, as this drives the hydrolysis of phosphocreatine^{2-} (equation 2). Adding equations 1 and 2 reveals that the net result is simply a stoichiometric conversion of phosphocreatine^{2-} to creatine^0 plus HPO_4^{2-}. Of note, there is no net production or removal of H^+ up to this point.

$$ATP^{4-} \rightarrow ADP^{3-} + HPO_4^{2-} + H^+ \tag{1}$$
$$ADP^{3-} + \text{phosphocreatine}^{2-} + H^+ \rightarrow ATP^{4-} + \text{creatine}^0 \tag{2}$$

There are three points to stress concerning the biochemistry of the hydrolysis of phosphocreatine^{2-}. First, the reaction is catalyzed by creatine kinase, an enzyme that has a very high activity, which allows its substrates and products to be interconverted at an extremely rapid rate. In other words, if there is a large rise in the concentration of one of its substrates, this will cause an enormous conversion of the other substrate to its products. Hence, as soon as the concentration of ADP^{3-} rises (and it rises enormously because the concentration of ADP^{3-} is so low in cells), phosphocreatine^{2-} is converted to ATP^{4-} plus creatine^0 (equation 2). Second, since the substrates of this reaction have a greater negative valence than its products, H^+ are consumed. Third, since the quantity of phosphocreatine^{2-} is very large (~25 mmol/kg skeletal muscle), there is an enormous production of HPO_4^{2-} (before exercise, the total HPO_4^{2-} and $H_2PO_4^-$ is ~4 mmol/L, and their concentrations are almost equal).

Removal of surplus HPO_4^{2-}, the donation of H^+ from carnosine

Since the cell pH is close to the pK for the phosphate buffer system, close to half of the HPO_4^{2-} formed from phosphocreatine^{2-} will be converted to $H_2PO_4^-$ (equation 3). For this to occur, a large source of H^+ is needed, and this comes from nonbicarbonate buffers as they donate H^+ when the concentration of H^+ declines (equation 4). The major donor of H^+ is those histidines, which have bound H^+ at the ICF pH. There are two sources of histidine, carnosine and proteins; carnosine is particularly abundant in skeletal muscle (*see margin note*). The equations describing the sequence of events that lead to alkalinization of skeletal muscle are the sum of equations 1, 2, 3, and 4. Note that there is now a much larger number of histidines without H^+ bound to them and a lower concentration of H^+ in skeletal muscle cells at the end of the phosphocreatine^{2-} hydrolysis stage of exercise, resulting in a large pool of potential H^+ acceptors.

$$HPO_4^{2-} + H^- \rightarrow H_2PO_4^{2-} \tag{3}$$

$$H \bullet Histidine^+ \rightarrow H^+ + histidine^0 \text{(a site for binding of future } H^+) \tag{4}$$

EXTRA HISTIDINE BUFFERS IN SKELETAL MUSCLE
- To minimize the number of H^+ that bind to histidine residues in proteins in the final phase of the sprint, these cells have "extra" histidines in an uncharged form—a dipeptide of β-alanine and histidine, called *carnosine*.
- The concentration of carnosine is high in skeletal muscle cells (~25 mmol/kg), which makes it an important buffer in these cells.

Acid phase of the sprint

There are two points to recognize in this stage of a sprint. First, when work is performed, ATP^{4-} is converted to ADP^{3-} (equation 5); the accumulation of ADP^{3-} initiates the conversion of glycosyl units of glycogen to L-lactate anions (equation 6). The sum of equations 5 and 6 causes the formation of a large H^+ load, which is generated when ATP^{4-} is converted to ADP^{3-}.

$$2\,ATP^{4-} \rightarrow 2\,ADP^{3-} + 2HPO_4^{2-} + 2\,H^+ \text{ (initiated by work)} \tag{5}$$

$$\text{"Glucose"} + 2\,ADP^{3-} + 2\,HPO_4^{2-} \rightarrow 2\,ATP^{4-} + 2\,L\text{-lactate}^- \tag{6}$$

The second issue concerns the fate of these H^+. The bicarbonate buffer system of skeletal muscle cannot remove many H^+ at this time because virtually all of the O_2 in each liter of blood in skeletal muscle capillaries is converted to CO_2, and this results in a high capillary and ICF P_{CO_2}, which prevents H^+ removal by the bicarbonate buffer system. Therefore, these H^+ will react quickly with histidines that had donated their H^+, and the driving force for this binding of H^+ is a rise in the concentration of H^+ in skeletal muscle cells. Because anaerobic glycolysis continues to occur at a very rapid rate, carnosine and the remaining HPO_4^{2-} must continue to remove some of these new H^+. Eventually, however, the concentration of H^+ will rise dramatically (pH falls), and this forces H^+ to bind to intracellular proteins, which may have deleterious effects (e.g., inhibition of phosphofructokinase-1, thereby diminishing the flux in glycolysis and the regeneration of ATP). Therefore, the subject is forced to stop running.

Recovery from the sprint, an important role for the bicarbonate buffer system

- This change in bicarbonate buffer availability is due to a large fall in the P_{CO_2} in capillaries of skeletal muscle.

When the sprint is over, there is no longer a need for a large regeneration of ATP, and the consumption of O_2 by muscle declines somewhat, yet there is still a large blood flow rate. Moreover, the runner is hyperventilating because of the acidemia and the continued adrenergic drive. As a result, there is a marked fall in the P_{CO_2} in capillary blood. When creatine^0 is converted back to phosphocreatine^{2-}, H^+ are released (*see margin note*). Of great importance, the bicarbonate buffer system can now operate effectively in skeletal muscle cells and

CONCENTRATIONS OF PHOSPHOCREATINE AND HCO$_3^-$
It is more than a coincidence that the concentration of phosphocreatine is double that of HCO$_3^-$ in skeletal muscle cells.

in its interstitial fluid to remove enough of these H^+ to avoid cell damage by this very large H^+ load.

QUESTIONS

(Discussion on pages 36 and 37)

1-7   *What is the major function of phosphocreatine in aerobic exercise?*

1-8   *Examine the data in Figure 1-22 for changes in the concentrations of phosphocreatine^{2-} and H^+ in skeletal muscle before and after performing vigorous aerobic exercise.*

   A   *Why did the ICF pH fall at the end of ischemic exercise?*

   B   *Why did the ICF pH not fall when phosphocreatine^{2-} was synthesized in the first 15 seconds of recovery?*

   C   *Why did the ICF pH rise between 30 and 45 seconds of recovery?*

DISCUSSION OF QUESTIONS

1-1   *In certain locations in the body, H^+ remain free and are not bound. What is the advantage in having such a high concentration of H^+?*

A high concentration of H^+ causes a large number of H^+ to bind to proteins, which change their charge and shape. Although this is generally undesirable, because it may lead to a change in function, it has certain biologic advantages. For example, this binding of H^+ to dietary proteins in the lumen of the stomach changes their shape so that pepsin can gain access to sites that permit hydrolysis of these proteins. Accordingly, the anion secreted by the stomach along with H^+ is Cl^- because Cl^- do not bind H^+ until the pH is very low. HCl dissociates completely in aqueous solutions, and there are no major buffers in gastric fluid; thus, the H^+ concentration is high and H^+ bind avidly to dietary proteins and denature them.

A second example of when it is beneficial to have a high H^+ concentration involves "stripping" of hormones from their protein receptors. This happens when the receptor plus its bound hormone is gathered into a sac (called an *endosome* [*endo-* means *in* and *-some* means *body*]) where its membrane secretes H^+ using a H^+-ATPase, raising the concentration of H^+ in this local environment. As a result, this makes the protein receptor and the hormone itself more positively charged, which alters their shape, and decreases the affinity of binding of the receptor to that hormone. The hormone is then sent to a site where there are proteolytic enzymes that destroy it (proteasome) while the receptor recycles back to the cell membrane. This diminishes the need for continuing resynthesis of receptor proteins (e.g., this recycling of receptors in cell membranes occurs almost 180 times in the lifetime of the insulin receptor).

1-2   *What is the rationale for the statement, "In biology only weak acids kill"?*

Chemistry books classify acids as strong or weak based on their dissociation constants (or pK, the pH at which the acid is 50% dissociated); strong acids have a much lower pK. This difference is of little importance in biology because the dissociation of virtually all weak and strong acids is much greater than 99% at pH values of close to 7. In addition, most acids encountered in physiology are weak acids (e.g., lactic acid and ketoacids).

1-3 *Does consumption of citrus fruit, which contains a large quantity of citric acid and its K⁺ salt, cause a net acid and/or a net alkali load?*

Before citrate anions are metabolized, there is an initial H^+ load because citric acid dissociates into H^+ and citrate anions. Later, when all citrate anions are removed by metabolism to neutral end products, there is a net alkali load as some citrate anions are added to the body with K^+ and not H^+.

$$\text{Citric acid} \rightarrow \text{citrate}^{3-} + 3\ H^+$$

$$\text{Citrate}^{3-} + 3\ H^+ + 4.5\ O_2 \rightarrow 6\ CO_2 + 4\ H_2O$$

1-4 *Why is the L-lactic acidosis observed during cardiogenic shock so much more devastating than the L-lactic acidosis observed during a sprint if the $P_{L\text{-lactate}}$, arterial pH, and P_{HCO3} are identical?*

There are two components to the answer. First, cells in vital organs in the patient with cardiogenic shock suffer from a lack of ATP as they are deprived of oxygen. In contrast, the brain and the heart are not undergoing anaerobic metabolism during a sprint. Hence, only skeletal muscle has a very large demand for anaerobic conversion of ADP to ATP to enable the performance of useful work. Second, there is also a major difference with respect to buffering of H^+. Only the patient with poor cardiac function has a *very* slow blood flow rate to vital organs. As a result, the P_{CO_2} in brain cells rises markedly and now H^+ *cannot* be eliminated by their bicarbonate buffer system. Accordingly, more H^+ bind to intracellular proteins and, as a result, these vital organs fail to function in an optimal fashion.

In summary, to answer this question, one must not focus solely on the production of H^+ and L-lactate anions. Rather, a broader and more integrative view is necessary, considering the function of individual organs, their ability to regenerate ATP, and whether they can buffer the H^+ produced by their bicarbonate buffer system.

1-5 *The heart extracts close to 70% of the oxygen from each liter of coronary artery blood. What conclusions can you draw about buffering of H^+ in the heart? Might there be advantages owing to this high extraction of O_2 per liter of blood flow?*

Because so much O_2 is extracted from each liter of blood delivered to the heart, cardiac myocytes add a large amount of CO_2 to each liter of coronary sinus blood. Accordingly, the venous P_{O_2} is low and the venous P_{CO_2} is high—each has potentially important effects.

Low venous P_{O_2}: There are two opposing factors to consider.
- *Risk*: A low capillary P_{O_2} slows the rate of diffusion of O_2 and thus its rate of delivery to cardiac mitochondria. On the other hand, the beating of the heart "stirs" its interstitial fluid, which accelerates diffusion.
- *Benefits*: First, a low interstitial P_{O_2} is advantageous if it leads to new blood vessel formation and thus the formation of collaterals with interweaving connections. Second, in conjunction with the high P_{CO_2}, a low P_{O_2} produces a vasodilatory ambiance that leads to an ability of the arterioles of the heart to vasodilate in response to less robust stimuli that accompany a need for increased cardiac work.

High venous P_{CO_2}: There are two opposing factors to consider.
- *Risk*: A high venous and cellular P_{CO_2} reduces the effectiveness of the bicarbonate buffer system of the heart. This should not be a problem as long as the heart maintains its aerobic state because the rate of H^+ formation is equal to the rate of H^+ removal.

- *Benefits*: First, a high capillary P_{CO_2} in the heart causes a rightward shift in the O_2/hemoglobin dissociation curve; this improves the diffusion of O_2 into cardiac myocytes (see Fig. 8-4, page 235). Second, the high interstitial P_{CO_2} enhances the response of arterioles of the heart to vasodilatory stimuli that are released in response to increased cardiac work (e.g., adenosine).

1-6 *What changes would you expect to find in the urine if the transport system that adds NH_3 to the lumen of the inner medullary collecting duct were to "disappear" (be knocked out) in a rodent?*

When this experiment was performed, there was little if any change in the pH in the blood or in the urine. The reason for these observations is that very little NH_4^+ enters the urine in mice consuming their usual diet, because the rate of excretion of NH_4^+ is very low (~150 µEq/day) as compared to their rate of excretion of organic anions (~3000 µEq/day), which reflects the large alkali load of their diet. Hence, it is not surprising that a small decrease in the rate of excretion of NH_4^+ could easily be overcome by a small decrease in the excretion of alkali in the form of organic anions in fed rodents. Moreover, it would be very difficult to find a small change in the urine pH given this large alkali load in their diet.

Therefore, we are very reluctant to conclude that knocking out the NH_3 channel in *fed* mice is strong evidence for its lack of importance in being an "adjuster" of the urine pH or the excretion of NH_4^+. To make this evaluation, we must await future studies where mice with this knockout have a *low* quantity of alkali in their diet (i.e., studies performed in mice consuming a diet with a low content of K^+ organic anions).

1-7 *What is the major function of phosphocreatine in aerobic exercise?*

- Creatine^0 and phosphocreatine^{2-} are used in an "energy shuttle" between contractile elements and mitochondria in muscle cells during aerobic exercise.

There is no net change in the concentrations of phosphocreatine^{2-}, creatine^0, HPO_4^{2-}, L-lactate$^-$, or H^+ during vigorous *aerobic* exercise. Hence, it may appear that there is no role for this phosphocreatine^{2-}/creatine^0 system as an energy reserve at this time. Notwithstanding, it would be erroneous to say that there is no important physiologic function of phosphocreatine^{2-} in this setting—rather, the more correct conclusion is that hydrolysis and resynthesis of phosphocreatine^{2-} occur at *equal* rates—in fact, these rates are very rapid indeed.

During heavy aerobic exercise, ATP is converted to ADP at very rapid rates in the vicinity of muscle contractile elements. Notwithstanding, the site where ADP is converted back to ATP is in mitochondria, and this is a large distance for diffusion. Diffusion is slow when concentration differences in absolute terms are low or if distances are large. Because the concentration of free ADP is extremely tiny (0.025 mmol/L) and the "distance" in skeletal muscle cells is large relative to the enormous amount of ATP required for vigorous exercise, there would be a *very* low rate of ATP synthesis unless this diffusion step could be accelerated or "bypassed." Nature's solution is to use a "bypass strategy"—to have creatine^0 and/or phosphocreatine^{2-} diffuse instead of ADP and ATP because the concentrations of the former pair are much more than 1000-fold higher than that of ADP (Fig. 1-21). To achieve these effects, there are two different creatine kinase enzymes. Hydrolysis of phosphocreatine^{2-} occurs

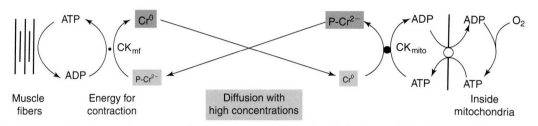

FIGURE 1-21 Phosphocreatine energy shuttle. Events are located in skeletal muscle (and heart) cells. To overcome the need for diffusion of ADP, the conversion of ADP to ATP near muscle contractile elements (shown to the *left*) leads to the conversion of phosphocreatine^{2-} (P-Cr^{2-}) to creatine^0. Because the sum of the concentrations of these latter compounds is close to 25 mmol/L, they can diffuse instead of ADP between these contractile elements and mitochondria (shown to the *right*). For emphasis, the sites where concentrations are higher are indicated by the *larger* and *darker green rectangles*. CK, creatine kinase; CK$_{mf}$, creatine kinase near muscle fibers; CK$_{mito}$, creatine kinase near mitochondria.

in one area of skeletal muscle cells, the region where the contractile elements exist. Resynthesis of phosphocreatine^{2-} occurs near the mitochondria. Diffusion is accelerated because the concentrations of phosphocreatine^{2-} and creatine^0 are very high. This way of accelerating diffusion is absolutely necessary during vigorous exercise. In fact, mice that lack these creatine kinase enzymes in their heart are fine at rest but are unable to perform even modest exercise.

1-8   *Examine the data in Figure 1-22 for changes in the concentrations of phosphocreatine^{2-} and H$^+$ in skeletal muscle before and after performing vigorous aerobic exercise.*

A   *Why did the ICF pH fall at the end of ischemic exercise?*

This fall in ICF pH implies that more H$^+$ were produced in anerobic glycolysis than HCO$_3$ was produced after the hydrolysis of phosphocreatine^{2-}.

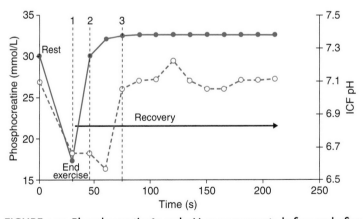

FIGURE 1-22 Phosphocreatine^{2-} and pH measurements before and after vigorous ischemic exercise. ^{31}Phosphorus magnetic resonance spectroscopy (^{31}P-MRS) data were obtained in a trained athlete who performed vigorous ischemic exercise for 30 seconds by repetitive leg kicking. Time is shown on the horizontal axis. The *filled circles connected by a solid line* depict the concentration of phosphocreatine^{2-} in exercising muscle (*left* y-axis), and the *white circles connected by a dashed line* depict the intracellular fluid (ICF) pH in muscle (*right* y-axis). Exercise began at zero time. *Vertical dashed line 1* indicates the end of ischemic exercise. *Vertical dashed line 2* indicates the first 15 seconds of recovery. *Vertical dashed line 3* indicates 45 seconds of recovery.

B *Why did the ICF pH not fall when phosphocreatine²⁻ was synthesized in the first 15 seconds of recovery?*

Although there was a large production of H^+ when phosphocreatine²⁻ was regenerated, there was no change in the ICF pH. Hence, all of these H^+ were removed, but not by nonbicarbonate (histidine) buffers. In more detail, for histidines to serve as H^+ acceptors, there must be an increase in the concentration of H^+ in cells, and this did not occur. Rather, the bicarbonate buffer system can remove these H^+, but only if the capillary P_{CO_2} falls.

C *Why did the ICF pH rise between 30 and 45 seconds of recovery?*

There was a marked rise in the ICF pH (a fall in the concentration of H^+ in the ICF), indicating that there was a large removal of H^+. In fact, H^+ are also *released* from nonbicarbonate buffers when the concentration of H^+ falls in the ICF compartment. There are three possible reasons for this fall in the concentration of H^+ in the ICF compartment. First, the P_{CO_2} in venous blood draining this muscle could have fallen even more as a result of a decline in muscle metabolic work and/or a rise in blood flow rate. Second, there was no change in this venous P_{CO_2}, as its initial fall was large, which caused H^+ removal by the bicarbonate buffer systems in both the ICF and ECF compartments, but there was a delay in the export of H^+ and/or entry of HCO_3^- into muscle cells. Third, there could be a sudden export of H^+ (L-lactic acid) on the monocarboxylic acid transporter. If this were the case, there would be a rise in the $P_{\text{L-lactate}}$ and in the venous P_{CO_2}. Unfortunately, the data to resolve this are not available at this time.

Summary: The bicarbonate buffer system in exercising muscle cells *and* in their ECF compartment does *not* remove an appreciable number of H^+ *during* ischemic exercise, as both areas are exposed to the same very high capillary P_{CO_2}. This preserves the bicarbonate buffer system for use when ischemic exercise stops, as there will be a very large H^+ load when phosphocreatine²⁻ is regenerated and nonbicarbonate buffers already have a large quantity of bound H^+. Therefore, the P_{CO_2} in capillaries of exercising skeletal muscle should fall at this point, and the likely mechanism is the reduced consumption of O_2 and possibly a continuing high blood flow rate.

2

Tools to Use to Diagnose Acid-Base Disorders

Introduction

There are four primary acid-base disturbances, two metabolic and two respiratory; each has an expected response. These expected responses are considered under two headings: buffering of H^+ by the bicarbonate buffer system and the response of the kidneys to return the concentration of H^+ in plasma toward the normal range. For buffering, the goal is to have only tiny changes in the concentration of H^+ in the intracellular fluid (ICF) compartment to minimize the binding of H^+ to intracellular proteins; this is achieved by ensuring that there is effective H^+ removal by the bicarbonate buffer system in the interstitial and intracellular spaces of skeletal muscle (see Fig. 1-7, page 13). The role of the kidney in chronic metabolic acidosis is to generate new HCO_3^- by increasing the rate of excretion of NH_4^+.

When metabolic alkalosis is secondary to a deficit of HCl or NaCl, the appropriate renal response is to excrete as little Cl^- as possible.

In patients with respiratory acid-base disorders, the expected change in P_{HCO3} differs depending on whether the disorder is acute or chronic. These expected responses, unfortunately, must be memorized. Nevertheless, knowing these expected responses helps identify mixed acid-base disorders.

Overall, one must integrate all the information from the medical history and the physical examination together with the laboratory data to make an acid-base diagnosis. If just one of these areas suggests that there is an inconsistency, there is something missing, so the evidence should be reviewed.

ABBREVIATIONS

P_{HCO3}, concentration of HCO_3^- in plasma

$P_{Anion\ gap}$, anion gap in plasma

$P_{Albumin}$, concentration of albumin in plasma

OBJECTIVES

- To illustrate the tools needed to identify whether there is an acid-base disorder and also to determine why it is present. In this chapter, our emphasis is on metabolic acidosis.
- To determine whether metabolic acidosis is present. When the extracellular fluid (ECF) volume is significantly contracted, a quantitative estimate of the ECF volume is needed to assess the *content* of HCO_3^- in the ECF compartment.
- To determine whether metabolic acidosis is due to the over-production of acids, one should detect the appearance of new anions in plasma (high value for the $P_{Anion\ gap}$ adjusted for the concentration of albumin in plasma [$P_{Albumin}$]) and/or in the urine.
- To illustrate how to assess whether H^+ were removed appropriately by the bicarbonate buffer system. The clues are that the arterial P_{CO_2} is appropriately reduced and that the P_{CO_2} in the venous drainage of skeletal muscle is sufficiently low to ensure that the P_{CO_2} is low in the interstitial and in the ICF compartments of skeletal muscle.
- To illustrate that the rate of excretion of NH_4^+ reflects the renal response to chronic metabolic acidosis. The urine osmolal gap provides the best indirect estimate of the concentration of NH_4^+ in the urine.

NORMAL ACID-BASE VALUES IN PLASMA

pH: 7.40 ± 0.02

[H^+]: 40 ± 2 nmol/L

P_{HCO3}: 25 ± 2 mmol/L

Arterial P_{CO_2}: 40 ± 2 mm Hg

Venous P_{CO_2}: Brachial venous P_{CO_2} is usually <10 mm Hg higher than arterial P_{CO_2}.

Anion gap: 12 ± 2 mEq/L

Case 2-1: Does This Man Really Have Metabolic Acidosis?

(Case discussed on page 57)

A 25-year-old man was perfectly healthy until he developed diarrhea 24 hours ago. He had no intake of food or water and currently has no urine output. His blood pressure is 90/60 mm Hg, pulse rate is 110 beats per minute, and his jugular venous pressure is low. Acid-base measurements in *arterial* blood reveal a pH of 7.39, a P_{HCO3} of 24 mmol/L, and a P_{CO_2} of 39 mm Hg. His $P_{Anion\ gap}$ is 24 mEq/L (*see margin note*). His diarrhea volume is estimated to be 5 L; the concentration of HCO_3^- in diarrhea fluid is 40 mmol/L. His hematocrit on admission is 0.60, and his $P_{Albumin}$ is 8.0 g/dL (80 g/L).

Questions

Does this patient have a significant degree of metabolic acidosis?

What is the basis for the high $P_{Anion\ gap}$?

Does the patient have respiratory acidosis?

PART A
DIAGNOSTIC ISSUES
DISORDERS OF ACID-BASE BALANCE

- The P_{HCO3} is also influenced by changes in the ECF volume.
- There is a tissue form of respiratory acidosis.

Before the discussion of each of the acid-base disorders, there are two points with regard to definitions that require emphasis (*see margin note*).

1. *Concentrations can be altered by changing their numerator and/ or their denominator.* The concentration of HCO_3^- in the ECF compartment can be influenced by the amount of HCO_3^- in the ECF compartment and/or the ECF volume. Therefore, a patient can have metabolic acidosis with a near normal P_{HCO3} if the ECF volume is very contracted (called a *mixture of metabolic acidosis* due to the deficit of HCO_3^- and a contraction type of metabolic alkalosis; see the discussion of Case 2-1, page 57).

2. *There is a "tissue" form of respiratory acidosis.* The traditional definition of respiratory acidosis focuses on only the *arterial* P_{CO_2}, which is influenced predominantly by regulation of ventilation. The arterial P_{CO_2} indicates that H^+ were removed by the bicarbonate buffer system, but only in arterial blood; it also sets the lower limit for the P_{CO_2} in all cells of the body. The arterial P_{CO_2} reflects the P_{CO_2} in brain cells in normal individuals because brain blood flow is autoregulated and the production of CO_2 by the brain undergoes only minor variations from minute to minute. Having a low arterial P_{CO_2} does *not* ensure that the P_{CO_2} is low in the interstitial fluid compartment of the ECF of muscles and in muscle cells where the bulk of bicarbonate buffer system exists because this P_{CO_2} is also influenced by both the rate of production of CO_2 and the blood flow rate to muscles. When muscle *venous* P_{CO_2} is high, buffering of H^+ by HCO_3^- in these areas is compromised; hence, a smaller proportion of the H^+ load is titrated by the bicarbonate buffer system, and, as a result, the blood pH falls. Consequently, more H^+ bind to intracellular proteins in vital organs (e.g., the brain)—we call this a "tissue" form of respiratory acidosis. In summary, if autoregulation of the blood flow to the brain fails or if the venous P_{CO_2} draining skeletal muscles rises, more H^+ bind to proteins in brain cells with possible untoward effects. See Table 2-1 for further information.

DEFINITIONS
- Acidemia is a low pH or a high concentration of H^+ in plasma.
- Acidosis is a *process* that adds H^+ to or removes HCO_3^- from the body.

Disorders with a high concentration of H^+ in plasma

There are two types of acid base disorders:
- Those where the primary change is in the P_{HCO3} (metabolic disorders).
- Those where the primary change is in the P_{CO_2} (respiratory disorders).

TABLE 2-1 **MODIFICATIONS TO THE DEFINITIONS OF PRIMARY ACID-BASE DISORDERS**

DISORDER	COMMON DEFINITION	REVISED DEFINITION
Metabolic acidosis	• Relies only on concentration terms (i.e., $\downarrow P_{HCO_3}$ and $\downarrow$ pH)	• Includes *content* of HCO_3^- in the ECF compartment when the ECF volume is contracted
Respiratory acidosis	• Relies only on a high arterial P_{CO_2}	• Includes venous P_{CO_2} to detect a "tissue" form of respiratory acidosis
Metabolic alkalosis	• Relies only on $\uparrow P_{HCO_3}$ and $\uparrow$ pH	• Includes *content* of HCO_3^- in the ECF compartment
Respiratory alkalosis	• Relies only on a low arterial P_{CO_2}	• Includes venous P_{CO_2} to detect a "tissue" form of respiratory acidosis

ECF, extracellular fluid.

If the concentration of H^+ in plasma is higher (pH is lower) than normal, the patient has acidemia. There are two potential disorders—metabolic acidosis or respiratory acidosis.

Metabolic acidosis

This is a process that adds H^+ to or removes HCO_3^- from the body and therefore will lead to a decrease in the *content* of HCO_3^- in the ECF compartment. One of the expected physiologic responses to acidemia of metabolic origin is to lower the arterial P_{CO_2}. On the other hand, the P_{HCO3} may be close to normal if there is a very contracted ECF volume, and hence there may be no changes in the arterial pH and P_{CO_2}.

Respiratory acidosis

When this is due to impaired ventilation, it is characterized by an increased *arterial* P_{CO_2} and $[H^+]$. The expected physiologic response is an increased P_{HCO3}, but this is tiny in acute respiratory acidosis and much larger in chronic respiratory acidosis. The definition of respiratory acidosis should also include the "tissue" form of respiratory acidosis as revealed by a high brachial or femoral venous P_{CO_2}.

Disorders with a low concentration of H^+ in plasma

If the concentration of H^+ in plasma is lower (pH is higher) than normal, the patient has alkalemia. Again, there are two potential causes—metabolic alkalosis or respiratory alkalosis.

Metabolic alkalosis

This is a process that raises the P_{HCO3} and lowers the concentration of H^+ in the ECF compartment and therefore in plasma. Although the expected physiologic response is hypoventilation (an increase in the arterial P_{CO_2}), this is usually modest because the resultant hypoxemia stimulates ventilation. If metabolic alkalosis is associated with a very contracted ECF volume, the patient could also have a "tissue" form of respiratory acidosis with binding of H^+ to intracellular proteins because of a high venous P_{CO_2}.

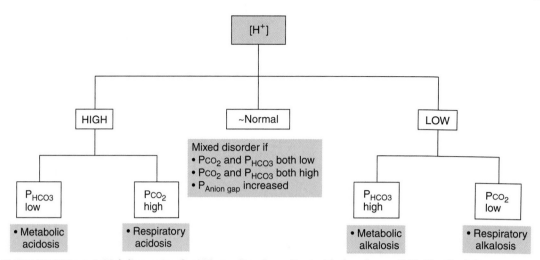

FLOW CHART 2-1 Initial diagnosis of acid-base disorders. Start with the plasma [H$^+$]. The final diagnoses are shown as statements headed by bullets below the boxes. For simplicity, changes in the brachial venous P_{CO_2} were not included in the flow chart. In addition, it is important to assess both the concentration of HCO$_3^-$ and its content in the extracellular fluid (ECF) compartment when the ECF volume is contracted.

Respiratory alkalosis

This is present when the *arterial* P_{CO_2} and concentration of H$^+$ are both low in plasma (*see margin note*). The expected physiologic response is a reduction in the P_{HCO3}. As in respiratory acidosis, this response is modest in acute disorders and more significant in chronic disorders.

Disorders with a normal concentration of H$^+$ in plasma

A normal concentration of H$^+$ in plasma implies that there is either no acid-base disorder or that more than one acid-base disorder is present—one that increases the concentration of H$^+$ and another that decreases the concentration of H$^+$ (Flow Chart 2-1).

MAKING AN ACID-BASE DIAGNOSIS

- Integrate the clinical picture and the laboratory values.
- Examine the following parameters in plasma: the concentration of H$^+$ or the pH (*see margin note*), P_{HCO3}, arterial P_{CO_2}, brachial or femoral venous P_{CO_2}, and the $P_{Anion\ gap}$.
- Assess not only the P_{HCO3} but also the content of HCO$_3^-$ in the ECF compartment if the ECF volume is significantly contracted.

One must integrate the clinical picture and the laboratory data to make a proper acid-base diagnosis. For example, the finding of acidemia, a high arterial P_{CO_2}, and an elevated P_{HCO3} does not indicate that chronic respiratory acidosis is present if that patient does *not* have a chronic problem with ventilation; rather, the patient may have metabolic alkalosis with an acute respiratory acidosis.

In addition to all the parameters mentioned above, the authors rely heavily on the hematocrit and/or total protein concentration to determine if the ECF volume is contracted and to obtain

COMMENT REGARDING FLOW CHART 2-1
- The $P_{Anion\ gap}$ must be "adjusted" for the $P_{Albumin}$.
- We did not include a "tissue" form of respiratory acidosis in this flow chart for simplicity; a high brachial or femoral venous P_{CO_2} is needed to establish this diagnosis.

MIXED RESPIRATORY ACID-BASE DISORDERS
A patient may have a respiratory alkalosis as defined by low arterial P_{CO_2} but a "tissue" form of respiratory acidosis as defined by a high brachial or femoral venous P_{CO_2} (e.g., when the rate of blood flow to skeletal muscle is very low).

pH VERSUS [H$^+$]
The authors prefer to think in terms of the [H$^+$] rather than the pH, but the principles are the same: A low [H$^+$] is a high pH, and vice versa.

a quantitative estimate of its content of HCO_3^- (see discussion of Case 2-1, page 57).

LABORATORY TESTS USED IN A PATIENT WITH METABOLIC ACIDOSIS

In this section we provide the rationale for some tests that can provide additional information at the bedside (Table 2-2). The specific questions to be addressed are shown in the following list; the importance of each becomes clear as the specific disorders are discussed.

1. Is the content of HCO_3^- in the ECF compartment low?

Calculate the content of HCO_3^- in the ECF compartment ($P_{HCO3} \times$ ECF volume) when the ECF volume is appreciably low. The hematocrit or total protein levels in plasma are very useful to obtain a quantitative estimate of the ECF volume.

2. Have new acids accumulated?

The presence of new anions in plasma can be detected by a rise in the $P_{Anion\ gap}$. New anions in the urine can be detected by calculating the anion gap in the urine (*see margin note*); for this calculation, the concentration of NH_4^+ in the urine (U_{NH4}) should be estimated using the urine osmolal gap ($U_{Osmolal\ gap}$).

3. Have toxic alcohols accumulated in the body?

Calculate the osmolal gap in plasma ($P_{Osmolal\ gap}$) to reveal whether many new uncharged particles are present in plasma ($P_{Osmolal\ gap}$ = measured $P_{Osm} - [2\ P_{Na} + P_{Glucose} + P_{Urea}]$, all in mmol/L units).

4. Has the bicarbonate buffer system in skeletal muscle removed an adequate quantity of H^+?

To make this assessment, we measure the brachial venous P_{CO_2}. A value that is more than 10 mm Hg higher than the arterial P_{CO_2} suggests that there is defective buffering of H^+ by the bicarbonate buffer system in the interstitial and intracellular compartments of muscles in its drainage bed. Thus, there is an increased risk of H^+ binding to intracellular proteins in vital organs (e.g., the brain).

URINE ANION GAP
When searching for new anions, use the formula: $U_{Na} + U_K + U_{NH4} - U_{Cl}$

ABBREVIATIONS
FE_{HCO3}, fractional excretion of HCO_3^-
$U_{Citrate}$, concentration of citrate in the urine

TABLE 2-2 TOOLS USED IN THE CLINICAL APPROACH TO PATIENTS WITH METABOLIC ACIDOSIS

QUESTION	PARAMETER ASSESSED	TOOLS TO USE
• Is the content of HCO_3^- low in the ECF?	• ECF volume	• Hematocrit or total plasma proteins
• Have new acids accumulated?	• Appearance of new anions in the body or the urine	• $P_{Anion\ gap}$ • Urine anion gap
• Are toxic alcohols present?	• Detect alcohols as unmeasured osmoles	• $P_{Osmolal\ gap}$
• Has H^+ removal by HCO_3^- been adequate?	• Buffering of H^+ by HCO_3^- in muscle interstitial fluid and in its intracellular fluid compartment	• Brachial venous P_{CO_2}
• Is the renal response to chronic acidemia adequate?	• Examine the rate of excretion of NH_4^+	• Urine osmolal gap
• What is the basis for a low excretion of NH_4^+?	• Low distal H^+ secretion • Low NH_3 availability • Both defects	• Urine pH > 6.5 • Urine pH ~ 5.0 • Urine pH ~ 6.0
• Where is the defect in H^+ secretion?	• Distal H^+ secretion • Proximal H^+ secretion	• P_{CO_2} in alkaline urine • FE_{HCO3}, $U_{Citrate}$
• If NH_4^+ excretion is high, which anion is excreted with NH_4^+?	• GI loss of $NaHCO_3$ • Acid added, but the anion is excreted in the urine	• Urine Cl^- is high • Urine anion gap

5. *In a patient with chronic hyperchloremic metabolic acidosis, is the rate of excretion of NH_4^+ high enough so that the kidneys are not the sole cause of the disorder?*

The $U_{Osmolal\ gap}$ is the best indirect test to estimate the U_{NH4}. To convert the U_{NH4} into an excretion rate, divide it by the concentration of creatinine in the urine ($U_{Creatinine}$) and multiply the $U_{NH4}/U_{Creatinine}$ ratio by an estimate of the rate of creatinine excretion (20 mg or 200 μmol per kg body weight).

6. *What is the basis for a low NH_4^+ excretion rate?*

The urine pH is most valuable to identify the pathophysiology of the low rate of excretion of NH_4^+ (*see margin note*). If the urine pH is greater than 6.5, the low rate of excretion of NH_4^+ is due to a reduced net rate of H^+ secretion in the distal nephron. To determine the basis of this lesion, measure the P_{CO2} in alkaline urine. In contrast, if the urine pH is close to 5, the low rate of excretion of NH_4^+ is usually due to a disease leading to a diminished production of NH_4^+. On the other hand, if urine pH is close to 6, there is a defect that lowers the availability of both H^+ and NH_3 in the lumen of the distal nephron (see Chapter 4, page 91, for further discussion).

LOW EXCRETION OF NH_4^+
A low rate of excretion of NH_4^+ is the hallmark of a group of diseases called *renal tubular acidosis.*

7. *Is there a defect in H^+ secretion in the proximal tubule?*

A fractional excretion of HCO_3^- that is greater than 15% after giving a $NaHCO_3$ load that raises the P_{HCO3} to close to 24 mmol/L indicates a defect in H^+ secretion in the proximal convoluted tubule. A high rate of excretion of citrate in these patients could be due to an alkaline proximal convoluted tubule cell pH (see Chapter 4, page 87 for further discussion) or a component of a generalized proximal convoluted tubule cell dysfunction (i.e., Fanconi syndrome).

8. *If the rate of excretion of NH_4^+ is high, what anion accompanies NH_4^+ in the urine?*

In a patient with metabolic acidosis and a high rate of excretion of NH_4^+, if the urine anion is Cl^-, the cause of the metabolic acidosis is usually loss of $NaHCO_3$ via the gastrointestinal tract (diarrhea). In contrast, if the anion is not Cl^-, suspect that the cause of metabolic acidosis is overproduction of an organic acid, the anion of which is excreted in the urine at a rapid rate (e.g., hippuric acid in the patient with glue sniffing; see Chapter 3, page 71.)

The anion gap in plasma

The $P_{Anion\ gap}$ ($P_{Na} - [P_{Cl} + P_{HCO3}]$) is a calculation that is useful for diagnostic purposes.
- The normal value is 12 ± 2 mEq/L, but it must be adjusted for the $P_{Albumin}$.
- It is helpful to detect metabolic acidosis owing to the gain of acids if the anion of the added acid is largely retained in plasma.
- It is helpful to detect mixed metabolic acidosis and metabolic alkalosis.
- It, along with the P_{HCO3}, is useful to follow the patient's response to therapy.

Metabolic acidosis owing to addition of acids can be detected from the accumulation of new anions in plasma. The concept of $P_{Anion\ gap}$ is based on the principle of electroneutrality—that is, the number of positive charges in plasma must equal the number of negative charges.

The major cation in plasma is Na^+, and the major anions are Cl^- and HCO_3^-. In quantitative terms (and ignoring K^+), the difference between the P_{Na} and $(P_{Cl} + P_{HCO3})$ is 12 ± 2 mEq/L; it reflects the other major negative charges in plasma, which are due primarily to the net negative valence on albumin—this is referred to as the $P_{Anion\ gap}$. Clearly, there is no "electrical" gap in plasma; therefore, if the $P_{Na} - (P_{Cl} + P_{HCO3})$ is greater than 12 mEq/L, another unmeasured anion is present in plasma. Note that this calculation must be adjusted for the $P_{Albumin}$.

Although other cations and anions in plasma were ignored in this calculation, this does not pose a problem for clinical purposes, either because their ion concentrations are relatively low (e.g., Ca^{2+}, Mg^{2+}, HPO_4^{2-}, SO_4^{2-}) or do not vary substantially (e.g., K^+). In quantitative terms, it is widely held that the rise in the concentration of new anions, as reflected by a higher value for the $P_{Anion\ gap}$, should be equal to the fall in the P_{HCO3}. Nevertheless, this underestimates the deficit of HCO_3^-, as this calculation is based on concentrations and does not take changes in the ECF volume into account.

An example

When L-lactic acid dissociates into H^+ and L-lactate anions in the ECF compartment, H^+ are removed virtually exclusively by reacting with HCO_3^-, leaving L-lactate anions as the "footprint" of the L-lactic acid that was added to the ECF compartment. These events are depicted in the following table, with values before and after the addition of 10 mmol of L-lactic acid to each liter of ECF; for this calculation to be valid, there must be no change in the ECF volume (for simplicity, events in cells are ignored). See Figure 2-1.

Using the values in Figure 2-1, one must assume that there is no change in the ECF volume or $P_{Albumin}$.

PLASMA (mEq/L)	P_{Na}	P_{Cl}	P_{HCO_3}	$P_{Anion\ gap}$
Normal	140	103	25	12
L-Lactic acid (10 mmol/L)	140	103	15 = 25 − 10	22 = 12 + 10

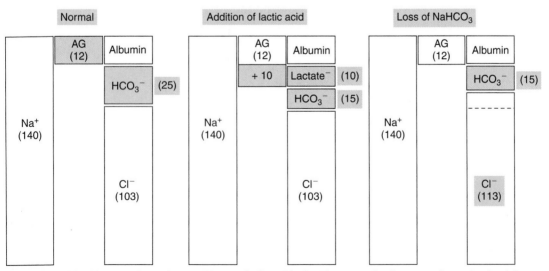

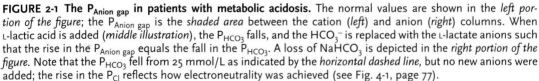

FIGURE 2-1 The $P_{Anion\ gap}$ in patients with metabolic acidosis. The normal values are shown in the *left portion of the figure*; the $P_{Anion\ gap}$ is the *shaded area* between the cation (*left*) and anion (*right*) columns. When L-lactic acid is added (*middle illustration*), the P_{HCO_3} falls, and the HCO_3^- is replaced with the L-lactate anions such that the rise in the $P_{Anion\ gap}$ equals the fall in the P_{HCO_3}. A loss of $NaHCO_3$ is depicted in the *right portion of the figure*. Note that the P_{HCO_3} fell from 25 mmol/L as indicated by the *horizontal dashed line*, but no new anions were added; the rise in the P_{Cl} reflects how electroneutrality was achieved (see Fig. 4-1, page 77).

The patient begins with a normal $P_{Anion\,gap}$ of 12 mEq/L ($140 - [103 + 25]$). The protons accompanying 10 mmol/L of L-lactate anion in the ECF react with HCO_3^-; the result is a decline in P_{HCO3} to 15 mmol/L and an increase in the $P_{Anion\,gap}$ to 22 mEq/L. This value is best thought of as the increment over the normal baseline $P_{Anion\,gap}$ (i.e., $12 + 10$ mEq/L), because this forces one to think of the normal value for the $P_{Anion\,gap}$ and to ask whether there is any reason for the patient not to have a normal baseline $P_{Anion\,gap}$. Thus, the increase in the $P_{Anion\,gap}$ (10 mEq/L) reflects the presence of the 10 mEq/L of L-lactate per liter of ECF because there was no change in its volume. If, in the preceding example, the increase in the $P_{Anion\,gap}$ was the same 10 mEq/L, but the concentration of L-lactate in plasma was only 5 mmol/L, L-lactic acidosis would not be the sole cause of the metabolic acidosis; the patient must have also accumulated unmeasured anions of other acids (e.g., ketoacid anions).

Pitfalls in the use of the plasma anion gap

Issues related to $P_{Albumin}$

> • The $P_{Albumin}$ can be very low or very high, and this changes the expected baseline value for the $P_{Anion\,gap}$.
> • The net anionic charge on $P_{Albumin}$ (or total plasma proteins) is not constant.

There are two pitfalls related to the $P_{Albumin}$. First, in some clinical situations, the $P_{Albumin}$ can be low (e.g., cirrhosis of the liver or nephrotic syndrome), whereas in others, the $P_{Albumin}$ can be high (e.g., a patient with a very contracted ECF volume). Hence, the baseline value for the $P_{Anion\,gap}$ must be adjusted for the $P_{Albumin}$ (*see margin note*). A rough guide for correcting the baseline value of $P_{Anion\,gap}$ for $P_{Albumin}$ is that at $P_{Albumin}$ of 4.0 g/dL (40 g/L), the $P_{Anion\,gap}$ including the P_K is 16 mEq/L; hence, for every 1.0-g/L (10-g/L) decrease in $P_{Albumin}$, the $P_{Anion\,gap}$ is lower by close to 4 mEq/L. The converse is true for a rise in the $P_{Albumin}$.

The second point is that the valence or net anionic charge on $P_{Albumin}$ (or total plasma proteins) is not constant. For example, when the effective arterial blood volume is low, it appears that the valence on $P_{Albumin}$ becomes more negative (*see margin note*).

RISE IN $P_{Albumin}$ OWING TO A LOW ECF VOLUME
• The higher $P_{Albumin}$ "defends" the plasma volume because there is a higher colloid osmotic pressure.
• The higher negative charge on albumin also causes interstitial fluid to enter capillaries owing to the Gibbs-Donnan effect (see Chapter 9, page 252 for discussion).

CHANGE IN CHARGE ON ALBUMIN
When the effective arterial blood is contracted, the $P_{Anion\,gap}$ is higher than expected for changes in the concentration of albumin, the change in its valence due to a rise in pH, or the gain of new anions.

Issues related to P_{Cl}

> • The pitfall to be aware of with respect to the P_{Cl} depends on the method used.

Owing to the use of different methods for the measurement of P_{Cl}, some laboratories report higher values for the P_{Cl}; hence, the value for the $P_{Anion\,gap}$ must be adjusted for the method used in each hospital. P_{Cl} is overestimated in patients with bromide ingestion, leading to a low or even negative value for the $P_{Anion\,gap}$.

Issues related to other cations

Some patients with multiple myeloma have cationic proteins present in plasma that cause the $P_{Anion\,gap}$ to be lower; usually Cl^- balances the valence of these unmeasured cations.

Issues related to other anions

The concentration of phosphate in plasma can rise in patients with renal failure or transiently after an enema using phosphate salts. In that setting, the $P_{Anion\ gap}$ is higher than the usual value of 12 mEq/L if the $P_{Albumin}$ is 4 g/dL (40 g/L).

The osmolal gap in plasma

- The $P_{Osmolal\ gap}$ is a way to detect the presence of alcohols in plasma.
- The $P_{Osmolal\ gap}$ is the measured P_{Osm} minus the calculated P_{Osm} (2 $[P_{Na}]$ + $P_{Glucose}$ [mmol/L] + P_{Urea} [mmol/L]).

The osmotic pressure of a solution is directly related to the concentration of its dissolved solutes. Hence, a molecule of protein, glucose, or Na^+ makes a virtually equal contribution to the osmotic pressure even though each varies greatly in molecular weight. Because the numbers of anions and cations must be equal, the value of $2 \times P_{Na}$ accounts for the vast majority of the osmotic pressure owing to cations plus anions in plasma (*see margin note*).

Glucose and urea are the two major nonionized molecules in plasma that are likely to change significantly in concentration. Hence, the calculated osmolality is $2\ (P_{Na})$ + $P_{Glucose}$ + P_{Urea} (the latter two measurements are in mmol/L; see Table 2-3 for conversion of concentrations in mg/dL to mmol/L). The difference between the measured and the calculated osmolality is the $P_{Osmolal\ gap}$. A high $P_{Osmolal\ gap}$ indicates the presence of an unmeasured compound; because the unmeasured compound is not charged, it is usually an alcohol (*see margin note*).

Tests used to estimate the rate of excretion of NH_4^+

- Because most clinical laboratories do not routinely measure U_{NH4}, clinicians must use indirect tests to estimate its rate of excretion in a patient with metabolic acidosis.

Although these tests provide only semiquantitative estimates of the rate of excretion of NH_4^+, this is adequate in most clinical settings with metabolic acidosis. The information needed is whether NH_4^+ excretion is low enough to be the sole cause of acidosis or is appropriately high for the presence of chronic metabolic acidosis. Normal subjects consuming a typical Western diet excrete 20 to 40 mmol of NH_4^+ per day, whereas normal subjects who are given

TABLE 2-3 **CONVERSION BETWEEN mg/dL AND mmol/L**

To convert mg/dL to mmol/L, multiply mg/dL by 10, and then divide by the molecular weight.

Sample calculations

CONSTITUENT	MOLECULAR WEIGHT	mg/dL	mmol/L
Glucose	180	90	5
Urea	60	30	5
Urea nitrogen	28 (2 × 14)	14	5

a large acid load for several days increase their rate of excretion of NH_4^+ to greater than 200 mmol/day. Therefore, in a patient with chronic metabolic acidosis and normal renal function, the expected rate of NH_4^+ excretion is greater than 200 mmol/day. Similarly, if a patient has chronic hyperchloremic metabolic acidosis, and the rate of NH_4^+ excretion is appreciably less than 40 mmol/day, the renal lesion could be the sole cause of the metabolic acidosis—that is, renal tubular acidosis (Flow Chart 2-2; *see margin note*). In contrast, if the rate of excretion of NH_4^+ is 100 mmol/day, there is still a renal component to the metabolic acidosis. Nevertheless, one must look for another important cause for the metabolic acidosis (such as loss of $NaHCO_3$ via the gastrointestinal tract or the addition of an acid with the excretion of its accompanying anion in the urine).

APPROPRIATE RATE OF EXCRETION OF NH_4^+ IN NORMAL SUBJECTS
To define the adequacy of NH_4^+ excretion if it appears to be low, compare the NH_4^+ and sulfate excretion rates in mEq terms (usually there is a 1:1 stoichiometry).

Urine net charge

- In most circumstances, we do not rely on this test because it detects only NH_4^+ that is excreted with Cl^-.

The premise of this test is that if the U_{Cl} is appreciably greater than the $U_{Na} + U_K$, there is a high concentration of another cation (i.e., NH_4^+) in the urine.

There are two issues when the urine net charge is used to estimate the rate of excretion of NH_4^+ that diminish its utility. First, the calculation of the urine net charge to detect NH_4^+ is correct only if its accompanying anion is Cl^-. For example, there is a loss of $NaHCO_3$ in diarrhea fluid (see Flow Chart 2-2). Second, as shown in the equation that follows, in this calculation, the difference between the concentrations of unmeasured anions and cations in the urine is assumed to be a constant value of 80 mEq, but this is not necessarily true for two reasons. First, this "constant" of 80 mEq is based

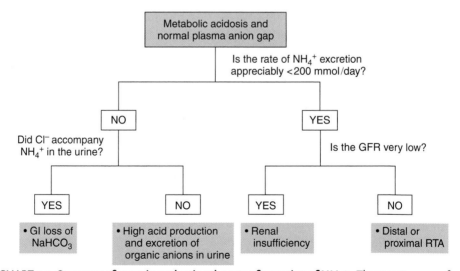

FLOW CHART 2-2 Sequence of steps in evaluating the rate of excretion of NH_4^+. These tests are performed in a patient with chronic hyperchloremic metabolic acidosis. The expected value for the urinary excretion of NH_4^+ is more than 200 mmol/day with metabolic acidosis and normal kidneys. If the rate of excretion of NH_4^+ is appreciably less than 40 mmol/day, the kidneys could be the sole cause of the acidosis. These tests provide estimates, not precise values; in addition, concentration terms must be converted to excretion rates. GFR, glomerular filtration rate; GI, gastrointestinal; RTA, renal tubular acidosis.

on a urine volume of 1 L/day. Second, the rate of excretion of these unmeasured anions varies considerably depending on dietary intake.

$$U_{NH4} = U_{Na} + U_K - U_{Cl} + 80 \text{ mEq/L}$$

Urine osmolal gap

> • The $U_{Osmolal\ gap}$ is the best indirect test to assess whether the U_{NH4} and thereby the rate of excretion of NH_4^+ is high enough in patients with chronic metabolic acidosis.

The $U_{Osmolal\ gap}$ is the best indirect test because it detects NH_4^+ regardless of the anion excreted with it. The formula for the $U_{Osmolal\ gap}$ is shown in the equation that follows; in this equation, all values are in mmol/L terms. The only difficulty is that one must measure the concentration of urea and sometimes that of glucose in the urine. The test is unreliable if other osmoles such as ethanol, methanol, ethylene glycol, or mannitol are present in the urine. To estimate the concentration of NH_4^+, divide the $U_{Osmolal\ gap}$ by 2, because the anions in the urine excreted with this cation are mainly monovalent ones. To estimate the rate of excretion of NH_4^+, use the ratio of the $U_{NH4}/U_{Creatinine}$, and multiply this ratio by the expected rate of excretion of creatinine (*see margin note*).

$$U_{Osmolal\ gap} = \text{measured } U_{Osm} - \text{calculated } U_{Osm}$$
$$\text{Calculated } U_{Osm} = 2(U_{Na} + U_K) + U_{Urea} + U_{Glucose}$$
$$U_{NH4} = U_{Osmolal\ gap}/2$$

CREATININE EXCRETION
• In normal subjects, this is approximately:
  −20 mg/kg body weight
  −200 μmol/kg body weight
• Be careful if obesity or marked muscle wasting exists when extrapolating per kg body weight.

Tests used to evaluate the basis for a low rate of excretion of NH_4^+

The urine pH

> • One cannot deduce the urinary concentration of NH_4^+ from the urine pH; the urine pH is most useful *after* you know that the rate of excretion of NH_4^+ is low; it helps to determine the pathophysiology for the low rate of excretion of NH_4^+.

When the urine pH is higher than 6.5 in a patient with chronic metabolic acidosis and a low rate of excretion of NH_4^+, its basis is a low *net* rate of distal H^+ secretion. Conversely, in a patient with chronic metabolic acidosis and a low rate of excretion of NH_4^+, a urine pH close to 5 suggests that the basis for the low rate of excretion of NH_4^+ is a low entry of NH_3 into the medullary collecting duct caused by a low rate of production of NH_4^+. Both of these groups of disorders are discussed in more detail in Chapter 4, page 89.

The Pco_2 in alkaline urine

> • The Pco_2 in alkaline urine permits one to examine net H^+ secretion in the distal nephron.
> • It is most useful when the low rate of NH_4^+ excretion is associated with a urine pH greater than 6.5.

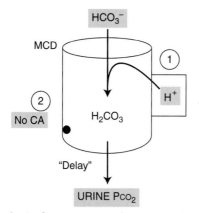

FIGURE 2-2 The basis for an increased P_{CO_2} in alkaline urine. When NaHCO₃ is given, there is a large delivery of HCO_3^- to the distal nephron, which makes HCO_3^- virtually the only H^+ acceptor in its lumen. Because there is no luminal carbonic anhydrase (CA), the H_2CO_3 formed is delivered downstream and forms CO_2 plus H_2O. Thus, if the urine P_{CO_2} is not appreciably higher than the plasma P_{CO_2}, this provides evidence for impaired distal H^+ secretion. The urine P_{CO_2} can be high despite decreased net distal H^+ secretion if there is H^+ back-leak or secretion of HCO_3^- in the distal nephron. MCD, medullary collecting duct.

The test begins after enough NaHCO₃ is administered to achieve a second-voided urine with a pH that is greater than 7.0 (*see margin note*). The secretion of H^+ (or HCO_3^-) by the collecting duct leads to the formation of luminal H_2CO_3. Because there is no luminal carbonic anhydrase in these nephron segments, H_2CO_3 is dehydrated slowly to $CO_2 + H_2O$ in the medullary collecting duct and in the lower urinary collecting system. The result is a urine P_{CO_2} that is considerably greater than the blood P_{CO_2} (Fig. 2-2).

The patient with normal secretion of H^+ in the collecting ducts should have a P_{CO_2} in alkaline urine that is close to 70 mm Hg. Patients with a defect in distal secretion of H^+ have a P_{CO_2} in alkaline urine that is close to that of their blood. A caveat here, however, is that the urine P_{CO_2} may be low despite a normal rate of distal secretion of H^+ if there is a major defect in renal concentrating ability. In contrast, the P_{CO_2} in alkaline urine is high in patients with disorders where HCO_3^- are secreted (e.g., some patients with Southeast Asian ovalocytosis; *see margin note* and see Case 4-2, page 89 for further discussion) or if H^+ back-diffuse in the distal nephron (e.g., owing to drugs such as amphotericin B).

The fractional excretion of HCO_3^-

- The fractional excretion of HCO_3^- permits one to examine net H^+ secretion in the proximal convoluted tubule.

In this test, NaHCO₃ is given to raise the P_{HCO3} to the normal range so that one can measure the rate of excretion of HCO_3^- and compare it with the filtered load of HCO_3^- (see the equation that follows and the *margin note* above entitled "Caution"). If more than 15% of filtered HCO_3^- is excreted, there is a defect in proximal reabsorption of HCO_3^-.

$$FE_{HCO3} = 100 \times (U/P)_{HCO3} / (U/P)_{Creatinine}$$

CAUTION
The patient with a low [K⁺] in plasma (P_K) is at risk of developing a more severe degree of hypokalemia and perhaps a cardiac arrhythmia if given NaHCO₃. Hence, the patient's K⁺ deficit must be corrected before this test is performed.

HIGH URINE P_{CO_2} IN RENAL TUBULAR ACIDOSIS OWING TO DISTAL SECRETION OF HCO_3^-
When HCO_3^- is secreted in the distal nephron, the luminal pH rises and H⁺ are released from $H_2PO_4^-$. When these H⁺ react with luminal HCO_3^-, CO_2 is formed. An example is the patient with Southeast Asian ovalocytosis *and* a second mutation in the gene encoding for the Cl^-/HCO_3^- anion exchanger (AE-1) that causes it to be mistargeted to the luminal membrane of intercalated cells in the collecting ducts.

ARTERIAL AND VENOUS
P$_{CO_2}$ VALUES
Note that in all of these disorders, the emphasis is on the arterial P$_{CO_2}$. On the other hand, the brachial venous P$_{CO_2}$ reflects the P$_{CO_2}$ in the interstitial compartment and in skeletal muscle cells and indicates whether H$^+$ will be removed by the bicarbonate buffer system in muscle cells and in their ECF compartment. Thus, the brachial venous P$_{CO_2}$ reflects whether many of the H$^+$ will bind to intracellular proteins in vital organs (e.g., the brain and the heart).

CONDITIONS WITH A VERY LOW EXTRACELLULAR FLUID VOLUME
In patients with metabolic acidosis, and a markedly reduced ECF volume, the P$_{HCO_3}$ might be close to normal even though the content of HCO$_3^-$ in the ECF compartment is low. Because these patients do not have acidemia, there is no expected respiratory response. Nevertheless, these patients have a "tissue form" of respiratory acidosis (high venous P$_{CO_2}$). As a result, they are at risk of more H$^+$ binding to intracellular proteins as previously discussed (see Fig. 1-8, page 14).

HENDERSON EQUATION
- This equation has three parameters; if two are known, the third can be calculated. If all three are measured, the equation can be useful to detect whether there may be a laboratory error in the measurements.

$$[H^+] \text{ (nmol/L)} = P_{CO_2} \text{ (mm Hg)} \times (24)/P_{HCO_3}$$

- To make the mathematics easier at the bedside, one can use 25 or 24 as the constant in this equation.

PART B
IDENTIFYING MIXED
ACID-BASE DISORDERS

EXPECTED RESPONSES TO PRIMARY ACID-BASE DISORDERS

- These expected values are largely empirical; they permit one to determine whether more than one acid-base disorder is present in a patient (*see margin note*)

It has been observed that when a patient has one of the four primary acid-base disturbances, a predictable response occurs to return the plasma pH (concentration of H$^+$ in plasma) toward the normal range (Table 2-4). Only in chronic respiratory alkalosis might the plasma pH actually return to the normal range as a result of the expected response to raise the P$_{HCO_3}$.

HOW TO RECOGNIZE MIXED ACID-BASE DISORDERS

I. Evaluate the accuracy of the laboratory data

There are two ways to detect laboratory errors in the measured values for acid-base parameters. The first way is to calculate the P$_{Anion\ gap}$. If it is very low or negative, there is probably an error in one of the electrolyte values unless the patient has multiple myeloma, has ingested bromide salts, or has a very low P$_{Albumin}$. The second way to evaluate the laboratory results is to insert the arterial [H$^+$], P$_{CO_2}$, and P$_{HCO_3}$ (from the plasma electrolyte values) into the Henderson equation (*see margin note*). If the latter is done, be careful if you use the

TABLE 2-4 **EXPECTED RESPONSES TO PRIMARY ACID-BASE DISORDERS**

DISORDER	EXPECTED CHANGE
Metabolic acidosis	For every mmol/L fall in P$_{HCO_3}$ from 25, the arterial P$_{CO_2}$ falls by ~1 mm Hg from 40.
Metabolic alkalosis	For every mmol/L rise in P$_{HCO_3}$ from 25, the arterial P$_{CO_2}$ rises by ~0.7 mm Hg from 40.
Respiratory acidosis	
Acute	For every mm Hg rise in the arterial P$_{CO_2}$ from 40, the plasma [H$^+$] rises by ~0.8 nmol/L from 40.
Chronic	For every mm Hg rise in arterial P$_{CO_2}$ from 40, the plasma [H$^+$] rises by ~0.3 nmol/L from 40 and the P$_{HCO_3}$ rises by ~0.3 mmol/L from 25.
Respiratory alkalosis	
Acute	For every mm Hg fall in arterial P$_{CO_2}$ from 40, the plasma [H$^+$] falls by ~0.8 nmol/L from 40.
Chronic	For every mm Hg fall in arterial P$_{CO_2}$ from 40, the P$_{HCO_3}$ falls by ~0.5 mmol/L from 25.

pH and P_{CO_2} from arterial blood and the P_{HCO3} from venous blood because the latter can be as much as 5 to 6 mmol/L higher than the arterial P_{HCO3} when most of the oxygen delivered is extracted from the arterial blood. If the discrepancy is large enough to change the diagnosis, the test should be repeated and the error identified.

2. Calculate the HCO_3^- content in the ECF volume

This requires a quantitative assessment of the ECF volume; use the hematocrit or the concentration of total proteins in plasma for this purpose (see the discussion of Case 2-1, page 57).

3. Examine the arterial P_{CO_2} in the patient with metabolic acidosis or alkalosis to identify the presence of a respiratory acid-base disturbance due to altered ventilation

If the arterial P_{CO_2} is much higher than expected (see Table 2-4), there is a coexistent "ventilation type" of respiratory acidosis. In contrast, if the arterial P_{CO_2} is much lower than expected, respiratory alkalosis is also present.

4. Determine the quantitative relationship between the fall in P_{HCO3} and the rise in the $P_{Anion\ gap}$

- This relationship can be useful to detect mixed acid-base disorders. On the other hand, it might be a misleading indicator of the magnitude of deficit of HCO_3^- if one does not adjust for changes in the ECF volume.
- Be careful to adjust baseline $P_{Anion\ gap}$ for the $P_{Albumin}$ and its valence.

The relationship between the rise in $P_{Anion\ gap}$ and the fall in P_{HCO3} is used to detect the presence of coexisting metabolic alkalosis and metabolic acidosis (the rise in $P_{Anion\ gap}$ is larger than the fall in P_{HCO3}) and/or the presence of both an acid overproduction type and a $NaHCO_3$ loss type of metabolic acidosis (the rise in $P_{Anion\ gap}$ is smaller than the fall in P_{HCO3}). There are several pitfalls in using this relationship that must be recognized.

Pitfall 1: Failure to adjust for changes in the extracellular fluid volume

As an example, consider a 50-kg patient with diabetic ketoacidosis who has a P_{HCO3} of 10 mmol/L and the expected 1:1 relationship between the rise in $P_{Anion\ gap}$ and the fall in the P_{HCO3}. We shall assume that this patient had a normal ECF volume of 10 L before diabetic ketoacidosis developed, but as a result of the glucose-induced osmotic diuresis, his current ECF volume is 8 L. Now, examine Table 2-5 when the fall in the P_{HCO3} and the rise in the concentration of ketoacid anions are equal to see whether indeed the deficit of HCO_3^- is quantitatively equal to the amount of ketoacids in the ECF compartment. In fact, the deficit of HCO_3^- is 170 mmol, but the quantity of new anions in the ECF is only 120 mEq. This discrepancy is revealed only when the content of HCO_3^- and of the new anions in the ECF volume is calculated. There was another component of the loss of HCO_3^- when ketoacids were added; some of the ketoacid anions were excreted in

TABLE 2-5 **QUANTITATIVE DESCRIPTION OF THE FALL IN THE P_{HCO_3} AND RISE IN THE CONCENTRATION OF KETOACID ANIONS IN PATIENTS WITH DIABETIC KETOACIDOSIS**

For simplicity, we disregarded changes in the $P_{Anion\,gap}$ due to changes in the $P_{Albumin}$ in these calculations.

CONDITION	ECF VOLUME	HCO$_3^-$		KETOACID ANIONS	
		CONCENTRATION (mmol/L)	*CONTENT (mmol)*	*CONCENTRATION (mmol/L)*	*CONTENT (mmol)*
Normal	10 L	25	250	0	0
DKA	8 L	10	80	15	120
Balance	− 2 L		− 170		+120

DKA, diabetic ketoacidosis.

the urine with Na^+, which is an indirect form of $NaHCO_3$ loss (see Chapter 5, page 120). This would not be reflected by an increase in $P_{Anion\,gap}$. Hence, the rise in $P_{Anion\,gap}$ did not reveal the actual quantity of ketoacids that were added, and the fall in P_{HCO_3} did not reflect the actual magnitude of the deficit of HCO_3^-. With expansion of the ECF volume with saline, the degree of deficit of HCO_3^- becomes evident. In addition, the fall in the $P_{Anion\,gap}$ will not be matched by a rise in P_{HCO_3} because some ketoacid anions will be lost in urine as their filtered load is increased with the increase in the glomerular filtration rate owing to expansion of effective arterial blood volume.

Pitfall 2: Failure to correct for the net negative valence attributable to $P_{Albumin}$

When calculating the $P_{Anion\,gap}$, one must adjust the value for changes in charge of plasma albumin. When the $P_{Albumin}$ is 40 g/L (4.0 g/dL), the net negative voltage attributed to all the plasma proteins is close to 16 mEq/L. Accordingly, when the $P_{Albumin}$ decreases from 4.0 g/dL (40 g/L) to 3.0 g/dL (30 g/L), the baseline value for the $P_{Anion\,gap}$ should fall close to 4 mEq/L. If this is not taken into consideration, the presence of new anions in plasma could be underestimated. We emphasize that the converse is true for a rise in $P_{Albumin}$ (see Case 3-1, page 70).

5. Detect the "tissue" form of respiratory acidosis

It is essential to measure the brachial venous P_{CO_2} to evaluate whether the removal of H^+ could occur by the bicarbonate buffer system in skeletal muscle. At the usual blood flow rate, the brachial venous P_{CO_2} is close to 46 mm Hg when the arterial P_{CO_2} is 40 mm Hg. The venous P_{CO_2} may be considerably higher than the arterial P_{CO_2} when a larger quantity of CO_2 is produced and/or when there is a reduced blood flow.

6. Assess the responses to respiratory acid-base disorders, differentiating between acute and chronic disorders on clinical grounds

With all the respiratory disturbances, if the P_{HCO_3} is unexpectedly high, metabolic alkalosis is present; if the P_{HCO_3} is lower than expected, metabolic acidosis is present. Decide whether the respiratory disorder is acute or chronic on clinical grounds, not on the basis of laboratory tests. In *acute* respiratory acidosis or alkalosis, there should be only a slight change in P_{HCO_3}, whereas in chronic respiratory acidosis or alkalosis, the slope of $[H^+]$ versus the arterial P_{CO_2} is much flatter because of a larger change in the P_{HCO_3} (see Table 2-4).

PART C
INTEGRATIVE PHYSIOLOGY

OTHER DIAGNOSTIC APPROACHES: THE STRONG ION DIFFERENCE

- Although the strong ion difference approach to acid-base diagnosis is popular with some clinicians, the authors do *not* believe that it adds worthwhile new information.
- Both the strong ion difference and the $P_{Anion\ gap}$ approaches must be modified for two reasons: (1) They ignore the Pco_2 in venous blood draining skeletal muscle and rely *solely* on the arterial Pco_2 to assess buffering of H^+ by the bicarbonate buffer system, and (2) they do not assess the content of HCO_3^- in the ECF compartment.

In 1981, Peter Stewart introduced a calculation to improve the ability to make accurate acid-base diagnoses as well as our understanding of the basis for these disorders. In this formulation, he discarded the traditional definitions of acids and bases and introduced two new terms from measurements in plasma, the strong ion difference (SID) ($Na^+ + K^+ - Cl^-$, which ignores HCO_3^-) and the sum of the net valence attributable to albumin plus phosphate in mEq/L (called A_{tot}). Based on these two new terms, the arterial pH and Pco_2, he solved six equations and created one "master equation." The implication is that this would provide unique and valuable information to understand acid-base disorders in patients. Both this approach and that based on the $P_{Anion\ gap}$, however, suffer from two major faults that must be overcome before either can be helpful in the clinical approach to all the patients with metabolic acidosis.

Reliance on the arterial Pco_2

The *arterial* Pco_2 is important in order to assess the adequacy of buffering by the bicarbonate buffer system in plasma and in red blood cells, but *only* in the arterial compartment. The arterial Pco_2 can help assess the bicarbonate buffer system in the brain if the patient does not have an increased production of CO_2 caused by a higher cerebral metabolic rate or a decrease in cerebral blood flow rate as its autoregulation fails. In contrast, one must know the brachial (or femoral) *venous* Pco_2 to evaluate the capillary Pco_2 and thereby the effectiveness of the bicarbonate buffer system in the interstitial compartment and in the ICF of skeletal muscles, where the bulk of this buffer system operates in a patient with metabolic acidosis.

Amendment
- Measure the brachial (or femoral) venous Pco_2 to gauge how dangerous a given H^+ load is for vital organs and to guide the response to therapy to restore perfusion of skeletal muscle and thereby the effectiveness of its bicarbonate buffer system.

Reliance on the *concentration* of HCO_3^- in plasma

Both methods again fail to provide important information in patients with an appreciable degree of ECF volume contraction because they rely on *only* concentration terms. In a patient with a major degree of contraction of the ECF volume, the P_{HCO3} may be in the normal range even though a severe degree of metabolic acidosis is present (e.g., a large loss of saline and $NaHCO_3$ in diarrhea fluid). To determine the *content* of HCO_3^- in the ECF compartment, one must also know what the ECF volume is in *quantitative* terms (use the hematocrit or total proteins for this purpose as described on page 57).

Amendment

- Because a large deficit of HCO_3^- would *not* be detected with either the SID or the $P_{Anion\ gap}$ approach in a patient with a severe degree of ECF volume contraction, one should measure the hematocrit, hemoglobin, and/or total protein in plasma to obtain quantitative data concerning the plasma volume and thereby the ECF volume and calculate the content of HCO_3^- in the ECF compartment.

Correction for the $P_{Albumin}$

A critical issue for both the SID and the $P_{Anion\ gap}$ methods is to detect the addition of acids to plasma by finding "new anions." To achieve this aim, one estimates the concentration of these new anions using the difference in mEq/L terms between the major cations and anions in plasma (slightly different premises are used, but largely similar results are obtained). The next step is to subtract the net negative valence attributable to $P_{Albumin}$ from that of all the unmeasured anions. This step is done automatically with the SID approach, whereas, although taken into account by many clinicians, it is not automatically included in the "casual" calculation of the $P_{Anion\ gap}$. This is an advantage of the SID approach but a rather minor one considering the complexity of the equations used and that routine correction for $P_{Albumin}$ can be easily incorporated into the $P_{Anion\ gap}$ approach.

There is another issue with regard to the valence that one attributes to plasma proteins. For example, both methods ignore changes in valence of albumin in patients with a contracted ECF volume *and* the change in valence of other circulating protein (e.g., the cationic globulins in plasma in patients with multiple myeloma).

Some advocates of the SID approach make an additional error because they believe that there would be a H^+ load when there is a rise in the $P_{Albumin}$. This would be the case only if enough salt-free albumin (albumin with H^+ bound to remove its net anionic valence) was infused to raise the $P_{Albumin}$. Even if this were to occur, the resulting H^+ load is modest (*see margin note*). This, however, virtually never occurs in clinical medicine; the rise in $P_{Albumin}$ is almost always due to a lower ECF volume. In this setting, one would *not* have a gain of an appreciable H^+ load. Hence, it is *not* correct to attribute a H^+ gain to a rise in $P_{Albumin}$ unless one knows that this rise was due to the administration of a sufficient quantity of salt-poor albumin.

CALCULATION:
H+ LOAD FROM INFUSION
OF SALT-FREE ALBUMIN
- For this calculation, we shall assume that enough salt-free albumin is infused to double the concentration of albumin in plasma and the interstitial portion of the ECF compartment.
- Albumin has close to 16 mEq/L of negative charge at a concentration of 4.0 g/dL (40 g/L) and a plasma pH of 7.40. The content of albumin in plasma and the interstitial space are roughly equal (e.g., ~120 g each when the plasma volume is 3 L).
- If enough salt-poor albumin were added to double the concentration of albumin in the *entire* ECF compartment, the number of H+ added would be only 96 mEq (16 mEq/L × 3 L × 2).

CASE 2-2: LOLA KAYE NEEDS YOUR HELP

(Case discussed on page 58)

Lola Kaye, an 18-year old woman, is brought to the emergency department because of severe weakness. Her blood pressure is low (80/50 mm Hg), and her pulse rate is high (124 beats per minute). Her respiratory rate is *not* low (20 breaths per minute). Her jugular venous pressure is low. The only laboratory values available at this time are *arterial* blood gas values: pH 6.90 ($[H^+]$ = 125 nmol/L), arterial P_{CO_2} = 30 mm Hg. *(See margin note.)* She does not have a history of diabetes mellitus and denies any ingestion of methanol or ethylene glycol.

RATIONALE
This case is provided to illustrate how a diagnosis of acid-base disorders is made while information becomes available at the bedside.

Questions

What is/are the major acid-base diagnosis/diagnoses?
What is the most likely basis for the metabolic acidosis?
What is the most likely basis for the respiratory acidosis?

DISCUSSION OF CASES

CASE 2-1: DOES THIS MAN REALLY HAVE METABOLIC ACIDOSIS?

(Case presented on page 40)

Does this patient have a significant degree of metabolic acidosis?

There are several ways to decide whether metabolic acidosis is present, but not all of them yield the correct answer for the correct reasons.

- *Laboratory data:* If one used a definition of metabolic acidosis that relies *solely* on concentration terms (pH = 7.39, P_{HCO3} = 24 mmol/L, and arterial P_{CO_2} = 39 mm Hg), the answer is "No." On the other hand, because the $P_{Anion\ gap}$ is 24 mEq/L, one might conclude (without careful thought) that this patient has two simultaneous acid-base disorders: metabolic acidosis owing to added acids and a second condition causing the high P_{HCO3} (metabolic alkalosis).
- *Clinical picture:* He lost 5 L of diarrhea fluid, and each liter contained 40 mmol of $NaHCO_3$; thus there was a loss of 200 mmol of HCO_3^- (5 L × 40 mmol/L). Hence, he does have a serious degree of metabolic acidosis even though he does not have acidemia. Moreover, there is no evidence of a gain of HCO_3^- because he did not ingest $NaHCO_3$, there was no history of significant vomiting, and there was little excretion of NH_4^+ (little urine output and an acute illness). Recall that the concentration of HCO_3^- is the quantity of HCO_3^- in the ECF compartment divided by the ECF volume. Hence, we must determine whether there was an "occult" source of HCO_3^- and/or a large decrease in the ECF volume.
- *Correlating the clinical and laboratory information:* One must distinguish between a process leading to a deficit of HCO_3^- (as suggested from history and the $NaHCO_3$ loss in diarrhea fluid) and a process that caused the addition of acids (as suggested by the rise in $P_{Anion\ gap}$) because of different implications for therapy. To confirm that there is a deficit of HCO_3^-, its *content* in the ECF compartment must be calculated. The hematocrit of 0.60 provides a quantitative, minimum estimate that his plasma volume was reduced from 3.0 L to

USE OF THE HEMATOCRIT TO ESTIMATE THE PLASMA VOLUME
In a patient with a blood volume of 5 L (3 L plasma and 2 L red blood cells [RBCs]), the hematocrit is 0.40.

$$Hematocrit = \frac{RBC\ volume\ 2\ L}{Blood\ volume\ (2\ L\ RBC + 3\ L\ plasma)}$$

When the hematocrit is 0.60, the new plasma volume can be calculated as follows:

0.60 = 2 L RBC/(X L blood volume)

Rearranging: 0.6 x = 2.0 L; X = 3.3 L

Assume no change in RBC volume

∴ Plasma volume =
3.3 L blood − 2 L RBC = 1.3 L

1.3 L (i.e., >50%; *see margin note*). There was probably a greater reduction in his ECF volume (10 to 4 L) because his $P_{Albumin}$ was 8.0 g/dL (80 g/L; see *margin note*). Therefore, it is safe to conclude that he has metabolic acidosis with a large deficit of HCO_3^- in his ECF compartment (24 mmol/L × 4 L = 96 mmol versus the usual 240 mmol [24 mmol/L × 10 L]).

What is the basis for the high $P_{Anion\ gap}$?

The high $P_{Anion\ gap}$ is mainly due to a very high $P_{Albumin}$ (because of the profoundly contracted plasma volume) rather than the addition of new acids. This is confirmed by the findings that there were only minor elevations in the $P_{L\text{-lactate}}$ while the $P_{Ketoacid\ anion}$ and $P_{D\text{-lactate}}$ were each less than 1 mmol/L.

Does the patient have respiratory acidosis?

Because the arterial blood pH and Pco_2 are in the normal range, he does not have a *ventilation form of respiratory acidosis*. His current brachial venous Pco_2 is much higher than usual because the blood flow rate to tissues is very low owing to the significant degree of ECF volume contraction. Although the uptake of O_2 is likely to be low, more O_2 is extracted per liter of blood flow and almost an identical amount of CO_2 is added to capillary blood, raising the brachial venous Pco_2. Accordingly, the higher concentration of CO_2 in interstitial space and in cells of muscles makes the bicarbonate buffer system ineffective in removing the H^+ load (i.e., a *tissue* form of respiratory acidosis).

There is another point to consider. When CO_2 is converted to $H^+ + HCO_3^-$, virtually all H^+ produced bind to ICF proteins and the HCO_3^- produced are added to the ECF compartment, raising the P_{HCO3} (see Fig. 3-1, page 66). This may account for the difference between the estimated loss of HCO_3^- (~200 mmol) in diarrhea fluid and the estimated content of HCO_3^- in the ECF compartment (now 96 instead of ~40 mmol of HCO_3^-).

CASE 2-2: LOLA KAYE NEEDS YOUR HELP

(Case presented on page 57)

What is/are the major acid-base diagnosis/diagnoses?

Lola has a very low blood pH, or a high H^+ concentration, because of the following:

Metabolic acidosis: Calculating the P_{HCO3} using the Henderson equation (*see margin note*) reveals that the P_{HCO3} is 6 mmol/L. Therefore, Lola has a severe degree of metabolic acidosis.

Respiratory acidosis: With such a low P_{HCO3}, the expected arterial Pco_2 should be less than 20 mm Hg. The effect of a Pco_2 of 30 versus 20 mm Hg on the H^+ concentration or pH in blood is very large (*see margin note*). Therefore, there is a second acid-base diagnosis, respiratory acidosis of the ventilation type. One might also suspect that a "tissue form" of respiratory acidosis is present because of the low ECF volume. This is confirmed; her brachial venous Pco_2 is 45 mm Hg. This is an important factor contributing to the danger of a high H^+ concentration, because it reduces the ability to buffer most of the H^+ load by the bicarbonate buffer system in the major site where this buffering occurs: skeletal muscle. Therefore, the degree of acidemia is more severe, and more of the H^+ load binds to intracellular proteins in vital organs (e.g., brain cells).

Additional information about Case 2-2

On history, there was no evidence to suspect that she had chronic lung disease. On physical examination, she was conscious, but somewhat obtunded. Her ECF volume appeared to be very low (blood pressure = 80/50 mm Hg, pulse rate = 124 beats per minute). Of importance, her respiratory rate was 20 breaths per minute. On laboratory testing, she did not have elevated values for the $P_{Anion\ gap}$ or $P_{Osmolal\ gap}$. Her P_K was 1.8 mmol/L and there were prominent U waves on electrocardiography.

ABBREVIATION
P_K, $[K^+]$ in plasma

What is the most likely basis for the metabolic acidosis?

Because the $P_{Anion\ gap}$ and $P_{Osmolal\ gap}$ were not elevated, the presence of ketoacidosis, L- or D-lactic acidosis, or alcohol ingestion are unlikely causes of the metabolic acidosis. Therefore, the most likely basis for the metabolic acidosis is a deficit of $NaHCO_3$, which could be due to its loss in a direct or indirect form (see Chapter 4, pages 79 and 84 for further discussion). Estimating the rate of excretion of NH_4^+ in the urine is needed to make a more specific diagnosis for the basis of the metabolic acidosis. The rate of excretion of NH_4^+ was high, and the accompanying anion was not Cl^-. The underlying disorder, glue sniffing, is discussed in Chapter 3, page 71.

What is the most likely basis for the respiratory acidosis?

She has no evidence of chronic lung disease. Although she may have consumed drugs that caused depression of her central nervous system, the fact that her respiratory rate is *not low* leads to a suspicion that the depth of breathing might be reduced, possibly because of weakness of respiratory muscles—the most obvious cause is a very low P_K (1.8 mmol/L; *see margin note*).

CAUTION
In this patient, do not give glucose or $NaHCO_3$ before dealing with the hypokalemia.

chapter 3

Metabolic Acidosis: Clinical Approach

Introduction

In this chapter, our goal is to provide a bedside approach to the patient with metabolic acidosis. This approach focuses not only on diagnosis but also on identifying and handling emergencies while anticipating and preventing risks that are likely to develop during therapy. An important component of our approach is to deduce whether there is a risk of excessive binding of H^+ to intracellular proteins in vital organs (e.g., the brain and the heart). We discuss how this may occur and how it can be reversed.

OBJECTIVES

- To emphasize the following issues in the approach to the patient with metabolic acidosis:
  1. *Treat emergencies first*: The first step is to recognize and deal with threats to the patient's life and to anticipate and prevent risks that may arise owing to therapy.

2. *Assess the effectiveness of the bicarbonate buffer system:* The brachial or femoral venous P_{CO_2} is needed to evaluate the effectiveness of the bicarbonate buffer system in skeletal muscle, where the bulk of this buffer system exists. When the bicarbonate buffer system is compromised, more H^+ bind to proteins in cells of vital organs (e.g., brain and heart).

■ To illustrate how to determine whether the basis of the metabolic acidosis is due to added acids and/or a deficit of sodium bicarbonate: Look for new anions in plasma and urine, and assess the rate of excretion of NH_4^+.

CASE 3-1: THE TRUTH WILL BE TOLD IN THE END

(Case discussed on page 70)

A 25-year-old man was perfectly healthy until he developed diarrhea 24 hours ago *(see margin note)*. He has had no intake of food or water and currently has no urine output. His blood pressure is 90/60 mm Hg, his pulse rate is 110 beats per minute, and his jugular venous pressure is low. Acid-base measurements in *arterial* blood reveal pH of 7.39, P_{HCO_3} of 24 mmol/L, and P_{CO_2} of 39 mm Hg. He has lost 5 L of diarrhea fluid, which contained Na^+ 140 mmol/L, K^+ 15 mmol/L, Cl^- 115 mmol/L, and HCO_3^- 40 mmol/L. On admission, his hematocrit is 0.60, $P_{Albumin}$ is 8.0 g/dL (80 g/L), and P_K is 4.8 mmol/L.

This case is also presented in Chapter 2 with a different title; the points emphasized there are how the diagnostic tests should be interpreted. In this chapter, the major emphasis is to recognize current threats to the patient and anticipate those that may develop during therapy. A more detailed description of the biochemistry and pathophysiology of cholera is provided in Chapter 4, Part D, page 106.

Questions

Is there a major threat to life on admission?
What dangers might be created by therapy?
Why is his P_{HCO_3} 24 mmol/L in the face of such a large loss of $NaHCO_3$?

ABBREVIATION
$P_{Albumin}$, [albumin] in plasma

CASE 3-2: STICK TO THE FACTS

(Case discussed on page 71)

A 28-year-old man had been sniffing glue on a chronic but intermittent basis. Over the past 3 days, he had become profoundly weak and had a very unsteady gait. On physical examination, his blood pressure was 100/60 mm Hg and his pulse rate was 110 beats per minute while lying flat. When he sat up, his blood pressure fell to 80/50 mm Hg and his pulse rate rose to 130 beats per minute. His *arterial* blood pH was 7.20, P_{CO_2} was 25 mm Hg, and P_{HCO_3} was 10 mmol/L. His $P_{Glucose}$ was 3.5 mmol/L (63 mg/dL), his $P_{Albumin}$ was 6.0 g/dL (60 g/L), and his hematocrit was 0.50.

ABBREVIATION
$P_{Glucose}$, concentration of glucose in plasma

		VENOUS BLOOD	URINE
pH		7.00	6.0
P_{CO_2}	mm Hg	60	—
HCO_3^-	mmol/L	15	<5
Na^+	mmol/L	120	50
K^+	mmol/L	2.3	30
Cl^-	mmol/L	90	0
Creatinine	mg/dL (μmol/L)	1.7 (150)	3.0 mmol/L
BUN (urea)	mg/dL (mmol/L)	14 (5.0)	150 mmol/L
Osmolality	mOsm/kg H_2O	250	500

Questions

Is metabolic acidosis present?
What dangers are present before therapy begins?
What dangers might be created by therapy?
What is the basis of the metabolic acidosis?

PART A
CLINICAL APPROACH

- The first step in the approach to the patient with metabolic acidosis is to identify threats for that patient.
- The next two steps are as follows: (1) Determine whether H^+ were buffered appropriately by the bicarbonate buffer system. (2) Determine whether the basis of the metabolic acidosis is due to added acids and/or a deficit of $NaHCO_3$.

Our initial approach to the patient with metabolic acidosis is provided in Flow Chart 3-1. Metabolic acidosis must be present to enter this flow chart. This diagnosis is based on one of the following criteria: (1) a low plasma pH and P_{HCO3}; (2) an increase in the anion gap in plasma ($P_{Anion\ gap}$) corrected for the $P_{Albumin}$; or (3) an appreciable decrease in the content of HCO_3^- in the extracellular fluid (ECF) compartment in the patient who has a history suggesting that the ECF volume may be contracted. For the third criterion, a *quantitative* estimate of the ECF volume is needed. Because one

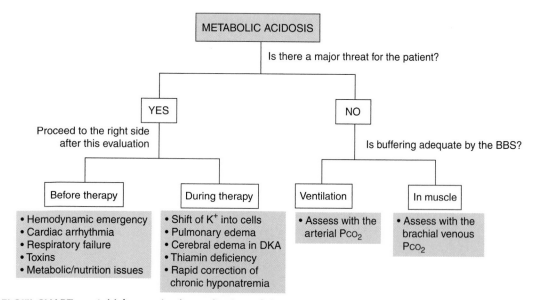

FLOW CHART 3-1 Initial steps in the evaluation of the patient with metabolic acidosis. One must use a definition of metabolic acidosis that is based not only on the P_{HCO_3} but also on the content of HCO_3^- in the ECF compartment if its volume is significantly contracted. The initial step is to determine threats for the patient that may be present and anticipate those that may develop during therapy (*left side of the flow chart*). The next step is to assess buffering by the bicarbonate buffer system (BBS) in the ECF and ICF of skeletal muscle to deduce whether more H^+ are bound to brain proteins (*right side of the flow chart*). DKA, diabetic ketoacidosis.

cannot obtain accurate quantitative data about the ECF volume with the physical examination, we recommend using the hematocrit or total protein level in plasma to obtain this information (see the discussion of Case 2-1, page 57).

1. *Identify threats.* The first step is to identify and deal with threats that are present before therapy begins *and* anticipate and prevent dangers that may develop during the course of the illness or with therapy.

2. *Determine whether H^+ are removed appropriately by HCO_3^-.* After the emergencies are considered and dealt with, the arterial P_{CO_2} and the brachial (or femoral) venous P_{CO_2} should be assessed, as the latter helps reveal to the effectiveness of the bicarbonate buffer system in the ECF and ICF compartments in skeletal muscle. If the *brachial* venous P_{CO_2} is high, the bicarbonate buffer system in skeletal muscle is compromised. Hence, more of the H^+ load binds to intracellular proteins in vital organs (e.g., brain cells). If autoregulation of cerebral blood flow fails, more H^+ will bind to intracellular proteins in the brain because of a marked decrease in the effective arterial blood volume.

ABBREVIATIONS
ECF, extracellular fluid
ICF, intracellular fluid

EMERGENCIES IN THE PATIENT WITH METABOLIC ACIDOSIS

Although it is common practice to begin the assessment of a patient with metabolic acidosis with an emphasis on diagnosis, we recommend a different approach for the critically ill patient with metabolic acidosis—begin with data that are most important to answer the question "How can I prevent this patient from dying?" The risks to the patient can be divided into those that are present when the patient seeks medical attention and those that may develop during therapy (Table 3-1).

TABLE 3-1 **THREATS TO LIFE ASSOCIATED WITH METABOLIC ACIDOSIS**

On admission

- Hemodynamic instability
  - Marked decrease in myocardial contractility (e.g., cardiogenic shock)
  - Very low intravascular volume (e.g., NaCl loss, hemorrhage)
  - Decreased peripheral vascular resistance (e.g., sepsis)
- Cardiac arrhythmia
  - Most frequently seen in patients with hyperkalemia or hypokalemia
- Failure of ventilation (e.g., respiratory muscle weakness due to hypokalemia)
- Presence of toxins (e.g., methanol, ethylene glycol)
- Presence of reactive oxygen species (e.g., pyroglutamic acidosis)
- Nutritional deficiency (especially B vitamins)

During therapy

- Development of cerebral edema during therapy of diabetic ketoacidosis in children
  - Overly rapid infusion of isotonic saline
  - Failure to prevent a fall in the effective plasma osmolality during therapy
- Pulmonary edema (e.g., in patients with severe diarrhea if the ECF volume is expanded, but $NaHCO_3$ is not given)
- Too rapid a rise in P_{Na} in patients with chronic hyponatremia
- Development of a severe degree of acidemia in a patient with metabolic acidosis (see discussion of Case 3-1, page 70)
- Acute shift of K^+ into cells (e.g., administration of glucose to patients with hypokalemia, administration of insulin to patients with DKA and hypokalemia, administration of $NaHCO_3$ to patients with a low P_K)
- Wernicke's encephalopathy due to failure to give thiamin (vitamin B_1) to chronic alcoholics with alcoholic ketoacidosis

The diagnostic category of metabolic acidosis is made up of two major subgroups, one where the basis of the disorder is the addition of acids and the other where the basis is a major loss of $NaHCO_3$. Although the emergencies may be different within each of the causes for the disorder, nevertheless, we start this discussion by emphasizing the importance of detecting, anticipating, and dealing with threats to life.

Risks prior to therapy

Hemodynamic emergency

> • The most common example is a patient with L-lactic acidosis owing to cardiogenic shock (e.g., myocardial infarction) because survival at this point depends on whether the cardiac output can be improved very quickly.

In most of the other settings of metabolic acidosis due to added acids, true hemodynamic emergencies are not common, with the possible exception of some patients with sepsis and others with alcoholic or diabetic ketoacidosis. Although a significant degree of contraction of the effective arterial blood volume is usually present in children with diabetic ketoacidosis (i.e., caused by the glucose-induced osmotic diuresis) a true hemodynamic emergency is usually not present. Hence, overly rapid and excessive administration of saline should be avoided because of the risk of inducing cerebral edema (see Chapter 5, page 128 for more discussion).

Conversely, patients with a *very* significant degree of contraction of the effective arterial blood volume that causes an inadequate delivery of oxygen to tissues and the production of an appreciable quantity of L-lactic acid require the urgent administration of a large volume of isotonic saline. In contrast, if the patient is not hemodynamically compromised, aggressive therapy is not warranted because, at times, serious complications related to this infusion might arise (see the discussion of Case 3-1, page 70).

Cardiac arrhythmia

Patients with metabolic acidosis may develop a cardiac arrhythmia when there is a severe degree of hyperkalemia (e.g., owing to renal failure) or hypokalemia (e.g., certain patients with distal renal tubular acidosis, patients with metabolic acidosis due to glue sniffing). In addition, hypokalemia may develop after therapy is initiated (see Cases 3-1 and 3-2). The emergency treatment of hypokalemia and of hyperkalemia is discussed in Chapters 14 and 15.

Failure of adequate ventilation

Respiratory muscle weakness due to a severe degree of hypokalemia could lead to respiratory failure and a more severe degree of acidemia in patients with metabolic acidosis. Enough KCl should be given to raise the P_K to 3.0 mmol/L in this setting; mechanical ventilation might also be needed.

Toxin-induced metabolic acidosis

Ingestion of methanol or ethylene glycol should always be suspected in a patient with metabolic acidosis, an elevated $P_{Anion\ gap}$, and no obvious cause for these findings, especially if the ECF volume is not significantly contracted (see Chapter 6, page 178). Failing to make this diagnosis can be devastating. If ingestion of these alcohols is suspected, one must calculate the $P_{Osmolal\ gap}$ (see Chapter 2, page 48). If the $P_{Osmolal\ gap}$ is considerably greater than 10 mOsm/kg H_2O, the diagnosis should be confirmed by direct measurements of methanol and of ethylene glycol in plasma because ethanol also contributes to the $P_{Osmolal\ gap}$. Because it is the products of the metabolism of these toxic alcohols that create the danger rather than the parent compounds, administer ethanol to prevent their metabolism until the facts become clear.

ABBREVIATION
$P_{Osmolal\ gap}$, osmolal gap in plasma

Dangers to anticipate after commencing therapy

Several threats are anticipated in a patient with metabolic acidosis.

Dangers related to overly aggressive administration of saline

Although enough saline should be given if there is evident hemodynamic instability, an excessive rate of administration of saline has its dangers. In absence of hemodynamic instability, we use the brachial venous P_{CO_2} and the hematocrit to guide decisions about intravenous fluid therapy (*see margin note*). If oliguria develops during therapy, a more vigorous restoration of intravascular volume may be needed. Several complications may arise from overly aggressive administration of saline.

A very severe degree of acidemia. There is a fall in the P_{HCO_3} when a large volume of saline without $NaHCO_3$ is given to a patient who has a severe degree of ECF volume contraction (e.g., the patient with a large loss of $NaHCO_3$ and saline in diarrhea fluid; see Case 3-1, page 70). When saline is infused *very* rapidly, some patients with metabolic acidosis caused by $NaHCO_3$ loss due to diarrhea and a severe degree of contraction of the effective arterial blood volume develop pulmonary edema before their ECF volume is sufficiently reexpanded. This may be the result of the severe degree of acidemia that develops, which leads to the redistribution of blood from the peripheral to the central circulating blood volume. It is important to recognize this complication, because pulmonary edema can be prevented and/or treated successfully with an infusion of fluid that contains $NaHCO_3$ (or an anion that can be metabolized to produce HCO_3^- [e.g., L-lactate$^-$]). See the discussion of Case 3-1, page 70.

CAUTION
The hematocrit on admission is not useful in patients who have anemia.

Three mechanisms may lead to a more severe degree of acidemia with the infusion of a large amount of saline in these patients.

1. *Dilution of the HCO_3^- in the ECF compartment*: These patients have metabolic acidosis with a large deficit of HCO_3^- even though their P_{HCO_3} might not be very low because of the marked degree of contraction of their ECF volume. Hence, the concentration of HCO_3^- in the ECF compartment declines when a large volume of saline is infused because of the rise in the denominator of the HCO_3^-:ECF volume ratio.
2. *Loss of more $NaHCO_3$ in diarrhea fluid*: Reexpansion of the effective arterial blood volume increases splanchnic blood flow. This permits a much larger quantity of Na^+ and Cl^- to be secreted in the small intestine. When a large volume of luminal fluid containing Na^+ and Cl^- reaches the colon, more Cl^- is reabsorbed in exchange for HCO_3^- compared with the absorption of Na^+ in exchange for secreted H^+; hence, the loss

of $NaHCO_3$ in diarrhea fluid may rise markedly (see Fig. 4-4, page 82).

3. *Back-titration of HCO_3^- by H^+ that were bound to intracellular proteins*: Assume that muscle cells have a constant consumption of oxygen and production of CO_2. Now when the blood flow rate rises, the same amount of oxygen is consumed, but less oxygen is extracted from *each liter* of blood. Because almost the same amount of CO_2 is produced as O_2 consumed, less CO_2 is added *per liter* of blood. Hence, the venous PCO_2 and the tissue PCO_2 decline. As a result of the decline in PCO_2, the concentration of H^+ in cells falls and fewer H^+ are bound to proteins in cells. Many of these H^+ that are released combine with HCO_3^- in the ICF and ECF compartments; hence, the concentration of HCO_3^- in the ECF compartment declines (Fig. 3-1).

Cerebral edema in children with diabetic ketoacidosis. Children with diabetic ketoacidosis, especially those with a long delay before arriving in hospital for therapy, are prone to develop cerebral edema during therapy (see Chapter 5, page 127 for more details). One of the factors that might predispose a patient to this dreaded complication is the administration of a large volume of saline. Enough saline should be given to restore systemic hemodynamics if there is evident hemodynamic instability. Conversely, in the absence of hemodynamic instability, one should avoid giving too much saline or giving it too quickly. The brachial venous PCO_2, hematocrit, and urine flow rate are parameters that can be used to guide the decision concerning the rate of administration of saline. Measures must also be taken to prevent a fall in the $P_{Effective\ osm}$ (*see margin note*).

Rapid correction of chronic hyponatremia. Another important risk factor for the patient with a markedly contracted effective arterial blood volume is removal of the stimulus for the release of vasopressin and an increase in the distal delivery of filtrate once the effective arterial blood volume is reexpanded. If that patient has chronic hyponatremia, the ensuing water diuresis may lead to a rapid rise in P_{Na} and thereby increase the risk for developing osmotic demyelination, especially in the patient with poor nutrition and/or hypokalemia.

ABBREVIATION

$P_{Effective\ osm}$, effective osmolality in plasma = $2\ P_{Na} + P_{Glucose}$ in mmol/L terms

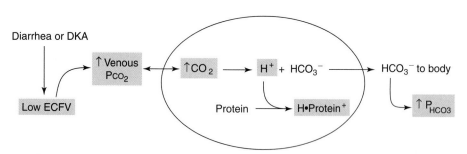

FIGURE 3-1 Fall in the P_{HCO_3} when the venous PCO_2 declines in a patient with metabolic acidosis. The *oval* represents a muscle cell with membrane containing its HCO_3^- and protein buffer systems. Owing to the diarrhea or DKA, the effective arterial blood volume is very contracted and the rate of blood flow to muscle is reduced. The subsequent enhanced O_2 extraction from each liter of blood flowing through the capillaries raises both the capillary and the ICF PCO_2. The higher PCO_2 in the interstitial fluid and in these cells drives the synthesis of H^+ and HCO_3; the H^+ bind to intracellular proteins while the HCO_3^- is exported to the ECF. The net result is a rise in the P_{HCO_3}. After the infusion of a large volume of saline and a decline in the PCO_2, in capillaries and in cells, these events are reversed, and this contributes to the fall in the P_{HCO_3}. DKA, diabetic ketoacidosis; ECFV, extracellular fluid volume.

Administering dDAVP at the outset should be considered to prevent a water diuresis and minimize the risk of developing this devastating complication.

Hypokalemia. A sudden shift of K^+ into cells causes hypokalemia and thus an increased risk of developing a cardiac arrhythmia and/or respiratory muscle weakness. Risk factors are the administration of insulin, a stimulator of its release (glucose), removal of the α-adrenergic–induced inhibition of the release of insulin (e.g., reexpanding the effective arterial blood volume by infusing saline), and/or administration of drugs that may increase β_2-adrenergic activity (see Chapter 14, page 477 for more discussion).

ABBREVIATION
dDAVP, desmopressin, or desamino, D-arginine vasopressin

Metabolic or nutritional issues

One must always suspect a deficiency of vitamin B family members in patients who have metabolic acidosis who are malnourished. Thiamin (vitamin B_1) deficiency is not uncommon in chronic alcoholics; these patients need therapy with this vitamin at the outset to prevent the development of Wernicke-Korsakoff encephalopathy (see Chapter 6, page 172). Other patients may have L-lactic acidosis if they are deficient in riboflavin (vitamin B_2). Patients who take isoniazid to treat tuberculosis are at risk for mini-seizures and L-lactic acidosis; these patients should be given vitamin B_6 (pyridoxine).

Another example of a metabolic threat is in patients with pyroglutamic acidosis (see Chapter 6, page 183). In this disorder, the threat to life is due to depletion of reduced glutathione and thus compromised ability to detoxify reactive oxygen species. Metabolic acidosis is a "red flag" that warns the physician about this pathophysiology.

ASSESS THE EFFECTIVENESS OF THE BICARBONATE BUFFER SYSTEM

There must be a low P_{CO_2} to ensure that HCO_3^- remove H^+.
- The arterial P_{CO_2} must be low.
- The P_{CO_2} in venous blood draining skeletal muscle must be low.

The *arterial* P_{CO_2} reflects the physiologic respiratory response to metabolic acidosis. It is also similar to the P_{CO_2} in brain cells because the metabolic rate in the brain is virtually constant; hence, there is little change in its rate of oxygen consumption and CO_2 production. In addition, its blood supply is autoregulated. The arterial P_{CO_2} sets the lower limit for the capillary P_{CO_2} in other organs.

Because most of the bicarbonate buffer system in the ECF and ICF compartments is in skeletal muscle, we use the P_{CO_2} in the brachial or femoral venous blood to indicate whether the bicarbonate buffer system in this location is effective in buffering the H^+ load (see Fig. 1-8, page 14). The bicarbonate buffer system in skeletal muscle is ineffective if the brachial or femoral venous P_{CO_2} is too high; hence, acidemia is more pronounced and more of the H^+ load is titrated in vital organs (e.g., brain and heart). Furthermore, if autoregulation of the blood supply to the brain fails because of a marked degree of contraction of the effective arterial blood volume, the brain venous P_{CO_2} rises and more H^+ bind to intracellular proteins in brain cells. The major clinical setting for failure of the bicarbonate buffer system in muscle is a low blood flow rate owing to a contracted effective arterial blood volume. At the usual blood flow rates at rest, the brachial venous P_{CO_2} is 46 mm Hg, whereas the arterial P_{CO_2} is 40 mm Hg. Hence, enough saline should be administered to restore the effective arterial blood volume and ensure that the brachial venous P_{CO_2} remains less than 10 mm Hg above the arterial P_{CO_2}.

DETERMINE THE BASIS OF METABOLIC ACIDOSIS

Three steps remain in the clinical approach:
1. Detect added acids by finding new anions in plasma or in excreted fluids.
2. If acids were added very rapidly, suspect hypoxia or ingestion of an acid.
3. Assess the renal response by estimating the rate of excretion of NH_4^+.

The basis of metabolic acidosis could be a gain of an acid or the loss of $NaHCO_3$ (Flow Chart 3-2). There are three important additional

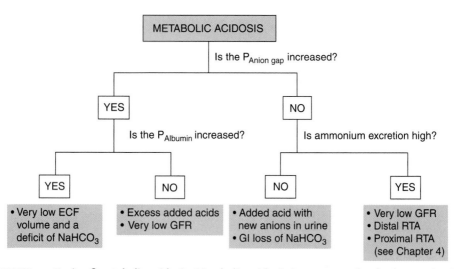

FLOW CHART 3-2 Basis of metabolic acidosis. Metabolic acidosis is a process that leads to a rise in the H^+ concentration in plasma and a fall in the P_{HCO_3}. The goal for this flow chart is to identify whether its cause is the net addition of acids and/or the net loss of Na^+ (or K^+) plus HCO_3^-. Hence, the first step is to identify whether the *footprints* of added acids (the anions that accompany the H^+) are present in plasma and thereby in the ECF compartment (detected by finding a high $P_{Anion\ gap}$; see the *left portion* of the flow chart). Be careful if the concentration of albumin is low. Notwithstanding, if there is a higher negative charge associated with the $P_{Albumin}$, there will be an increased $P_{Anion\ gap}$ that may not reflect added acids (e.g., a patient with a marked degree of contraction of the ECF volume owing to severe diarrhea with large losses of $NaCl$ and $NaHCO_3$ in diarrhea fluid). As shown in the *right portion* of the flow chart, a net loss of $NaHCO_3$ is present if the $P_{Anion\ gap}$ is not increased. If the rate of excretion of NH_4^+ is high along with an anion other than Cl^-, suspect that the cause of metabolic acidosis is the addition of an acid that has an accompanying anion that is excreted rapidly in the urine. If the rate of excretion of NH_4^+ is low, on the other hand, seek the basis for the renal defect that compromises the rate of excretion of NH_4^+. ECF, extracellular fluid; GFR, glomerular filtration rate; GI, gastrointestinal; RTA, renal tubular acidosis.

considerations that improve the diagnostic approach to the patient with metabolic acidosis.

Detect addition of acids by finding new anions

- Search for new anions in plasma, in urine, and at times in diarrhea or drainage fluids.

An increase in the $P_{Anion\ gap}$ is used to detect the addition of new acids. Nevertheless, there are two pitfalls to avoid in this context. First, the baseline value for the $P_{Anion\ gap}$ should be lower if the $P_{Albumin}$ is reduced; the converse is also true (*see margin note*). Second, there is a much smaller rise in the $P_{Anion\ gap}$ if the anions of the added acids are excreted in the urine at a rapid rate (e.g., hippurate anions in a patient with metabolic acidosis due to glue sniffing; see the discussion of Case 3-2, page 71). To detect new anions in the urine, we calculate the urine anion gap ($U_{Na} + U_K + U_{NH_4} - U_{Cl}$). The concentration of NH_4^+ in the urine is estimated from the $U_{Osmolal\ gap}$.

ADJUST $P_{Anion\ gap}$ FOR $P_{Albumin}$
As a rough approximation, the $P_{Anion\ gap}$ should decrease by 4 mEq/L for each 1.0-g/dL (10-g/L) decrease in the $P_{Albumin}$. The converse is also true.

Detect conditions with fast addition of H^+

- If metabolic acidosis develops over a short period of time, the likely causes are overproduction of L-lactic acid (e.g., shock) or ingested acids.

ABBREVIATIONS
$U_{Osmolal\ gap}$, osmolal gap in the urine
U_{NH_4}, concentration of NH_4^+ in the urine
$U_{Creatinine}$, concentration of creatinine in the urine

The first one is obvious: hypoxic L-lactic acidosis (i.e., when the supply of oxygen is too low to match the demand for ATP regeneration by aerobic fuel oxidation). The other setting where H^+ input can be very fast is the ingestion of a large quantity of an acid (e.g., metabolic acidosis due to ingestion of citric acid; see Chapter 6, page 184).

Assess the renal response to metabolic acidosis

The expected renal response to chronic metabolic acidosis is the excretion of 200 to 250 mmol of NH_4^+ per day in an adult. The calculation of the $U_{Osmolal\ gap}$ provides the most reliable indirect estimate of the concentration of NH_4^+ in the urine (see Chapter 2, page 48). This U_{NH_4} can be converted to an excretion rate by dividing the U_{NH_4} by $U_{Creatinine}$ and multiplying this ratio by expected rate of excretion of creatinine.

QUESTIONS

(*Discussions on pages 73 and 74*)

3-1 *In a patient with cholera and metabolic acidosis due to the loss of $NaHCO_3$ in diarrhea fluid, the ECF volume is contracted by close to 50%, yet O_2 delivery to tissues is adequate to avoid anaerobic metabolism. Should this patient have an elevated value for the $P_{Anion\ gap}$?*

3-2 *Why might pulmonary edema develop before the ECF volume is fully reexpanded in this patient with cholera?*

PART B
DISCUSSIONS
DISCUSSION OF CASES

CASE 3-1: THE TRUTH WILL BE TOLD IN THE END

(Case presented on page 61)

Is there a major threat to life on admission?

The following threats are present:

Low effective arterial blood volume: There is a very severe degree of plasma volume contraction (~60%) as judged from the hematocrit (0.60). The decision that the clinician must make in this context is how fast saline should be administered. On one hand, there are potential dangers from such a severe degree of effective arterial blood volume contraction, including acute tubular necrosis, venous thrombosis due to high blood viscosity because of slow blood flow rate, and a "tissue" form of respiratory acidosis. On the other hand, this patient does *not* have a significant degree of decreased tissue perfusion because there is no appreciable rise in the $P_{\text{L-lactate}}$; thus, one *need not* reexpand the ECF volume with *very great* haste if there is a potential danger in doing so (see the discussion of the next question).

High venous Pco_2*, a tissue form of respiratory acidosis*: This is particularly relevant when dealing with a patient with poor tissue perfusion due to either severe cardiac disease or ECF volume contraction. The very low ECF volume in this patient suggests that a "tissue" form of respiratory acidosis might be present; this was confirmed by the high Pco_2 in brachial venous blood (69 mm Hg) compared with the arterial Pco_2 (39 mm Hg). This high venous Pco_2 indicates that the buffering by the bicarbonate buffer system in skeletal muscles is compromised and thus that there is a more severe degree of acidemia and more H^+ binding to intracellular protein in vital organs (e.g., brain, especially if the autoregulation of its blood flow is compromised; see Fig. 1-8, page 14).

The venous Pco_2 should fall once tissue perfusion improves; this provides the clinician with a tool to guide the rate of administration of saline. As a rough guide, enough saline should be given to lower brachial venous Pco_2 to a value that is less than 10 mm Hg higher than the arterial Pco_2.

What dangers might be created by therapy?

These dangers should be anticipated and prevented:

A more severe degree of acidemia: Reexpanding his ECF volume by infusing a saline solution that does not contain HCO_3^- might cause a severe degree of acidemia because this patient has a large deficit of HCO_3^- and little opportunity to add new HCO_3^- to the body (no available anions that can be converted into HCO_3^-). The other mechanisms that would cause a fall in the P_{HCO3} when saline is administered include accelerated loss of $NaHCO_3$ in diarrhea fluid and titration of HCO_3^- with H^+ that are bound to intracellular proteins and are released from cells when the venous Pco_2 falls (see Fig. 3-1, page 66). The administration of saline to such patients and development of a severe degree of acidemia are associated with the appearance of pulmonary edema (see the discussion of Question 3-2, page 74 for more information).

Hypokalemia: Despite an important degree of K^+ depletion, hypokalemia was not present on admission, presumably because K^+ had shifted out of cells. The mechanism for this K^+ shift is probably a deficiency of insulin, which is the result of inhibition of its release by the α-adrenergic surge in response to the very contracted effective arterial blood volume. Hence, one should expect a significant drop in the P_K with reexpansion of the ECF volume because this leads to a fall in circulating α-adrenergic hormone, which causes a rise in the $P_{Insulin}$. One should also be aware that the degree of hypokalemia may become more severe with the infusion of $NaHCO_3$ and thus more aggressive therapy with KCl may be needed.

ABBREVIATION
$P_{Insulin}$, concentration of insulin in plasma

If a severe degree of K^+ depletion with hypokalemia develops, bowel motility may diminish to a degree such that intestinal secretions are pooled in the gut and diarrhea is no longer observed; this serious complication is called *cholera sicca*.

Why is his P_{HCO_3} 24 mmol/L in the face of such a large loss of $NaHCO_3$?

- The concentration of HCO_3^- in the ECF compartment is equal to its content divided by the ECF volume.

First, this patient had a very severe degree of contraction of his ECF volume, as reflected by the hematocrit of 0.60; this raises his P_{HCO3} 2.5-fold compared with the value if his ECF volume were normal. Second, there is added HCO_3^- to his ECF compartment because of the very high venous P_{CO_2} draining muscle (see Fig. 3-1, page 66).

Of interest, the high value for his $P_{Anion\ gap}$ may suggest that there were added acids, which would lower his P_{HCO3}. In this context, the acid to suspect is L-lactic acid due to the very markedly contracted effective arterial blood volume. Nevertheless, the fact that the high $P_{Anion\ gap}$ is due to a very high $P_{Albumin}$ secondary to the profoundly contracted ECF volume and not to the addition of new acids was confirmed by failing to find an appreciably elevated $P_{L\text{-}lactate}$. In addition, $P_{Ketoacid\ anions}$ and $P_{D\text{-}lactate}$ were not elevated.

At this point, our attention turns to the need to reexpand his effective arterial blood volume despite an ongoing and increasing volume of diarrhea fluid because expansion of his effective arterial blood volume results in a marked increase in the secretion of Na^+ and Cl^- in the small intestine. Notwithstanding, the positive balance for Na^+ and Cl^- can be maintained by promoting the absorption of Na^+ and Cl^- in the intestinal tract by giving large volumes of a solution containing equimolar amounts of glucose and Na^+ with Cl^- plus some citrate anions by the oral route (this is called *oral rehydration therapy*; see Fig. 4-6, page 83).

CASE 3-2: STICK TO THE FACTS

(Case presented on page 61)

Is metabolic acidosis present?

Yes, he has metabolic acidosis because his arterial pH is 7.20, P_{HCO_3} is 10 mmol/L, and arterial P_{CO_2} is 25 mm Hg.

What dangers are present before therapy begins?

Cardiac arrhythmia and/or hypoventilation: The low P_K can cause both of these complications. The K^+ deficit is due to an excessive excretion of K^+ in the urine in this patient because the urine contains a large quantity of the organic anion, hippurate, which is excreted at a faster rate than NH_4^+.

Because of the danger of causing a shift of K^+ into cells that would aggravate an already severe degree of hypokalemia, one should not administer $NaHCO_3$ or give glucose (unless the patient also has hypoglycemia) until the P_K is raised to a safe level. Treatment of hypokalemia is discussed in detail in Chapter 14, page 500.

Binding of more H^+ to proteins in cells: His brachial *venous* PCO_2 is 60 mm Hg and the *arterial* PCO_2 was 25 mm Hg; this PCO_2 difference suggests that there was a significantly reduced blood flow rate to muscle owing to the very contracted effective arterial blood volume. This high brachial venous PCO_2 suggests that the buffering by the bicarbonate buffer system in muscles is compromised and thus there is a risk of binding of more H^+ to intracellular proteins in vital organs (e.g., brain and heart; see Fig. 1-8, page 14).

What dangers might be created by therapy?

These are listed with a few comments because most of the dangers were discussed in Case 3-1. The dangers to anticipate are a fall in the P_K, a further fall in the P_{HCO3}, and too rapid a rise in the P_{Na}. There could also be nutritional issues.

Further fall in the P_K: Just as in the previous case, reexpansion of the effective arterial blood volume can lead to a fall in α-adrenergics and thereby to a rise in insulin levels. In addition, as renal perfusion improves, the excretion of hippurate at a rate faster than NH_4^+ could lead to very high rates of excretion of K^+. Again, if HCO_3^- and/or glucose is administered, this could further aggravate the degree of hypokalemia owing to a shift of K^+ into cells.

Further fall in the P_{HCO3}: Just as in the previous case, the P_{HCO3} falls for a number of reasons when isotonic saline is administered. The dilemma is balancing the need for giving exogenous HCO_3^- versus the danger of causing an acute fall in the P_K. In the opinion of the authors, K^+ replacement should take precedence. If there is a need to administer HCO_3^- early on, give $NaHCO_3$ with sufficient KCl to prevent a fall in the P_K; this should be done in a setting where cardiac and respiratory monitoring can be carried out.

Too rapid a rise in the P_{Na}: This is very important in a patient who is poorly nourished and/or K^+ depleted, because these are risk factors for the development of osmotic demyelination during therapy. Our rationale for administering dDAVP at the outset of therapy is discussed in Chapter 10, page 331.

What is the basis of the metabolic acidosis?

Because the $P_{Anion\ gap}$ is in the normal range, one might have thought that the metabolic acidosis was not due to a gain of acids. Nevertheless, the rate of excretion of NH_4^+ was high (*see margin note*), and the accompanying anions were not Cl^-. This case represents the overproduction of an organic acid with the rapid excretion of its anion in the urine. Metabolic acidosis develops because some of the anions are excreted in the urine with Na^+ and K^+ (not NH_4^+ or

DISTAL RENAL TUBULAR ACIDOSIS
This diagnosis is excluded because the rate of excretion of NH_4^+ is not low. This information is deduced using the $U_{Osmolal\ gap}$ as follows:

- Calculated U_{Osm} = 2 (U_{Na} [60 mmol/L] + U_K [20 mmol/L]) + (U_{Urea} [100 mOsm/L]) = 260 mOsm/L
- U_{NH4} = ½ (Measured U_{Osm} − calculated U_{Osm}) (i.e., [0.5 (566 − 260 mOsm/L)]) = 153 mmol/L
- Because the $U_{Creatinine}$ is 8 mmol/L, the $U_{NH4}/U_{Creatinine}$ is close to 20. If we assume that the urine creatinine excretion is 10 mmol/day, this represents a 24-hour NH_4^+ excretion of 200 mmol.

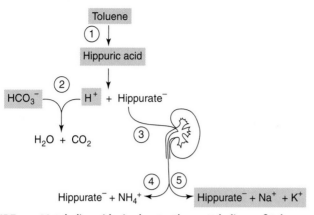

FIGURE 3-2 Metabolic acidosis due to the metabolism of toluene. The metabolism of toluene occurs in the liver, where benzoic acid is produced via alcohol and aldehyde dehydrogenases. Conjugating benzoic acid with glycine produces hippuric acid (all represented as *site 1* for simplicity). The H^+ are titrated by HCO_3^- for the most part (*site 2*). The hippurate anions are filtered and also secreted in the proximal convoluted tubule (*site 3*). Therefore, instead of accumulating in blood and increasing the $P_{Anion\ gap}$, they are excreted in the urine. Some of the hippurate anions are excreted in the urine with NH_4^+ (*site 4*) and others with Na^+ and K^+ (*site 5*), when the capacity to excrete NH_4^+ is exceeded. The excretion of hippurate anions with Na^+ and/or K^+ (and not NH_4^+) leads to the persistence of the metabolic acidosis, extracellular fluid volume contraction, and hypokalemia.

H^+), and hence there is an indirect loss of $NaHCO_3$ (see Fig. 4-2, page 78). The most likely basis for the metabolic acidosis in this patient is glue sniffing with the production of hippuric acid and the excretion of hippurate anions in the urine at a rate that exceeds that of NH_4^+ (Fig. 3-2).

DISCUSSION OF QUESTIONS

3-1 *In a patient with cholera and metabolic acidosis due to the loss of $NaHCO_3$ in diarrhea fluid, the ECF volume is contracted by close to 50%, yet O_2 delivery to tissues is adequate to avoid anaerobic metabolism. Should this patient have an elevated value for the $P_{Anion\ gap}$?*

The oversimplified and incorrect answer is that there is no change in the $P_{Anion\ gap}$ when there is a net loss of Na^+ and HCO_3^-. Notwithstanding, because most of the $P_{Anion\ gap}$ is due to the net negative charge on albumin, the value for this gap would be higher if the $P_{Albumin}$ were to rise because of a contracted plasma volume. In quantitative terms, the net valence on albumin is close to 16 mEq/L per 4.0 g albumin/dL. When the $P_{Albumin}$ is 8.0 g/dL, the expected rise in the $P_{Anion\ gap}$ is close to 16 mEq/L above the usual 12 ± 2 mEq/L (*see margin note*). Moreover, there appears to be a rise in value for the negative valence on albumin when the effective arterial blood is contracted. Therefore, the rise in $P_{Anion\ gap}$ in this setting does not represent the addition of new acids.

$P_{Anion\ gap}$
In this calculation for the rise in the $P_{Anion\ gap}$, we assumed that the P_K did not change.

3-2 *Why might pulmonary edema develop before the ECF volume is fully reexpanded in this patient with cholera?*

The clinicians who treated severely ill patients with cholera were very surprised when 5 of their first 40 patients developed pulmonary edema when they received isotonic saline at a rapid rate. In fact, the positive balance of saline was significantly *less* than what would be needed to fully reexpand the ECF volume. Even more surprising was the fact that pulmonary edema was ameliorated when isotonic $NaHCO_3$ was infused at a rapid rate, whereas other treatments for pulmonary edema were not successful. One speculation to explain these observations was that the more severe degree of acidemia that developed following partial reexpansion of the ECF volume with isotonic saline led to a more intense constriction of the peripheral venous capacitance vessels and thus a larger increase in the central blood volume. Because pulmonary edema could be reversed by the administration of a solution that contains HCO_3^-, these patients should receive an isotonic solution (to the patient) that contains close to 40 mmol $NaHCO_3$ or its equivalent (e.g., sodium L-lactate) to match the concentration of HCO_3^- in diarrhea fluid. As mentioned previously, one must be extremely cautious if the patient has hypokalemia.

chapter 4

Metabolic Acidosis due to a Deficit of NaHCO$_3$

Introduction

DEFINITION
Low rate of excretion of NH_4^+: This is present when the rate of NH_4^+ excretion is less than that found when a person with normal kidneys is given an acid load that is larger enough to cause acidemia for more than 3 days (i.e., low is defined as less than 200 mmol/day in an adult).

The central theme of this chapter is the type of metabolic acidosis that is caused by a deficit of $NaHCO_3$. There are two categories of this type of metabolic acidosis: (1) the direct loss of Na^+ and HCO_3^- via a single route, either the gastrointestinal (GI) tract or the urine; and (2) the indirect loss of $NaHCO_3$, in which the Na^+ and the HCO_3^- are lost by different routes. In the latter group, the process begins when an acid is added, its H^+ removes HCO_3^-, and the resulting CO_2 is exhaled while the conjugate base of the acid is excreted in the urine or in feces with a cation other than NH_4^+ or H^+ (i.e., Na^+ and/or K^+). In these latter settings, if the loss of Na^+ is large and leads to a very contracted extracellular fluid (ECF) volume, this may dominate the clinical picture (e.g., the patient with secretory diarrhea). If the ECF volume is significantly contracted, the P_{HCO3} may not be very low and thus the deficit of HCO_3^- may be underestimated unless one has a quantitative assessment of the ECF volume.

If the kidneys are normal in a patient who has acidemia, the expected renal response is to excrete as much NH_4^+ as possible. If the rate of excretion of NH_4^+ is high, suspect that there is a loss of $NaHCO_3$ via the GI tract (e.g., diarrhea) or that there is overproduction of an acid while its anion is being excreted faster than NH_4^+ (e.g., hippuric acid in the glue sniffer). Because the anion is lost rapidly in the urine, there is little rise in the $P_{Anion\ gap}$.

If the rate of excretion of NH_4^+ is low in a patient who has chronic acidemia, the diagnostic category is the group of disorders called *renal tubular acidosis* (RTA). One subgroup of patients has a metabolic disorder in which the kidneys are responsible for losing $NaHCO_3$ (called *proximal renal tubular acidosis*). A second subgroup of patients is a heterogeneous one in which the likely basis for this disorder is a low rate of excretion of NH_4^+. In some patients, the basis is a low rate of production of NH_4^+ due to a very low glomerular filtration rate (GFR). In others, the basis for the low rate of excretion of NH_4^+ is a low rate of H^+ secretion or a low availability of ammonia (NH_3), called *distal renal tubular acidosis*. In these settings, the kidneys cannot generate enough new HCO_3^- to replace that lost while titrating the H^+ load produced from usual intake of dietary proteins.

OBJECTIVES

- To explain how a deficit of $NaHCO_3$ might develop.
- To provide an approach to the diagnosis of the patient with metabolic acidosis due to a deficit of $NaHCO_3$, emphasizing the importance of assessing the rate of excretion of NH_4^+ in the urine.
- To describe the settings where therapy with $NaHCO_3$ is required and emphasize where it might be dangerous.

PART A
OVERVIEW

DEFINITIONS OF METABOLIC ACIDOSIS

Several terms should be defined clearly when making a diagnosis of metabolic acidosis.

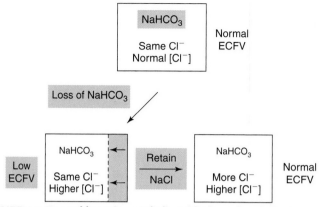

FIGURE 4-1 Hyperchloremic metabolic acidosis, a descriptive term. The *green shading in the rectangles* represents the extracellular fluid (ECF) compartment. As shown in the *top rectangle*, the patient has a normal ECF volume (ECFV) and then develops a deficit of NaHCO₃ (e.g., owing to diarrhea). As shown in the *lower left rectangle*, the ECFV is contracted because of the loss of Na⁺. Since the content of Cl⁻ in the ECF compartment does not change, the P_{Cl} rises because of the contracted ECFV. Hence, there is a low ECFV, a higher P_{Cl}, a lower P_{HCO_3}, and a decreased content of HCO₃⁻ in the ECF compartment. As shown in the *lower right rectangle*, if NaCl is ingested, it is retained because of the low effective arterial blood volume. As a result, the ECFV returns to normal and its content of Cl⁻ increases. Hence, there is a normal ECFV, a higher P_{Cl}, and a lower P_{HCO_3}.

ABBREVIATIONS
P_{Cl}, concentration of Cl⁻ in plasma
P_{HCO_3}, concentration of HCO₃⁻ in plasma
$P_{Osmolal\ gap}$, osmolal gap in plasma
$U_{Osmolal\ gap}$, osmolal gap in urine

Acidemia: This is a low pH or a high H⁺ concentration in plasma. When acidemia is due solely to metabolic acidosis, both the blood pH and the P_{HCO_3} are low.

Metabolic acidosis: This describes a process that leads to the accumulation of H⁺ and a decrease in the content of HCO₃⁻ in the body. Nevertheless, the concentration of H⁺ and HCO₃⁻ might be close to normal if there is another condition present that raises the P_{HCO_3}. For example, this second process might add new HCO₃⁻ to the body (e.g., the loss of HCl from the stomach; see page 198, Fig. 7-2) or the P_{HCO_3} may rise because the ECF volume is very contracted (the P_{HCO_3} is the content of HCO₃⁻ in the ECF compartment divided by the ECF volume).

Hyperchloremic metabolic acidosis (HCMA): HCMA refers to the presence of metabolic acidosis that is due to a deficit of NaHCO₃ (*see margin note*); it is simply a descriptive term based on an observed associated rise in the P_{Cl}. Nevertheless, there is no primary role for Cl⁻ in the pathogenesis of the metabolic acidosis. There are two possible mechanisms that explain the higher value for the P_{Cl} in these patients (Fig. 4-1).

HCMA
Another name given to the subgroup of disorders that cause metabolic acidosis where there is a near-equivalent fall in the P_{HCO_3} and rise in the P_{Cl} is a *nonanion-gap type of metabolic acidosis*.

1. *Same content of Cl⁻ but a contracted ECF volume*: The first step is a loss of NaHCO₃. As a result of the deficit of Na⁺, the ECF volume declines. If there is no intake of NaCl, the content of Cl⁻ in the ECF compartment remains unchanged, but as the ECF volume is contracted, the concentration of Cl⁻ rises (bottom left portion of Fig. 4-1).

2. *Higher content of Cl⁻, but a normal ECF volume*: The first step is also a loss of NaHCO₃. As a result of the deficit of Na⁺, the ECF volume declines. In response to the low ECF volume, there is renal retention of Na⁺ and Cl⁻ if the diet provides NaCl. The net result is a normal ECF volume and a positive balance of Cl⁻; hence, the P_{Cl} rises (bottom right portion of Fig. 4-1).

PATHOGENESIS OF METABOLIC ACIDOSIS DUE TO NaHCO$_3$ LOSS

There are two ways to create a deficit of NaHCO$_3$:
- Direct loss of NaHCO$_3$: occurs via the GI tract or in the urine.
- Indirect loss of NaHCO$_3$: there is a gain of an acid and the excretion of its anion with Na$^+$ in the urine or in the feces.

There are two ways to create a deficit of NaHCO$_3$ while preserving electroneutrality (Fig. 4-2). A direct loss of NaHCO$_3$ occurs if both Na$^+$ and HCO$_3^-$ are lost via one route (e.g., via the GI tract or in the urine). An indirect loss of NaHCO$_3$ occurs in two steps as follows:

1. *Addition of an acid*: The H$^+$ of the added acid react with HCO$_3^-$, resulting in the formation of CO$_2$ + H$_2$O; this CO$_2$ is exhaled via the lungs. At this point, there is a deficit of HCO$_3^-$ together with an equivalent gain of new anions in the ECF compartment.

$$HA \rightarrow H^+ + A^-$$
$$H^+ + HCO_3^- \rightarrow H_2O + CO_2 \,(\text{lost via lungs})$$

2. *Excretion of the A$^-$ with Na$^+$*: The second step is the excretion of the anion in the urine with a cation other than H$^+$ or NH$_4^+$ (i.e., with Na$^+$ and/or K$^+$). The net effect is a loss of NaHCO$_3$ from the body.

$$A^- + Na^+ \text{ in ECF} \rightarrow A^- + Na^+ (\text{lost in urine})$$

There are two subgroups of disorders that cause metabolic acidosis due to the indirect loss of NaHCO$_3$; the basis for this division is the rate of excretion of NH$_4^+$ in these patients (*see margin note*).

1. *Acid overproduction with a higher rate of excretion of the new anions than NH$_4^+$*: In this subgroup, the major lesion is an overproduction of acids with a high rate of excretion of their anions in the urine. Even though the rate of excretion of NH$_4^+$ may be

EXPECTED RATE OF EXCRETION OF NH$_4^+$
- The rate of excretion of NH$_4^+$ in adults consuming a typical Western diet is 20 to 40 mmol/day.
- In a patient with chronic metabolic acidosis and normal renal function, the expected rate of excretion of NH$_4^+$ is ~200 mmol/day, which is ~200 mmol NH$_4^+$/g creatinine (~20 mmol NH$_4^+$/mmol creatinine).

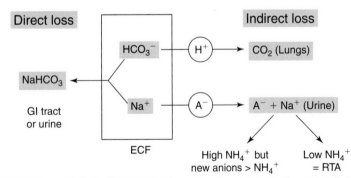

FIGURE 4-2 Deficit of NaHCO$_3$. The *rectangle* represents the extracellular fluid (ECF) compartment; for convenience, it contains only Na$^+$ and HCO$_3^-$. As shown in the *left portion of the figure*, NaHCO$_3$ can be lost directly in gastrointestinal (GI) fluids or in the urine. As shown in the *right portion of the figure*, there is an indirect loss of NaHCO$_3$ when an acid (depicted as H$^+$ + A$^-$) is added and the rate of excretion of new anions (A$^-$) exceeds that of NH$_4^+$; there are two subgroups here, based on the rate of excretion of NH$_4^+$. Individuals with a high rate of excretion of NH$_4^+$ have a primary high acid load, whereas those with a low rate of excretion of NH$_4^+$ have renal tubular acidosis (RTA) or renal insufficiency.

TABLE 4-1 **THE DEVELOPMENT OF METABOLIC ACIDOSIS DUE TO AN INDIRECT LOSS OF NaHCO$_3$**

Acid overproduction with a higher rate of excretion of new anions than NH$_4^+$

- Glue-sniffing (hippuric acid overproduction)
- Diabetic ketoacidosis with ketonuria that exceeds NH$_4^+$ excretion

Normal acid production, but a low urinary excretion of NH$_4^+$

- Low glomerular filtration rate
- Renal tubular acidosis
  - Low NH$_3$ type
  - Low net distal H$^+$ secretion type
  - Low NH$_3$ *and* low net distal H$^+$ secretion type

appropriately high, the rate of excretion of new anions exceeds that of NH$_4^+$; hence, some of the anions are excreted with Na$^+$ or K$^+$. These new anions are excreted at a high rate primarily because they are secreted by the proximal convoluted tubule (e.g., hippurate$^-$ produced during the metabolism of toluene in a glue sniffer; see the discussion of Case 3-2, page 71) or because they are filtered and a sufficient quantity is not reabsorbed in the proximal convoluted tubule (e.g., ketoacid anions early in the course of diabetic ketoacidosis).

2. *Normal acid production but a low rate of excretion of NH$_4^+$*: The basis of the metabolic acidosis in this subgroup of patients is failure of the kidneys to regenerate "new" HCO$_3^-$ owing to a low rate of NH$_4^+$ excretion relative to their dietary acid load. This is the hallmark of a group of disorders called *renal tubular acidosis* (RTA; discussed in Part C in this chapter). A list of causes for an indirect loss of NaHCO$_3$ is provided in Table 4-1.

PART B
CONDITIONS THAT CAUSE
A DEFICIT OF NaHCO$_3$

- The rate of excretion of NH$_4^+$ is key to determining the pathophysiology of metabolic acidosis in these patients.

ANION GAP IN PLASMA
- This calculation is used to detect the conjugate base (new anions) in plasma in a patient who has metabolic acidosis.
- The value must be adjusted for changes in the concentration and the valence on albumin in plasma.

Before proceeding with the clinical approach, two points are worthy of emphasis. First, do not rely *solely* on the P$_{HCO3}$ to make a diagnosis of metabolic acidosis because in patients with a very low ECF volume, the P$_{HCO3}$ may not be low even though there is a deficit of NaHCO$_3$. Second, the P$_{HCO3}$ may be higher if the patient has had a recent episode of vomiting.

The initial steps to take to define why a patient might have metabolic acidosis without the accumulation of new anions is outlined in Flow Chart 4-1 (*see margin note*).

DIRECT LOSS OF NaHCO$_3$

INGESTION OF HCl
Ingestion of HCl is not included in the flow chart, as it is a rare cause of HCMA.

In these conditions, both Na$^+$ and HCO$_3^-$ are lost via the same route leading to metabolic acidosis (a deficit of HCO$_3^-$ and possibly a low P$_{HCO3}$). NaHCO$_3$ may be lost via the GI tract (e.g., in a patient with diarrhea) or via the urine (e.g., in a patient with proximal RTA).

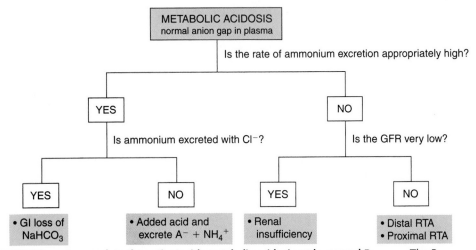

FLOW CHART 4-1 Approach to the patient with metabolic acidosis and a normal $P_{Anion\ gap}$. The $P_{Anion\ gap}$ should be adjusted for the concentration of albumin in plasma ($P_{Albumin}$). Patients with proximal renal tubular acidosis (RTA) who are in a steady-state acid-base balance have a low rate of excretion of NH_4^+; this is discussed in detail later in the chapter. GFR, glomerular filtration rate; GI, gastrointestinal.

Loss of $NaHCO_3$ in the gastrointestinal tract

There are two major sites where HCO_3^- is added to the lumen of the GI tract and thus possible sites for its loss.

Secretion of HCO_3^- by the pancreas and small intestine

NaHCO$_3$ is secreted by the pancreas and small intestine; this secretion is stimulated by the load of H^+ from the stomach (~100 mmol/day). Somewhat more than 100 mmol of $NaHCO_3$ are secreted to ensure neutralization of this H^+ load. Hence, there is only a modest daily net deficit of $NaHCO_3$ if most of these upper GI secretions are lost (*see margin note*); therefore, metabolic acidosis in these patients is likely to be mild unless the duration of these losses is prolonged and/or there is also another disorder that diminishes the rate of excretion of NH_4^+ in the urine. At times, the fluid rich in $NaHCO_3$ is retained in the lumen of the intestine (e.g., ileus), and hence metabolic acidosis develops.

Secretion of HCO_3^- by the late small intestine and the colon

Two luminal transport mechanisms are involved in this process, a Na^+/H^+ exchanger (NHE) and a Cl^-/HCO_3^- anion exchanger (AE; Fig. 4-3). Whether the net result is a loss of $NaHCO_3$ depends on the rate of delivery of Na^+ and Cl^- and the maximum transport capacity of each exchanger.

Low delivery of Na^+ and Cl^- to the colon. In this setting, virtually all of the Na^+ and Cl^- are reabsorbed while the secreted H^+ and HCO_3^- are converted to $CO_2 + H_2O$. There is no loss of $NaHCO_3$ in this setting.

Very large delivery of Na^+ and Cl^- to the colon. There are two possible outcomes to consider depending on the maximum transport capacity of these two ion exchangers; there could be a loss of $NaHCO_3$ (*see margin note*) or an indirect loss of HCl.

Loss of NaCl and $NaHCO_3$. Normally, the maximum transport capacity of NHE is less than that of AE. The net effect is to reabsorb as much of the NaCl as possible and to convert some of the remaining NaCl in the lumen to $NaHCO_3$ as more Cl^- are exchanged with

LOSS OF NaHCO₃ DURING VOMITING
- This is common in children or adults who have a patent pyloric sphincter; hence, vomited fluid contains $NaHCO_3$ that is secreted by the pancreas and small intestine.
- The net loss of $NaHCO_3$ is larger in patients with achlorhydria or patients who take drugs that block the secretion of HCl in the stomach.

COMPOSITION OF DIARRHEA FLUID IN A PATIENT WITH SEVERE DIARRHEA

HCO_3^-	40 to 45 mmol/L
Cl^-	110 to 115 mmol/L
K^+	15 mmol/L
Na^+	140 mmol/L

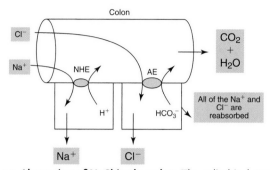

FIGURE 4-3 Absorption of NaCl in the colon. The *cylindrical structure* represents the colon; *two rectangles* representing cells are drawn for convenience. H$^+$ and HCO$_3^-$ are formed from CO$_2$ + H$_2$O by a reaction that is catalyzed by the enzyme carbonic anhydrase. When Na$^+$ and Cl$^-$ are delivered to the colon, both are absorbed using separate, electroneutral ion exchangers (Na$^+$ is absorbed in exchange for H$^+$ [Na$^+$/H$^+$ exchanger; NHE] while Cl$^-$ is absorbed in exchange for HCO$_3^-$ [Cl$^-$/HCO$_3^-$ anion exchanger; AE]). In normal physiology, virtually all the Na$^+$ and Cl$^-$ are absorbed and CO$_2$ + H$_2$O are produced. Notice that AE has a larger V$_{max}$ than NHE.

HCO$_3^-$ in severe diarrhea (Fig. 4-4). The composition of diarrhea fluid in a patient with cholera is shown in the margin note.

Loss of NaCl and an indirect loss of HCl. There are circumstances when diarrhea fluid contains little or no HCO$_3^-$ and thus the patient may not develop metabolic acidosis. The underlying defect is a decrease in the transport capacity of the Cl$^-$/HCO$_3^-$ anion exchanger in the colon (Fig. 4-5). This was noted in patients with certain colonic adenomas and adenocarcinomas (hence, the name *down-regulated in adenoma* [DRA]). This low transport capacity of AE may also be due to an inborn error (e.g., patients with congenital chloridorrhea) or in certain inflammatory disorders that involve the lower intestinal tract (e.g., some patients with ulcerative colitis). In this setting, the diarrhea fluid consists primarily of NaCl and usually an indirect loss of HCl (*see margin note*).

Renal loss of NaHCO$_3$

Renal loss of NaHCO$_3$ may occur as a result of a proximal tubular malfunction that impairs the normal reabsorption of filtered NaHCO$_3$; this is called *proximal RTA*. This topic is discussed in more detail in Part C.

CLINICAL APPROACH TO A PATIENT WITH DIRECT NaHCO$_3$ LOSS

The patient with NaHCO$_3$ loss via the GI tract

The clinical history is usually obvious, although some patients may deny the use of laxatives. Urine electrolytes may provide a helpful clue in this setting. The concentration of Na$^+$ in the urine should be low owing to decreased effective arterial blood volume, but the concentration of Cl$^-$ in the urine may be high owing to the enhanced rate of excretion of NH$_4^+$ in response to chronic metabolic acidosis. The ECF volume becomes contracted if the loss of Na$^+$ significantly exceeds its intake. Hence, the P$_{HCO3}$ may be close to normal despite a significant deficit of HCO$_3^-$. In this setting, this presence of metabolic acidosis and the magnitude of the deficit of HCO$_3^-$ is detected only if the content of HCO$_3^-$ in the ECF compartment is calculated;

EXCRETION OF WATER IN DIARRHEA FLUID
- Water crosses the cell membranes of the colon and achieves osmotic equilibrium. Therefore, for every 300 mOsm in the lumen of the colon, there is a loss of 1 L of water in stool.
- In normal conditions, the stool contains close to 30 mosmol/day and thus daily stool water volume is ~0 1 L.

INDIRECT LOSS OF HCl IN DIARRHEA FLUID
- The diarrhea fluid never has a high concentration of HCl because the colonic NHE cannot raise the concentration of H$^+$ in luminal fluid above 0.1 mmol/L (or below pH 4).
- If the luminal fluid in the colon does not have H$^+$ acceptors that bind H$^+$ at pH 4 or higher, there will be an insignificant addition of HCO$_3^-$ to the body.
- Conversely, if the luminal fluid has histidines without bound H$^+$ (e.g., in proteins of bacterial origin), secreted H$^+$ will bind to the H$^+$ acceptors and HCO$_3^-$ will be added to the body while the concentration of Cl$^-$ in the diarrhea fluid will exceed that of Na$^+$ + K$^+$.

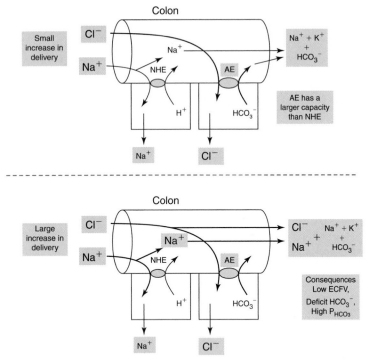

FIGURE 4-4 Loss of NaHCO₃ from the colon. The *cylindrical structure* represents the colon; *two rectangles* representing cells are drawn for convenience. The *portion of the figure above the horizontal dashed line* reflects the effects of a modest increase in the delivery of Na⁺ and Cl⁻ to the colon. Notice that the NHE cannot absorb as much Na⁺ as the AE can absorb Cl⁻. Therefore, not all of the Na⁺ is absorbed by NHE, whereas all the Cl⁻ delivered is absorbed by AE. Hence, the diarrhea fluid contains Na⁺ and HCO₃⁻, but virtually no Na⁺ and Cl⁻. In contrast, *the portion of the figure below the horizontal dashed line* reflects the effects of a very large increase in the delivery of Na⁺ and Cl⁻ to the colon. In this setting, only a small proportion of Na⁺ is absorbed and somewhat more of the Cl⁻ delivered is absorbed in exchange for HCO₃⁻. Hence, the diarrhea fluid contains a very large quantity of Na⁺ and Cl⁻ and some Na⁺ and HCO₃⁻.

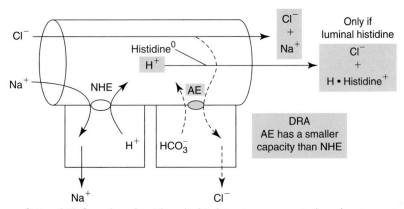

FIGURE 4-5 Loss of H⁺ and Cl⁻ from the colon. The *cylindrical structure* represents the colon; *two rectangles* representing cells are drawn for convenience. When a large quantity of Na⁺ and Cl⁻ is delivered to the colon, more Na⁺ than Cl⁻ are absorbed if there is down-regulation of its Cl⁻/HCO₃⁻ AE. In contrast, if the luminal fluid contains histidines without bound H⁺, NHE secretion can be much larger, as the free concentration of H⁺ is not high enough to inhibit flux through NHE. In this setting, the diarrhea fluid contains Na⁺ and Cl⁻. DRA, down-regulated in adenoma.

this requires a quantitative assessment of the ECF volume (using the hematocrit; see the discussion of Case 2-1, page 57).

When the degree of ECF volume contraction is very marked, there is a rise in the $P_{Anion\ gap}$ even in absence of overproduction of acids (i.e., owing to an increased $P_{Albumin}$ and perhaps its anionic valence). Acidemia becomes more severe after the ECF volume is reexpanded with the administration of a saline solution that does not contain enough HCO_3^- or potential HCO_3^- (e.g., citrate).

Three factors can make the degree of metabolic acidosis more severe in a patient with diarrhea. First, the loss of $NaHCO_3$ can be enormous when diarrhea volume is very large. Second, in some patients who have diarrhea, there may be overproduction of organic acids in the colon, such as D-lactic acid. Third, there may be a low rate of excretion of NH_4^+ if the GFR is low—owing primarily to the very contracted effective arterial blood volume.

Patients with diarrhea may have a severe degree of K^+ depletion. Nevertheless, hypokalemia may not be evident on presentation because of a shift of K^+ out of cells owing to a deficiency of insulin (secondary to inhibition of its release by an α-adrenergic surge due to marked effective arterial blood volume contraction). A severe degree of hypokalemia may develop when the effective arterial blood volume is reexpanded.

Treatment

One must first identify and treat emergencies that may be present on admission(e.g. hemodynamic instability) as well as anticipate and avoid those that might develop with therapy (e.g., hypokalemia). Enhancing the absorption of NaCl secreted in the intestinal tract diminishes the volume of diarrhea fluid. This can be achieved by giving an equimolar mixture of glucose and NaCl by mouth (Fig. 4-6); this is called *oral rehydration therapy* (*see margin note*). In more modern versons of this solution, a form of alkali is added (e.g., replace 25 to 50 mEq of Cl^- with citrate anions).

EARLY EFFECT OF ORT
Since the effective arterial blood volume is very low, there is a small delivery of blood to the intestine, and a very small volume is secreted. Hence ORT leads to partial reexpansion of the ECF volume.

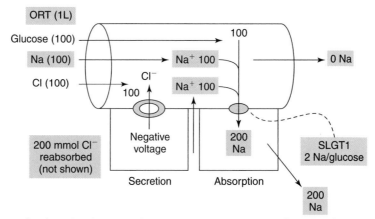

FIGURE 4-6 Effects of early oral replacement therapy (ORT) on the volume of diarrhea fluid. The rehydration fluid (ORT) is shown in the *top left portion of this figure*; it contains 100 mmol of glucose, Na^+, and Cl^- per liter. The structure is the early small intestine where the cholera toxin induces the secretion of Cl^- (shown in the *enlarged green shaded oval*) due to insertion of a cystic fibrosis transmembrane conductance regulator (CFTR) Cl^- channel in its luminal membrane, which adds 100 mmol of Cl^- and negative voltage to the lumen. This lumen-negative voltage provides the driving force for 100 mmol of Na^+ to enter the lumen through the tight junctions between these cells (shown as the *vertical arrow*). These 100 mmol of Na^+ plus another 100 mmol of Na^+ from the ORT are reabsorbed with the 100 mmol of glucose provided in the ORT via the Na^+-linked glucose transporter (SLGT1), as SLGT1 requires 2 Na^+/glucose. Although not shown (for simplicity), 200 mmol of Cl^- are absorbed, driven by the lumen-negative voltage. As a result, the volume of diarrhea fluid declines initially and the ECF volume is partially reexpanded.

LATER EFFECT OF ORT
The absorbed NaCl and water partially reexpands the ECF volume, which increases the splanchnic blood flow rate. As a result, the diarrhea volume rises despite ORT, but the hemodynamic state in the patient has improved.

SOURCE OF Na⁺ FOR THE INTESTINAL SLGT
- Glucose intake is close to 270 g or 1500 mmol/day.
- Because the SLGT stoichiometry is 2 Na⁺/glucose, there is a need for 3000 mmol of Na⁺ per day to absorb this amount of glucose; the diet supplies only ~150 mmol/day.
- Therefore, there is a need to recycle Na⁺ to allow for the reabsorption of the daily intake of glucose (see Part D for more discussion).

Oral rehydration therapy

The Na^+-linked glucose transporter (SLGT1) mediates the absorption of glucose from the lumen of the small intestine (see Fig. 4-6). Its stoichiometry is critically important—2 Na^+ per glucose absorbed (*see margin note*). This stoichiometry permits some of the NaCl secreted in the intestinal tract to be reabsorbed when oral rehydration therapy is given because the rehydration solution contains equal amounts of glucose and NaCl (e.g., 100 mmol of each of Na^+, Cl^-, and glucose in 1 L of water). The absorption of 100 mmol of glucose on SLGT leads to the absorption of 200 mmol of Na^+. The source of the second 100 mmol of Na^+ is intestinal secretions (equivalent to two thirds of a liter of secreted isotonic NaCl fluid). The negative voltage created by the electrogenic absorption of Na^+ via SLGT provides the driving force for reabsorption of 200 mmol of Cl^-.

INDIRECT LOSS OF NaHCO₃

Patients with an indirect loss of $NaHCO_3$ (see Fig. 4-2) can be subdivided into two major categories.

1. *Those with overproduction of an acid with a high rate of excretion of its anion*: Although the rate of excretion of NH_4^+ may be appropriately high, the rate of excretion of the anion exceeds that of NH_4^+; hence, some of the anion is excreted with Na^+ and/or K^+. The $P_{Anion\ gap}$ will not be appreciably increased despite this high rate of acid production if the kidneys readily excrete the anions that were produced (i.e., via secretion). Similarly, the acidemia will not be corrected despite a high rate of excretion of NH_4^+ and in fact it will become more severe as long as the rate of anion excretion (which reflects H^+ addition) exceeds the rate of NH_4^+ excretion.

2. *Those with a normal acid production and a low rate of excretion of NH_4^+*: In this subgroup of patients, the rate of production of acids is *not* increased. Rather, the major defect is a low rate of excretion of NH_4^+ (low is defined as a rate that is insufficient to dispose of the daily acid load produced in metabolism of sulfur-containing amino acids). Patients in this subgroup are heterogeneous with regard to the pathophysiology of their disorder (low net H^+ secretion and/or low NH_3 availability); nevertheless, these patients are grouped together under the diagnostic category of RTA; this is discussed in detail in the next section.

PART C
DISEASES WITH LOW RATE OF EXCRETION OF NH₄⁺

- The cardinal features of RTA are metabolic acidosis, a normal $P_{Anion\ gap}$, and a low rate of NH_4^+ excretion.
- There are two types of RTA, proximal and distal. Although both types have impaired NH_4^+ excretion, in proximal RTA, there is also a decreased capacity for the reabsorption of HCO_3^- in the proximal convoluted tubule.

Patients with metabolic acidosis of renal origin have a low rate of net acid excretion. In practical terms, however, there are three clinical groups of disorders that merit emphasis: first, those with proximal RTA; second, those with distal RTA; and third, those with a very low GFR. From a pathophysiologic perspective, the renal defect results in a low rate of excretion of NH$_4^+$. Proximal RTA is also characterized by a decreased capacity to reabsorb NaHCO$_3$.

PROXIMAL RENAL TUBULAR ACIDOSIS

- The pathophysiology of metabolic acidosis in patients with proximal RTA has two components.

1. *Decreased reabsorption of HCO$_3^-$ in the proximal convoluted tubule*: Although renal HCO$_3^-$ wasting and bicarbonaturia are present at the onset of disease, this is not a feature of its chronic steady state in most patients. In more detail, a decrease in the rate of H$^+$ secretion in the proximal convoluted tubule diminishes the reabsorption of HCO$_3^-$ in the initial phase of the disease. As a result, delivery of HCO$_3^-$ to distal nephron segments suddenly exceeds their capacity to secrete H$^+$, and HCO$_3^-$ is lost in the urine. As the P$_{HCO3}$ falls, the filtered load of HCO$_3^-$ decreases until a point is reached where the distal delivery of HCO$_3^-$ matches the rate of distal H$^+$ secretion and thus there is no further bicarbonaturia; in fact, the urine pH is characteristically low in patients with isolated proximal RTA (Table 4-2). There are times, however, during the day (the alkaline tide; *see margin note*) when the P$_{HCO3}$ may rise and this may cause bicarbonaturia with a urine pH close to 7.0.

2. *A low rate of excretion of NH$_4^+$:*

- The rate of excretion of NH$_4^+$ is low in patients with proximal RTA despite the presence of chronic metabolic acidosis.

This low rate of excretion of NH$_4^+$ is due to an alkaline proximal cell pH (discussed later) in patients with the isolated form of proximal RTA and to a generalized proximal convo-

ALKALINE TIDE
This is a term to describe a transient rise in the P$_{HCO3}$ and/or the urine pH owing to the secretion of HCl in the stomach with the subsequent addition of HCO$_3^-$ to the ECF compartment (along with a loss of Cl$^-$; see Fig. 7-2, page 198).

NORMAL FILTERED LOAD OF HCO$_3^-$

= GFR × P$_{HCO3}$

= 180 L/day × 25 mmol/L

= 4500 mmol/day

TABLE 4-2 **RENAL HANDLING OF HCO$_3^-$ IN PATIENTS WITH PROXIMAL RENAL TUBULAR ACIDOSIS**

In all of the examples, the glomerular filtration rate is 180 L/day. The normal filtered load of HCO$_3^-$ is 4500 mmol/day (*see margin note*). The lesion in proximal renal tubular acidosis is a reduced proximal H$^+$ secretion so the proximal reabsorption of HCO$_3^-$ falls (lines 2 and 3). Because distal H$^+$ secretion has a much lower capacity (600 mmol/day of HCO$_3^-$ per day in this example), all the extra HCO$_3^-$ delivered to the distal nephron that escapes distal reabsorption is excreted. As the filtered load of HCO$_3^-$ declines to the limit of the tubular reabsorption of HCO$_3^-$, all the filtered HCO$_3^-$ is reabsorbed and the urine pH is low in steady state.

STATE	FILTERED HCO$_3^-$	PROXIMAL HCO$_3^-$	DISTAL HCO$_3^-$	HCO$_3^-$ EXCRETION
		REABSORBED	*DELIVERY*	
Normal	4500	4000	500	<5
Low H$^+$ secretion in proximal convoluted tubule				
Initial phase	4500	3000	1500	900
Steady state	3600	3000	600	<5

luted tubule cell dysfunction in patients with the Fanconi-syndrome type of disorder. Although there is direct evidence to support this notion in patients with the familial form of isolated proximal RTA, the low rate of excretion of NH_4^+ in other patients with proximal RTA could be deduced by the absence of bicarbonaturia in the steady state of the disease. For if the kidneys were able to generate the expected close to 200 mmol/day of HCO_3^- in these patients, the capacity for HCO_3^- reabsorption would be exceeded and this would result in bicarbonaturia.

FANCONI SYNDROME
This is a generalized defect in proximal tubular function that leads to glucosuria and aminoaciduria as well as to an increased excretion of urate, phosphate, citrate, and $NaHCO_3$ (proximal RTA).

Clinical subtypes of proximal renal tubular acidosis: Fanconi syndrome

In addition to a defect in $NaHCO_3$ reabsorption, patients with this syndrome exhibit defects in other Na^+-linked transport functions in the proximal convoluted tubule (*see margin note*). This syndrome might be due to a genetic defect or it might be acquired in a number of disorders (Table 4-3). The most common cause in pediatric populations is cystinosis, whereas common causes in adult populations are paraproteinemias and autoimmune disorders. Chinese herb ingestion is a common cause of Fanconi syndrome in Asian patients; the toxin implicated is aristolochic acid. If not stopped quickly, damage to the proximal tubules will be extensive and may ultimately result in renal failure. Fanconi syndrome is also associated with the use of drugs such as the cyclophosphamide analogue ifosfamide.

Possible basis of the findings in isolated proximal renal tubular acidosis

- Patients with isolated proximal RTA have both a reduced capacity to reabsorb HCO_3^- in their proximal convoluted tubule and a low rate of excretion of NH_4^+.

One possible explanation for this combination of defects would be if the proximal tubular cells were more alkaline. This hypothesis

TABLE 4-3 **CONDITIONS LEADING TO PROXIMAL RENAL TUBULAR ACIDOSIS (RTA)**

Conditions causing Fanconi syndrome

- Genetic disorders: e.g., cystinosis, galactosemia, hereditary fructose intolerance, Wilson's disease, Lowe's syndrome, tyrosinemia
- Toxin-induced: e.g., Chinese herbs containing aristolochic acid, heavy metals such as lead
- Unclear mechanisms: e.g., dysproteinemias including multiple myeloma, autoimmune diseases such as Sjögren syndrome, chronic active hepatitis, post-renal transplantation

Isolated proximal RTA

- Genetic disorders: e.g., mutations in the gene encoding the basolateral $Na(HCO_3)_3{}^{2-}$ cotransporter, familial isolated proximal RTA
- Acquired disorders: e.g., hyperparathyroidism, hypocalcemia, vitamin D deficiency
- Drug induced: e.g., carbonic anhydrase IV inhibitors

Combined proximal and distal RTA

- Genetic disorders: carbonic anhydrase II deficiency

could also explain the high rate of excretion of citrate observed in these patients (*see margin note*).

Molecular lesions causing isolated proximal renal tubular acidosis

> • There are three possible targets for a molecular lesion to cause isolated proximal RTA: the basolateral membrane, the intracellular enzyme systems controlling proximal tubular H⁺ secretion, and the NHE in the luminal membrane of the proximal convoluted tubule.

In fact, only two of these possible lesions have been demonstrated to be associated with proximal RTA (Fig. 4-7).

Basolateral membrane

HCO_3^- reabsorbed in the proximal convoluted tubule exits the cell as an ion complex containing 1 Na^+ and the equivalent of 3 HCO_3^- (or 1 HCO_3^- and 1 CO_3^{2-}; $Na[HCO_3]_3^{2-}$), via a coupled $Na(HCO_3)_3^{2-}$ cotransporter (NBC). Mutations in the gene encoding NBC have been reported in children with isolated proximal RTA associated with ocular abnormalities. These mutations result in either a decreased maximum velocity (V_{max}) or a lower affinity for $HCO_3)_3^{2-}$ (higher K_m) such that a higher concentration of HCO_3^- and a more alkaline intracellular fluid (ICF) pH is needed in the proximal tubule to export all HCO_3^- that are reabsorbed. It is also possible (but not confirmed in patients) that drugs or abnormal proteins might decrease the activity of NBC.

Intracellular defect

The H⁺ to be secreted are derived from H_2O. The OH^- formed in proximal convoluted tubule cells are removed as HCO_3^- in a reaction that is catalyzed by carbonic anhydrase II (second equation). Mutations involving carbonic anhydrase II lead to a more alkaline proximal tubule cell pH because the OH^- is a stronger base than HCO_3^- (*see margin note*).

$$H_2O \rightarrow H^+(\text{secreted}) + OH^-(\text{in cells})$$

$$OH^- + CO_2 \rightarrow HCO_3^- \text{ (if } CA_{II} \text{ is active)}$$

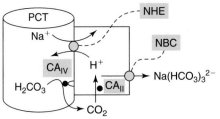

FIGURE 4-7 Molecular lesions causing proximal renal tubular acidosis (RTA). The structure represents the proximal convoluted tubule (PCT). The identified sites of lesions causing proximal RTA are inactivating mutations involving the $Na(HCO_3)_3^{2-}$ cotransporter (NBC) in the basolateral membrane or carbonic anhydrase II (CA_{II}) in PCT cells. There is no known single lesion that might affect the different Na^+-linked transport functions of the cells of the PCT and cause the Fanconi syndrome. Possible candidate lesions are listed in the margin note. NHE, Na^+/H^+ exchanger.

Margin notes

EXCRETION OF CITRATE
- The rate of excretion of citrate provides a "window" on the pH in proximal convoluted tubule cells. An acidified proximal convoluted tubule cell pH is associated with an enhanced reabsorption of citrate. Therefore, patients with metabolic acidosis have a very low rate of excretion of citrate.
- The sole exception to the previous statement is in patients with isolated proximal RTA who, despite metabolic acidosis, have a high rate of excretion of citrate. This suggests that there is an alkaline proximal cell pH in these patients.
- In patients with Fanconi syndrome, citraturia can be part of the generalized proximal convoluted tubule cell transport dysfunction.
- Because the high rate of excretion of citrate decreases the urinary concentration of ionized calcium, calcium stones are not usually seen in patients with proximal RTA.

CARBONIC ANHYDRASE II DEFICIENCY
- This enzyme is present in cells of the proximal convoluted tubule and in the late distal nephron segments. It is involved in the process of H⁺ secretion in both locations. Hence patients lacking this enzyme develop both proximal RTA and distal RTA.
- Carbonic anhydrase II is also involved in bone reabsorption. Hence these patients have more frequent bone fractures, as their bones are more fragile (called osteopetrosis).

FANCONI SYNDROME: POSSIBLE CANDIDATE LESIONS
- Multiple separate defects (unlikely)
- A membrane defect
- A defect in the trafficking of transporters
- An energy metabolism defect that may limit the availability of ATP for the Na-K-ATPase

Luminal membrane. Although, in theory, a molecular defect in the major luminal H^+ pump, NHE-3, could cause proximal RTA, mutations in the gene encoding this transporter have not been reported in patients with isolated proximal RTA. Perhaps the reason is that this Na^+/H^+ exchanger catalyzes the absorption of close to 10-fold more HCO_3^- (4000 mmol/day) compared with HCO_3^- in the ECF compartment (375 mmol). Therefore, even a relatively moderate defect in its transport activity would lead to a profound degree of acidemia. In fact, when NHE-3 was knocked out in mice, virtually all of them died at an early age.

Diagnostic issues in the patient with proximal renal tubular acidosis

> • The diagnosis of proximal RTA is rarely a problem because these patients have metabolic acidosis without an elevated $P_{Anion\ gap}$ and even large doses of $NaHCO_3$ fail to correct the acidemia.

There are other features of proximal RTA, including a low rate of excretion of NH_4^+ and the absence of a low rate of excretion of citrate (compare these two parameters to those expected during *chronic* metabolic acidosis).

One may wish to confirm that there is a reduced capacity to reabsorb HCO_3^- in the proximal convoluted tubule by measuring the fractional excretion of HCO_3^- (FE_{HCO3}) after enough $NaHCO_3$ is given to raise the P_{HCO3} to 25 mmol/L (*see margin note*). Before discussing the use of the FE_{HCO3} for the diagnosis of proximal RTA, there are several points about the excretion of HCO_3^- in patients with proximal RTA that merit emphasis. First, the absence of bicarbonaturia does not rule out proximal RTA. In fact, the urine is usually HCO_3^- free and the urine pH is well below 6.0 in many of these patients in the chronic steady state. Second, if a patient with proximal RTA does have bicarbonaturia, suspect one of the following:

1. A recent ingestion of alkali
2. A disease process that is in evolution and currently destroying proximal convoluted tubular cells and thus a steady state has not been yet achieved (e.g., recent intake of Chinese herbs containing aristolochic acid)
3. A disease that also causes decreased distal H^+ secretion (e.g., a mutation involving carbonic anhydrase II)
4. Intake of a drug (e.g., acetazolamide) that inhibits carbonic anhydrase IV, the enzyme in the luminal membrane of proximal convoluted tubular cells—this enzyme is needed to reabsorb $NaHCO_3$ at the usual rapid rate (see Fig. 4-7)

In patients with proximal RTA, the FE_{HCO3} is generally greater than 15% at a P_{HCO3} of 25 mmol/L. In addition, the P_{HCO3} should fall promptly when the infusion of $NaHCO_3$ is stopped. It is not always necessary to measure the FE_{HCO3} to confirm this diagnosis because failure to correct the metabolic acidosis with large doses of alkali strongly suggests a proximal tubular lesion. There is a caution here. Administration of $NaHCO_3$ can be dangerous if the patient has hypokalemia because it may cause a significant fall in the P_K (*see margin note*). Therefore, if you wish to perform this test, give the $NaHCO_3$ only after the K^+ deficit is replaced.

FRACTIONAL EXCRETION OF HCO_3^-

$$\frac{100 \times U_{HCO3}/P_{HCO3}}{U_{Creatinine}/P_{Creatinine}}$$

K^+ AND PROXIMAL RTA
- Most patients with isolated proximal RTA do not have significant hypokalemia unless they are treated with high doses of $NaHCO_3$, because the resultant bicarbonaturia and/or high urine pH can augment the rate of excretion of K^+.
- If the patient has significant hypokalemia on presentation, look for other problems such as combined proximal and distal RTA.

In patients with proximal RTA, there is usually no defect in distal H^+ secretion so the urine P_{CO_2} in alkaline urine is not low. A low P_{CO_2} in alkaline urine is observed in patients with combined proximal and distal RTA due to CA_{II} deficiency. The molecular lesion that produces this dual-site lesion is a defect in carbonic anhydrase II. It is also possible that paraproteinemias or autoimmune disorders may involve both these proximal and distal nephron sites.

To determine whether the patient has isolated proximal RTA or Fanconi syndrome, look for other findings of a generalized proximal tubule dysfunction (*see margin note on page 87*).

Treatment of the patient with proximal renal tubular acidosis

This depends on the specific cause. If the patient is taking an agent capable of causing proximal RTA (see Table 4-3), this intake should, of course, be stopped. In general, do not be overaggressive with treatment with $NaHCO_3$—the P_{HCO3} is rarely maintained near the normal range in patients with proximal RTA because bicarbonaturia ensues when the distal capacity for HCO_3^- reabsorption is exceeded. Bicarbonaturia may lead to the development of hypokalemia and may increase the risk of formation of $CaHPO_4$ kidney stones. Conversely, $NaHCO_3$ seems to be beneficial in some patients with proximal RTA and growth retardation.

DISTAL RENAL TUBULAR ACIDOSIS

CASE 4-1: A MAN DIAGNOSED WITH TYPE IV RENAL TUBULAR ACIDOSIS

(Case discussed on page 108)
A 51-year-old man has a long-standing history of type 2 diabetes mellitus that is relatively poorly controlled and persistent hyperchloremic metabolic acidosis (HCMA). On physical examination, his blood pressure is 160/100 mm Hg, his pulse rate is 80 beats per minute, and there is no evidence of a contracted ECF volume. He is noted to have hyperkalemia. Further investigation revealed a low plasma renin activity and a somewhat low plasma aldosterone level. His current laboratory results are summarized in Table 4-4.

Questions

What is the basis of the metabolic acidosis?
What is the cause of the low rate of excretion of NH_4^+?

CASE 4-2: WHAT IS THIS WOMAN'S "BASIC" LESION?

(Case discussed on page 109)
A 23-year-old woman suffers from Southeast Asian ovalocytosis. She is referred for assessment of HCMA and hypokalemia. Her physical examination was not remarkable, and her laboratory results are summarized in Table 4-4.

Questions

What is the basis of the metabolic acidosis?
What is the cause of the low rate of excretion of NH_4^+?

TABLE 4-4 **VALUES IN PLASMA AND A SPOT URINE SAMPLE**

		CASE 4-1		CASE 4-2	
		PLASMA	*URINE*	*PLASMA*	*URINE*
Na^+	mmol/L	140	140	140	75
K^+	mmol/L	5.5	60	3.1	35
Cl^-	mmol/L	112	130	113	95
HCO_3^-	mmol/L	16	0	15	—
pH		7.30	5.0	7.30	6.8
Pco_2	mm Hg	30	—	30	—
Anion gap	mEq/L	12	—	12	—
Glucose	mg/dL (mmol/L)	180 (10)	2+	90 (5.0)	0
Creatinine	mg/dL (µmol/L)	2.3 (200)	6 mmol/L	0.7 (60)	5 mmol/L
BUN (urea)	mg/dL (mmol/L)	28 (10)	700 (250)	14 (5.0)	560 (200)
Osmolality	mOsm/kg H_2O	295	700	290	450

Nomenclature

Numeric terms are currently used to describe patients who have metabolic acidosis caused by a low rate of excretion of NH_4^+ (i.e., type I, type II, type IV RTA). These terms, however, do not provide insights into the etiology of the disorder in each type; moreover, patients with a different reason for the low rate of excretion of NH_4^+ are grouped into a single type of RTA. Furthermore, terms such as *distal* or *proximal* may not reflect the site of the lesion in an individual patient. Hence, we prefer a classification of RTA based on the pathophysiology of the disorder (Table 4-5).

Clinical approach: Initial steps

> • In a normal adult subject, the rate of excretion of NH_4^+ should rise to close to 200 mmol/day during chronic metabolic acidosis.

The expected renal response to chronic metabolic acidosis is to increase the rate of excretion of NH_4^+ markedly. Two steps are involved. First, metabolic acidosis stimulates the production of NH_4^+ in the cells of the proximal convoluted tubule. Second, metabolic acidosis enhances the transfer of NH_3 and augments the rate of distal H^+ secretion in the late distal nephron. A detailed discussion of the physiology of the excretion of NH_4^+ is provided in Chapter 1, page 20.

HETEROGENEITY OF PATIENTS WITH RTA AND A HIGH P_K
In some patients, a high P_K might cause the low rate of excretion of NH_4^+. In other patients, however, separate lesions may cause the high P_K and the low rate of NH_4^+ excretion.

TYPE III RENAL TUBULAR ACIDOSIS
This diagnostic category was never clearly defined and did not stand the test of time.

TABLE 4-5 **NOMENCLATURE USED IN THE CLASSIFICATION OF RENAL TUBULAR ACIDOSIS**

We prefer a classification based on the pathophysiology of the disorder rather than numerical labels.

COMMONLY USED	SUGGESTED CHANGE
Type I RTA or distal RTA	Low NH_4^+ excretion disease
Type II RTA or proximal RTA	Renal HCO_3^- wasting disease
Type IV RTA (*see margin note*)	Low NH_4^+ excretion associated with hyperkalemia

Assess the rate of NH$_4^+$ excretion

The hallmark of RTA is a *low rate* of NH$_4^+$ excretion in a patient with chronic metabolic acidosis. Hence, assessment of the rate of excretion of NH$_4^+$ is the first diagnostic step in these patients. Because the urine pH does *not* provide reliable information about the rate of excretion of NH$_4^+$, it is wrong to use the urine pH to make the diagnosis of RTA (*see margin note*). To evaluate the rate of excretion of NH$_4^+$, the concentration of NH$_4^+$ in the urine should be estimated by calculating the U$_{Osmolal\ gap}$ (see Chapter 2, page 48). If the U$_{NH4}$/U$_{Creatinine}$ is less than 3 in a random urine sample while acidemia is present, the rate of NH$_4^+$ excretion is low enough to be the sole cause of the metabolic acidosis.

URINE pH GREATER THAN 7 AND THE RATE OF EXCRETION OF NH$_4^+$
- When the urine pH is greater than 7, it is usually safe to assume that the rate of excretion of NH$_4^+$ is low.
- A possible exception is the presence of a lower urinary tract infection with bacteria that release the enzyme urease; this adds HCO$_3^-$ and NH$_4^+$ to the urine.

Determine the basis of the low rate of excretion of NH$_4^+$

Once it has been established that the rate of excretion of NH$_4^+$ is low in a patient with HCMA, examining the urine pH permits one to determine the *basis* of this low rate of NH$_4^+$ excretion. When H$^+$ secretion in the distal nephron occurs but little NH$_3$ is available to bind these H$^+$, the urine pH is close to 5.0. Conversely, if H$^+$ secretion in the distal nephron is low in the presence of ample NH$_3$, the urine pH is greater than 6.5. A urine pH close to 6.0 suggests that there is a lesion causing defects in both NH$_3$ availability and distal H$^+$ secretion (Flow Chart 4-2).

Subtypes of disorders causing low NH$_4^+$ excretion

Subtype with low NH$_3$

Pathophysiology

- The hallmark of this subtype is a urine pH close to 5.0. The most common cause is a low rate of production of NH$_4^+$ in cells of the proximal convoluted tubule owing to hyperkalemia.

There are two subgroups of disorders that can cause this pathophysiology:
  1. *Low production of NH$_4^+$ in the proximal convoluted tubule*: The usual causes of a low production of NH$_4^+$ are an alkaline proximal cell pH due to hyperkalemia and/or a low availability of ADP in proximal cells due to a very low GFR (Table 4-6). Less

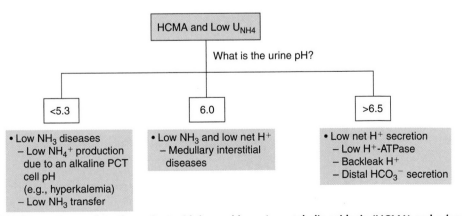

FLOW CHART 4-2 Approach to the patient with hyperchloremic metabolic acidosis (HCMA) and a *low* rate of excretion of NH$_4^+$. In a patient with HCMA *and* a low rate of excretion of NH$_4^+$, the next step is to measure the urine pH to determine the basis for the low rate of excretion of NH$_4^+$. PCT, proximal converted tubule.

TABLE 4-6 **CAUSES OF A LOW RATE OF PRODUCTION OF NH$_4^+$ IN THE PROXIMAL CONVOLUTED TUBULE**

High proximal cell pH
• Hyperkalemia
• Carbonic anhydrase II deficiency
• Some subtypes of proximal RTA

A low rate of metabolism of glutamine
• Low glomerular filtration rate causing low availability of ADP in proximal cells
• Low availability of glutamine (e.g., malnutrition)
• Provision of alternate fuels that compete with glutamine for oxidation (e.g., fatty acids in patients given parenteral nutrition)

common causes include an alkaline proximal cell pH due to a genetic disorder or a disease process that causes a defect in the exit step for HCO$_3^-$ (which also results in a renal HCO$_3^-$ wasting disease; proximal RTA), decreased availability of glutamine due to malnutrition, and/or high levels of other fuels that proximal cells can oxidize instead of glutamine to regenerate its requisite ATP (e.g., during total parenteral nutrition)

2. *Low transfer of NH$_3$ into the collecting duct*: There is uncertainty concerning the *quantitative* significance of the shunt of NH$_4^+$ across the renal medullary compartment in the process of excretion of NH$_4^+$. On the one hand, experimental evidence in rats with chronic metabolic acidosis suggests that the quantitative contribution of this shunt pathway to achieve a high rate of excretion of NH$_4^+$ is relatively small. On the other hand, diseases involving the renal medullary interstitial compartment are the most common cause of chronic metabolic acidosis due to a low rate of excretion of NH$_4^+$ (*see margin note*).

RTA IN PATIENTS WITH MEDULLARY INTERSTITIAL DISEASES
- There is no clear explanation for the pathophysiology of this group of disorders in our opinion.
- Notwithstanding, data from microcatheterization of the medullary collecting duct (MCD) in the fed rat, which suggests that little NH$_3$ is added to the MCD, might not be applicable to humans in quantitative terms, owing to marked differences in the diet alkali load (see the discussion of Question 4-1, on page 109).

QUESTION

(Discussion on page 109)

4-1 *How different are the rat and the human with respect to their rate of excretion of NH$_4^+$ per kg of body weight?*

Clinical features

- The two most common causes of a low production of NH$_4^+$ are hyperkalemia and a low GFR.

Hyperkalemia. The term *type IV RTA* is used by some authorities to describe the constellation of findings of hyperkalemia and metabolic acidosis due to a low rate of excretion of NH$_4^+$ (see Table 4-5). Nevertheless, there are two distinct ways that hyperkalemia and a low rate of excretion of NH$_4^+$ may coexist.

1. *Hyperkalemia is responsible for the low rate of excretion of NH$_4^+$.* Hyperkalemia may cause a low rate of NH$_4^+$ excretion by inhibiting either ammoniagenesis (hyperkalemia causes an alkaline proximal cell pH) and/or the transfer of NH$_3$ in the loop of Henle (K$^+$ competes with NH$_4^+$ on the Na$^+$, K$^+$, 2 Cl$^-$ cotransporter). In these patients, the urine pH is low (~5). If this is the case, the patient should have a sufficient increase in the rate of excretion of NH$_4^+$ to correct the metabolic acidosis once the P$_K$ returns to the normal range. In some patients, however, it might be difficult to establish a "cause and effect" relationship if there is another factor that may also contribute to the low rate

of excretion of NH$_4^+$ (e.g., a low GFR due to a very contracted effective arterial blood volume as in a patient with adrenal insufficiency) because this will also be corrected during therapy.

2. *Hyperkalemia is **not** the major reason for the low rate of excretion of NH$_4^+$.* In this subgroup of patients, the low rate of excretion of NH$_4^+$ is not causally linked to the hyperkalemia as indicated by the fact that the rate of excretion of NH$_4^+$ remains low after the P$_K$ has returned to the normal range. In general, the basis of the low excretion of NH$_4^+$ in this subgroup is a combination of low NH$_3$ availability and low distal H$^+$ secretion; hence, the urine pH would be close to 6. For chronic hyperkalemia to be present, the disease process must involve the late cortical distal nephron, the site of K$^+$ secretion.

In the absence of hyperkalemia or a low GFR, look for a disorder that leads to an alkaline proximal tubular cell pH. The diagnostic criteria for this lesion are discussed on page 95.

Consequences of a persistently low urine pH. If a patient with a very low urine pH also has a low urine volume, the risk of forming uric acid stones rises appreciably. Because there are only modest variations in total urate excretion, one should focus on measures to raise the urine pH by administering alkali to minimize the risk of recurrent uric acid stone formation.

Treatment

Emergency management. The most important threat to the patient is a cardiac arrhythmia due to hyperkalemia. If an electrocardiographic abnormality or a severe degree of hyperkalemia is present, this should be dealt with first. In the longer term, one must seek the basis for the hyperkalemia; its treatment is discussed in Chapter 15, page 532. Obviously, if the patient has a significant degree of ECF volume contraction, this must be treated as well.

Acid-base management. If the P$_K$ returns to the normal range and this is sufficient to raise the rate of excretion of NH$_4^+$ and correct the acidosis, one can suspect that hyperkalemia was the cause of the disorder. In other patients, treatment with NaHCO$_3$ may be necessary, because the chronic metabolic acidosis may lead to catabolism of lean body mass and the persistently low urine pH may lead to uric acid stones. Significant bicarbonaturia, however, should be avoided because it might predispose to the formation of CaHPO$_4$ kidney stones should the urine pH rise excessively. Therefore, the dose of NaHCO$_3$ should be distributed throughout the day to ensure that the urine pH is not much greater than 6.0 throughout a 24-hour period. Once the P$_{HCO3}$ is in the normal range, the dose of NaHCO$_3$ needed to maintain a normal P$_{HCO3}$ is expected to be less than 30 mmol/day (i.e., match the usual rate of NH$_4^+$ excretion).

Subtype with low net distal H$^+$ secretion

Pathophysiology

- The hallmark of this subtype is a urine pH greater than 6.5. The urine P$_{CO_2}$ in alkaline urine and the rate of excretion of citrate help define the pathophysiology.

These patients have a low rate of excretion of NH$_4^+$ because of a low *net* addition of H$^+$ into the lumen of the distal nephron. The potential causes of this low net distal H$^+$ secretion are listed in Table 4-7. The possible etiologies can be distinguished by examining the P$_{CO_2}$ in alkaline urine and the rate of citrate excretion (Flow Chart 4-3).

TABLE 4-7 **CAUSES OF A LOW RATE OF EXCRETION OF NH$_4^+$ DUE TO DECREASED NET H$^+$ SECRETION**

Low H$^+$-ATPase activity (Pco$_2$ in alkaline urine is low)

- Mutations involving the H$^+$-ATPase (± sensory-neuronal deafness)
- Alkaline distal cell pH due to carbonic anhydrase II deficiency or acquired disorders causing an alkaline distal cell pH (e.g., autoimmune diseases and hypergammaglobulinemic states such as Sjögren disease and systemic lupus erythematosus)

High distal secretion of HCO$_3^-$ in α-intercalated cells (Pco$_2$ in alkaline urine is high)

- Some patients with Southeast Asian ovalocytosis (these patients have two mutations in the gene encoding AE-1: the usual one that leads to ovalocytosis and a second one that causes the AE-1 to be targeted abnormally to the luminal membrane of α-intercalated cells)
- Possibly in some patients with autoimmune disorders

Backleak of H$^+$ (Pco$_2$ in alkaline urine is high)

- Drugs (e.g., amphotericin B)

Low number of H$^+$-ATPase pumps in the distal nephron

- This group includes rare inborn errors affecting the H$^+$-ATPase and some autoimmune diseases that may cause secondary damage to the H$^+$-ATPase.

In some patients with low distal H$^+$ secretion, the H$^+$-ATPase is not detected in luminal membranes of α-intercalated cells by immuno-histologic staining in renal biopsy specimens. Nevertheless, there can be more than one reason for a low H$^+$-ATPase in the patients with an acquired defect. Although it is possible that circulating antibodies may damage the H$^+$-ATPase, it is also possible that the low amount of H$^+$-ATPase is secondary to a persistently alkaline α-intercalated cell pH (discussed later). If the defect compromises the H$^+$-ATPase sufficiently, the Pco$_2$ in alkaline urine should be close to 40 mm Hg. Citrate excretion in these patients is low because of enhanced reabsorption of citrate in the proximal convoluted tubule stimulated by acidemia.

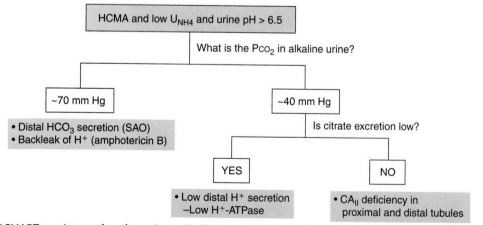

FLOW CHART 4-3 Approach to the patient with distal renal tubular acidosis (RTA) and a urine pH greater than 6.5. RTA is present because the rate of excretion of NH$_4^+$ is low; its basis is a low net rate of H$^+$ secretion in the distal nephron when the urine pH is greater than 6.5. The steps to define the underlying mechanisms are summarized here. CA$_{II}$, carbonic anhydrase; HCMA, hyperchloremic metabolic acidosis; SAO, Southeast Asian ovalocytosis.

Inhibition of existing H⁺-ATPase pumps by an alkaline cell pH

- There is a diminished exit of HCO_3^- from α-intercalated cells, which leads to a low rate of distal secretion of H⁺ because of inhibition of the H⁺-ATPase by the high ICF pH in these cells (Fig. 4-8).

There are two subgroups of patients in this category. The first consists of patients with autoimmune disorders that lead to an inhibited basolateral Cl^-/HCO_3^- anion exchanger. The second subgroup consists of patients with a lesion that compromises CA_{II} (see proximal RTA, page 85). In both subgroups, the P_{CO_2} in alkaline urine would be close to 40 mm Hg because of a low rate of distal secretion of H⁺. The rate of excretion of citrate, however, would be low in the first subset of patients but could be high in patients with CA_{II} deficiency because this disorder causes proximal cells to have a high pH.

Backleak of H⁺ in the distal nephron

- It is commonly thought that amphotericin B may cause a low *net* H⁺ secretion in the distal nephron because of a backleak of H⁺ into α-intercalated cells.

The reason for this is that amphotericin B makes pores in the cell membranes facing the lumen through which there is a backleak of cations, including H⁺. Nevertheless, with a large backleak of H⁺, there would be a continuously high rate of distal H⁺ secretion with a considerable expenditure of energy in an area of the kidney with a low blood flow rate and thereby marginal supply of oxygen, which might predispose this area of the kidney to hypoxic damage. Therefore, although the defect in net H⁺ secretion may initially be due to a backleak of H⁺, this might be followed by a longer-term defect, owing in large part to medullary damage.

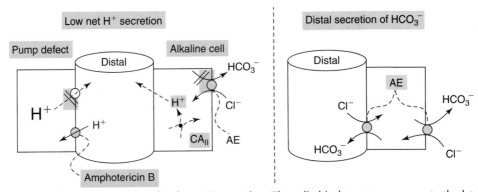

FIGURE 4-8 Lesions compromising distal net H⁺ secretion. The *cylindrical structure* represents the late distal nephron; the *rectangles* represent α-intercalated cells. Lesions causing a decrease in net H⁺ secretion are shown *to the left of the dashed line*, whereas those causing the secretion of HCO_3^- are shown *to the right of the dashed line*. The major causes for low net H⁺ secretion are a H⁺ pump defect (deficient H⁺-ATPase), backleak of H⁺, or an alkaline intercalated cell (i.e., failure to remove OH⁻ via CA_{II} or failure to export HCO_3^- via the anion exchanger [AE] on their basolateral membrane). Enhanced distal secretion of HCO_3^- is shown in the *right portion of the figure*; this secretion of HCO_3^- occurs due to mistargeting of AE to the luminal membrane of α-intercalated cells.

DISTAL RENAL TUBULAR
ACIDOSIS AND AUTOIMMUNE
DISEASE

- In some patients with autoimmune disorders, the antibodies may be directed against the H^+-ATPase pump or the HCO_3^- exit step. If this is the case, the P_{CO_2} in alkaline urine would be low. Nevertheless, one would need to explain how circulating antibodies entered these cells and remained intact in the process to affect the H^+-ATPase.
- In other patients, however, the P_{CO_2} in alkaline urine is high, suggesting that some of the basolateral Cl^-/HCO_3^- anion exchangers are misdirected to the luminal membrane, which induces the secretion of HCO_3^-, akin to the lesion in Southeast Asian ovalocytosis.

Distal secretion of HCO_3^-

- The usual basis for this disorder is a molecular defect in Cl^-/HCO_3^- anion exchanger.

The best example is seen in rare patients with Southeast Asian ovalocytosis who have a second mutation in the Cl^-/HCO_3^- anion exchanger, which results in some of the exchanger being targeted abnormally to the luminal membrane of α-intercalated cells (see Fig. 4-8; *see margin note*). In this setting, the secretion of HCO_3^- causes the luminal pH to increase, liberating H^+ from $H_2PO_4^-$, which raises the P_{CO_2} in alkaline urine to greater than 70 mm Hg. Because proximal cells do not have this anion exchanger as their alkali exit step, their ICF pH is reduced owing to the acidemia; hence, these patients have a low rate of excretion of citrate.

Voltage defect in H^+ secretion in the distal nephron

- It is not clear whether a high lumen-negative voltage in the distal nephron is important for a high rate of excretion of NH_4^+.

On the one hand, although there is an abundance of H^+-ATPase pumps in the luminal membrane of the medullary collecting duct, there is no appreciable lumen-negative voltage in this nephron segment; hence, this nephron segment does not have voltage-driven H^+ secretion. On the other hand, although there is an appreciable lumen-negative voltage in the cortical collecting duct (CCD), its primary function is to control the net secretion of K^+. Therefore, if this lumen-negative voltage is also required for H^+ secretion in the CCD, one would expect to see a link between hyperkalemia and metabolic acidosis due to a low rate of excretion of NH_4^+, *with a high urine pH, but this is not a common presentation (see margin note on page 90).*

Clinical features. The diagnostic approach is outlined in Flow Chart 4-3 and a list of possible causes is provided in Table 4-7.

Associated findings

Hypokalemia. Hypokalemia is often a feature of distal RTA that is due to a low rate of H^+ secretion or secretion of HCO_3^- in the late cortical distal nephron. The renal loss of K^+ is due to an unexpectedly high rate of K^+ secretion because of an effect of bicarbonaturia and/or an alkaline luminal pH to increase the lumen-negative voltage in the CCD or perhaps to an increase in the number of open K^+ channels in the luminal membrane of principal cells (see Chapter 14, page 466).

Hypokalemia may be severe and cause muscle weakness. At times, this may be the symptom that brings the patient to clinical attention.

Nephrocalcinosis. Patients with distal RTA that is accompanied by hypokalemia have an increased incidence of calcium deposition in the medullary interstitial compartment—this is called *nephrocalcinosis*. The reasons that calcium salts are more likely to precipitate in this region are higher concentrations of ionized calcium and/or of the anions it might precipitate within the medullary interstitial compartment. Medullary alkalinization is required to form a precipitate of calcium with phosphate or carbonate anions. We provide a more detailed discussion of possible mechanisms in Part D, page 103.

Consequences of a high urine pH

- The major consequence of a high urine pH is a higher concentration of HPO_4^{2-} in the urine and thereby, the formation of a precipitate of calcium phosphate ($CaHPO_4$).

There are two major factors that permit $CaHPO_4$ stones to grow: a higher concentration (really higher activity) of ionized calcium and a higher concentration (i.e., activity) of divalent phosphate anions (HPO_4^{2-}) in the urine. The major risk factor for the former is a low rate of excretion of citrate because this anion chelates ionized calcium. The low rate of excretion of citrate can be due to acidemia and/or hypokalemia, both of which are present in this group of patients with distal RTA. The major reason to have a high concentration of HPO_4^{2-} in the lumen is a high urine pH, which converts $H_2PO_4^-$ to HPO_4^2. Although alkali therapy with K^+ citrate may be beneficial in these patients if it increases the excretion of citrate, it may, however, cause a further rise in the urine pH, thereby increasing the risk of precipitation of $CaHPO_4$ in the urine (*see margin note*). Nevertheless, the effect of a rise in urine pH on increasing the concentration of divalent phosphate becomes progressively smaller as the urine pH rises above 6.8 (Table 4-8).

PRECIPITATION OF CaHPO₄
CaHPO₄ deposits form at the mouth of the terminal medullary collecting duct, which leads to obstruction and ultimately to progressive renal insufficiency. Hence, treatment is much more important for these patients to prevent the development of renal insufficiency.

Treatment

Emergency issues

- NaHCO₃ should *not* be given until the P_K rises to a safe level (~3 mmol/L) to avoid a dangerous decline in the P_K owing to a shift of K^+ into cells.

The most important threat to the patient is a cardiac arrhythmia due to hypokalemia. Hypokalemia may also cause respiratory muscle weakness and thus severe acidemia due to superimposed respiratory acidosis. The emergency treatment of hypokalemia is discussed in Chapter 14.

Acid-base issues. Alkali therapy is usually needed in patients with distal RTA and a urine pH greater than 6.5 because they are unable to excrete enough NH_4^+ to regenerate the HCO_3^- consumed by the dietary acid load. Bicarbonaturia, however, should be minimized, because it might predispose to excessive renal K^+ loss and $CaHPO_4$ kidney stone formation. Therefore, the dose of NaHCO₃ should be as small as possible and be distributed throughout the day. After

TABLE 4-8 **EFFECT OF RAISING THE URINE pH ON THE URINARY DIVALENT PHOSPHATE CONCENTRATION**

For this calculation, we used a total 24-hour excretion of inorganic phosphate of 30 mmol, a urine volume of 1 L/day, and a pH of 6.8. At a urine pH of 7.1, two thirds of the total phosphate in the urine is in the divalent form. There is a small percent increase in HPO_4^{2-} concentration when the urine pH rises from 7.1 to 7.5.

URINE pH	$H_2PO_4^-$ (mmol/L)	HPO_4^{2-} (mmol/L)
6.8	15	15
7.1	10	20
7.3	7.5	22.5
7.4	6	24
7.5	5	25

the P_{HCO3} is corrected, the dose of $NaHCO_3$ needed to maintain P_{HCO3} in the normal range is usually less than 30 to 40 mmol/day (i.e., enough to titrate the acid load produced from the metabolism of dietary sulfur-containing amino acids).

Subtype with lesions involving both distal H⁺ secretion and NH₃ availability

Pathophysiology

> • The hallmark of this subtype is a urine pH in the low 6 range.

Diseases involving the renal medulla can compromise collecting duct cells and thereby cause a low H^+-ATPase activity and also diminish NH_3 availability in the medullary interstitium. Hence, the rate of excretion of NH_4^+ is low and the urine pH is usually close to 6.0.

Clinical features. These patients have HCMA with a low rate of excretion of NH_4^+ and a urine pH close to 6.0. Because of the presence of acidemia, the rate of excretion of citrate is low. The defect in distal H^+ secretion can be confirmed by finding a P_{CO_2} in alkaline urine close to 40 mm Hg.

Because of the medullary interstitial disorder, these patients may also have a reduced urinary concentrating ability. Hyperkalemia may be present if the disease process also involves the cortical collecting duct. Nevertheless, when the P_K returns to the normal range, the acidemia persists. The list of causes of disorders that affect the renal medullary interstitial compartment is long and includes infections, drugs, infiltrations, precipitations, inflammatory disorders, and sickle cell anemia, among others.

Treatment. Administration of alkali is needed to correct the acidemia. The issues for alkali therapy that were discussed in the subgroup with diminished net H^+ secretion apply here.

INCOMPLETE RENAL TUBULAR ACIDOSIS

> • This diagnostic category is based on finding a high urine pH and the absence of metabolic acidosis. Notwithstanding, it includes more than one pathophysiologic entity. Ruling out other causes of a high urine pH should improve our understanding of this group of disorders.

Background physiology

The label "incomplete RTA" originated in an era when the linch-pin in the diagnosis of distal RTA was a high urine pH in patients with HCMA. Hence, it is not surprising that when patients present with recurrent $CaHPO_4$ stones, especially at a young age, and they have a *high* urine pH in the *absence* of HCMA, the name given to this constellation of findings was *incomplete RTA* (*see margin note*). This combination of findings, however, may be found in three circumstances, which are discussed in the paragraphs that follow. Only the third one represents distinct renal lesions; hence, the term *incomplete RTA* should be reserved for this last subgroup.

INCOMPLETE RTA
- While the historical basis for the definition of *incomplete RTA* has been explained, the authors believe that this misleading terminology should be abandoned, as RTA is a disorder with the principal finding of a low rate of excretion of NH_4^+, and this disorder has a high rate of excretion of NH_4^+.
- A more correct definition of this group of disorders is "increased urine pH in a patient with a high rate of excretion of NH_4^+."

Conditions that are not true "incomplete renal tubular acidosis"

Distal renal tubular acidosis due to low net distal secretion of H⁺

> • Although these patients usually have a degree of acidemia, a low blood pH may not be present if they ingest a *low net H⁺ load*.

If their diet were to have more alkali (e.g., more fruit and vegetables [see Fig. 1-5, page 10]) and/or fewer precursors of H_2SO_4 (e.g., low protein intake; see Fig. 1-3, page 9), acidemia may be absent. Accordingly, the key diagnostic step in this setting is to find a low rate of excretion of NH_4^+ after chronic acidemia is induced by the administration of an acid load (e.g., NH_4Cl) for several days.

Large intermittent intake of alkali in a normal subject

> • To exclude this subgroup of patients from those with "true incomplete RTA," they should be studied on a diet that more closely reflects the composition of typical Western diet.

The diet in this category of patients provides a large episodic load of alkali (e.g., fruit and vegetables). These patients have a normal plasma pH and P_{HCO3} along with a high urine pH. Additional clues to suggest that this is the basis for the high urine pH are the following: (1) The rate of excretion of NH_4^+ is low when compared with that of SO_4^{2-} in mEq terms (diet alkali load titrates H⁺ from H_2SO_4) and (2) the calculated dietary *net* alkali intake is large (e.g., as reflected by the rate of excretion of organic anions including citrate in the urine; *see margin note*). The patients in this subgroup resemble the patients with distal RTA due to low net H⁺ secretion described previously, except that they do not develop acidemia when they consume a typical Western diet, and they are able to increase their rate of excretion of NH_4^+ appropriately when given a large and chronic acid (NH_4Cl) load.

Patients with true "incomplete renal tubular acidosis"

> • These patients also come to medical attention because they have recurrent $CaHPO_4$ kidney stones.
> • To assess the expected rate of excretion of NH_4^+, compare this value to the excretion of SO_4^{2-} in mEq terms. In incomplete RTA, the U_{NH4} is higher than the U_{SO4}.

The initial diagnostic workup reveals a persistently high urine pH for much of the day (>6.5 for at least 12 out of 24 hours, an admittedly arbitrary definition). The key diagnostic feature in this group of patients is a *high* rate of excretion of NH_4^+ when compared with that of SO_4^{2-}. In contrast, normal subjects have near-equal daily excretions of NH_4^+ and SO_4^{2-}, and patients with distal RTA excrete less NH_4^+ than SO_4^{2-}. We envisage two subtypes of "true incomplete RTA" as discussed in the following paragraphs.
  1. *Patients with an acidified proximal cell pH*: The lesion begins with a higher than expected rate of production of NH_4^+ in cells of the proximal convoluted tubule owing to a high concentration of H⁺ in these cells. In the absence of hypokalemia, an acidified proximal cell pH could be due to a lesion that causes activation

CALCULATION OF DIET ALKALI INTAKE

• A high rate of excretion of organic anions (including citrate) is suspected when their "electrical shadow" is present in the urine ($U_{Na} + U_K + U_{NH4} + U_{Ca} + U_{Mg}$) is much greater than ($U_{Cl} + U_{HPO4} + U_{SO4}$), all in mEq/L terms.

• To change concentrations into excretion rates, divide the difference in concentration between urinary cations and urinary anions in mEq/L terms by the $U_{Creatinine}$ and multiply this ratio by the expected rate of excretion of creatinine (20 mg/kg or 0.2 mmol/kg).

Shorter calculation:

• Because the major source of Na⁺ and Cl⁻ in the urine comes from NaCl, the rate of excretion of these ions is virtually always equal in mEq terms and they can be removed from the preceding calculation.

• In most patients, the rates of excretion of NH_4^+ and SO_4^{2-} are virtually equal in mEq terms, so they too can be removed from the calculation.

• Overall, the calculation becomes the difference of rates of excretion of K⁺ and inorganic phosphate in the urine (i.e., the K⁺ from meat, which is largely balanced by organic monovalent phosphate) and the remaining extra K⁺, which is accompanied by organic anions in the urine.

$U_{OA} = U_K - U_{PO4}$ in mEq terms

of the exit step for the $Na(HCO_3)_3^{2-}$ complex in the basolateral membrane of these cells. As a result of the low intracellular pH, there is a greater rate of production of NH_4^+ and thus a higher concentration of NH_3 in the renal medullary interstitial compartment. If this were to lead to a greater rate of NH_3 entry into the lumen of the medullary collecting duct, the urine pH would be greater than 6.5 and the rate of excretion of NH_4^+ would also be unusually high.

As a result of the low pH in the proximal cells, the rate of reabsorption of citrate should rise and the excretion of citrate would be extremely low. This contributes in a major way to the likelihood of forming kidney stones that contain calcium because of the low content of this chelator of ionized calcium in the urine.

There is also an interesting potential long-term issue in this diagnostic category—a high medullary NH_3 concentration may activate the complement system and thereby lead to secondary medullary interstitial damage. If this were to lead to a decrease in excretion of NH_4^+, the patient would develop distal RTA later in life. These findings would now be those in the subtype of distal RTA with a urine pH that is close to 6.0.

2. *Patients with a primary increase in the medullary NH_3 shunt*: It is also possible to have a high excretion of NH_4^+ ($U_{NH4} > U_{SO4}$ in mEq terms) and a high urine pH if there were a higher rate of entry of NH_3 into the lumen of the medullary collecting duct (see Fig. 1-17, page 27). Although these findings are similar to those in the subtype of patients with true "incomplete RTA" discussed earlier, patients with this disorder would lack the findings directly attributable to a low pH in proximal cells. This, in effect, means that this subgroup would *not* have a low rate of excretion of citrate. Hence, they would form $CaHPO_4$ stones owing to the high urine HPO_4^{2-} concentration, especially if they had another lesion that leads to a high rate of excretion of calcium and/or a low urine flow rate (this may raise the concentration of calcium and HPO_4^{2-} in the urine).

Diagnostic approach

The first step in patients who present with $CaHPO_4$ kidney stones is to compare the rates of excretion of NH_4^+ and SO_4^{2-}. If the excretion of NH_4^+ exceeds that of SO_4^{2-} by an appreciable amount, this rules out patients with "occult" distal RTA due to decreased distal net H^+ secretion who consume a low net dietary H^+ load (i.e., those with a high alkali intake). Hence, the diagnosis in this setting is "incomplete RTA" (see Flow Chart 4-4). Nevertheless, this diagnostic category represents a heterogeneous group with regard to pathophysiology. We highlight the following two groups of disorders with a high urine pH and a higher NH_4^+ than SO_4^{2-} excretion rate: (1) a higher than usual production of NH_4^+ in proximal cells due to an acidified proximal cell pH and (2) a primary increase in the medullary NH_3 shunt. Examining the rate of excretion of citrate permits one to distinguish between these two disorders.

Understanding the pathophysiology in the individual patient may have implications for therapy to prevent the recurrence of kidney stones once these separate diagnostic categories can be studied in more detail. This is particularly important because of recent findings that patients with this type of kidney stone develop progressive parenchymal damage and nephron loss owing to plugging of the terminal collecting duct with $CaHPO_4$ crystals.

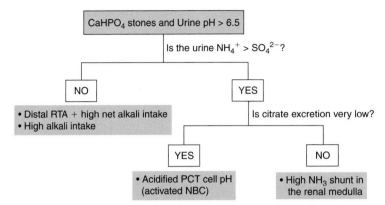

FLOW CHART 4-4 Approach to the patient with a high urine pH and CaHPO₄ kidney stones. To be considered for a diagnosis of incomplete renal tubular acidosis (RTA), hyperchloremic metabolic acidosis (HCMA) must *not* be present. Patients with recurrent CaHPO₄ stones have a high urine pH for most of the day. The diagnostic subgroups of true incomplete RTA are distinguished after examining the rate of excretion of citrate. NBC, Na(HCO₃)²⁻ cotransporter; PCT, proximal convoluted tubule.

METABOLIC ACIDOSIS IN RENAL FAILURE

- The rate of H^+ accumulation is influenced by the dietary intake of acid and alkali precursors as well as the rate of excretion of NH_4^+.
- The $P_{\text{Anion gap}}$ is increased because of the low GFR (no overproduction of acids).
- The major danger to the patient is usually due to hyperkalemia rather than to the acidemia.

When the GFR is markedly reduced, the following changes could be expected.

$H_2PO_4^-$ excretion: This still matches the input of $H_2PO_4^-$ because the urine pH is well below 6.8, the pK of $HPO_4^{2-}/H_2PO_4^-$. Hence, this form of dietary H^+ plays a trivial role in the development of metabolic acidosis in these patients (see Chapter 1, page 8).

Ammonium excretion: The excretion of NH_4^+ declines markedly because of low availability of ADP in proximal cells (less filtered Na^+ so less renal work; see Fig. 1-12, page 21). The quantity of H^+ retained depends on how much protein is ingested and thereby how much H_2SO_4 is produced and to what degree the excretion of NH_4^+ is reduced. The retention of H^+ can be as high as 30 to 40 mEq/day if the dietary protein intake is not reduced and the excretion of NH_4^+ is very low.

Diet alkali: This is often ignored because of an *"unbalanced"* view of acid versus base balance. The alkali load is derived mainly from dietary fruit and vegetables (e.g., K^+ + citrate anions), and it is normally eliminated as K^+ plus organic anions in the urine (see Fig. 1-5, page 10). Notwithstanding, once metabolic acidosis develops, the excretion of alkali as potential HCO_3^- declines and the dietary HCO_3^- load is retained. In this setting, these HCO_3^- titrate many of the H^+ from H_2SO_4 produced in metabolism of sulfur-containing amino acids and thereby diminish the net H^+ load that must be eliminated each day by the excretion of NH_4^+. Because patients with renal insufficiency are usually placed on a

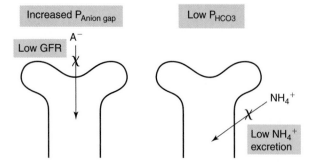

FIGURE 4-9 Basis of high plasma anion gap and acidosis in patients with renal failure. The basis of the increased $P_{Anion\ gap}$ is the low glomerular filtration rate (GFR) with reduced excretion of anions, such as phosphate or sulfate (*left side*). The acidosis is due to a low rate of excretion of NH_4^+ (*right side*).

low K^+ diet, they eat less alkali and, as a result, are more likely to become acidemic. On the other hand, if their intake of fruit and vegetables were not restricted, the degree of acidemia is less, but the large price to pay is hyperkalemia.

The high $P_{Anion\ gap}$ in patients with renal insufficiency does not represent the production of an unusually high amount of new acids; rather, it is due to the low GFR with the accumulation of SO_4^{2-} and HPO_4^- anions (Fig. 4-9). Usually the $P_{Anion\ gap}$ does not rise appreciably until the GFR has fallen to less than 20 mL/min.

Experimental evidence from studies in rats strongly suggests that acidemia is a catabolic signal in uremia. Although the evidence from human data is less robust, we recommend that metabolic acidemia in patients with chronic kidney disease be corrected. Once this is done, the dose of $NaHCO_3$ required to maintain a normal P_{HCO3} is likely to be less than 30 to 40 mmol/day. This salt load should not represent a problem to most patients with chronic kidney disease.

PART D
INTEGRATIVE PHYSIOLOGY

STEADY-STATE ACID-BASE BALANCE IN PATIENTS WITH RENAL TUBULAR ACIDOSIS

Patients with RTA are in acid-base balance year in and year out, despite having a low rate of excretion of NH_4^+ ($U_{NH4} < U_{SO4}$). Hence, there appears to be other factors that permit them to achieve acid-base balance. The possible mechanisms are discussed subsequently.

Generate new HCO_3^- by dissolving the alkaline salts in bone

If this were the case, there would be very close to 1 mEq of calcium excreted per mEq of HCO_3^- produced (*see margin note*). A modest increase in calcium excretion is noted in human subjects during *acute* acidosis, but this is transient and there is no evidence for an appreciable increase in calcium excretion in patients with *chronic* acidosis. Moreover, this is unlikely to be a source for a significant amount of alkali for a sustained period of time without a very substantial loss of bone mass.

DISSOLVING ALKALINE BONE SALTS
- Calcium salts in bone are $CaCO_3$ and $Ca_3(PO_4)_2$. When they dissolve, there is a net addition of Ca^{2+} and HCO_3^- in the body.
- For this to represent a gain of alkali, the Ca^{2+} must be lost without forming a precipitate in the body (e.g., excreted in the urine). If it were to precipitate again as $CaCO_3$ and $Ca_3(PO_4)_2$ in bone or in other sites, the HCO_3^- load would be removed.

Excrete less potential HCO₃⁻ in the urine so dietary alkali titrate some of the dietary acid load

In normal physiology, dietary alkali is disposed of by excreting organic anions in the urine (see Fig. 1-5, page 10). Hence, when there is an acid load, much less citrate (and other organic anions) will be excreted in the urine, and thus gain from dietary alkali will be used to titrate some of the dietary acid load. In quantitative terms, the decline in NH_4^+ excretion is matched by the decline in the urinary excretion of potential HCO_3^- and thereby, acid-base balance is preserved.

NEPHROCALCINOSIS IN PATIENTS WITH DISTAL RENAL TUBULAR ACIDOSIS

The subgroup of patients with distal RTA, a urine pH greater than 6.5, and a low P_K are prone to deposit calcium salts in the renal medullary interstitial compartment. The factors that increase the likelihood of deposition of calcium salts are those that raise the activity of ionized calcium and/or the anion that precipitates with calcium. Hypokalemia plays a central role, but other factors might also be important.

Mechanisms

Raise the medullary interstitial ionized calcium concentration

- The most important risk factor for the development of nephrocalcinosis is the addition of calcium without water to the medullary interstitial compartment.
- There are factors that diminish the likelihood of developing nephrocalcinosis.

Absence of a risk for nephrocalciosis during the absorption of calcium in the proximal convoluted tubule. Calcium absorption in this nephron segment, although large in magnitude, does not increase the risk for interstitial calcification because the proximal convoluted tubule has AQP1 water channels, and thus the nephron segment is *permeable* to water. Moreover, the absorption of water is the initial step to absorb calcium, as it creates the driving force for this process (a rise in the concentration of ionized calcium in its lumen).

Presence of a risk for nephrocalcinosis during the absorption of calcium in the medullary thick ascending limb of the loop of Henle (mTAL). In this water-*impermeable* nephron segment, there is also a passive reabsorption of calcium, but there is a different driving force, a lumen-positive voltage. This voltage is created by the entry of K^+ into its lumen via ROMK channels. The greatest risk for a large rise in the interstitial calcium concentration is immediately adjacent to the basolateral membrane of the mTAL. Although a low rate of blood flow and a countercurrent exchange in the vasa recta should increase the risk of precipitation of calcium salts, there are four major defense mechanisms that diminish this risk. First, there is inhibitory control of reabsorption of Ca^{2+} (and Na^+) via the interstitial calcium activity, which acts via basolateral calcium-sensing receptors that are linked to the number of open luminal ROMK channels. Second, there is a process of urea recycling in the renal inner medulla, which leads to the delivery of water without calcium to this interstitial region and hence lowers the interstitial calcium concentration. Third, the ascending vasa recta have holes (fenes-tra), which carry the very small precipitates of calcium carbonate out of the medulla. Fourth, the high ionic strength in the renal medullary interstitial compartment leads to a diminished activity of ionized calcium. Fifth, high interstitial magnesium concentrations may decrease the precipitation of calcium salts.

QUESTION

(Discussion on page 110)

4-2 *Why is nephrocalcinosis so common in patients with antenatal Bartter's syndrome (a total defect in the reabsorption of NaCl and calcium in the medullary thick ascending limb of the loop of Henle)?*

Raise the medullary interstitial concentration of HPO_4^{2-} and CO_3^{2-}

This requires alkalinization of the medullary interstitium. In a patient with hypokalemia, the H^+/K^+-ATPase activity in the medul-lary collecting duct is increased. The net effect of this H^+ secretion into the lumen of the medullary collecting duct is an addition of K^+ and HCO_3^- to the interstitial compartment (Fig. 4-10). As a result, the pH in this compartment rises, converting $H_2PO_4^-$ to HPO_4^{2-}.

Nevertheless, the rise in pH is too small to raise the concentration of PO_4^{3-} appreciably. Notwithstanding, although the P_K for carbonate is also very high (~10), there is a large pool of precursor for carbonate in the form of bicarbonate.

The ability to have supersaturated solutions

It is possible that other factors may operate to promote or retard the development of nephrocalcinosis. There could be inhibitors of crystal formation in this interstitial compartment that permit supersaturation of calcium salts without precipitation. On the other

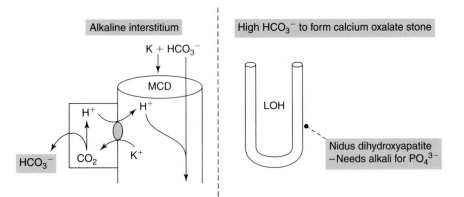

FIGURE 4-10 Alkalinization of the renal inner medullary interstitial compartment. The *larger structure in the left portion of the figure* is the medullary collecting duct (MCD), whereas *the smaller thin loop in the right portion* represents the thin limbs of the loop of Henle (LOH) in the inner medulla. When more K^+ are reabsorbed by the H^+/K^+-ATPase in the MCD, HCO_3^- are added to the inner medullary interstitial compartment. As shown in the *right portion*, this alkalinization raises the concentration of CO_3^{2-} and thereby PO_4^{3-} (see Chapter 13, page 452 for more discussion), which can lead to local precipitation of apatite on the basolateral aspect of the thin limb of the LOH.

hand, there may be other promoters present in this location, and thus if a nidus of calcium phosphate is formed, the likelihood of precipitate formation from supersaturated solutions would increase.

ABSORPTION OF NUTRIENTS IN THE INTESTINAL TRACT

- A challenge for the designer of the GI tract is to *prevent* water entry into the lumen of the intestine despite the large daily osmole load that is present in the lumen from digestion of dietary proteins and carbohydrates.
- Each day 3000 mmol of Na^+ are added to the lumen of the intestinal tract to absorb the 1500 mmol of dietary-derived glucose; this quantity of Na^+ is close to 150% of the entire content of Na^+ in the ECF compartment. In addition, amino acids must also be absorbed by a Na^+-linked process.
- A high concentration of Na^+ at the tip of the intestinal villus is required for this purpose.

One might ask, "Why use 2 Na^+ to absorb one glucose on SLGT when one Na^+ should suffice?" The downside in using 2 Na^+ per glucose is that more ATP molecules are hydrolyzed (two thirds instead of one third of an ATP per glucose absorbed). Therefore, there should be an advantage for the use of more Na^+ because this consumes more energy. To answer this question, focus on events in the tip of the villus of the small intestine (Fig. 4-11; *see margin note*).

Events in the tip of the villus

Consumption of one liter of fruit juice yields close to 750 mmol of glucose plus fructose when its carbohydrate load is hydrolyzed by the enzyme sucrase. This load of osmoles in the lumen of the small intestine creates a strong osmotic force (15,000 mm Hg) to draw water from the body (each mosmol exerts an osmotic pressure of ~20 mm Hg). A sudden shift of water into the intestinal lumen causes the P_{Na} to rise in the portal vein and shortly thereafter in arterial plasma. This rise in P_{Na} causes thirst, and a viscous cycle is created if one were to try to quench this thirst by drinking more fruit juice. Thus the question becomes, "How can the body avoid this unwanted shift of water?" There are several possible solutions, but the first two in Table 4-9 would cause more harm than good, so it is not surprising that they do not occur.

Strategy used: Raise the osmolality at the tip of the villus

By raising the osmolality at the tip of the villus in the small intestine, an osmotic difference that would favor the movement of water into the lumen is minimized. This is achieved because the hairpin loop of the capillaries of the villus functions as a countercurrent exchanger. The active absorption of Na^+ provides the single effect for countercurrent multiplication (see Fig. 4-11). One possible advantage of a stoichiometry of 2 Na^+/glucose is provided in the *margin note* next to Figure 4-11. With a finite permeability for Na^+ through tight junctions between intestinal cells, a high local interstitial Na^+ (and Cl^-) concentration

ABBREVIATION
SLGT1, the Na^+-linked glucose transporter in the small intestine

PHYSIOLOGIC ROLE OF THE STOICHIOMETRY OF SLGT1
- This transporter requires transport of 2 Na per glucose absorbed.
- When this transport occurs, more ATP is utilized; thus more ADP is formed.
- Since ADP is a glycolytic substrate, the rate of glycolysis is accelerated.
- When pyruvate is formed faster than the oxidation of pyruvate in mitochondria, more L-lactic acid is formed.
- The higher production of L-lactate helps the liver remove dietary K^+ and thereby prevents hyperkalemia after a meal (see Chapter 13, page 433 for more discussion).

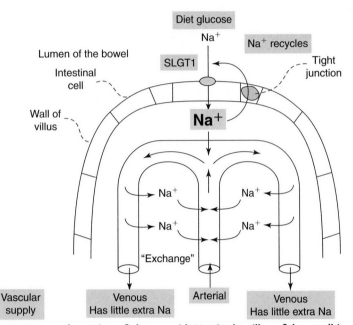

FIGURE 4-11 Absorption of glucose with Na⁺ in the villus of the small intestine. The major structure is an intestinal villus, which faces into the lumen of the intestine at the *top portion of the figure.* Sugar (glucose) from the diet diffuses into the unstirred layer outside cells at the tip of the villus, which has a high concentration of Na⁺. Two molecules of Na⁺ and one molecule of glucose are absorbed via the Na⁺-linked glucose transporter 1 (SLGT1). Most of the Na⁺ diffuses into the lumen through the tight junctions to drive the absorption of glucose. Some of the Na⁺ is absorbed and enters the subepithelial capillaries; this Na⁺ recycles by entering the central capillary, completing a countercurrent exchanger, which sustains the high concentration of Na⁺ at the tip of the villus as long as glucose is being absorbed (*see margin note*).

MOVEMENT OF WATER IN THE INTESTINAL TRACT

- Water is absorbed, driven by the osmotic pressure difference between the luminal fluid and the interstitial fluid in the tip of the villus.
- The goal is to prevent water entry into the lumen of the absorptive area of the small intestine driven by its large daily osmole load (~1500 mOsm of glucose and ~1000 mOsm of amino acids after digestion of dietary carbohydrate and proteins).
- A high osmolality in the tip of the villus prevents the secretion of an excessive quantity of water.

TABLE 4-9 **POTENTIAL STRATEGIES TO DEAL WITH THE OSMOLE LOAD IN INTESTINAL TRACT AFTER THE INGESTION OF FRUIT JUICE**

POTENTIAL STRATEGY	COMMENT
1. Absorb glucose very quickly	Could cause acute severe hyperglycemia and then, rebound hypoglycemia
2. Limit water permeability to avoid a shift of water into the intestinal tract	Problem occurs when water is needed in the body
3. Raise the osmolality at the tip of the villus	Should occur only when the lumen has a high glucose concentration

(~400 mmol/L) is generated when glucose is being absorbed. This creates a local osmolality of 800 mOsm/kg H_2O so there is no longer an osmotic driving force to draw water into the lumen of the intestine.

CHOLERA: FROM BACTERIA TO DISEASE

Recent discoveries have led to a better understanding of the pathophysiology of this disease.

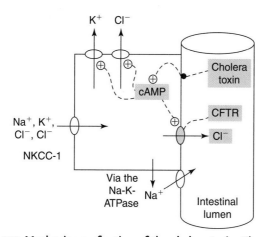

FIGURE 4-12 Mechanisms of action of the cholera toxin. The *cylindrical structure* represents the small intestine and *the rectangle to its left* represents a crypt cell. The cholera toxin binds irreversibly to the luminal membrane of this cell as illustrated by the *dashed line to the solid dot*, and as a result, more cyclic AMP (cAMP) is formed. This rise in cAMP leads to the insertion of a cystic fibrosis–related Cl⁻ ion channel (CFTR) in the luminal membrane, and the negative voltage in cells drives the secretion of Cl⁻. Na⁺ enter the lumen of the intestine between cells, drawn in by the luminal negative voltage. The source of Na⁺, K⁺, and Cl⁻ is via the Na⁺, K⁺, 2 Cl cotransporter type 1 (NKCC-1 cotransporter) on the basolateral side of the cell. The rise in cAMP also leads to the exit of K⁺ and Cl⁻ via their respective ion channels in the basolateral membrane of these cells, which leads to intracellular electrical and chemical balance (details are not provided in this figure).

ABBREVIATION
CFTR, cystic fibrosis transmembrane conductance regulator.

Source of cholera bacteria in nature

Cholera epidemics occur with a dramatic suddenness in certain parts of the world and then disappear, only to resurface in another region. There is a surprising source for cholera bacteria: ocean water. This insight helps explain why cholera appears in epidemics when there is a flood of ocean water in countries where drinking water is easily contaminated, whereas the disease virtually disappears at other times.

The ocean's salinity is not an impediment for the survival of cholera bacteria; in fact, a high NaCl concentration is a requirement for this bacterial species to survive (*see margin note*). There is also a strong direct correlation between the number of these bacteria and the warming of ocean water. There is an increased supply of bacteria when warm but not hot ocean water floods a region; hence, there is a seasonal feature to epidemics of cholera.

There is one more piece in this puzzle: the vector that delivers cholera bacteria to the human small intestine. There is a symbiosis between these bacteria and a family of oceanic zooplankton (*see margin note*). These copepods have a tough outer shell, which is an ideal location for cholera bacteria to live while in the ocean. At the appropriate time, these bacteria hydrolyze the outer shell of the zooplankton, releasing the ova of the host, and thus aiding their survival.

Reducing the incidence of cholera

There is now a simple way to diminish the cholera bacteria load, even where water purification methods are inadequate, because of knowledge about the natural history of the cholera bacteria described

CHOLERA BACTERIA AND NaCl
It is intriguing to think that the site of action of these bacteria in humans is in an environment where there is a high concentration of Na⁺ and Cl⁻ owing to Cl⁻-driven NaCl secretion using the CFTR Cl⁻ channel (Fig. 4-12).

DETECTING THE ZOOPLANKTON
By studying satellite images of the oceans, the abundance of zooplankton can be recognized by the characteristic color of the ocean. In addition, if the ocean water level is high, cholera bacteria in copepods can move up river deltas, contributing to epidemics. Therefore, public health workers can have advance warnings to minimize the hazards of cholera outbreaks.

previously. It may be potentially devastating to try to eradicate the cholera bacteria in the ocean because of its important role in the food chain. An old sari folded four times across the inlet of a drinking vessel, however, prevents most of the copepods (and their cholera bacteria) from entering the drinking container. This is sufficient to dramatically reduce the incidence of cholera infections, because the severity of the disease is "dose dependent" for cholera bacteria (*see margin note*).

BIOCHEMISTRY OF THE CHOLERA TOXIN

When cholera bacteria are ingested, they do *not* enter the circulation; they exert their harmful effects by releasing a toxin. The first step in this toxin action is to make an irreversible linkage with the exterior of small intestinal cells in the crypt area of the villus (see Fig. 4-12). This is accomplished by the five β-units of the toxin (akin to the ricin toxin and the strategy used by certain other bacterial toxins such as the shiga toxin that causes hemolytic-uremic syndrome). The two α-subunits of the toxin can now have a portion of their protein enter crypt cells of the small intestine. Once inside these cells, they catalyze the formation of the second messenger, cyclic AMP. Cyclic AMP activates protein kinase A, which ultimately leads to more open Cl^- channels in the luminal membrane; these Cl^- channels are the same ones that are defective in patients with cystic fibrosis. The net secretion of Cl^- is driven by the negative voltage in cells; it initiates the net secretion of NaCl because Na^+ can enter the lumen through the tight junctions between cells, which are permeable for Na^+. The source of secreted Na^+ and Cl^- is the Na^+, K^+, 2 Cl^- cotransporter on the basolateral membrane. For electrical balance, K^+ and Cl^- exit across their basolateral membrane through specific ion channels. This exit of K^+ is driven by the high K^+ concentration in cells because the rise in cAMP also permits these K^+ channels to have a higher open-probability (see Fig. 4-12). Conversely, the negative voltage drives the diffusion of Cl^- through their basolateral (and luminal) Cl^- channels.

DISCUSSION OF CASES

Both patients have metabolic acidosis of the normal $P_{Anion\ gap}$ type. After ensuring that the patients are at no immediate risk of a cardiac arrhythmia or a hemodynamic emergency, the first diagnostic step is to establish whether they have a low rate of excretion of NH_4^+ (see Flow Chart 4-1).

CASE 4-1: A MAN DIAGNOSED WITH TYPE IV RENAL TUBULAR ACIDOSIS

(Case presented on page 89)

What is the basis of the metabolic acidosis?

The measured U_{Osm} (700 mOsm/kg H_2O) is very close to the calculated U_{Osm} (720 mOsm/kg H_2O; *see margin note*); hence, his U_{NH4} is very low. The $U_{NH4}/U_{Creatinine}$ is close to 2, and thus the rate of excretion of NH_4^+ is very low. Because his GFR (creatinine clearance) is *not* very low, RTA is the correct diagnostic category.

What is the cause of the low rate of excretion of NH_4^+?

The urine pH of 5.0 suggests that the basis for the low rate of NH_4^+ excretion is a low availability of NH_3, probably owing to a low production of NH_4^+ in proximal convoluted tubule cells. The next step is to examine Table 4-7 to identify a possible cause for a low rate of NH_4^+ production. An alkaline proximal convoluted tubular cell pH due to a high P_K is the most likely basis for his low rate of NH_4^+ excretion; the pathophysiology of hyperkalemia is discussed in detail in Chapter 15, page 515). Because his metabolic acidosis resolved when hyperkalemia was corrected, a causal role for hyperkalemia is likely.

CASE 4-2: WHAT IS THIS WOMAN'S "BASIC" LESION?

(Case presented on page 89)

What is the basis of the metabolic acidosis?

Because her measured U_{Osm} (450 mOsm/kg H_2O) is very close to the calculated U_{Osm} (420 mOsm/kg H_2O), her U_{NH4} is low. In fact, her $U_{NH4}/U_{Creatinine}$ is close to 3, confirming that her NH_4^+ excretion rate is low. Because the GFR is *not* very low, she has RTA.

What is the cause of the low rate of excretion of NH_4^+?

Because the urine pH is 6.8 (see Table 4-8), the basis for the low rate of NH_4^+ excretion is a low *net* secretion of H^+ in the distal nephron. Because her rate of excretion of citrate is low (due to hypokalemia and acidemia), there is no evidence to suggest that she also has an alkaline pH in her proximal convoluted tubule cells.

After hypokalemia was corrected, the Pco_2 in alkaline urine was measured. It was 70 mm Hg; this suggests that there is no major defect in the H^+-ATPase or an alkaline pH in her distal tubule cells. Hence, either HCO_3^- was secreted or there was a backleak of H^+ in the distal nephron. The patient was not treated with amphotericin B, which may cause backleak of H^+ in the distal nephron. Because she suffers from Southeast Asian ovalocytosis, her lesion seems to be a problem with mistargeting of the Cl^-/HCO_3^- anion exchanger to the luminal membrane of the distal nephron. Because the P_{HCO3} remained in the normal range after the infusion of $NaHCO_3$, proximal RTA is ruled out.

DISCUSSION OF QUESTIONS

4-1 *How different are the rat and the human with respect to their rate of excretion of NH_4^+ per kg of body weight?*

The impression that the medullary shunt pathway for NH_3 plays a minor role in the excretion of NH_4^+ comes from data obtained by micropuncture of cortical nephron segments and microcatheter insertion into the medullary collecting duct of rats with high rates of excretion of NH_4^+ (see the discussion of Question 1-6, page 36 for more information). To extrapolate from these data in the rat in *quantitative* terms to humans, the question is, "How different are the rat and the human in their need for the excretion of NH_4^+?"

As shown in the following table, the rat has a large net daily alkali load and excretes very little NH_4^+, whereas the human has near-equal acid and alkali loads and the excretion of NH_4^+ plays a much more important role in daily acid-base balance. Therefore, it would not be a great surprise if the medullary shunt pathway for NH_3 is *quantitatively* much more important in the human for the excretion of NH_4^+ to maintain acid balance. If so, amputation of the medullary shunt pathway for NH_3 in humans could compromise the rate of excretion of NH_4^+ sufficiently to cause distal RTA.

SPECIES	EXCRETION OF NH_4^+	EXCRETION OF ORGANIC ANIONS	EXCRETION OF HCO_3^-
Rat	180 µEq/day	3600 µEq/day	Low
Human	40 mEq/day	40 mEq/day	Low

4-2 *Why is nephrocalcinosis so common in patients with antenatal Bartter's syndrome (a total defect in the reabsorption of NaCl and calcium in the medullary thick ascending limb of the loop of Henle)?*

Nephrocalcinosis is a condition in which precipitates of calcium salts accumulate in the renal outer medullary interstitial compartment for the most part. On the one hand, we would have expected less risk of nephrocalcinosis because there should be substantially less Ca^{2+} reabsorption in the loop of Henle in patients with antenatal Bartter's syndrome, as they have a defective NKCC-2 or ROMK. On the other hand, it appears that hypokalemia leading to medullary alkalinization, less water addition to the medullary interstitium due to lower medullary interstitial osmolality, and reduced urea recycling are likely to be important risk factors, as the incidence of nephrocalcinosis is high in this setting. These issues are discussed in more detail in the following list.

CONDITIONS ASSOCIATED WITH NEPHROCALCINOSIS
- There is an association between chronic hypokalemia and nephrocalcinosis.
- Examples include antenatal Bartter's syndrome, distal RTA where there is a defective H^+-ATPase, and animal models of metabolic alkalosis with a deficit of KCl.

1. If anions that can precipitate with ionized calcium are added to the interstitial compartment, this could increase the risk of nephrocalcinosis. In fact, the only anion with this property is carbonate, as there is no absorption of phosphate from nephron segments that traverse the medulla.

2. If the interstitial pH could rise appreciably, monovalent phosphate ($H_2PO_4^-$), which does not form a precipitate with ionized calcium, would be converted to divalent phosphate (HPO_4^{2-}), which may precipitate with Ca^{2+} to form $CaHPO_4$. Nevertheless, because the plasma and interstitial pH are close to 7.4, there can only be a small rise in the concentration of HPO_4^{2-} in the medullary interstitium (see Table 4-8). Notwithstanding, since chronic hypokalemia is virtually universally present in these patients (*see margin note*), they should have up-regulated the H^+/K^+ ATPase in their medullary collecting ducts, and thereby, there is an enhanced net addition of K^+ and HCO_3^- to the interstitial compartment (see Fig. 4-10, page 104). This could have an important effect on the likelihood of precipitating $CaCO_3$.

3. If much less water is reabsorbed from the medullary collecting duct, the concentrations of divalent phosphate and carbonate will be higher in this location. Furthermore, because these patients cannot raise the concentration of urea in the lumen of the inner medullary collecting duct owing to less water reabsorption from the late cortical distal nephron and the outer medullary collecting duct, there will be much less addition of water to this region and hence there will be a higher interstitial concentration of calcium.

Ketoacidosis

Introduction

KETOACIDS
Although acetoacetic acid,
β-hydroxybutyric acid, and acetone
are commonly called *ketoacids*, this
is technically incorrect for the
following reasons:
- β-hydroxybutyric acid is a
  hydroxyacid.
- Acetone is not an acid.
- Only acetoacetic acid is a ketoacid.

Before discussing the clinical aspects of diabetic ketoacidosis (DKA), we provide a synopsis of the metabolic background of ketoacidosis (*see margin note*). This information should allow the reader to understand the metabolic setting required for high rates of formation of ketoacids and what limits their rate of production. Notwithstanding, it is arguably more important to understand what controls the rate of removal of ketoacids because it is a diminished rate of removal of ketoacids that makes a modest degree of acidemia become a serious one. Therefore, we emphasize the *quantitative* aspects of the rates of production and removal of ketoacids.

COMMENT
While ketoacidosis is a form of metabolic acidosis due to added acids, it is discussed separately in this chapter because metabolic and biochemical issues are required to understand the clinical aspects of this disorder.

Once these principles and quantitative aspects are understood, the clinician should be able to deduce why ketoacidosis may develop, why an excessive amount of H^+ may accumulate, and where the emphasis should be placed in therapy.

OBJECTIVES

- To emphasize that an understanding of the principles of energy metabolism helps reveal the pathophysiology of ketoacidosis, when ketoacids will accumulate, and when this may lead to a medical emergency.
- To describe the biochemical basis, the clinical presentation, the threats to life that may be present on admission to the hospital, and the dangers to anticipate during therapy for patients with the two major clinical types of ketoacidosis, diabetic and alcoholic ketoacidosis.
- To describe some aspects of integrative physiology where ketoacids play a central role.

ABBREVIATIONS
β-HB, β-hydroxybutyrate
AcAc, acetoacetate

CASE 5-1: A MAN IS ANXIOUS TO KNOW WHY HE HAS KETOACIDOSIS

(Case discussed on page 152)

CONTENT OF SOFT DRINKS
Relevant to the pathophysiology of this case, the soft drinks the patient consumed contained a large quantity of glucose, fructose, and caffeine, but little Na^+ or K^+.

This is the fourth similar hospital admission for a 22-year-old man with mild cerebral palsy. Like the other episodes, this illness began with a "panic attack" that lasted for several days. During that period, he drank many liters of sweetened soft drinks on a daily basis (*see margin note for a clue*). He developed crampy lower abdominal pain that became prominent in the 24 hours prior to coming to the hospital. He denied the intake of alcohols (including methanol or ethylene glycol). He was normal between episodes, taking only medications for control of mild depression. He had no history suggestive of diabetes mellitus. On physical examination, there was an odor of acetone on his breath, but his effective arterial blood volume was not contracted. Arterial blood gas revealed a blood pH of 7.20, an arterial P_{CO_2} of 22 mm Hg, and a P_{HCO3} of 8 mmol/L. Of note, his plasma osmolal gap ($P_{Osmolal\ gap}$) was not elevated. The following additional laboratory data were obtained on admission:

Anion gap	mEq/L	26
Glucose	mg/dL (mmol/L)	92 (5)
K^+	mmol/L	4.2
Creatinine	mg/dL (μmol/L)	1.0 (88)
Albumin	g/dL (g/L)	4.1 (41)
β-HB	mmol/L	4.5
L-lactate	mmol/L	1.0
Osmolality	mOsm/kg H_2O	285

His initial in-hospital therapy consisted of 1 L of isotonic saline and 1 L of water containing 50 g of glucose (D_5W). Within 24 hours, all his laboratory values returned to the normal range. Later, the results of extra blood tests become available; hemoglobin A_1C level was not elevated (4.4%) and the plasma insulin level was in the normal range.

Questions

What makes DKA an unlikely diagnosis?

What makes alcoholic ketoacidosis an unlikely diagnosis?

What makes ketoacidosis due to starvation or hypoglycemia an unlikely diagnosis?

How may the patient's intake of sweetened soft drinks contribute to the development of ketoacidosis?

What other factors might have increased the degree of keto-acidosis?

Is ketoacidosis the only cause of metabolic acidosis in this patient?

PART A
BIOCHEMICAL BACKGROUND
METABOLIC PROCESS ANALYSIS

- A "metabolic process" consists of a series of metabolic pathways that carry out a specific function; its control can be deduced by examining its function.
- To determine the acid-base impact of a metabolic process, count the net valence of all of its substrates and all of its final products.

Metabolic processes often consist of more than one metabolic pathway, and these pathways usually exist in more than one organ. In the metabolic process involving ketoacids, there are segments in adipose tissue, liver, brain, and kidneys (Fig. 5-1); each of them is regulated, but control of the whole metabolic process is in keeping with its overall function.

The function of the metabolic process involving ketoacids is to supply the brain with a water-soluble, fat-derived fuel when its major fuel in the fed state, glucose, is in short supply. The blood-brain barrier limits the entry of free fatty acids into the brain; however, there is a transport system that allows ketoacids to enter the brain at a rapid rate.

An important element in the control of each metabolic process is to block all alternative pathways for the metabolism of its intermediates to ensure that the desired products are formed. Therefore, during ketoacid production, alternative pathways for metabolism of its substrate, free fatty acids, in the liver must be inhibited (i.e., oxidation and conversion to storage fat; see Fig. 5-1).

To determine the H^+ balance in a metabolic process, examine the net valences of *all* of its substrates and end products. H^+ are produced if the products of a metabolic process have a greater net anionic valence than its substrates; H^+ are removed if the products have a less net anionic valence than its substrates. In the metabolic process that involves ketoacids during prolonged fasting, there is

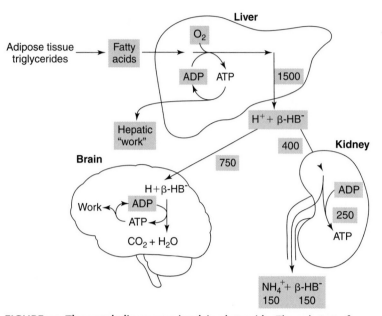

Liver

Brain

Kidney

TRIGLYCERIDES
- Triglycerides in adipose tissue are the major storage form of fat. Three fatty acids are each linked by an ester bond to one of the three OH groups of glycerol.

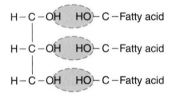

- Ester bonds form when the H and OH in the green shading are removed.

FIGURE 5-1 The metabolic process involving ketoacids. The substrate for this metabolic process is storage triglyceride in adipose tissue (*see margin note*). When the concentration of the usual brain fuel—glucose—is low in plasma, this provides a signal (low net actions of insulin) to cause the release of fatty acids from adipose tissue. The liver extracts many of these fatty acids and converts them to ketoacids when signals are present to block alternate metabolic pathways for their metabolism and when the other substrate in their metabolism, NAD^+ and/or ADP, is (are) present in adequate amounts. Ketoacid removal is restricted largely to the brain and the kidneys. The concentration of ketoacids in plasma does not vary if their rate of formation is equal to their rate of removal. Moreover, there is no net production or removal of H^+, because this metabolic process is electroneutral (the net valences of all substrates and products are equal). When ketoacid anions are excreted in the urine, H^+ balance is maintained if the cations excreted with the ketoacid anions are H^+ and/or NH_4^+.

no net production or removal of H^+ because the net valence of all substrates (triglycerides in adipose tissue) and products (CO_2 + H_2O) is equal. If this metabolic process does not proceed to completion, however, the rate of production of ketoacids exceeds their rate of removal and H^+ accumulate (see Fig. 5-1).

> **Clinical pearl**
> A large accumulation of ketoacids is usually due to a decreased rate of ketoacid removal rather than an increased rate of their production.

FUNCTION/CONTROL ANALYSIS

Hormonal signals

- The major physiologic function of the metabolic process involving ketoacids is to provide a water-soluble, fat-derived fuel for the brain when the concentration of its other fuel, glucose, is low in plasma.

When the diet contains glucose, signals are generated to prevent the production of ketoacids in the liver. The signal system centers on the stimulation of β-cells of the pancreas by glucose to release the hormone insulin. In contrast, during prolonged starvation, insulin is not released because of a low $P_{Glucose}$. This leads to the release of fatty acids from adipose tissue and the formation of ketoacids in the liver to provide the brain with a fuel that it *can* oxidize to regenerate a sufficient quantity of ATP to carry out its essential functions. Hence, it is not surprising that the central control factor in the metabolic process involving ketoacids is a relative lack of insulin (*see margin note*).

RELATIVE LACK OF INSULIN
This term describes the combination of low levels of insulin and high levels of the hormones that oppose the actions of insulin (e.g., glucagon, cortisol, adrenaline, and the pituitary hormones adrenocorticotropic hormone and growth hormone).

NAD⁺ and ADP as substrates

To understand this concept, one must think in terms of metabolic processes.

Metabolic process of glucose oxidation
- This metabolic process begins with work, which converts ATP to ADP plus inorganic phosphate. In glycolysis, ADP is the "essential" substrate because NADH is converted back to NAD⁺ when L-lactic acid is formed (*see margin note*).

Metabolic process of ketoacid formation and removal
- This metabolic process of ketoacid formation begins with the supply of fatty acids to the liver; NAD⁺ is a substrate for the oxidation of fatty acids and the formation of ketoacids.
- This hepatic pathway does not have an obligatory step to convert NADH back to NAD⁺. Hence ADP must be converted to ATP in mitochondria to convert NADH to NAD⁺. Therefore, ADP is also an indirect substrate of this metabolic process.
- For ketoacid removal, anything that decreases the rate of work in the brain and kidneys will diminish the availability of ADP, and hence lowers the rate of removal of ketoacids and thereby leads to a more severe degree of ketoacidosis.

NAD⁺ AND NADH
- These are cofactors in the removal of H and electrons during the oxidation of fuels (e.g., glucose or fatty acids).
- It is critical to recognize that NAD⁺ is a substrate for oxidation of fuels, which means that when NAD⁺ is not formed, oxidation of these fuels must stop.
- Chemistry:
  N, nicotinamide
  A, adenine
  D, dinucleotide
- For more information about the relationship between NAD⁺ and ADP, see page 146 in this chapter.

The availability of NAD⁺ and/or ADP, which in turn depends on the rate of utilization of ATP to perform work, can set an upper limit on rate of fuel oxidation (see Chapter 6, Figure 6-4, page 166, and *margin note*). During a state of relative insulin lack, the liver must regenerate a sufficient quantity of ADP to produce enough ketoacids for the brain and the kidneys to carry out their work. Nevertheless, as we discuss in Part D, the amount of hepatic work, the degree of uncoupling of oxidative phosphorylation, and ultimately the rate of hepatic blood flow (supply of oxygen to the liver) may limit the rate of ketoacid formation in DKA. Similarly, factors that affect the rate of oxygen consumption in the brain and kidney and hence the availability of ADP can modulate their rate of ketoacid removal.

ADP AND NAD⁺ ARE RELATED
- NAD⁺ and ADP are present in tiny amounts.
- When NAD⁺ is the cofactor for the oxidation of fuels, NADH is produced.
- When NADH is converted back to NAD⁺ in coupled respiration, ADP is consumed, thereby linking these two metabolites (this topic is discussed in more detail in Part D, page 146).

Hierarchy of fuel selection in a metabolic process

- Glucose is oxidized at an appreciable rate only when fatty acids and ketoacids are absent.
- Metabolic removal of glucose is very low in a patient with DKA until circulating fat-derived fuels are removed.

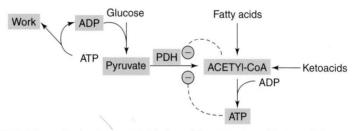

FIGURE 5-2 Fuel selection: Oxidation of fat prevents oxidation of glucose. Oxidation of fat-derived fuels inhibits oxidation of glucose because the products of the oxidation of fat-derived fuels inhibit pyruvate dehydrogenase (PDH). Key to this control is the availability of ADP, which is a substrate in both processes.

Fuels compete to be oxidized using the available quantity of ADP. When fat-derived fuels are present, they will have first priority to use the available ADP, which prevents the cell from oxidizing glucose. An important aspect of this control is exerted at the key crossroad in energy metabolism, the conversion of pyruvate—the last compound that can still be made back into glucose—into acetyl-CoA, a metabolic intermediate that *cannot* be made into glucose. This reaction is catalyzed by pyruvate dehydrogenase, an enzyme that is tightly regulated by the products of oxidation of fat-derived fuels (Fig. 5-2).

There is a lag period before ketoacids are produced at a rapid rate when there is a relative lack of insulin actions, although its underlying mechanism is not completely understood. Nevertheless, since oxidation of fat-derived fuels inhibits the oxidation of glucose, it would have been an error to have a high rate of production of ketoacids when carbohydrates are ingested because this leads to hyperglycemia and a glucose-induced osmotic diuresis.

PRODUCTION OF KETOACIDS IN THE LIVER

- The rate of consumption of O_2 in the liver sets an upper limit on the rate of ketogenesis (O_2 consumption includes coupled [the availability of ADP] and uncoupled respiration).
- Production of ketoacids requires that alternative pathways of acetyl-CoA removal be inhibited (e.g., inhibition of fatty acid synthesis at the acetyl-CoA carboxylase step).

The process of production of ketoacids in the liver can be divided into two major steps: first, the formation of acetyl-CoA; second, the conversion of acetyl-CoA to ketoacids.

Formation of acetyl-CoA in the liver

There are three different extrahepatic substrates and thus three different metabolic processes from which acetyl-CoA can be made rapidly enough in the liver to lead to an appreciable rate of formation of ketoacids (Fig. 5-3). Owing to the tight regulation of pyruvate dehydrogenase by acetyl-CoA, dietary fuels that can be converted to pyruvate are not important substrates for ketoacid formation.

The only important physiologic substrate for hepatic ketogenesis is free fatty acids derived from storage fat. During prolonged fasting, the function of this metabolic process is to produce a water-soluble,

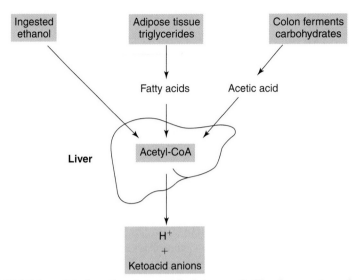

FIGURE 5-3 Extrahepatic substrates for ketogenesis. The three major substrates for the production of a large quantity of acetyl-CoA in the liver are long-chain fatty acids, ethanol, and acetic acid. The regulation of each of these metabolic pathways differs, however, as described in the text.

ETHANOL AS A SUBSTRATE FOR KETOGENESIS
- The function of ethanol metabolism in the liver is to remove the vast majority of ethanol produced during fermentation in the intestinal tract in a single pass. To achieve this aim, ketoacids must be the final product.
- Removing all of this ethanol avoids its effect to cause a disturbance in cerebral function.
- Ingested ethanol "takes advantage" of this biochemistry to produce a serious degree of ketoacidosis.

fat-derived brain fuel when the $P_{Glucose}$ is low; hence, the hormonal setting is a relative lack of insulin. In the patient with DKA, there is also a relative lack of insulin, but this is due to damage of β-cells of the pancreas. In either case, the relative lack of insulin provides the signal to activate the enzyme hormone-sensitive lipase, which catalyzes the release of free fatty acids from triglycerides in adipose tissues.

The second substrate for ketoacid formation is ethanol. This is not a physiologic pathway, because a very small quantity of ethanol is produced from fermentation in the colon in normal physiology, and it does not yield an appreciable rate of ketogenesis (*see margin note*). Nevertheless, the ingestion of ethanol may provide enough substrate for an appreciable rate of ketogenesis when there is a relative lack of insulin.

The substrate for the third metabolic process in which ketoacids are formed is a group of short-chain organic acids—the most abundant one is acetic acid. These compounds are produced during the fermentation of poorly absorbed carbohydrates (fiber and fructose) by bacteria in the colon. A large quantity of these short-chain organic acids are produced, released into the portal vein, and delivered to the liver each day.

In the metabolic process where ketoacids are formed from storage fat and/or ethanol, the maximum rate is set by the rate of consumption of oxygen in hepatocytes (see Part D, page 145, for further discussion of this topic).

The metabolic fates of acetyl-CoA

To have a metabolic process that results in the formation of ketoacids in the liver, the most important issue for regulation is to inhibit the removal of acetyl-CoA by the two major alternative pathways for its metabolism: first, the oxidation of acetyl-CoA to produce ATP (and CO_2), and second, the conversion of acetyl-CoA to long-chain fatty acids (Fig. 5-4).

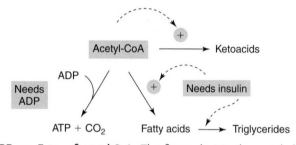

FIGURE 5-4 Fates of acetyl-CoA. The figure depicts the metabolism of acetyl-CoA in a liver cell in an oversimplified form. When the concentration of acetyl-CoA rises, this cannot "force" liver cells to burn it to make more ATP, largely because there is not enough ADP. The other major fate of acetyl-CoA is conversion into fatty acids, but this occurs only when net insulin actions are high. Accordingly, in states with a relative lack of insulin, ketoacids are formed, driven by the high concentration of acetyl-CoA and a limited rate of generation of ADP that prevents acetyl-CoA oxidation.

Inhibition of the oxidation of acetyl-CoA in the tricarboxylic acid cycle

This oxidation pathway is limited by the rate of generation of ADP during the performance of hepatic work (biosynthesis, ion pumping).

Inhibition of the conversion of acetyl-CoA to long-chain fatty acids

The other metabolic fate of acetyl-CoA is its conversion to fatty acids. Fatty acid synthesis is controlled by insulin, which activates the first committed enzyme involved in the conversion of acetyl-CoA to fatty acids (acetyl-CoA carboxylase; Fig. 5-5). Fatty acid synthesis is inhibited under conditions of relative lack of insulin; it can also be inhibited if there are high levels of β-adrenergic hormones.

Conversion of acetyl-CoA to ketoacids

When the oxidation of acetyl-CoA and fatty acid synthesis are inhibited, acetyl-CoA is converted to ketoacids (see Fig. 5-4). In this setting, the maximum possible rate of ketogenesis may be set by availability of ADP (hepatic work). This limitation can be overcome by uncoupling of oxidative phosphorylation (*see margin note*). In this setting, the maximum possible rate of ketogenesis is set by availability of the substrates, fatty acids, and oxygen.

NEED FOR UNCOUPLED RESPIRATION TO AUGMENT KETOGENESIS

- As discussed on pages 143 and 146 in Part D, the amount of ADP formed during the performance of hepatic work is insufficient to permit the observed rates of ketoacid formation (~1 mmol/min). Hence, there is a need for a degree of uncoupling of oxidative phosphorylation.
- The degree of uncoupling, however, must be modest to avoid the dangers of inducing a very rapid rate of glycolysis and thereby L-lactic acidosis owing to a much higher concentration of ADP.

AN UNCONVENTIONAL FORM OF UNCOUPLING

- In uncoupling of oxidative phosphorylation, NADH is converted to NAD+ *without* causing the conversion of ADP to ATP.
- When acetoacetate (AcAc) is converted to β-hydroxybutyrate (β-HB), NADH is converted to NAD+. This has the same net effect as uncoupling except that it does not need direct consumption of O_2. The NAD+ formed will permit the oxidation of more fatty acids and thereby the production of more AcAc and NADH, which increases the total production of ketoacids.

AcAc + NADH → β-HB + NAD+

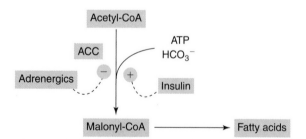

FIGURE 5-5 Acetyl-CoA carboxylase (ACC) in the liver. The *long vertical arrow* represents the enzyme, acetyl-CoA carboxylase. This enzyme is activated by insulin and inhibited by β-adrenergics, which operate by different mechanisms. High β-adrenergic activity may play an important role in the pathogenesis of alcoholic ketoacidosis.

REMOVAL OF KETOACIDS

There are two major sites of ketoacid oxidation, the brain and the kidneys. It is equally important that other organs with a high rate of oxygen consumption (e.g., skeletal muscle) are prevented from oxidizing ketoacids during prolonged fasting to ensure an adequate quantity of fuel for the brain. Nevertheless, the detailed mechanisms involved are still not perfectly clear to the authors.

Oxidation of ketoacids in the brain

The brain can oxidize close to 750 mmol of ketoacids per day, almost half the quantity of ketoacids that is produced when ketogenesis is most rapid (see Fig. 5-1). The brain oxidizes ketoacids preferentially if their levels are high, because the products of their metabolism (NADH, acetyl-CoA) inhibit pyruvate dehydrogenase (see Fig. 5-2). If the rate of generation of ADP declines in the brain because of less biologic work (e.g., owing to coma, intake of sedatives including ethanol, effect of anesthesia), fewer ketoacids can be oxidized, and the degree of acidemia becomes more severe.

Removal of ketoacids by the kidney

The kidneys remove close to 400 mmol of ketoacids per day. If renal work (largely the reabsorption of Na^+) is at its usual rate, the kidneys oxidize close to 250 mmol of ketoacids per day. Because more ketoacids are filtered than reabsorbed, close to 150 mmol of ketoacid anions are excreted daily during the ketoacidosis of prolonged fasting. Because virtually all of these anions are excreted along with NH_4^+ (major) and H^+ (minor) during prolonged fasting, acid-base balance is maintained (Fig. 5-6, lower portion).

In DKA, the filtered load of Na^+ declines (owing to a low GFR secondary to loss of Na^+ in the glucose-induced osmotic diuresis). Accordingly, renal removal of β-HB^- and H^+ declines because the rates of NH_4^+ excretion and β-HB^- oxidation are both reduced. From an energy point of view, oxidation of β-HB^- or glutamine is equivalent in terms of ADP utilization.

Ketoacid oxidation in other organs

The intestinal tract oxidizes ketoacids when it performs work. If digestion and absorption are proceeding at a usual rate, the intestinal tract oxidizes 200 to 300 mmol of ketoacids per day. Notwithstanding, intestinal work is extremely low during prolonged fasting and in most patients with DKA. Skeletal muscle does not oxidize an appreciable quantity of ketoacids when fatty acid levels are high.

Production of acetone from ketoacids

When the level of acetoacetic acid is high, this ketoacid is converted to acetone and CO_2 in a reaction that does not require enzyme actions (Fig. 5-7). To have high levels of acetoacetic acid, both a high level of total ketoacids and a low level of NADH are required.

BASIS FOR THE METABOLIC ACIDOSIS

- In the early stage, there is a small rise in the concentration of β-HB in the ECF and therefore no large increase in $P_{Anion\ gap}$.
- In the later stage, there is a steady-state high concentration of β-HB in plasma and a large excretion of β-HB plus NH_4^+ in the urine.

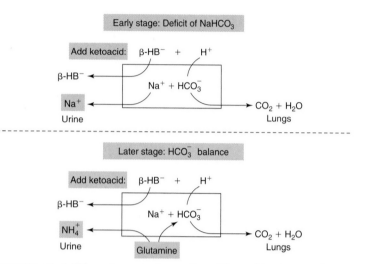

FIGURE 5-6 Acid-base impact of excretion of ketoacid anions early and later during prolonged fasting. The liver produces H^+ with β-HB⁻ (*top line*). H^+ are removed after reacting with HCO_3^- to form $CO_2 + H_2O$; the result is a deficit of HCO_3^- and a gain of β-HB⁻ anions in the extracellular fluid compartment (*central rectangle*). Early in ketoacidosis, the kidneys have not yet increased their rate of excretion of NH_4^+; hence, β-HB⁻ anions are excreted with Na^+ (*upper portion*), and a deficit of HCO_3^- develops (i.e., metabolic acidosis develops). When the rate of production of NH_4^+ and HCO_3^- by the kidney rises (*lower portion*), NH_4^+ and β-HB⁻ are excreted in the urine while HCO_3^- are added to the body to remove the H^+ that were produced. Hence, there is a nil balance for the sum of H^+ and HCO_3^-.

Clinical messages

1. The ultimate fate of the ketoacid anions (oxidation or excretion in the urine) determines the acid-base impact of this metabolic process.
2. If the rate of fuel oxidation declines in either of the two major organs involved in the metabolic removal of ketoacids (the brain and the kidneys), a more serious degree of acidemia may develop.
3. H^+ also accumulates if ketoacid anions are excreted in the urine with a cation other than NH_4^+ (or H^+; see Fig. 5-6).

NADH AND KETOACID FORMATION

When the NADH:NAD^+ ratio is elevated (a high NADH:NAD^+ is usually present when the supply of oxygen is very low or when ethanol is oxidized), acetone formation declines, its odor in exhaled air may not be detected at the bedside, and there may be a false-negative nitroprusside test (this bedside test detects acetoacetate and acetone, but not β-HB).

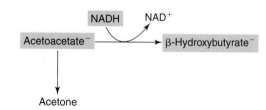

FIGURE 5-7 Conversion of acetoacetic acid to acetone or β-hydroxybutyric acid. There are two major fates for acetoacetic acid when its concentration is high. First, this ketoacid can be converted to acetone by a mechanism that does not depend on enzyme actions. Second, acetoacetic acid can be converted to β-hydroxybutyric acid when the NADH:NAD^+ ratio is high; this removes NADH and generates NAD^+ (*see margin note*).

(Discussions on pages 156 and 157)

5-1 *How many extra H^+ would be added to the body in 24 hours in a 70-kg patient with DKA if that patient had a 25% reduction in the rate of oxygen consumption in the brain (e.g., due to sedation or development of a decreased level of consciousness)?*

5-2 *What are the risks and benefits of excreting ketoacid anions plus NH_4^+ in the urine during prolonged fasting?*

5-3 *If dialysate fluids contain acetate as the source of alkali, acetate anions are converted to β-hydroxybutyric acid. Does this process alter the balance of H^+?*

CLINICAL ASPECTS OF KETOACIDOSIS

The differential diagnosis of ketoacidosis is listed in Table 5-1. The causes of a relative deficiency of insulin are listed in Table 5-2—two groups are evident, those with normal β-cells of the pancreas that either lack a stimulus or are inhibited and those with damage to these beta cells (diabetes mellitus). Diabetic and alcoholic ketoacidosis are discussed in detail in the next two sections.

TABLE 5-1 **CAUSES OF KETOACIDOSIS**

TYPES	SPECIAL FEATURES	DANGERS
Diabetic ketoacidosis	Common in children with type 1 DM; uncommon in type 2 DM. Low EABV, very high $P_{Glucose}$. P_K ~ 5.5 mmol/L, K^+-depleted	Cerebral edema in children. Cardiac arrhythmia. Initially hyperkalemia; then hypokalemia >2 hours after insulin given. Neuroglucopenia ~6 hours after insulin given
Alcoholic ketoacidosis	Alcohol binge, some have low EABV, prominent gastrointestinal complaints; $P_{Glucose}$ not very high, P_{HCO_3} not very low	K^+ depletion might be large. In a chronic alcoholic, possible thiamin deficiency
Hypoglycemic ketoacidosis including starvation	$P_{Glucose}$ < 3 mmol/L (54 mg/dL). Past or family history might be positive; look for drugs that inhibit glucose production or fatty acid oxidation	Give enough glucose to raise $P_{Glucose}$ to 5 mmol/L (90 mg/dL). Seek basis of an underlying disorder
Other type of ketoacidosis	Fermentation of poorly absorbed carbohydrate plus inhibition of acetyl-CoA carboxylase	Usually there are no dangers once intake of poorly absorbed carbohydrate is discontinued

DM, diabetes mellitus; EABV, effective arterial blood volumes; $P_{Glucose}$, concentration of glucose in plasma.

TABLE 5-2 **CAUSES OF RELATIVE LACK OF INSULIN**

With normal β-cells

- Lack of stimulators for β-cells (e.g., low $P_{Glucose}$)
- Inhibitors of insulin release (e.g., high α-adrenergics)
- Hormones that oppose the actions of insulin (e.g., glucagon, α-adrenergics, cortisol, growth hormone, thyroid hormone)

With abnormal β-cells

- Damage or destruction of pancreatic islets (e.g., type 1 diabetes mellitus, pancreatitis, hemochromatosis)

PART B
DIABETIC KETOACIDOSIS

- DKA develops when there is a lack of actions of insulin. Nevertheless, the pathophysiology is not that simple.
- The major medical emergency in children with DKA is cerebral edema; this complication may be the result of less than optimal current recommendations for treatment in these patients.

CASE 5-2: HYPERGLYCEMIA AND ACIDOSIS

(Case discussed on page 154)

Andy, age 14, weighs 50 kg; he has been feeling well until he had the "flu" 2 weeks ago. During this period, his urine output increased markedly, and he felt thirsty; he drank a large volume of fruit juice. He had a 4-kg weight loss. This morning, he was confused and difficult to rouse, and he was brought to the hospital. On physical examination, respirations were rapid and deep, the odor of acetone was detected on his breath, and his effective arterial blood volume was very contracted. On laboratory examination, he had metabolic acidosis with a high value for the anion gap in plasma ($P_{Anion\ gap}$), a strongly positive serum test for ketone bodies, and a hematocrit of 0.60, and the concentration of glucose in his urine was 300 mmol/L. Other values in blood are provided below.

PLASMA				PLASMA		
pH		7.25		HCO_3^-	mmol/L	10
Arterial P_{CO_2}	mm Hg	25		Venous P_{CO_2}	mm Hg	50
Glucose	mg/dL	900		Glucose	mmol/L	50
Creatinine	mg/dL	2.8		Creatinine	μmol/L	250
BUN	mg/dL	56		Urea	mmol/L	20
Na^+	mmol/L	130		K^+	mmol/L	5.5
Cl^-	mmol/L	93		Anion gap	mEq/L	27

Questions

Are there any other tests that you need to obtain to confirm the diagnosis of DKA?

What are the major threats to Andy's life?

How does his depressed sensorium contribute to the degree of ketoacidosis?

Should the physician administer $NaHCO_3$?

DIAGNOSIS OF DIABETIC KETOACIDOSIS

DIABETES MELLITUS
- Type 1 diabetes mellitus is the form that occurs most commonly in young patients. These patients are prone to develop DKA.
- Type 2 diabetes mellitus is the form that is most common in older, obese patients. DKA is rare in these patients.

Although DKA occurs most often in patients with previously diagnosed type 1 diabetes mellitus (often with a precipitating event), it may be the initial mode of presentation in young patients with this disorder. The most important parameters that indicate that the likely diagnosis is DKA are a typical history of polyuria and polydipsia, the presence of a low effective arterial blood volume, rapid and deep respirations, an odor of acetone on the breath, together with hyper-glycemia, metabolic acidosis with a high value for the $P_{Anion\ gap}$, and a strongly positive test for ketones in serum and in urine.

Hormonal basis

Failure of a patient with known type 1 diabetes mellitus to take insulin is a common reason for the development of DKA. An associated stress due to an illness can lead to elevated concentrations of hormones with actions that oppose those of insulin (e.g., adrenaline and glucocorticoids).

Consequences of hyperglycemia

The major complaints are polyuria (secondary to the glucose-induced osmotic diuresis) and thirst (owing to the effective arterial blood volume contraction), fatigue, and malaise. Catabolism of lean body mass contributes to the excessive weight loss (*see margin note*). The severity of hyperglycemia is influenced mainly by the degree of contraction of the effective arterial blood volume and the resultant low glomerular filtration rate (GFR) because this decreases the excretion of glucose (see Chapter 16, page 553). Other factors that can influence the $P_{Glucose}$ are the quantity of glucose ingested (usually in the form of fruit juice and sweetened soft drinks to quench thirst) and the rate of stomach emptying (see Chapter 16, page 562).

WEIGHT LOSS IN PATIENTS WITH DIABETIC KETOACIDOSIS
Some clinicians rely on weight loss to indicate the degree of contraction of the extracellular fluid volume. Nevertheless, there are usually confounding issues such as the degree of catabolism and the volume of fluid retained in the lumen of the gastrointestinal tract.

Signs associated with ketoacidosis

The major signs are a contracted effective arterial blood volume owing to the excretion of ketoacid anions with Na^+, the smell of acetone on the breath, and an extreme degree of hyperventilation (Kussmaul respirations; *see margin note*).

KUSSMAUL RESPIRATIONS
This is deep and rapid breathing owing to stimulation of the respiratory center by acidemia. The pH should be low in the area of the respiratory center because of high brain venous Pco_2 owing to a very contracted effective arterial blood volume and thereby a low cerebral blood flow rate as autoregulation of cerebral blood flow fails.

Precipitating factors

The most common precipitating factor is an underlying infection (usually gastroenteritis, pneumonia, or a urinary tract infection). Nevertheless, the patient may not be febrile because hypothermia is frequently present in a patient with a severe degree of DKA. In the adult patient with DKA, precipitating factors also include myocardial infarction, stroke, trauma, pancreatitis, alcohol abuse, and the intake of drugs (e.g., corticosteroids).

Symptoms related to specific organs

The most important symptoms are those related to dysfunction of the central nervous system. As DKA becomes more severe, confusion and even coma may develop. Other common symptoms include blurring of vision, nausea, and vomiting. Abdominal pain with a picture that mimics an "acute abdomen" may be present.

Natural history

The patient who stops taking insulin does not feel well for a period of days to weeks, but the symptoms lack specificity at that time. The actual symptoms attributable to DKA develop very slowly with a lag time of many days. The onset may be more rapid, however, in settings with high levels of hormones with actions that oppose those of insulin

EXCRETION OF Na$^+$ PLUS KETOACID ANIONS

When ketoacids are formed, there is a net addition of H$^+$ to the body. If these ketoacid anions are excreted with NH$_4^+$, there is an addition of HCO$_3^-$ to the body. In contrast, if they are excreted with Na$^+$ or K$^+$, there is no addition of HCO$_3^-$ and therefore more severe acidemia.

EFFECT OF A LOW GFR

- *NH$_4^+$ production*: When the GFR falls, fewer Na$^+$ are filtered. Therefore, there is less renal work (ADP formation). This diminishes the availability of ADP during chronic metabolic acidosis, which means that less glutamine can be converted to NH$_4^+$, which is excreted, and HCO$_3^-$, which is added to renal venous blood.
- *Ketoacid anion excretion*: Ketoacid anion excretion is equal to the filtered ketoacid anions minus the reabsorption of these anions. Hence, when the GFR falls appreciably, there is a much lower filtered load of ketoacid anions and thereby a lower rate of excretion of these anions because the reabsorption of these anions is relatively small and it does not change appreciably during DKA.
- *Overall*: While both NH$_4^+$ and ketoacid anion excretion rates fall, they are still excreted in a 1:1 stoichiometry. Hence, their excretion rates will not contribute to acidemia unless:
  - There is another lesion present that results is an even lower rate of excretion of NH$_4^+$.
  - The body fails to oxidize the extra ketoacid anions + H$^+$ to CO$_2$ + water, and/or there is an increased rate of production of ketoacids.

CORRECTION OF THE P$_{Na}$ FOR THE P$_{Glucose}$

- Calculations that attempt to adjust the P$_{Na}$ for a change in the P$_{Glucose}$ are based on the assumption that glucose was added to the ECF compartment with little water, which causes a rise in the P$_{Effective Osm}$ and thereby a shift of water from the intracellular fluid (ICF) to the ECF compartment
- Because the addition of glucose is virtually always accompanied by the addition of an unknown volume of water, these "correction factors" are not correct. Hence, they should not be performed.

and/or the consumption of ethanol. When hyperglycemia and acidemia become prominent, a vicious cycle develops. As the patient starts to become confused, cerebral metabolism of ketoacids declines, and the degree of ketoacidosis suddenly becomes more severe. As the GFR also declines, renal work is reduced as a result of a low filtered load of Na$^+$, and this also contributes to the development of a more severe degree of acidemia because the rate of ketoacid oxidation by the kidney is diminished and fewer ketoacid anions are excreted with NH$_4^+$ (*see margin note*).

Changes in body composition owing to the osmotic diuresis

Sodium

> - The magnitude of the deficit of Na$^+$ depends on the number of liters of osmotic diuresis. This, in turn, depends on the quantity of glucose ingested for the most part (see Chapter 16, page 557 for a discussion of the role of ingestion of fruit juice on the P$_{Glucose}$ and the effective arterial blood volume).

A major feature of DKA is a significant degree of contraction of the effective arterial blood volume, which may dominate the clinical picture. Deficits of Na$^+$ are said to be 5 to 10 mmol Na$^+$/kg body weight unless renal failure is present (Table 5-3). The site of Na$^+$ loss is in the urine as there is an osmotic diuresis with a concentration of Na$^+$ in the urine that is often 40 to 50 mmol/L in this setting. In fact, the reason for this deficit of Na$^+$ is that this natriuresis largely exceeds the usual intake of Na$^+$.

It is important to have a quantitative estimate of the Na$^+$ deficit in each *individual* patient with DKA. This deficit of Na$^+$ can be calculated once one has a quantitative estimate of the ECF volume using the change in the hematocrit. Those patients who consume much more sugar (i.e., fruit juice or sweetened soda to quench thirst) will have a much greater deficit of Na$^+$ in their ECF compartment because of a larger osmotic diuresis. If a hemodynamic emergency is not present, it is important to avoid overzealous administration of saline even in the presence of a large deficit of NaCl, as this is a risk factor for the development of cerebral edema in children.

The P$_{Na}$ is the ratio of Na$^+$ to H$_2$O in the ECF compartment (*see margin note*). Although patients with DKA may have hyponatremia,

TABLE 5-3 TYPICAL DEFICITS IN A PATIENT WITH DIABETIC KETOACIDOSIS

	DEFICIT	COMMENT	DANGER
Na$^+$	5–10 mmol/kg	Restore quickly *only* if a hemodynamic emergency.	Rapid expansion of the ECF volume, which may induce cerebral edema in children
K$^+$	5–10 mmol/kg	K$^+$ will shift into cells when insulin acts.	Hyperkalemia on admission Hypokalemia > 1–2 hours after therapy
H$_2$O	Many liters	Do not administer hypotonic saline.	A large fall in P$_{Effective osm}$ may cause cerebral edema
HCO$_3^-$	Can be variable	Give NaHCO$_3$ only if the P$_{HCO3}$ and pH are *very* low.	Strong opinions, but data are lacking

ECF, extracellular fluid.

their P_{Osm} is usually high because of the hyperglycemia. Hyponatremia may be present in a patient with DKA for four major reasons:

1. *Deficit of Na+*: Na^+ is lost in the urine primarily owing to the glucose-induced osmotic diuresis and, to a lesser degree, the excretion of Na^+ with ketoacid anions early in the course of DKA.

2. *Gain of water*: Because of thirst, there is a large water intake in a patient with stimuli for the release of vasopressin and hence a diminished excretion of water (e.g., a very low effective arterial blood volume, pain, nausea, anxiety). Although the concentration of Na^+ in the urine is relatively low (~40 to 50 mmol/L) during the glucose-induced osmotic diuresis, hyponatremia develops because of the large intake of fluids with low salt content.

3. *Shift of water from cells to the ECF compartment*: Adding hypertonic glucose causes water to shift into the ECF compartment from cells that require insulin for glucose transport (*see margin note on page 555*; see also Chapter 16, page 556). Nevertheless, one cannot know whether ingested sugar will result in a hyperosmolar load, because the volume of water that was ingested is unknown.

4. *Laboratory error*: This is secondary to hyperlipidemia if the technique used to measure the P_{Na} requires dilution of plasma (see Chapter 10, page 317).

Potassium: Changes in the P_K and total body K^+

- The P_K is usually close to 5.5 mmol/L in most patients with DKA prior to therapy despite the fact that there is a large overall total body deficit of K^+ due to renal K^+ loss.

Hyperkalemia is due to insulin deficiency, which causes K^+ to shift out of cells; the degree of hyperkalemia may be more severe if there is excessive tissue catabolism (*see margin note*), a large K^+ intake (e.g., consumption of large amount of fruit juice), and/or a lower rate of excretion of K^+.

Some patients may have a P_K that is in the normal range, whereas others may be hypokalemic if they have had large prior losses of K^+ (vomiting or a prolonged osmotic diuresis with high rate of secretion of K^+ in the cortical collecting duct; *see margin note*) and/or a low intake of fruit juice (which contains close to 50 mmol/L of K^+). These patients are at risk for developing a more severe degree of hypokalemia and cardiac arrhythmia during therapy with the administration of insulin or $NaHCO_3$.

Creatinine and urea

Both are elevated in plasma, primarily reflecting the low GFR (*see margin note*).

Laboratory findings in a patient with diabetic ketoacidosis

- The diagnosis of DKA is usually not a difficult one; it should be ruled out in all patients with metabolic acidosis and an increase in the $P_{Anion\ gap}$.

K+ EXCRETION IN DIABETIC KETOACIDOSIS
- On admission, a patient with diabetes in poor control has a compromised ability to excrete K^+ even though aldosterone is present and there is sufficient delivery of Na^+ to the distal nephron.
- Within 1 to 2 hours after the administration of insulin, K^+ shifts into cells, and the P_K falls by close to 1 mmol/L.
- We observed in some patients that if insulin is administered intravenously for a protracted period of time, there is a further fall in the P_K even if K^+ is being administered, because there is now a very high K^+ excretion rate (~30 to 40 mmol K^+/mmol of creatinine). This may reflect the fact that actions of insulin on the cortical collecting duct have similar effects to aldosterone (see Chapter 13, page 555 for more discussion).

UREA PRODUCTION IN A PATIENT WITH DIABETIC KETOACIDOSIS
Although there is tissue catabolism in DKA, the rate of production of urea may not be substantially increased if the intake of protein is decreased.

METHODS TO MEASURE CREATININE AND THEIR PITFALLS
- Some enzyme-based assays may yield lower values for creatinine when hyperglycemia is present.
- The picric acid method may yield higher values for creatinine in presence of acetoacetate.

Typical findings in the patient with DKA include hyperglycemia, glucosuria, metabolic acidosis with an increase in the $P_{Anion\ gap}$, an elevated hematocrit (*see margin note*), and a strongly positive qualitative test for acetoacetate in serum. The diagnosis of DKA can be confirmed by measuring the concentration of β-hydroxybutyrate and acetoacetate in blood.

Cautions in the laboratory diagnosis of diabetic ketoacidosis

β-Hydroxybutyric acidosis but little acetoacetic acidosis

• If hyperglycemia and glycosuria are present with only a moderate degree of ketonemia in a patient with DKA, suspect coexistent ketoacidosis and L-lactic acidosis possibly owing to the ingestion of ethanol (*see margin note*).

β-Hydroxybutyrate$^-$ and acetoacetate$^-$ are in equilibrium because of the high activity of the enzyme β-hydroxybutyrate dehydrogenase in mitochondria. If NADH has accumulated in mitochondria (e.g., during alcohol metabolism), the equilibrium of this equation is displaced to the right and the concentration of acetoacetate$^-$ falls (see Fig. 5-7). Because the quick screening test for ketoacids (nitroprusside reaction) detects only acetoacetate$^-$ and acetone, it may be only weakly positive; thus, the degree of ketoacidosis may be underestimated in this setting. Enzymatic determinations for β-HB and L-lactate anions in plasma, the presence of a large increase in the $P_{Osmolal\ gap}$, and the measurement of ethanol in blood confirm the diagnosis.

$P_{Anion\ gap}$ that is not sufficiently increased

• The rise in the $P_{Anion\ gap}$ may be lower than expected for the drop in P_{HCO3} in a patient with DKA; the likely causes are a low $P_{Albumin}$ or a large degree of loss of ketoacid anions in the urine with Na$^+$ or K$^+$.

Hypoalbuminemia. This problem is avoided by adjusting the $P_{Anion\ gap}$ for the $P_{Albumin}$. As a rough approximation, the baseline $P_{Anion\ gap}$ (16 mEq/L, including the P_K) is lower by 4 mEq/L for every 1.0-g/dL (10-g/L) decrease in the $P_{Albumin}$.

Indirect loss of NaHCO₃ (see Chapter 4, page 84)

• When the content of HCO_3^- in the ECF compartment is calculated, there is evidence of both a gain of acids *and* an indirect loss of NaHCO₃ in most patients with DKA.

This loss is quite difficult to recognize because the fall in the P_{HCO3} may be equal to the rise in the $P_{Anion\ gap}$ in many patients with DKA on admission (Table 5-4). Nevertheless, this loss of NaHCO₃ can be identified if one has a quantitative estimate of the degree of contraction of the ECF volume on presentation (i.e., use the hematocrit). As shown in the far right column of Table 5-4, the decline in the content of HCO_3^- in the ECF compartment is 75 mmol greater than

TABLE 5-4 **CHANGES IN THE P$_{HCO_3}$ AND P$_{β-HB}$ AND THEIR CONTENT IN DIABETIC KETOACIDOSIS**

Examine the concentrations and contents of HCO_3^- and β-HB$^-$ in the ECF compartment during DKA and after successful therapy with insulin plus saline. The numbers that merit special emphasis before therapy are the contracted ECF (12 L vs. 15 L) *and* the diminished HCO_3^- + β-HB$^-$ content in the ECF compartment (75 mmol) during DKA. After therapy, the HCO_3^- + β-HB$^-$ content has remained unchanged, but the P$_{HCO_3}$ rises only to 18 mmol/L, even after conversion of all the β-HB$^-$ to HCO_3^-. For simplicity, in this example we ignored the ongoing loss of β-HB$^-$ in urine. Moreover, we assumed that β-HB$^-$ represents all the ketoacid anions and its concentration is equal to most of the rise in the P$_{Anion\ gap}$ (ignoring the component of the rise in P$_{Anion\ gap}$ due to a higher P$_{Albumin}$).

CONDITION	ECF VOLUME (L)	HCO$_3^-$ (mmol/L)	HCO$_3^-$ (mmol)	β-HB$^-$ (mmol/L)	β-HB$^-$ (mmol)	HCO$_3^-$ + β-HB$^-$ (mmol)
Normal	15	25	375	0.05	<1	375
DKA	12	10	120	15	180	300
Difference	−3	−15	−255	+15	+180	−75

DKA, diabetic ketoacidosis; ECF, extracellular fluid.

the rise in ketoacid anions in this example. Other evidence to support this interpretation is that when isotonic saline is infused without NaHCO$_3$ and the ECF volume is reexpanded, the rise in P$_{HCO_3}$ is always smaller than expected from the prior rise in the P$_{Anion\ gap}$, and the patient now has a P$_{HCO_3}$ that is about 18 mmol/L.

The next objective is to examine the mechanism responsible for the indirect loss of NaHCO$_3$ (i.e., the concentrations of Na$^+$ plus K$^+$ exceed that of Cl$^-$ in the urine). Because the urine pH is close to 6.0 at this time, it contains little HCO$_3^-$. Accordingly there is a net loss of Na$^+$ plus K$^+$ and ketoacid anions, an excretion that leads to a fall in the P$_{HCO_3}$ without an increase in the P$_{Anion\ gap}$. In patients who have a smaller decline in their effective arterial blood volume, the GFR is only minimally decreased. As a result, the filtered load of ketoacids is high, and because there is not a sufficient capacity to reabsorb the entire filtered load of these anions, more are excreted and this may result in a severe degree of acidemia with only a modest rise in the P$_{Anion\ gap}$. Another cause for an indirect loss of NaHCO$_3$ is provided in the margin note.

ANOTHER CAUSE OF INDIRECT LOSS OF NaHCO$_3$

If a patient has impaired proximal tubular reabsorption of ketoacid anions (e.g., because of high salicylates levels), the P$_{Anion\ gap}$ may not be very high in the presence of ketoacidosis. The clue to the diagnosis is the presence of metabolic acidosis and a large positive urine anion gap (Na$^+$ + K$^+$ > Cl$^-$; see Chapter 2, page 48). To confirm the diagnosis, measure the concentration of β-HB$^-$ in the urine.

TREATMENT OF THE PATIENT WITH DIABETIC KETOACIDOSIS

The therapeutic approach to the patient with DKA involves attention to six major issues:
1. Reexpand the ECF volume to maintain hemodynamic stability.
2. Avoid cerebral edema: prevent an appreciable fall in the P$_{Effective\ osm}$; avoid an overzealous infusion of saline.
3. Diminish the net rate of H$^+$ production.
4. Replace the deficit of K$^+$; timing is critical.
5. Identify and deal with underlying events that may have precipitated DKA.
6. Anticipate and prevent complications that may arise during therapy.

Cerebral edema during treatment of diabetic ketoacidosis in children

- Cerebral edema is a clinical diagnosis; it is largely preventable with well-planned therapy.

- Even though most children with cerebral edema survive, many may be left with neurologic deficits. Moreover, those who seem to be neurologically intact may have subtle cognitive and behavioral deficits.

Because the major serious complication that may develop during therapy of DKA in children is the development of cerebral edema, we discuss this topic before addressing the other aspects of therapy.

Clinically evident cerebral edema occurs in close to 0.5% of cases of DKA in children; it is the major cause of mortality and morbidity in these patients. It occurs more commonly in younger children during the first episode of DKA, which is often more severe, possibly because of a long delay before making the diagnosis. It usually becomes evident at the bedside 5 to 15 hours after therapy is instituted and often with little warning. Cerebral edema should be suspected when there is complaint of headache, vomiting, deterioration in neurologic status, the persistence of a comatose state without an obvious cause, or an unexpected rise in blood pressure and a fall in heart rate—signs that may suggest an increased intracranial pressure. Therefore, children with DKA should be admitted to a unit where they can be observed closely, because therapy must commence without delay to minimize the risk of permanent brain damage.

Cerebral edema is primarily a clinical diagnosis. The presumptive diagnosis of cerebral edema is supported if there is a rapid improvement in neurologic status in response to intravenous administration of 3% NaCl or hypertonic mannitol solution. Making and acting on a clinical diagnosis should take precedence over performing a computed tomography scan or a magnetic resonance imaging study (*see margin note*).

Pathophysiology

- Because water cannot be compressed and the skull is a rigid box, it is obvious that if the volume of one of the brain compartments (ECF or ICF) were to expand and if this were not accompanied by an equivalent decrease in the volume of the other, there would be a rise in intracranial pressure with potentially devastating results.
- The risk factors for the development of cerebral edema can be thought of as those that increase the ECF volume within the skull and those that lead to an increase in the volume of cells in the brain.

There is some evidence to suggest that the blood-brain barrier is somewhat compromised (or leaky) in some patients with DKA, as judged by the fact that the brain appears to be swollen on admission at a time when both the ECF and ICF compartment volumes of the brain should be decreased. There can also be more fluid retained in brain cells before therapy if there is a sudden fall in the $P_{Effective\ osm}$ due to stomach emptying and the absorption of water that was ingested recently.

For cerebral edema to become life threatening, intracranial pressure must rise appreciably. Five potentially important risk factors that may help explain why an increase in the brain ICF and/or ECF compartment volumes may occur are emphasized (Fig. 5-8). Each risk factor

CAUTION
- Provision of care may suffer if the patient is transported to an area of the hospital where continuous monitoring may be less than ideal.
- Changes of cerebral edema using these studies frequently do not keep pace with the clinical course and may not be detected after therapy is instituted.

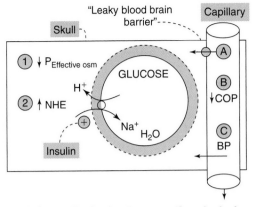

FIGURE 5-8 Risk factors for the development of cerebral edema. The *large rectangle* represents the skull and the circle represents a brain cell. The two factors that might contribute to swelling of brain cells are shown on the *left*: a fall in the $P_{Effective\ osm}$ (*site 1*) and activation of Na^+/H^+ exchanger (NHE) by a bolus of insulin (*site 2*). The factors causing expansion of the ECF volume in the brain are shown on the *right*: they include a less restrictive blood-brain barrier (*site A*), an excessive administration of saline, which can lead to a fall in the colloid osmotic pressure (COP) in plasma (*site B*), and/or a rise in hydrostatic pressure (BP) across the blood-brain barrier (*site C*).

must be considered with respect to its magnitude, the risks imposed by therapy, and what other risk factors may be also present at that time to understand why a devastating rise in intracranial pressure may occur.

Intracellular fluid issues. Water moves rapidly across cell membranes to achieve equal concentrations of effective osmoles in the ICF and ECF compartments. There are two major factors that could cause the ICF volume to expand, a rise in the number of solute molecules that are restricted to the ICF compartment (effective osmoles) and/or a fall in the concentration of effective osmoles in the ECF compartment (i.e., a fall in the $P_{Effective\ osm}$; *see margin note*).

Extracellular fluid issues. The interstitial compartment of the ECF can expand if there is a higher capillary hydrostatic pressure, a lower plasma colloid osmotic pressure, or an increase in permeability of capillaries such that they no longer effectively restrict the movement of albumin.

> $P_{Effective\ osm}$
> $P_{Effective\ osm} = 2\ (P_{Na}) + (P_{Glucose})$, all in mmol/L terms. Urea is not included in this calculation because it is not an effective osmole.

QUESTIONS

(Discussions on page 157; see margin note)

5-4 *How might stomach emptying increase the likelihood of developing cerebral edema in a patient with DKA?*

5-5 *How might protein catabolism increase the likelihood of developing cerebral edema in a patient with DKA?*

> The purpose of Questions 5-4 and 5-5 is to illustrate when factors other than those related to therapy can increase the risk of developing cerebral edema.

Risk factors for cerebral edema early in the therapy of DKA

Administration of a large bolus of saline

- With a less restrictive blood-brain barrier, dangers associated with a large intravenous bolus of saline can be understood by an analysis of the Starling forces across capillary membranes.

An intravenous bolus of saline distributes initially in the plasma volume and reaches the brain with little mixing with the large interstitial volume of the entire ECF compartment. There are two major reasons for a saline bolus to cause fluid movement across the blood-brain barrier into the brain. First, capillary hydrostatic pressure may rise owing to the expansion of the plasma volume. Second, the plasma colloid osmotic pressure may fall because of lowering of the $P_{Albumin}$ by dilution. Based on this reasoning, we suggest that a bolus of saline should *not* be given to children with DKA unless there is a hemodynamic emergency.

Administration of a bolus of insulin. The Na^+/H^+ exchanger (NHE-1) in cell membranes is normally inactive (see Chapter 13, page 431). Following a large intravenous bolus of insulin in the presence of intracellular acidosis, NHE-1 may be active. This leads to a gain of Na^+ and a loss of H^+, which increases the number of solute molecules in cells because the bulk of H^+ exported from the cell were bound to ICF proteins. An intravenous bolus of insulin could have a more dramatic effect on NHE-1 in brain cell membranes if it is given early in therapy when the blood-brain barrier may be less restrictive to the passage of insulin.

Risk factors for cerebral edema later in therapy for diabetic ketoacidosis

Fall in the $P_{Effective\ osm}$

- Because the $P_{Glucose}$ falls quickly in the first 6 hours of therapy, the $P_{Effective\ osm}$ will decline unless the P_{Na} rises by an appropriate amount.

This is particularly important because there may be a slower decline in the concentration of glucose and related metabolites in brain cells (see Fig. 5-8). To avoid a fall in $P_{Effective\ osm}$, the P_{Na} must rise by an amount that is one half of the fall in the $P_{Glucose}$ (both Na^+ and its anion contribute to the $P_{Effective\ osm}$; Fig. 5-9; *see margin note*). Raising the P_{Na} by this amount is not common in adults with DKA because they usually present with a low P_{Na} when they are hyperglycemic; the target for the P_{Na} is often close to 140 mmol/L when the $P_{Glucose}$ falls to 15 mmol/L. In contrast, there may be a therapeutic dilemma in children in whom the initial P_{Na} on admission is often close to

FALL IN $P_{Glucose}$ AND THE TARGET P_{Na}

- If the $P_{Glucose}$ on admission was 50 mmol/L (900 mg/dL) and it fell to 20 mmol/L (360 mg/dL) during therapy, the P_{Na} must be raised by 15 mmol/L (half the fall in $P_{Glucose}$ [30 mmol/L]) to avoid a fall in the $P_{Effective\ osm}$.
- Beware of "occult" water that is generated when glucose is metabolized, because water without effective osmoles is left behind.
- Beware of an unknown volume of "hidden" water (± glucose) in the large dilated stomach, because this will eventually be absorbed.
- Another source of water later during therapy is the excretion of urine with a very high concentration of Na^+ plus K^+, which causes desalination of body fluids (i.e., the generation of electrolyte-free water; see Chapter 10, Fig. 10-4, page 325 for more discussion).
- Hypotonic solutions (e.g., one-half isotonic saline) should *not* be infused to treat this hyperosmolar state.

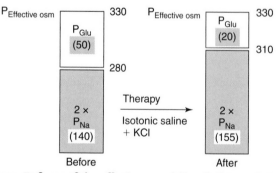

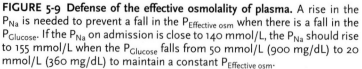

FIGURE 5-9 Defense of the effective osmolality of plasma. A rise in the P_{Na} is needed to prevent a fall in the $P_{Effective\ osm}$ when there is a fall in the $P_{Glucose}$. If the P_{Na} on admission is close to 140 mmol/L, the P_{Na} should rise to 155 mmol/L when the $P_{Glucose}$ falls from 50 mmol/L (900 mg/dL) to 20 mmol/L (360 mg/dL) to maintain a constant $P_{Effective\ osm}$.

140 mmol/L when the $P_{Glucose}$ is close to 50 mmol/L. Because the goal of therapy is to prevent a significant fall in the $P_{Effective\ osm}$ over the initial 15 hours, the P_{Na} should be raised to 155 mmol/L when the $P_{Glucose}$ falls to 20 mmol/L. Although this may make clinicians uncomfortable, it is what is needed to defend the $P_{Effective\ osm}$ in this population, which is at a high risk of developing cerebral edema (*see margin note*).

Avoiding a fall in the $P_{Effective\ osm}$ when insulin acts

There are two components to this threat in children with DKA.

1. In 5 to 10 hours after the administration of insulin, its antilipolytic actions cause a marked decline in circulating fatty acids ($P_{Fatty\ acids}$) and its antiketogenic actions lead to the virtual disappearance of circulating ketoacid anions. As a result, the signals to inhibit glucose oxidation by the metabolic products of these fat-derived fuels will be removed, leading to a faster rate of glucose oxidation. In addition, after a lag period of about 10 hours, actions of insulin will induce the enzymes required for the synthesis of glycogen in muscle and in liver. Overall, there will be a much faster rate of removal of glucose by metabolism in this setting.
2. The second component of the threat is the addition of glucose and water to the ECF compartment. In more detail, it is recommended that the intravenous infusion of saline should be switched to glucose in water (D_5W) when the $P_{Glucose}$ has declined to about 250 mg/dL (15 mmol/L) to prevent the development of neuroglucopenia. While this is necessary, one must recognize that when 50 g of glucose in 1 L of D_5W are removed by oxidation or glycogen synthesis, this "generates" 1 L of solute-free water, which causes the P_{Na} to fall and as a result, cells will swell (including brain cells). There is also a second and less obvious source of added intravenous glucose and water: the absorption of water plus sugar that was retained in the stomach. In addition to enhanced removal of glucose by metabolic means, if some of this added glucose was excreted in an osmotic diuresis, it would cause a loss of Na^+, which also would cause the P_{Na} to fall (the concentration of Na^+ and K^+ in this urine will usually be ~70 mmol/L).

Two final points merit emphasis. First, the absence of a rise in the $P_{Glucose}$ following the administration of D_5W is a warning sign of the generation of solute-free water secondary to removal of glucose. Second, the generation of even a small degree of brain cell swelling can induce brain herniation if there were prior reasons for the retention of water in the skull (*see margin note*). Infusing less water with the glucose (e.g., $D_{10}W$) or adding the infused glucose to isotonic saline rather than water may minimize this danger.

Goals of intravenous therapy

- Hemodynamic emergencies are rarely present in children with DKA.
- There are three issues that need to be considered with respect to intravenous fluids: the *tonicity*, the *rate* of infusion, and the *volume* to infuse.

Treat a hemodynamic emergency if present

A true hemodynamic emergency is *not* common in children with DKA. A bolus of intravenous saline can be a risk factor for the development of cerebral edema because it increases the hydrostatic pressure

CHANGE IN THE $P_{Effective\ osm}$ PRIOR TO THERAPY FOR DKA
- Approximately 5% of young patients with DKA develop cerebral edema prior to therapy.
- It is possible that a large volume of water was ingested and was in the stomach. After a variable time, the stomach contracted and the water entered the intestine, where it was absorbed rapidly. This could cause a large fall in the $P_{Effective\ osm}$ in arterial blood. If this is suspected, raise the $P_{Effective\ osm}$ quickly by infusing hypertonic saline.

DANGERS FOR CEREBRAL EDEMA
- Intravenous bolus of saline and/or insulin
- A fall in the $P_{Effective\ osm}$
- Absorption of stomach contents
- Infusion of D_5W when insulin acts

and diminishes the colloid osmotic pressure in capillaries in the blood-brain barrier. Nevertheless, if a hemodynamic emergency is present, enough saline should be given to restore hemodynamic stability. If a large infusion of saline fails to elicit expected response, consider causes for the hemodynamic instability other than ECF volume depletion (*see margin note*). We use 3 mmol Na^+/kg body weight as a ceiling for the amount of saline to administer in the first 120 minutes in most patients.

In the absence of a hemodynamic emergency, we use the brachial venous P_{CO_2} as a guide to the rate of infusion of saline. Enough saline should be administered to lower the brachial or femoral venous P_{CO_2} to a value that is no more than 10 mm Hg above the arterial P_{CO_2}. This is important to allow effective buffering of H^+ by the bicarbonate buffer system to occur in muscle and thus decreased binding of H^+ to intracellular proteins in vital organs (e.g., brain and heart; see Fig. 1-8, page 14).

Avoid a large fall in the $P_{Effective\ osm}$

- An important objective is to prevent a rise in brain cell volume—this occurs if the $P_{Effective\ osm}$ falls.
- The cause of a large fall in the $P_{Effective\ osm}$ is the large decrease in the $P_{Glucose}$ early during therapy.

To prevent a fall in the $P_{Effective\ osm}$, the effective osmolality of the infusate should be equal to that of the urine in this polyuric state (*see margin note*). Therefore, infuse isotonic saline with 10 to 40 mmol KCl added per liter when K^+ needs to be infused—this results in an effective osmolality of the fluid infused of 320 to 380 mOsm/L.

There are a number of cautions. First, although one may be tempted to switch to hypotonic saline to treat the hyperosmolar state, this is very dangerous because it increases the risk of developing cerebral edema. Second, one should not adjust the P_{Na} for the degree of hyperglycemia (*see margin note on page 124*). Third, beware of occult water retained in the gastrointestinal (GI) tract that may be absorbed when stomach emptying and intestinal motility improve. Fourth, when the fluid in the stomach contains glucose, this can be converted to water following stomach emptying if insulin is acting and the concentration of fat-derived fuels (ketoacids, fatty acids) is not elevated in plasma. Electrolyte free water may be generated by desalination of body fluids when the urine contains little glucose, and therefore its concentration of Na^+ plus K^+ rises considerably above the sum of the P_{Na} plus P_K.

Replace the Na^+ deficit

- A quantitative estimate of the ECF volume is required to determine the total deficit of Na^+ that should ultimately be replaced; this can be done using the hematocrit or the total plasma protein concentration.
- Because hyperglycemia helped maintain the effective arterial blood volume early on, a portion of the loss of glucose in the urine should be replaced by giving different effective osmoles for the ECF compartment, Na^+ and Cl^-.
- The goal should not be to replace the Na^+ deficit rapidly because of a risk of cerebral edema (*see margin note*).

Margin notes

EXPRESSING VOLUME TO INFUSE PER KILOGRAM OF BODY WEIGHT
Because patients with DKA differ in size, it is better to express the volume to infuse per kilogram of body weight rather than to infuse an absolute volume. An infusion of 3 mmol Na^+/kg body weight is equivalent to a volume that is 10% of the normal ECF volume in a given subject.
- The normal ECF volume in a 50-kg patient is 10 L.
- 3 mmol Na^+/kg body weight = 150 mmol Na^+ because 1 L of isotonic saline has 150 mmol Na^+.

EFFECTIVE URINE OSMOLALITY DURING GLUCOSE-INDUCED OSMOTIC DIURESIS
- In a polyuric state, the effective osmolality of the infusate should be similar to that in the urine.
- In these patients, the infusate is 150 mmol NaCl/L plus 20 ~ 30 mmol KCl/L (~350 mOsm/kg H_2O) whereas the $U_{Effective\ osm}$ is ~500 mOsm/kg H_2O (300–350 mmol glucose/L + 70 mmol Na^+ + K^+/L [140 mOsm/kg H_2O]).
- In patients with DKA, the $U_{Effective\ osm}$ is ~150 mOsm/kg H_2O greater than the $P_{Effective\ osm}$. Nevertheless, this should not be an issue because some of the urine glucose may have come from stomach emptying. In addition, the loss of these extra osmoles is small relative to the total osmoles in the ECF + ICF (~900 mosmol when total body water is 30 L and the $P_{Effective\ osm}$ is close to 300 mosmol/L).

NORMAL ECF VOLUME
- Subjects who consume a "typical" Western diet have an expanded ECF volume to provide the kidney with a signal to excrete the ingested Na^+ and Cl^-.
- Thus one should not aim initially to replace the entire negative balance for Na^+.

Having defined the safe rate and the tonicity of the fluid to infuse, the issue now is to define what is a reasonable total volume of saline to infuse. A guide to the total amount of Na^+ that is needed is obtained by defining the deficit of Na^+ in the ECF compartment on presentation from the P_{Na} and a quantitative assessment of the ECF volume (estimated from the hematocrit). Hence, overexpansion of the ECF volume, which is a common occurrence during therapy in these patients, can be avoided.

Replace the urine volume with saline that is isotonic to the urine early in therapy. To maintain the desired effective arterial blood volume early in therapy, ongoing losses of Na^+ in the urine must be replaced. Because hyperglycemia helped maintain the effective arterial blood volume early on, loss of glucose in the urine should be replaced by giving NaCl. Hence, one is, in effect, replacing the effective osmoles Na^+, Cl^-, and glucose that were present in the body and excreted in the urine with the infusion of isotonic saline. One must *not* replace *all* the glucose that is excreted during therapy because some of this is glucose that was in the lumen of the GI tract when the patient first arrived in the hospital. An example of how to decide how much of the glucose excreted should be replaced with Na^+ and Cl^- is provided (*see margin note*).

Replace the remainder of the deficit of Na^+

> • Na^+ is the major effective osmole in the ECF compartment. Hence, the quantity of Na^+ in the ECF compartment—and not its concentration—normally determines the ECF volume.

The quantity of Na^+ in the ECF compartment is the product of the P_{Na} and the ECF volume (see following equation). Therefore, to calculate the Na^+ deficit, a quantitative estimate of the ECF volume at the bedside is needed. Simply put, even the most careful clinical examination does not provide quantitative information about the ECF volume. Similarly, changes in body weight cannot be used for this purpose because patients with DKA have, on one hand, lean body mass catabolism and on the other hand, an unknown, but often large, volume of fluid retained in the lumen of the GI tract. Accordingly, we use the hematocrit (or hemoglobin concentration in plasma) or the concentrations of albumin or total proteins in plasma for this purpose (*see margin note*). If there are reasons to believe that the patient suffers from anemia, one could follow the change in hematocrit with therapy as a measure of the degree of reexpansion of the ECF volume.

Na^+ content in the ECF compartment (mmol)
$$= P_{Na} \text{ (mmol/L)} \times \text{ECF volume (L)}$$

Stop ketoacid production

> • Short-acting insulin is needed initially to stop the formation of ketoacids. Nevertheless, we strongly *caution* against giving a bolus of insulin to children with DKA (see the discussion of cerebral edema, page 127).

There is a lag period of several hours before there is a significant decline in the degree of ketoacidosis even though the correct dose of insulin is administered. The $P_{Anion\ gap}$ usually returns to normal in 8 to 10 hours. Furthermore, the P_{HCO3} does not return to the normal range, as the diminished content of HCO_3^- in the ECF compartment is revealed by the reexpansion of the ECF volume; the deficit of

QUANTITY OF GLUCOSE IN THE EXTRACELLULAR FLUID COMPARTMENT
In a patient with a $P_{Glucose}$ of 50 mmol/L (900 mg/dL) and an ECF volume that has fallen from 10 L to 7 L, the current content of glucose in the ECF compartment is 350 mmol (50 mmol/L × 7 L). Prior to developing DKA, the content of glucose in the ECF compartment was 50 mmol (5 mmol/L × 10 L). Therefore, 300 mmol of the glucose that is excreted in the urine should be replaced with 150 mmol NaCl to prevent a fall in the quantity of effective osmoles in the ECF compartment.

USE OF HEMATOCRIT TO ESTIMATE EXTRACELLULAR FLUID VOLUME
• Hematocrit of 0.60: Calculate the new blood volume (X) in a 50-kg person, assuming the normal RBC volume is 2 L and the plasma volume is 3 L.

Hematocrit = red blood cell volume /blood volume

0.60 = 2 L/X L blood volume

X = 3.3 L

• Because the red blood cell volume is 2 L, the plasma volume is 1.3 L (i.e., decreased by 60%).
• The following table relates the hematocrit to ECF volume. Of note, the percent decline in the ECF volume is larger than the decline in the plasma volume in the patient with DKA because of changes in Starling forces (hydrostatic pressure is lower and plasma oncotic pressure is higher when the $P_{Albumin}$ is increased), which increases the plasma volume at the expense of the interstitial volume.

HEMATOCRIT	% ↓ IN ECF VOLUME
40	0
50	33
60	60

HCO_3^- is due to the initial loss of ketoacid anions (potential HCO_3^-) in the urine with Na^+ and K^+ early in the course of DKA (see Table 5-4). Nevertheless, because saline without HCO_3^- is infused, expect little rise in the P_{HCO3} in the first several hours, despite the fact that insulin has acted and ketoacid anions were converted to HCO_3^-.

K^+ therapy

- The major parameter to guide K^+ replacement therapy is the P_K.
- Patients with DKA are usually quite severely K^+ depleted, but they have hyperkalemia prior to therapy owing to the insulin deficiency and thus a shift of K^+ out of cells.
- Later in therapy, there is a particularly high rate of excretion of K^+ in the urine.

If the P_K is greater than 5 mmol/L, wait at least 1 hour before adding K^+ to the infusate. KCl should be added to each liter of infusion once insulin is given if the P_K is less than 5 mmol/L. If the initial P_K is less than 4 mmol/L, the patient is profoundly K^+ depleted and special precautions should be taken (aggressive replacement of K^+, cardiac monitoring, attention to alveolar ventilation). Because the P_K will fall after insulin administration, do not administer a bolus of insulin, and strongly consider withholding insulin until the P_K exceeds 4.0 mmol/L. These patients are particularly at risk for the development of severe hypokalemia later during therapy as the rate of excretion of K^+ increases significantly.

Phosphate therapy

Patients with DKA are catabolic; they have a large deficit of RNA in cells. The usual deficit of phosphate and of K^+ is about 100 mmol. Because the plasma phosphate levels decline markedly once insulin acts, there is a rationale to administer phosphate to patients with DKA. On the other hand, there are no compelling data that this alters the course of recovery. Notwithstanding, if a decision is made to give phosphate, the maximum dose is 6 mmol/hr after insulin acts. The danger to avoid is the development of hypocalcemia due to precipitation of calcium with phosphate.

Search for underlying illness

Always look for an underlying illness (e.g., an infection) that initiated this metabolic emergency. One should also be on the lookout for complications that may arise during therapy such as venous thrombosis or aspiration pneumonia (Table 5-5).

TABLE 5-5 **POTENTIAL CAUSES OF DEATH IN PATIENTS WITH DIABETIC KETOACIDOSIS**

CAUSE	TIME	TREATMENT
Brain herniation	Usually 5–15 hours, but may occur earlier	Hypertonic saline; cerebral edema must be prevented
$P_K > 6.0$ mmol/L	Admission	Insulin
Hypokalemia	Develops early or late after insulin is given	KCl to maintain P_K near 4.0 mmol/L
Relative hypoglycemia	Usually occurs 6 to 8 hours later	IV glucose when $P_{Glucose}$ is ~15 mmol/L (270 mg/dL)*
Underlying illness and complications	All times	Specific measures needed for individual causes

*This can cause a fall in the $P_{Effective\ osm}$; see page 131.

PART C
ALCOHOLIC KETOACIDOSIS

Overview
- The liver is "programmed" to oxidize as much ethanol as possible when fatty acid synthesis is inhibited.
- There is no lag period before ketoacid production rises when the substrate is ethanol.
- Metabolism of ethanol in the liver yields acetyl-CoA, the precursor for ketoacid synthesis. To allow for a larger amount of ethanol to be removed, the final product must be β-hydroxybutyric acid.
- Decreased rate of removal of ketoacids is a critical factor in determining the severity of the ketoacidosis.
  - A lower rate of oxidation of ketoacids occurs in the brain owing to the sedative effect of ethanol.
  - A lower rate of oxidation of ketoacids occurs in the kidneys when the GFR is low (less renal work to reabsorb the lower filtered load of Na^+).

CASE 5-3: SAM HAD A DRINKING BINGE YESTERDAY

(Case discussed on page 155)

Sam is a chronic alcoholic; he does not have diabetes mellitus. After a large intake of only store-bought liquor, he had several bouts of vomiting. On physical examination, he responded only to painful stimuli. He had a low blood pressure and tachycardia. Acetone was not detected on his breath. The following laboratory values were obtained.

pH (arterial)		7.30
Glucose	mg/dL (mmol/L)	45 (2.5)
Na^+	mmol/L	116
K^+	mmol/L	3.5
Cl^-	mmol/L	66
P_{HCO_3}	mmol/L	15
P_{CO_2} (arterial)	mm Hg	30
Anion gap	mEq/L	35
Creatinine	mg/dL (μmol/L)	2.0 (175)
Osmolality	mOsm/kg H_2O	290
Albumin	g/dL (g/L)	4.5 (45)
BUN (Urea)	mg/dL (mmol/L)	10 (28)

Questions

What is Sam's acid-base disorder?
Why does he appear to have a low effective arterial blood volume?
What is the significance of his low $P_{Glucose}$?
What are the issues for therapy?

BIOCHEMISTRY OF ALCOHOLIC KETOACIDOSIS

- The liver must remove as much ethanol as possible from the portal venous blood (and it does so without a lag period).

KETOACIDOSIS

- There is no physiologic function when ketoacids are produced in both DKA and alcoholic ketoacidosis. Rather, both represent an abnormal state, which leads to excessive accumulation of ketoacids.
- There appears to be a degree of uncoupling of oxidative phosphorylation in the liver in patients with DKA (see page 148 for more discussion of this topic).

TABLE 5-6 **BIOCHEMICAL BACKGROUND FOR THE PRODUCTION OF KETOACIDS**

	PROLONGED FASTING	ETHANOL LOAD
Hepatic production		
Primary function	Produces fat-derived brain fuels	Removes as much ethanol as possible in a single pass
Lag period	A few days	None
Major control	ADP availability ± uncoupled oxidative phosphorylation	Ethanol concentration in portal venous blood and SIAM
Hormonal setting = low ACC	Inhibition of insulin release by hypoglycemia	Inhibition of ACC and insulin release by high adrenergics
Oxidation in		
Brain	Limit by brain work	Lower due to sedative effect
Kidneys	Limit set by GFR	Lower if the GFR falls

ACC, acetyl-CoA carboxylase; GFR, glomerular filtration rate; SIAM, swift initial accelerated metabolism (*see margin note*).

The biochemical features of ketoacid formation from ethanol are very similar to those of the physiologic process of ketoacid formation during prolonged fasting, even though the substrate for the formation of acetyl-CoA is different. For the production of ketoacids to proceed at a rapid rate, the usual metabolic fates of acetyl-CoA (fatty acid synthesis and oxidation in the tricarboxylic acid cycle; see Fig. 5-4, page 118) must be inhibited in the liver. Nevertheless, an upper limit on the rate of ketogenesis is set in large part by the rate of consumption of oxygen in the liver.

There are also important differences in ketoacid formation when fatty acids or ethanol are the major substrate—the most notable being how each pathway is regulated (Table 5-6). To gain insights into the control of each of these metabolic processes, one must focus on its function. In prolonged fasting, the substrate for ketogenesis is long-chain fatty acids and the function of the process is to produce a water-soluble, fat-derived brain fuel (ketoacids) at a rate that is equal to their rate of removal by the brain and the kidneys. Conversely, when ethanol is the substrate, the function is to remove as much ethanol as possible via alcohol dehydrogenase so that its depressant effect on the central nervous system is avoided. There is a lag period before ketoacids are produced at a rapid rate when long-chain fatty acids are the substrate but *not* when ethanol is the substrate. Simply put, the rate of formation of acetyl-CoA is regulated when fatty acids are the substrate but not when ethanol is the substrate. In alcoholic ketoacidosis, there is no regulation to speak of once the ethanol level rises other than that the rate of ethanol oxidation is limited by the rate of removal of NADH (its oxidation in mitochondria to yield NAD^+, which requires the consumption of oxygen and either the availability of ADP or uncoupled oxidative phosphorylation; *see margin note*). Quantitative aspects of this metabolism of ethanol to ketoacids are provided in Part D, page 151.

Removal of ketoacids in the patient with alcoholic ketoacidosis

- Ketoacids are oxidized primarily in the brain and the kidneys. To have high rates of oxidation in these organs, there must be a high rate of consumption of oxygen.

Brain: The consumption of oxygen in the brain can be diminished by the sedative effect of ethanol when there are very high levels of

ETHANOL AND THE UNCOUPLING OF OXIDATIVE PHOSPHORYLATION

- When rats were given a very large load of ethanol, a *swift initial accelerated metabolism* of ethanol (abbreviated as SIAM) was observed; this was accompanied by an increase rate of consumption of O_2 that persisted for a period of time after ethanol disappeared. This is consistent with a form of uncoupled oxidative phosphorylation in the liver (see Part D, page 151 for more discussion). It is not certain what triggers this accelerated metabolic rate.
- The conversion of acetoacetate + NADH to β-hydroxybutyrate + NAD^+ has a similar net effect as uncoupling of oxidative phosphorylation (convert NADH to NAD^+ without requiring the consumption of ADP).

ethanol in blood in the patient with alcoholic ketoacidosis. In addition, removal of ketoacids by the brain may be decreased because there appears to be a lag period before the transporter for ketoacids is induced in the blood-brain barrier.

Kidneys: The kidneys oxidize fewer ketoacids if the GFR falls; this is usually due to a low effective arterial blood volume.

Acetone: A minor pathway for H^+ removal during ketoacidosis is the nonenzymatic conversion of acetoacetic acid to acetone. Because of the high NADH:NAD$^+$ ratio in the liver secondary to the oxidation of ethanol by alcohol dehydrogenase, more acetoacetic acid is converted to β-hydroxybutyric acid and thus less is converted to acetone.

Associated biochemical findings

P$_{Glucose}$

- When ethanol is oxidized in the liver, there is a rise in the NADH:NAD$^+$ ratio, which converts pyruvate to L-lactate.
- A fall in the P$_{Glucose}$ to the hypoglycemic range occurs only in patients with alcoholic ketoacidosis who have little glycogen in their liver (i.e., patients who have a poor dietary carbohydrate intake).

The major metabolic consequence of this high NADH:NAD$^+$ ratio is a lower concentration of pyruvate and a higher concentration of L-lactate because these two metabolic intermediates can be interconverted by an NAD-linked dehydrogenase with a very large catalytic capacity (Fig. 5-10); this reduces the rate of formation of glucose from pyruvate. Nevertheless, well-fed patients who have had a large, acute alcohol intake are not likely to develop hypoglycemia because their liver contains an abundant amount of glycogen that can be converted to glucose.

β-Hydroxybutyric acidosis

- In a setting with a high NADH:NAD$^+$ ratio in the liver, the majority of the ketoacids that are formed from ethanol are released in the form of β-HB$^-$ anions plus H^+.

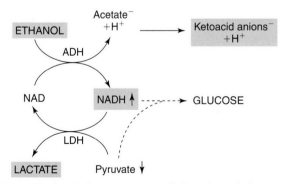

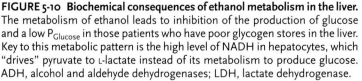

FIGURE 5-10 Biochemical consequences of ethanol metabolism in the liver. The metabolism of ethanol leads to inhibition of the production of glucose and a low P$_{Glucose}$ in those patients who have poor glycogen stores in the liver. Key to this metabolic pattern is the high level of NADH in hepatocytes, which "drives" pyruvate to L-lactate instead of its metabolism to produce glucose. ADH, alcohol and aldehyde dehydrogenases; LDH, lactate dehydrogenase.

This provides a pathway to regenerate NAD^+ that does not require the availability of ADP or the consumption of O_2 and thus a larger amount of ethanol can be removed. The price to pay is a more severe degree of acidemia, especially if the rate of removal of ketoacids is compromised (discussed previously).

Concentration of K^+ in plasma

There are two opposing forces on the P_K, owing to the high levels of adrenergic hormones that affect the distribution of K^+ between the ICF and ECF compartments in patients with alcoholic keto-acidosis. On the one hand, a β_2-adrenergic effect leads to a shift of K^+ into cells because it activates the Na-K-ATPase and this makes the cell interior more negative (see Chapter 13, page 432 for more discussion). On the other hand, a high α-adrenergic action leads to inhibition of the release of insulin. As a result, there is a shift of K^+ out of cells because the cell interior becomes less negative (see Chapter 13, page 433 for more discussion). Hence, the actual P_K observed can be low, normal, or high depending on which of these events predominates *and* on the body total K^+ status prior to this large intake of ethanol.

DIAGNOSIS OF ALCOHOLIC KETOACIDOSIS

Classification

There are two different subgroups of patients who develop alcoholic ketoacidosis; this classification is important because the emphasis in therapy is different for each subgroup.
- *Normal subjects with a binge intake of ethanol*: In this setting, the effective arterial blood volume is not markedly contracted, there is no significant deficit of K^+, the $P_{Glucose}$ is usually normal or somewhat elevated, and nutritional deficiencies are not present.
- *Patients with chronic alcohol abuse and a binge intake of ethanol*: There may be a decreased effective arterial blood volume, K^+ depletion (despite normokalemia or hyperkalemia on presentation), hypoglycemia, and nutritional deficiencies (e.g., vitamin B_1 [thiamin]).

The clinical story begins with a very large intake of ethanol. Ethanol levels in plasma can be measured directly or inferred from the $P_{Osmolal\ gap}$. An important point to keep in mind is that other alcohols (methanol, ethylene glycol) might also be present (see Chapter 2, page 48); the clinician must keep this in mind because of the toxicity of the metabolites of these alcohols, which requires a different emphasis for therapy.

In addition to the large intake of ethanol, a key to the development of ketoacidosis is a large release of catecholamines owing to a decreased effective arterial blood volume and/or repetitive bouts of vomiting secondary to gastric irritation. This adrenergic surge has important metabolic effects, including inhibition of the release of insulin, enhanced lipolysis, and inhibition of acetyl-CoA carboxylase, the enzyme that catalyzes the first committed step in fatty acid synthesis. Other factors that cause an adrenergic surge may be also present (e.g., a large intake of caffeine).

TABLE 5-7 **CLASSIFICATION OF PATIENTS WITH ALCOHOL KETOACIDOSIS**

For details, see text. In both subgroups, there is a large prior intake of ethanol that leads to a high rate of ketoacid formation. By normal subjects we mean those with no prior history of chronic alcohol abuse.

	NORMAL SUBJECTS	CHRONIC ALCOHOLIC
Clinical features		
Ethanol intake	Episodic	Chronic + acute
Gastritis and vomiting	Very prominent	Very prominent
EABV	Not obviously contracted	Usually very low
Laboratory features		
$P_{Glucose}$	High normal range	Usually not very high
P_K	Can be low, normal or high	Often low but can be normal or high
Metabolic acidosis and alkalosis	Yes	Yes
L-lactic acidosis	Should be mild	Can be more severe for a number of reasons
Respiratory alkalosis	May be present	Present if aspiration pneumonia, chronic liver disease, or alcohol withdrawal
Nutritional deficits		
Thiamin deficiency	No	May be present

EABV, effective arterial blood volume.

Patients with alcoholic ketoacidosis can be classified into two groups with regard to their clinical presentation (Table 5-7). The first group consists of normal subjects who consumed a large amount of ethanol, and the second group consists primarily of chronic alcoholics who had a large acute intake of ethanol. The $P_{Glucose}$ on admission may help identify each group. This point is emphasized because it has implications for therapy.

Importance of the $P_{Glucose}$

Alcoholic ketoacidosis in normal subjects

- These subjects have an appreciable store of glycogen in their liver when the ethanol is consumed.

As a result of hydrolysis of liver glycogen, there is an input of glucose into the circulation. In addition, oxidation of glucose is inhibited because of the high α-adrenergic surge from vomiting, which leads to low insulin levels, high levels of fatty acids, and high levels of ketoacids. Therefore, these patients have a modestly elevated $P_{Glucose}$ and they do *not* develop hypoglycemia with therapy.

Alcoholic ketoacidosis in subjects with chronic alcohol abuse

- Some of these patients may have depleted hepatic stores of glycogen owing to long periods of poor dietary intake.

As a result of a lack of glycogen in the liver, they are dependent on the conversion of protein to glucose in the liver (gluconeogenesis) to maintain a $P_{Glucose}$ in the normal range. These patients may present with hypoglycemia because when ethanol is being metabolized, the high hepatic $NADH:NAD^+$ ratio drives the metabolism of pyruvate to L-lactate rather than permitting its conversion to glucose (see Fig. 5-10).

Effective arterial blood volume

Alcoholic ketoacidosis in normal subjects

The effective arterial blood volume is not appreciably contracted in these patients even though they had protracted vomiting because little Na^+ is lost via the GI tract. Although there is little Na^+ in the gastric secretions, the contents of the stomach that are lost during vomiting could contain some Na^+ from swallowed saliva or from entry of intestinal secretions that are rich in $NaHCO_3$ through a patent pyloric sphincter. There could also be some loss of Na^+ in the urine because alkalemia caused by vomiting may increase the renal excretion of $NaHCO_3$ and/or the Na^+ salts of organic acids.

Alcoholic ketoacidosis in subjects with chronic alcohol abuse

- Many patients in this group present with a significant degree of effective arterial blood volume contraction; this may reflect a prior depletion of NaCl.

In addition, redistribution of the ECF volume owing to acute pancreatitis and/or paralytic ileus, or pooling of blood in venous capacitance vessels could also contribute to the low effective arterial volume. A decreased effective arterial blood volume may also be due to the presence of alcoholic cardiomyopathy.

Potassium

Alcoholic ketoacidosis in normal subjects

These patients, in general, do not have a K^+ deficit. Nevertheless, there could be a shift of K^+ across cell membranes, causing either hypokalemia or hyperkalemia. The factors to be considered include the adrenergic response, low insulin levels, and metabolic alkalosis, as well as a potential role of the intake of drugs and/or the ingestion of caffeine (see Chapter 14, page 506). These patients have normal P_K values once their ketoacidosis disappears.

Alcoholic ketoacidosis in subjects with chronic alcohol abuse

If vomiting occurred for a long period of time, there could be a large kaliuresis and K^+ depletion (see Chapter 7, page 199 for more discussion). On the other hand, hyperkalemia may be present if there is a deficiency of insulin (owing to an α-adrenergic surge) that has led to a shift of K^+ out of cells. Rhabdomyolysis is another possible cause for hyperkalemia in this group of patients.

Nutritional deficiencies

These are present only in the group of patients with chronic alcoholism; the treatment of these deficiencies is considered in Chapter 6, page 172. These patients should be given thiamin at the onset of therapy to avoid the development of Wernicke's encephalopathy.

Acid-base disorders

Mixed metabolic acidosis and metabolic alkalosis

- Even though ketoacidosis is present, the patient might not be acidemic because of the presence of metabolic alkalosis consequent to vomiting and also possibly a higher P_{HCO3} owing to a contracted ECF volume (see Chapter 7, page 195).

The key to the diagnosis of this mixed acid-base disturbance is an increase in the $P_{Anion\,gap}$ that is larger than the fall in the P_{HCO3}. A note of caution is important. A low $P_{Albumin}$ might mask the rise in the $P_{Anion\,gap}$; therefore, the baseline value for the $P_{Anion\,gap}$ must be adjusted for $P_{Albumin}$ (for every 1.0-g/dL [10-g/L] decline in the $P_{Albumin}$, the $P_{Anion\,gap}$ [including K^+] falls by 3 to 4 mEq/L). In addition, the content of HCO_3^- in the ECF compartment should be calculated as described earlier using the hematocrit and/or total plasma protein concentration. To the extent that some patients might have reduced gastric HCl secretion (e.g., owing to intake of drugs such as proton pump inhibitors because of gastritis), there is a low net addition of HCO_3^- to the body during vomiting, or in some patients there may be loss of $NaHCO_3$ during vomiting if the pyloric sphincter is patent (see Fig. 7-2, page 198).

L-Lactic acidosis

- There might be a mild degree of L-lactic acidosis because metabolism of ethanol raises the $NADH:NAD^+$ in the cytosol of hepatocytes, and this results in the conversion of pyruvate to L-lactate (see Fig. 5-10, page 137).

If a more severe degree of L-lactic acidosis is present, reasons in addition to ethanol metabolism should be suspected. Two of the most common causes of L-lactic acidosis are usually obvious; first, tissue hypoxia can be present if the effective arterial blood volume is very low; second, muscular contractions (the tremors in delirium tremens, or the presence of a recent seizure). The most important cause, however, is thiamin deficiency, which may also cause permanent cerebral damage (Wernicke's encephalopathy) if it is not recognized and treated promptly. Other B vitamin deficiencies (e.g., riboflavin) can also cause L-lactic acidosis (see Chapter 6, page 172).

Respiratory alkalosis

Given the high propensity for aspiration pneumonia in these patients, the fact that alcohol withdrawal may stimulate ventilation by an adrenergic overdrive and that patients with chronic liver disease often hyperventilate, it is not uncommon for respiratory alkalosis to be present in these patients.

TREATMENT OF ALCOHOLIC KETOACIDOSIS

- There can be several life-threatening components to the clinical picture of alcoholic ketoacidosis.

• This is especially the case in patients with chronic alcoholism who also have deficits of electrolytes and B vitamins.

Hypoglycemia

DOSE OF GLUCOSE NEEDED IN A 70-kg PATIENT WITH A P_{Glucose} OF 45 mg/dL (2.5 mmol/L)
To be safe, aim to raise the $P_{Glucose}$ by 5 mmol/L (90 mg/dL). Because the volume of distribution of glucose under conditions of lack of insulin is close to 20 L (ECF volume + 5 L of ICF), give 100 mmol of glucose (18 g) (= ⅓L of D_5W or 30 mL of $D_{50}W$). A larger amount of glucose will be needed later to permit the usual rate of glucose oxidation in the brain once the circulating level of ketoacids declines appreciably.

Glucose is needed *only* if hypoglycemia is present; a small amount of glucose is usually sufficient to maintain a normal $P_{Glucose}$ because metabolism of glucose is slow in this setting (*see margin note*). Avoid hyperglycemia because very high levels of insulin may lead to a sudden fall in P_K. In addition, inhibition of insulin release by α-adrenergic actions will no longer be present once the effective arterial blood volume is reexpanded.

Effective arterial blood volume contraction

• In patients with a very contracted effective arterial blood volume, isotonic saline can be infused rapidly to normalize the hemodynamic state.
• One must be cautious because some of these patients may have cardiomyopathy.

In the absence of hemodynamic instability, we infuse enough saline to lower brachial venous P_{CO_2} to a value that is not more than 10 mm Hg higher than arterial P_{CO_2} to allow for buffering of H^+ by HCO_3^- buffers in the interstitial space and ICF of muscles and prevent their binding to intracellular proteins in cells of vital organs (e.g., brain cells). One may not always be able to use the hematocrit or total plasma proteins concentration to estimate the total Na^+ deficit in the ECF compartment because some patients may not have had normal values to begin with; nevertheless, changes with therapy may provide rough guides to the degree of reexpansion of the ECF volume. Of great importance, if the patient has chronic hyponatremia and is malnourished, a rapid rise in the P_{Na} must be avoided because of the risk of developing osmotic demyelination. Administration of dDAVP to prevent a large water diuresis once the effective arterial blood volume is reexpanded should be considered (see Chapter 10, page 346 for more discussion). Water intake must be curtailed in this setting.

ABBREVIATION
dDAVP, desamino, D-arginine vasopressin, a long-acting form of vasopressin

K^+ deficit

• Once the effective arterial blood volume is reexpanded, the α-adrenergic surge disappears, insulin is released, and thus K^+ moves rapidly into cells.

Do not wait for hypokalemia to develop before administering KCl. The actual amount of KCl to give depends on the P_K during therapy; the deficit could exceed several hundred millimoles in the chronic alcoholic.

Nutritional deficiencies

Thiamin

It is critical that thiamin (and probably riboflavin) be added early in therapy in a chronic alcoholic and malnourished patient. This will permit aerobic oxidation of glucose in the brain once ketoacids disappear and prevent the development of Wernicke's encephalopathy (for more discussion, see Chapter 6, page 172).

Phosphate

Although phosphate depletion is quite marked, it takes time before anabolic reactions occur subsequent to the actions of insulin. Hence, as in DKA, replacing the majority of the phosphate deficit (with K^+) should be delayed.

Ketoacidosis

There is usually no specific therapy needed to deal with the keto-acidosis because excessive production of ketoacids falls once the alcohol disappears and the effective arterial blood volume is reexpanded (insulin is released from β-cells of the pancreas). Moreover, the utilization of ketoacids improves when the GFR rises owing to reexpansion of the effective arterial blood volume and when ethanol levels fall sufficiently to permit normal cerebral function. Therapy with $NaHCO_3$ is not needed in most cases.

QUESTION

(Discussion on page 158)

5-6 *Can ketoacidosis and/or L-lactic acidosis be present even though ethanol has disappeared from the plasma?*

PART D
INTEGRATIVE PHYSIOLOGY

CONTROL OF KETOGENESIS: A MORE DETAILED ANALYSIS

- Free fatty acids, ADP and/or NAD^+, and oxygen are substrates for the formation of ketoacids in the liver.
- In the partial oxidation of glucose, control is via availability of ADP (i.e., work).
- In ketogenesis, control is via availability of NAD^+ (i.e., rate of oxygen consumption in coupled and uncoupled oxidative phosphorylation).

Control of the maximum rate of production of ketoacids in the liver when there is hormonal permission for ketogenesis to occur (low net actions of insulin) can be due to limitations in the supply of extrahepatic and/or intrahepatic substrates to make these water-soluble brain fuels (Fig. 5-11). In this section, we provide a quantitative analysis to define whether the availability of any of the substrates for ketogenesis may limit the rate of ketoacid production during prolonged fasting and in patients with DKA.

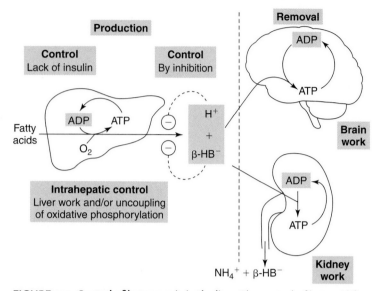

FIGURE 5-11 Control of ketogenesis in the liver. The control of ketoacid formation in the liver begins with a lack of insulin, which increases the supply of long-chain fatty acids *and* decreases the rate of fatty acid synthesis. The upper limit of ketoacid formation is set by the rate of O_2 consumption in hepatocytes, and part of this control most likely involves a form of uncoupling of oxidative phosphorylation. In addition, an increase in the concentration of β-HB⁻ and/or H⁺ in plasma owing to a decrease in the rate of their removal by the brain and/or the kidney may provide the signal for feedback inhibition of the production of ketoacids in the liver.

Control by extrahepatic substrates

Control by the supply of fatty acids to the liver

During prolonged fasting. When there is a relative lack of insulin, the content of fatty acids in 1 liter of plasma is close to 1 mmol, if the concentration of albumin in blood is normal (4.0 g/dL [40 g/L]) because the vast majority of circulating fatty acids are bound to albumin. The hepatic blood flow is close to 1 L/min; therefore, the delivery of fatty acids to the liver is about 0.6 mmol/min when the hematocrit is 0.40 (0.4 L red blood cells and 0.6 L plasma). Because 4 mmol of ketoacids are formed per 1 mmol of palmitate (16 carbons; see following equation), the liver could form 2.4 mmol of ketoacids per minute. Approximately half of this amount is more likely, however, because of a limited capacity of the uptake process of fatty acids into hepatocytes. Therefore, the delivery of fatty acids to the liver should be able to support the observed rate of ketogenesis in this setting.

$$\text{Palmitate } (C_{16}H_{32}O_2) + 6\ O_2 \rightarrow 4 \text{ ketoacids } (C_4H_7O_3) + 2\ H_2O$$

During diabetic ketoacidosis

- A possible reason why DKA may be more severe in children is that they have a higher supply of fatty acids from triglycerides that are stored in the liver.

In the patient with DKA, there is a slower rate of blood flow to the liver owing to the markedly contracted effective arterial blood volume, which may reduce the quantity of fatty acids that can be taken up by the liver sufficiently to lower the rate of ketogenesis in these patients. On the other hand, there could be a higher content of fatty acids in each liter of plasma in patients who develop DKA because of a higher $P_{Albumin}$ and that most of the fatty acids in plasma are bound to albumin. Therefore, only if the splanchnic blood flow rate is very low will the rate of production of ketoacids be limited by the supply of fatty acids. Nevertheless, the rate of ketogenesis will still be rapid enough to have a serious degree of metabolic acidosis and acidemia because the rate of ketoacid removal by the kidneys and possibly the brain will be reduced in this setting.

Control by the supply of oxygen to the liver

Each liter of arterial blood has close to 8 mmol of O_2 (see *margin note*). Although the liver receives 1 L of blood per minute, most of this blood arrives via the portal vein, where one fourth to one third of its oxygen was extracted by the intestinal tract. As a result, the liver receives close to 6 mmol of oxygen per liter of blood. If the liver extracted all 6 mmol of O_2, it could convert 1 mmol of palmitate to ketoacids (see previous equation). Notwithstanding, each liter of blood contains about 0.6 L of plasma with a concentration of palmitate of 1 mmol/L; thus, the liver receives only 0.6 mmol palmitate per minute. Hence, there is a surplus of O_2 delivered to the liver even if all of this palmitate were extracted and used only for the synthesis of ketoacids (an unlikely scenario). Therefore, the delivery of O_2 does *not* control the rate of ketoacid production by the liver.

O$_2$ CONTENT PER LITER OF BLOOD
- 140 g of hemoglobin/L equals 2 mmol/L (molecular weight ~70,000).
- 4 mmol O_2 bind to 1 mmol hemoglobin.
- Therefore, the content of O_2 in 1 L of arterial blood is 8 mmol.

Control by the supply of intrahepatic substrates (ADP and NAD⁺)

One of the intrahepatic substrates for the synthesis of ketoacids is NAD^+. It is present in a very tiny quantity, which means that there must be ways to regenerate NAD^+ very quickly to have a rapid flux in the pathway of ketogenesis. In fact, the rate of regeneration of NAD^+ can limit the rate of production of ketoacids. To understand how this regeneration occurs, it is important to think of this regulation in a "metabolic process" analysis (i.e., consider the true starting point and the true final product). To illustrate a way to think about this issue, we describe the pathways of oxidation of glucose and fatty acids in the context of having a need for NAD^+ and/or ADP as the substrates for the metabolic process. The interrelationship between ADP and NAD^+ is depicted in Figure 5-12.

NAD⁺ and ADP as substrates for the partial oxidation of glucose

- Because there is insufficient consumption of O_2 by mitochondria in skeletal muscle cells during a sprint, the availability of the substrate ADP, and not NAD^+, controls the rate of aerobic glycolysis.

Function. A high rate of anaerobic glycolysis is needed in a sprint because this is the most rapid way to regenerate ATP during glucose metabolism.

Metabolic process. The first step in the performance of work is the hydrolysis of ATP to yield ADP during the race. In the second step, glycogen is converted to L-lactic acid if one were to look at only the "carbon biochemistry." From an overall perspective, however, there are two other substrates to consider: NAD^+ and ADP (plus inorganic phosphate).

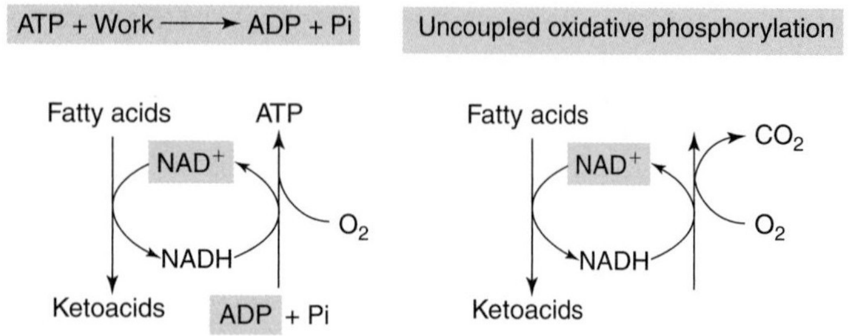

ATP + Work ⟶ ADP + Pi   Uncoupled oxidative phosphorylation

FIGURE 5-12 Central role of NAD⁺/ADP in the control of fatty acid metabolism in the liver. $NAD^+ + O_2$ are obligatory substrates for the oxidation of fatty acids to produce CO_2 and/or ketoacids (*see margin note*). One way to convert NADH to NAD^+ in mitochondria requires that ADP be converted to ATP. Therefore, ADP must be formed in the liver in sufficient quantity to permit this oxidation pathway to occur (shown to the *left*). The major source of this ADP is the hydrolysis of ATP when work is performed in the liver. If there is insufficient work, fewer ketoacids can be formed unless there is a way to bypass the need to generate ADP (i.e., uncoupling of oxidative phosphorylation; shown to the *right*).

As shown in Figure 5-12, NAD^+ is the actual substrate for fatty acid oxidation. Nevertheless, ADP is equivalent to NAD^+ as a substrate because it is needed to convert NADH back to NAD^+ in mitochondria. Hence, coupled oxidation of fatty acids requires that an appropriate amount of ADP be present.

NAD^+ biochemistry. NAD^+ is converted to NADH during the conversion of glucose to pyruvate. In the conversion of pyruvate to L-lactate, NADH is converted to NAD^+, so this cofactor is regenerated.

ADP biochemistry. ADP is formed when muscles work. ADP (plus inorganic phosphate) is (are) substrate(s) to regenerate ATP during the conversion of glucose to pyruvate. Because there is not enough consumption of O_2 in this setting, the rate of aerobic glycolysis is driven by work (availability of ADP; see following equations).

$$\text{Work} + \text{ATP} \rightarrow \text{ADP} + \text{inorganic phosphate}$$
$$\text{Glucose} + 2\ NAD^+ + 2\ (ADP\ [+\ \text{inorganic phosphate}])$$
$$\rightarrow 2\ \text{ATP} + 2\ \text{NADH} + 2\ \text{L-lactate}$$

Control. The availability of the substrate ADP, and not NAD^+, controls the rate of aerobic glycolysis.

NAD^+ and ADP as substrates for the conversion of fatty acids to ketoacids

- NAD^+ is a substrate for fatty acid oxidation. Because it is present in tiny amounts, the rate of this oxidation is dependent on the rate of conversion of NADH to NAD^+.
- Because the consumption of oxygen is needed to convert NADH to NAD^+, there is a link between the rates of consumption of oxygen and ketogenesis in liver cells.
- In coupled respiration, the availability of ADP (i.e., hepatic work) sets a limit on the rate of formation of ketoacids.
- Uncoupling of oxidative phosphorylation can permit higher rates of production of ketoacids as it bypasses the limiting step of the availability of ADP.

Function. A high rate of ketogenesis is needed when there is a decreased supply of glucose for the brain.

Metabolic process. The first step in ketogenesis is the hydrolysis of triglycerides to yield fatty acids. In the liver, control of ketogenesis is largely due to the blocking of other pathways in the metabolism of the carbon product of fatty acid oxidation, acetyl-CoA (oxidation and fat synthesis). The ketoacids formed become the main fuel for the brain.

In the process of ketogenesis, fatty acids are converted to ketoacids, if one were to look at only the "carbon biochemistry." From an overall perspective, there are two other substrates to consider: NAD^+ and ADP (+ inorganic phosphate).

NAD^+ biochemistry. NADH is converted to NAD^+ during the consumption of oxygen in mitochondria. There are two controls on the rate of oxygen consumption, conversion of ATP to ADP during hepatic work, and the rate of uncoupled oxidative phosphorylation (see Fig. 5-12; *see also accompanying margin note*). In addition, there can be some conversion of NADH to NAD^+ that does not involve control by the consumption of oxygen—this occurs in dehydrogenase reactions (i.e., when acetoacetate + NADH are converted to β-hydroxybutyrate and NAD^+).

$$Palmitate + NAD^+ + FAD$$
$$\rightarrow acetoacetate/\beta\text{-hydroxybutyrate} + NADH + FADH$$

$$NADH + ADP + O_2 \rightarrow NAD^+ + ATP$$

$$FADH + ADP + O_2 \rightarrow FAD + ATP$$

$$Sum: Palmitate + ADP + O_2 \rightarrow$$
$$acetoacetate/\beta\text{-hydroxybutyrate} + ATP$$

Control. The availability of the substrate NAD^+ via factors that determine the rate of consumption of oxygen (coupled and uncoupled oxidative phosphorylation) controls the rate of ketogenesis in the liver. More ketoacids are formed when β-hydroxybutyrate rather than acetoacetate is the final product of the pathway.

Control of intrahepatic substrates by uncoupled respiration

- Because there is very little biologic work performed in the liver in prolonged fasting or in DKA, a strategy is needed to bypass this limit set by availability of ADP on the conversion of NADH to NAD^+ to permit rapid rate of synthesis of ketoacids; this strategy involves uncoupling of oxidative phosphorylation.

Hepatic work consists primarily of biosynthesis and flux through the Na-K-ATPase. Notwithstanding, the liver does very little biosynthetic work or ion pumping when there are low net actions of insulin. Hence, this problem must be overcome when an augmented rate of ketogenesis is needed for the brain to have an alternate fuel when glucose is not available and for the kidney to excrete enough effective osmoles to avoid oliguria and the formation of precipitates in the urine. The process that is most likely to achieve this task is uncoupling of oxidative phosphorylation.

In coupled oxidative phosphorylation, H^+ are pumped out of mitochondria using the energy derived from the oxidation of fuels—these H^+ reenter mitochondria via special H^+ channels that are linked to the conversion of ADP (+ inorganic phosphate) to ATP (Fig. 5-13). In contrast, if H^+ reenter mitochondria through another H^+ channel that is *not* linked to the conversion of ADP to ATP, this results in an uncoupled oxidative phosphorylation. The net effect of this uncoupling

CONTENT OF ADP IN CELLS
- It is important to recognize that the concentration of free ADP in cells is very tiny—less than 1% of the total ATP + ADP. Therefore, liver cells need to hydrolyze a very large quantity of ATP to regenerate enough ADP and thereby NAD^+ to convert fatty acids to ketoacids at a rapid rate.
- The major way ADP is formed is when cells perform biologic work (mechanical, biosynthetic, electrical). If there is insufficient work, fewer ketoacids can be formed unless there is a way to bypass the need to generate ADP (i.e., uncoupling of oxidative phosphorylation)

ABBREVIATION
FAD, flavine-adenine-dinucleotide, a member of the electron transport system in mitochondria

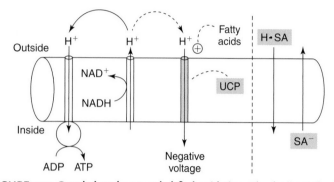

FIGURE 5-13 Coupled and uncoupled fuel oxidation. The *horizontal cylindrical structure* represents the inner mitochondrial membrane. In the presence of oxygen, NADH is converted to NAD^+ and H^+ are pumped out of mitochondria (*left portion*). The latter action creates a huge electrochemical driving force across the mitochondrial membrane to drive the entry of H^+ into mitochondria. During coupled metabolism, these exported H^+ reenter mitochondria through a pathway that leads to the conversion of ADP to ATP (*solid curved arrow above the mitochondrial membrane*). If availability of ADP is limited (less work and thus less regeneration of ADP from breakdown of ATP), there is less conversion of NADH to NAD^+ because fewer H^+ are transported out of mitochondria. This control can be bypassed in two ways: First (*central portion*), H^+ can enter mitochondria via the uncoupler type of H^+ channels (uncoupler protein; UCP). These UCPs are *not* linked to the machinery to regenerate ATP (*dashed curved arrow above the mitochondrial membrane*) and they are more active in the presence of fatty acids. Second (*right portion*), weak acids (e.g., salicylic acid [H•SA]) carry H^+ in, and because their conjugate bases are "lipid-soluble anions" (e.g., salicylate [SA^-]), they can exit from the mitochondria to complete the H^+ entry cycle.

is to increase the rate of oxidation of fuels in the presence of O_2 because this process removes the absolute need for ADP availability to convert NADH back to NAD^+ to permit fuel oxidation (NADH → NAD^+ without the consumption of ADP). These H^+ channels are called *uncoupler proteins* (UCPs; see Fig. 5-13).

Strategies to uncouple oxidative phosphorylation

- If the intrahepatic control system for ketoacid production truly involves a degree of uncoupled oxidative phosphorylation, more uncoupling of oxidative phosphorylation in the liver in children than in adults could explain why children readily develop DKA.

UNCOUPLER PROTEINS
- UCP-1 is induced in brown adipose tissue when there is a need for heat production (e.g., in the newborn, during cold exposure), especially in small animals where there is a much greater heat loss.
- UCP-2, which is important in skeletal muscle, helps to remove excess stores of fat in the fed state and to lower the concentration of reactive oxygen species after vigorous aerobic exercise (see Chapter 6, discussion of Case 6-3, page 185 for more discussion).

As shown in the central portion of Figure 5-13, one possible mechanism to increase the rate of H^+ entry into mitochondria without converting ADP to ATP (i.e., uncouple oxidative phosphorylation) is to insert UCPs into the inner mitochondrial membrane. There are many different UCPs, depending on which tissue is examined, and the regulation of their synthesis and/or insertion depends on the metabolic setting (*see margin note*). Nevertheless, it is difficult to have a precise regulation of the rate of synthesis of ketoacids with this mechanism of control.

There is a second mitochondrial mechanism to increase the rate of H^+ entry into the mitochondria without converting ADP to ATP. This occurs when weak acids enter mitochondria (H^+ entry) and have their anions exit the mitochondria without H^+ so this weak acid can, in effect, recycle. Two examples of this type of uncouplers of oxidative phosphorylation are metformin (discussed in more detail in Chapter 6, page 174) and salicylic acid (discussed in more detail in Chapter 8, page 232). Therefore, the ingestion of aspirin may augment the rate of hepatic ketogenesis in a patient with DKA. Another metabolic pathway that is equivalent to uncoupling is discussed in the margin (*see margin note*).

Risks associated with uncoupling of oxidative phosphorylation

There are two settings where the risks are apparent.

1. When the rate of uncoupling is very high, there may be a diminished ability to convert ADP to ATP. As a result, the concentration of ADP rises and this augments the rate of anaerobic glycolysis. Because the rate of glycolysis can easily exceed the rate of oxidation of pyruvate in mitochondria, L-lactic acidosis could develop.

2. When the brain has a limited activity of pyruvate dehydrogenase (e.g., owing to thiamin deficiency or inborn errors), the intake of a chemical uncoupler (e.g., salicylic acid) can lead to the generation of ADP at a rate that is faster than the rate of its conversion to ATP when ketoacids are absent (i.e., when ATP formation is dependent on pyruvate dehydrogenase activity). This may be the underlying pathophysiology for the development of Wernicke-Korsakoff encephalopathy (see Chapter 6, page 172 for more discussion).

Benefits associated with uncoupling of oxidative phosphorylation

• When flux in the pathways that lead to uncoupled oxidative phosphorylation is increased, the net effect is that more fuels plus O_2 are consumed, but ADP formation during work is not required.

Three examples of benefits of this process follow.

1. In the liver when there is low net insulin action, the rate of fatty oxidation will be increased somewhat as more NAD^+ becomes available and this permits the production of more ketoacids for oxidation by the brain and for excretion by the kidneys to avoid oliguria. In addition, when there is a large input of ethanol, its removal can be augmented by having uncoupled oxidative phosphorylation.

2. There is also a potential benefit of lowering the concentration of O_2 so that fewer reactive oxygen species (ROS) will be formed. In this context, ROS increase the rate of uncoupled oxidative phosphorylation in skeletal muscle as long as fatty acids are also present. This may be observed after exercise as discussed in the response to Question 5-7, page 158.

3. After a large meal, the oxidation of fatty acids rises in skeletal muscle even though there is little or no extra muscle work (*see margin note*). The signal may be swelling of adipocytes due to new stored triglycerides; the messengers are adiponectins and leptin released by cells, and the effector organ is skeletal muscle with its large capacity to oxidize more fatty acids if the existing uncoupler proteins permit more H^+ to traverse these channels and/or if the number of these channels is increased—this is may be an important strategy that may help prevent progressive obesity (Fig. 5-14).

METABOLIC EQUIVALENTS OF UNCOUPLING

• When fructose-6-phosphate (F6P) is converted to fructose-1,6-diphosphate (FDP), ATP is consumed; when the reverse reaction occurs simultaneously, inorganic phosphate (Pi) is formed (see following equations). The net effect is the conversion of ATP to ADP and Pi; this is called *futile cycling*, but it is not necessarily "futile" because it can permit a faster rate of conversion of fatty acids to ketoacids.

$$F6P + ATP \rightarrow FDP + ADP$$

$$FDP \rightarrow F6P + Pi$$

$$Net: ATP \rightarrow ADP + Pi$$

• In the reaction in which acetoacetate is converted to β-hydroxybutyrate (see Fig. 5-7), NADH is converted to NAD^+. Hence, the rate of oxidation of fatty acids in the liver can rise because the supply of NAD^+ is increased. Therefore, the net effect is the same as a mild degree of uncoupling of oxidative phosphorylation.

CAUTION
This proposed mechanism is our speculation.

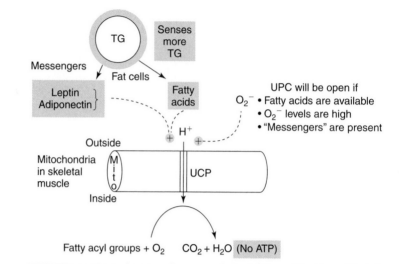

FIGURE 5-14 Control system for uncoupled oxidation of fat. The *solid circle in the top left portion of the figure* represents a fat cell. When stretched (*green shaded area*), both fatty acids and hormonal messengers are sent to uncouple oxidative phosphorylation in mitochondria in skeletal muscle. High levels of reactive oxygen species lead to a greater flux through the uncoupler protein (UCP) H^+ channels in these mitochondria, providing that fatty acids are present. This requirement for fatty acids avoids depleting the brain of its fuel in the fed state, glucose. TG, triglyceride.

UNCOUPLED OXIDATION OF FATTY ACIDS AND OBESITY

- This hypothesis is provided to stimulate thinking.
- Although we realize that both intake and energy expenditure can be controlled to some degree, some other control systems are undoubtedly in place.
- A diminished degree of uncoupling of oxidative phosphorylation of fatty acid oxidation may play a role in obesity.
- On the other side of the coin, excessive uncoupling may play a role in disorders characterized by cachexia.

QUESTION

(Discussion on page 158)

5-7 *What might be the biologic role of increased uncoupler proteins in skeletal muscle during prolonged fasting?*

Regulation of ketoacid formation in prolonged fasting

- Feedback control is required to have the rate of ketogenesis in the liver match the rate of removal of ketoacids in the brain and the kidney during prolonged fasting; the concentration of H^+ in plasma may provide the signal for feedback control.

QUANTITY OF KETOACIDS REQUIRED IN PROLONGED FASTING

- The brain oxidizes close to 750 mmol of ketoacids per day. The kidneys remove close to 400 mmol/day of ketoacids during prolonged fasting. Hence, the liver must synthesize this quantity of ketoacids each day in this setting.
- The quantity of ketoacids in the ECF compartment of a 50-kg fasted person is quite small (~50 mmol [5 mmol/L × 10 L]).

There is little variation in the concentrations of acetoacetic and β-hydroxybutyric acids in plasma during prolonged fasting. In addition, there is a fairly robust turnover of these metabolic intermediates (i.e., ~1 mmol/min; *see margin note*). Accordingly, regulatory mechanisms that exert tight control on the rate of ketoacid production are needed. When quantities are examined, the need for relatively precise control becomes obvious. First, close to 1500 mmol of ketoacids are produced each day during prolonged fasting (~1 mmol minute). Second, the content of ketoacid anions in the ECF compartment of a 50-kg (10-L) person is only 50 mmol. If the ketoacid anions were distributed in total body water, the overall content would be 150 mmol (5 mmol/L × 30 L). Hence, the concentration of ketoacids would double if ketoacid removal were zero for only one tenth of the day (2.4 hours). Based on these numerical considerations, feedback regulation of ketogenesis is very likely to be present.

Control by $P_{Ketoacid\ anions}$. Because a high level of glucagon and a low level of insulin are required for rapid rates of hepatic ketogenesis to occur, and because a high level of $P_{Ketoacid\ anions}$ can stimulate the secretion of insulin from β-cells of the pancreas in experimental animals, it is possible that secretion of insulin could be an important regulator of the rate of ketoacid production. Nevertheless, when subjects who have fasted for a prolonged period consumed a very small quantity of sugar (7.5 g), they had a marked *and* prolonged fall in $P_{β-HB}$. Hence, although possible, control via $P_{Ketoacid\ anions}$ by varying insulin secretion seems to lack the sensitivity for the desired control to match the rate of production of ketoacids to their rate of removal.

Control by the concentration of H⁺ in plasma

- There are data to suggest that the rate of ketogenesis in the liver might be regulated by changes in the pH and P_{HCO3}.

The administration of an acid load to obese subjects who fasted for a prolonged period led to a marked decline in the $P_{Ketoacid\ anions}$ and in the rate of ketoacid anion excretion. Conversely, both the $P_{Ketoacid\ anions}$ and the rate of ketoacid anion excretion rose appreciably when $NaHCO_3$ was administered to these subjects. Taken together, it is possible that changes in the pH and P_{HCO3} might play an important role in the control of hepatic ketogenesis in this setting. We are not certain about the mechanism(s) involved, but a change in the gating of uncoupler H⁺ channels and/or an increased intramitochondrial negative voltage to accelerate H⁺ entry into these organelles via uncoupler proteins in the presence of a high concentration of fatty acids are distinct possibilities.

QUANTITATIVE ASPECTS OF ETHANOL METABOLISM

- Ethanol is a minor product of fermentation of poorly absorbed carbohydrates by bacteria in the colon. The function of the liver is to remove virtually all the ethanol delivered via the portal vein in a single pass to avoid intoxication.

There is a high activity of alcohol dehydrogenase in the liver, and this enzyme has a high affinity for ethanol. Hence, the liver is poised to clear virtually all the ethanol it receives in a single pass. When ethanol is oxidized, NAD^+ is converted to NADH (see following equation). Hence, the maximum rate of oxidation of ethanol during coupled oxidative phosphorylation depends on the quantity of ADP produced in the liver, and this in turn depends on the carbon product of the pathway (*see margin note*). The stoichiometry for the metabolism of ethanol is shown in the following equations.

$$Ethanol + 2\ NAD^+ \rightarrow acetic\ acid + 2\ NADH$$
$$Acetic\ acid + CoASH + ATP \rightarrow acetyl\text{-}CoA + ATP + AMP$$
$$ATP + AMP \rightarrow 2\ ADP$$
$$2\ Acetyl\text{-}CoA \rightarrow acetoacetate + CoASH$$
$$Acetoacetate + NADH \rightarrow β\text{-}hydroxybutyrate + NAD^+$$

Uncoupling of oxidative phosphorylation is required for a higher rate of metabolism of ethanol. The limit is set by the rate of consumption of O_2 in the liver. NADH is also converted to NAD^+ when

ABBREVIATIONS

$P_{Ketoacid\ anions}$, concentration of ketoacid anions in plasma
$P_{β-HB}$, concentration of β-HB in plasma

QUANTITATIVE ANALYSIS OF ETHANOL METABOLISM IN COUPLED RESPIRATION

PRODUCT	ADP/ ETHANOL	ETHANOL/ 42 ADP*
Acetic acid	6	7
AcAc	3.5	12
β-HB	2	21

*We used the regeneration of 42 ADP to have results in whole numbers. The units are in mmol terms.
AcAc, acetoacetate.

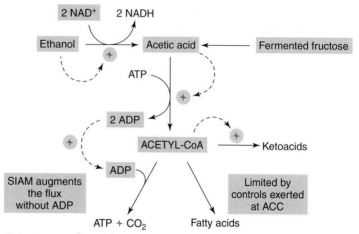

FIGURE 5-15   The production and oxidation of acetic acid. What is relatively unique about acetic acid is that there is no regulation by inhibitory controls for both its production and oxidation. Rather, each pathway exhibits positive feed-forward control, which means that a higher concentration of the substrate, ethanol, increases the formation of acetic acid no matter how high the concentration of acetate as long as NAD^+ is present. In addition, once acetic acid is formed, it promotes its own oxidation in the liver because the conversion of acetate to acetyl-CoA generates ADP, which allows the subsequent oxidation of acetyl-CoA (shown by the *dashed arrows* linked to a + sign). This minimizes the risk of releasing acetate into the systemic circulation.

acetoacetate is converted to β-hydroxybutyrate (see Fig. 5-7); hence, more ethanol can be removed without requiring an increase in O_2 consumption or the regeneration of ADP (Fig. 5-15).

DISCUSSION OF CASES

CASE 5-1: A MAN IS ANXIOUS TO KNOW WHY HE HAS KETOACIDOSIS

(Case presented on page 112)

What makes DKA an unlikely diagnosis?

DKA is unlikely because his $P_{Glucose}$ is in the normal range despite a large intake of sugar, he does not have a history of diabetes mellitus, his effective arterial blood volume is not contracted, and his ketoacidosis resolves without the administration of insulin. Moreover, his plasma insulin level, which was measured during this admission, is in the normal range.

What makes alcoholic ketoacidosis an unlikely diagnosis?

Alcoholic ketoacidosis is unlikely because the patient denies the intake of alcohol and his $P_{Osmolal\ gap}$ is not elevated (although he could have metabolized the alcohol by the time he presented).

What makes ketoacidosis due to starvation or hypoglycemia an unlikely diagnosis?

Starvation and hypoglycemic ketoacidosis are ruled out because he does not have a low $P_{Glucose}$ and he has a large intake of sugar.

How may the patient's intake of sweetened soft drinks contribute to the development of ketoacidosis?

• To develop ketoacidosis, one requires a source of carbon for the synthesis of acetyl-CoA in hepatic mitochondria at a rate that exceeds its removal via oxidation to CO_2 + ATP in the tricarboxylic acid cycle and mechanisms to inhibit the synthesis of long-chain fatty acids from acetyl-CoA.

The source for acetyl-CoA formation in the liver is not fatty acids (there is no lack of insulin) or ethanol. The patient, however, has ingested a large quantity of fructose in sweetened soft drinks and therefore has a very large delivery of acetic acid to his liver (Fig. 5-16). In more detail, fermentation of poorly absorbed carbohydrates by bacteria in the colon normally leads to the absorption of close to 200 mmol/day of acetic acid. Fructose is a major fuel for bacteria in the lower intestinal tract because there are no specific transporters to absorb fructose in the intestinal tract. Nevertheless, some absorption of fructose does occur on one of the intestinal glucose transporters, but this absorption is slow. Hence, a significant proportion of fructose is delivered to the colon, where it is fermented and a major product is acetic acid. The major metabolic fate of this acetic acid is its conversion to acetyl-CoA in the liver, a process that *produces* two ADP from ATP (see previous equations, page 151). In more detail, the first product of breakdown of ATP is AMP, which reacts with a second ATP to yield two ADP.

The usual site of regulation of formation of acetyl-CoA from long-chain fatty acids in the liver is their entry into mitochondria via a carnitine-dependent transport step; it is bypassed because it is not required for the entry of acetic acid into the mitochondria. Therefore, acetyl-CoA is produced at a rapid rate. If the rate of acetyl-CoA production exceeds its possible rate of removal via oxidation,

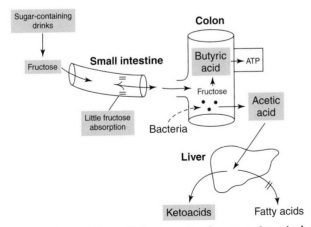

FIGURE 5-16 Fermentation of fructose in the gastrointestinal tract. Consumption of a large amount of sweetened soft drinks provides a very large quantity of fructose, an important substrate for colonic bacteria. Nevertheless, only a small proportion of the fructose is absorbed in the intestinal tract. The butyric acid produced is a fuel for colonic cells, whereas acetic acid is delivered to the liver, where it is converted to fatty acids in the fed state. If there is a large supply of acetic acid and the pathway for its conversion to fatty acids is inhibited, there can be a large production of ketoacids.

ketogenesis may occur if fatty acid synthesis is inhibited. The rate-limiting enzyme for fatty acid synthesis, acetyl-CoA carboxylase, may be inhibited when the level of adrenaline is high (see Fig. 5-5). In fact, this patient is suffering from an anxiety reaction; furthermore he has drunk excessive amounts of soft drinks that contain a large quantity of caffeine, which causes an adrenergic surge (*see margin note*). Therefore, acetyl-CoA carboxylase could have been inhibited.

What other factors might have increased the degree of ketoacidosis?

His brain might have a reduced rate of oxidation of ketoacids because he has cerebral palsy owing to a birth injury and he is also taking a sedative drug.

Is ketoacidosis the only cause of metabolic acidosis in this patient?

His metabolic acidosis is not simply due to ketoacidosis because the $P_{\beta\text{-HB}}$ is only 4.5 mmol/L, yet his $P_{\text{Anion gap}}$ is elevated by 14 mEq/L. Perhaps there is an unusually high concentration of acetoacetate. Alternatively, other short-chain fatty acids produced by bacterial fermentation in the colon could account for the remaining unmeasured anions in plasma.

CASE 5-2: HYPERGLYCEMIA AND ACIDOSIS

(Case presented on page 122)

Are there any other tests that you need to obtain to confirm the diagnosis of DKA?

This is DKA because the patient is in the appropriate age range, the history is strongly suggestive, the physical findings are characteristic, and the laboratory findings are all consistent with this diagnosis. Therefore, additional blood tests for diagnostic purposes are not needed. The possibility of an underlying illness that precipitated DKA should be evaluated further, however.

What are the major threats to Andy's life?

- Hemodynamic collapse and a cardiac arrhythmia are not present.
- The major complication to worry about is cerebral edema.

To minimize the risk of developing cerebral edema, avoid giving a bolus of insulin. Also, a bolus infusion of saline is not needed because Andy is not hemodynamically unstable. Ensure that the $P_{\text{Effective osm}}$ does not fall appreciably for at least the first 15 hours by infusing isotonic saline plus KCl as needed. The other issues in therapy include preventing a cardiac arrhythmia secondary to hypokalemia after insulin acts; neuroglucopenia can be a problem close to 6 hours after insulin acts owing to down-regulation of glucose transporters in the blood-brain barrier by hyperglycemia. Problems related to the underlying illness can be a threat at any time. Be sure to look for signs of stomach emptying. This should be more important once ketoacid anions have been oxidized.

How does his depressed sensorium contribute to the degree of ketoacidosis?

The depressed sensorium can lead to a more severe degree of keto-acidosis because the brain will oxidize fewer ketoacids (see the discussion of Question 5-1, page 156 for a quantitative example).

Should the physician administer NaHCO₃?

NaHCO₃ should not be given, because life-threatening acidemia is *not* present. Expect that the P_{HCO3} will be close to 18 mmol/L after 8 to 12 hours of therapy (see Table 5-5) and the P_{HCO3} will return to normal in 24 to 36 hours providing there is no other factor to diminish the rate of excretion of NH_4^+ in the urine.

CASE 5-3: SAM HAD A DRINKING BINGE YESTERDAY

(Case presented on page 135)

What is Sam's acid-base disorder?

Metabolic acidosis with a high $P_{Anion\ gap}$ is present; nevertheless, the rise in the $P_{Anion\ gap}$ (from 12 mEq/L) exceeds the fall in the P_{HCO3} (from 25 mmol/L). There are several reasons for the high $P_{Anion\ gap}$, ketoacid and possibly L-lactic acid accumulation and a rise in the $P_{Albumin}$ and its negative valence secondary to the contracted ECF volume. Of great importance, one should screen for other toxic alcohols. Metabolic acidosis has not caused acidemia because there is another acid-base disorder—metabolic alkalosis, owing to the loss of HCl in vomiting. The markedly contracted ECF volume also raises the P_{HCO3} because the same amount of HCO_3^- in the ECF compartment is now in a smaller volume (see Fig. 7-1, page 196).

Why does he appear to have a low effective arterial blood volume?

The appreciable degree of contraction of his effective arterial blood volume suggests that he has a deficit of Na^+. Gastric secretions, however, do not contain Na^+. Perhaps he has had a prior deficit of Na^+ and/or has lost Na^+ that had entered the stomach from saliva and/or intestinal secretions (if he has a patent pyloric sphincter). One should keep in mind that there might be redistribution of some of his ECF volume because of pancreatitis or an ileus.

What is the significance of his low $P_{Glucose}$?

The lower than expected $P_{Glucose}$ suggests that he has a chronic nutritional problem that led to a depletion of glycogen in his liver in addition to a metabolic effect of ethanol that led to inhibition of glucose production in the liver (see Fig. 5-10). This should alert the clinician that the patient is likely to have a history of chronic abuse of alcohol and other nutritional deficiencies that could lead to serious consequences during therapy may also be present (see next question).

What are the issues for therapy?

Thiamin deficiency: B vitamins must be added at the outset in therapy in a chronic alcoholic who may be malnourished so that energy metabolism in the brain is not compromised once ketoacids disappear (see Chapter 6, page 172 for more discussion).

ABBREVIATION
dDAVP, desamino, D-arginine Vasopressin

Hypovolemia: The effective arterial blood volume should be reexpanded to avoid a circulatory problem; this should be done rapidly only if there are signs of imminent hemodynamic collapse. The dangers of this therapy are raising the P_{Na} too rapidly (>4 mmol/L/day) and hypokalemia (see below). Administration of dDAVP should be considered at the outset to avoid the development of a water diuresis and thereby, a rapid rise in the P_{Na}. Sam is malnourished and K^+ depleted. Be vigilant about restricting the intake of water while dDAVP acts, which adds a risk of developing osmotic demyelination.

Potassium: Sam might have a large deficit of K^+ if there is a source for this loss together with a poor prior intake of K^+. Despite this deficit, a shift of K^+ out of cells owing to the low levels of insulin could have caused a higher P_K than otherwise expected. First, it is necessary to anticipate a significant shift of K^+ into cells, because restoring the effective arterial blood volume removes the α-adrenergic response, which inhibits the release of insulin from β-cells. Second, the administration of glucose to correct the hypoglycemia stimulates the release of insulin. Hence, sufficient K^+ must be administered to keep the P_K in the normal range. KCl is the preparation of choice. Phosphate will be needed later and it will be available in the diet during the anabolic phase of recovery.

DISCUSSION OF QUESTIONS

5-1 *How many extra H^+ would be added to the body in 24 hours in a 70-kg patient with DKA if that patient had a 25% reduction in the rate of oxygen consumption in the brain (e.g., due to sedation or development of a decreased level of consciousness)?*

The brain normally removes 750 mmol of ketoacids per day. Therefore, a 25% reduction in the rate of oxygen consumption in the brain would lead to an extra H^+ load of about 200 mmol. Comparing this to his normal and current contents of HCO_3^- in ECF compartment, one can quickly see how serious this would be for this patient.

Normal state: ECF volume $(15\,L) \times 25\,mmol/L = 375\,mmol\,HCO_3^-$

During DKA: ECF volume $(12\,L) \times 10\,mmol/L = 120\,mmol\,HCO_3^-$

5-2 *What are the risks and benefits of excreting ketoacid anions plus NH_4^+ in the urine during prolonged fasting?*

From an acid-base point of view, the oxidation of a ketoacid and the excretion of a ketoacid anion with NH_4^+ have the same net effect—there is no net gain or loss of H^+. Nevertheless, there are potential risks and benefits of NH_4^+ excretion in the ketoacidosis of chronic starvation and they are discussed subsequently.

Risk: The source of glutamine for NH_4^+ excretion is derived from endogenous proteins. This leads to the loss of lean body mass. Nevertheless, this does not pose a major problem if the period of starvation is not too long. In addition, by excreting somewhat less urea, there need not be a large loss of lean body mass.

Benefits: These relate to a decreased risk of forming kidney stones.

Raise the urine flow rate: The excretion of NH_4^+ and ketoacid anions increases the number of effective osmoles in the urine, and thus leads to an increase in the urine flow rate when vasopressin acts. Therefore, a judicious rise in the rate of excretion of NH_4^+ plus ketoacid anions prevents the development of excessive oliguria and minimizes the risk of kidney stone formation in a subject who is also deprived of water.

Maintain a urine pH close to 6: The excretion of NH_4^+ provides NH_3, the H^+ acceptor, to maintain urine pH close to 6 when distal H^+ secretion is stimulated by acidemia. Maintaining the urine pH close to 6 is important to minimize the risk of forming uric acid kidney stones (see Fig. 1-19, page 28).

5-3 *If dialysate fluids contain acetate as the source of alkali, acetate anions are converted to β-hydroxybutyric acid. Does this process alter the balance of H^+?*

The answer becomes clear after counting the valences of the substrate and the products; 2 mmol of acetate anions are converted to 1 mmol of β-hydroxybutyrate in the liver. In this process, the product has less anionic charge than its substrates, so H^+ are removed despite the fact that a ketoacid (β-hydroxybutyric acid) is the product.

$$2 \text{ Acetate}^- + 2 \text{ H}^+ \rightarrow \text{β-hydroxybutyrate}^- + \text{H}^+$$

5-4 *How might stomach emptying increase the likelihood of developing cerebral edema in a patient with DKA?*

Cerebral edema becomes a clinical emergency when there is a large gain of water in brain cells, as this represents the largest compartment of water inside the skull. This complication occurs prior to therapy (~5% of cases with cerebral edema) and 5 to 15 hours after therapy begins (~95% of cases with cerebral edema). In both instances, stomach emptying may make an "occult" contribution to this disorder.

Before therapy begins: When the stomach contains water with few effective osmoles (glucose, electrolytes) and some of the stomach contents are expelled into the intestinal tract where the water is absorbed, this will add water to the portal vein. This causes a large fall in the $P_{\text{Effective osm}}$ in the *arterial* plasma. Since the brain has a very rich blood supply (1 L/min) and weighs 1 kg in an adult, brain cells will receive a large water load per unit cell mass, causing them to swell more than other cells in the body. If the swelling is large enough, cerebral edema will develop. The P_{Na} in brachial venous blood will not be low, as muscles extract most of the extra water from arterial blood.

Cerebral edema 5 to 15 hours after therapy begins: Although water without effective osmoles may also be released at any time during therapy for DKA, leading to the development of cerebral edema, a second unique issue exists at this later time: the absorption of water with a high glucose concentration. Since insulin actions can accelerate the oxidation of glucose when fatty acid levels and ketoacid levels have markedly declined, some of this sugar water can be converted to water with few effective osmoles. In addition, since the liver can remove a large proportion of this absorbed glucose when glycogen synthesis is promoted by insulin actions, the net result would be a further fall in the effective osmolality of arterial plasma. As a result, the swelling of brain cells can trigger the development of cerebral edema, especially if the patient has received a bolus of insulin, which may raise intracellular effective osmoles (i.e., Na^+), and too much isotonic saline, which increases the volume of the ECF compartment in the skull (see *margin note*).

GLUCOSE ACTS AS AN EFFECTIVE OSMOLE
If glucose is present in the ECF compartment and cannot be metabolized quickly as a result of low net insulin actions, it behaves as an effective osmole.

GLUCOSE IS NOT AN EFFECTIVE OSMOLE
When glucose plus water is absorbed after stomach emptying, when insulin acts, some of the glucose will be converted to glycogen in liver cells or oxidized to CO_2 plus water in other cells in the body. Therefore, glucose disappearance turns the initial solution with effective osmoles released from the stomach into one that lacks effective osmoles. Under these circumstances, absorbed glucose plus water becomes a risk factor for cerebral edema.

5-5 *How might protein catabolism increase the likelihood of developing cerebral edema in a patient with DKA?*

A sudden rise in intracranial pressure occurs when the quantity of water in the skull increases to a greater extent than the water in the ventricles and cerebrospinal fluid can be "squeezed out" of the skull. We discussed the processes that lead to a gain of water in cells and in the ECF of the brain on page 129. The one compartment that was not considered is the vascular compartment. First, this can expand if there is mechanical obstruction of the veins but not the arteries (pressure on the veins as they cross the margin of bones [e.g., the foramen ovale]). Second, vascular engorgement can occur when there is a vasodilator present (e.g., CO_2 and/or nitric oxide). Focusing on the latter, nitric oxide levels rise when nitric oxide synthase is induced and/or if arginine levels rise in plasma ($P_{Arginine}$). A higher $P_{Arginine}$ in the systemic circulation occurs during a catabolic state. An example of a catabolic state is DKA, especially if it is associated with infection. Moreover, the danger of a rise in intracranial pressure becomes greater when brain cells have become swollen (e.g., a fall in the $P_{Effective\ osm}$ or a bolus of insulin is given) and/or a rise in the ECF volume of the brain (e.g., an excessive infusion of NaCl).

5-6 *Can ketoacidosis and/or L-lactic acidosis be present even though ethanol has disappeared from the plasma?*

Ketoacidosis: Although ethanol levels are elevated when ketoacids are formed initially, the source of acetyl-CoA to form ketoacids can switch to fatty acids if insulin levels remain low. In more detail, contraction of the effective arterial blood volume causes the release of adrenaline, which results in the stimulation of hormone-sensitive lipase and the subsequent release of more fatty acids. In addition, its α-adrenergic effect inhibits the release of insulin while its β-effects inhibit acetyl-CoA carboxylase and thereby, fatty acid synthesis.

L-Lactic acidosis: In the absence of other causes of L-lactic acidosis such as a deficiency of thiamin, the rate of production of L-lactic acid is not high in the liver once the oxidation of ethanol stops, because this causes the $NADH:NAD^+$ ratio in the liver to fall (see Fig. 5-10). Therefore, in the absence of other causes for L-lactic acidosis, L-lactic acidosis is *not* present in the absence of ethanol.

5-7 *What might be the biologic role of increased uncoupler proteins in skeletal muscle during prolonged fasting?*

A puzzling feature of uncoupler proteins in skeletal muscle is that it is increased 5- to 10-fold during prolonged starvation. On the one hand, this seems to be counterintuitive because energy is wasted when it is most needed. On the other hand, inducing UCPs in starvation could lead to a lower concentration of oxygen and electrons in cells (see Chapter 6, page 174 for more discussion). The beneficial effect of uncoupling in this setting would be to lower the concentration of reactive oxygen species when flux through the electron transport system is low and as a result, reduces damage to vital organs. The price to pay is a small increase in the catabolism of stored triglycerides. In the context of a system to minimize the toxicity of reactive oxygen species, the potential benefits would greatly outweigh the small decrease in fat mass because on average, more than a 2-month supply of triglycerides are stored in the human body.

There may be an important role for uncoupler proteins in skeletal muscle immediately after a sprint. The mechanisms involved include the large blood flow rate (increases "stirring" to accelerate diffusion of oxygen, as well as the delivery of oxygen) and a progressive decline in the rate of consumption of oxygen. As a result, the P_{O_2} in skeletal muscle cells should rise. In addition, there is a high availability of reduced members of the electron transport system, the most important one being the semialdehyde form of coenzyme Q. In this setting, the rate of production of reactive oxygen species can rise sufficiently to exceed their rate of removal. On the other hand, increased flux through these uncoupler H^+ channels could diminish this rate of formation of reactive oxygen species by lowering both the P_{O_2} and the semialdehyde form of coenzyme Q. Of interest, the concentration of urate in plasma is a component of this defense mechanism against reactive oxygen species (see the discussion of Case 6-3, page 188).

chapter

6

Metabolic Acidosis: Acid Gain Types

Introduction

The focus in this chapter is on metabolic acidosis due to the accumulation of acids. Two of the disorders causing this type of metabolic acidosis are not discussed in this chapter. First, ketoacidosis has been discussed in Chapter 5 because a very strong emphasis on basic biochemistry is needed to understand its pathophysiology. Second, although the metabolic acidosis due to toluene intoxication is caused by overproduction of hippuric acid, the hippurate anion is uniquely secreted into the urine, which results in an indirect loss of NaHCO$_3$. Therefore, it has been discussed along with other disorders that lead to hyperchloremic metabolic acidosis in Chapter 4, page 77.

OBJECTIVES

- To provide an understanding of the pathophysiology and an approach to the patient with metabolic acidosis due to the accumulation of new acids.
- To emphasize the importance of establishing the specific cause of the metabolic acidosis because the threats posed with each disorder and those that may arise during therapy are different.

CASE 6-1: PATRICK IS IN FOR A SHOCK

(Case discussed on page 186)

Patrick, a large muscular man, has a long history of alcohol abuse. He was perfectly well until he drank a solution containing an unknown substance close to 6 hours ago. In the past hour, he began to feel very unwell. He denied blood loss, excessive sweating, vomiting, or appreciable diarrhea. His clinical condition deteriorated very quickly. On admission to the hospital, his blood pressure was 80/50 mm Hg, pulse rate was 150 beats per minute, jugular venous pressure was very low, and respirations were rapid and deep. His electrocardiogram revealed changes due to hyperkalemia with tall, peaked T waves. Laboratory data are provided in the following table. Shortly after he was given intravenous calcium gluconate for the emergency treatment of hyperkalemia, his blood pressure rose and he felt much better.

pH	([H$^+$] nmol/L)	7.20 (64)	Na$^+$	mmol/L	143
Pco$_2$ (arterial)	mm Hg	25	K$^+$	mmol/L	6.3
HCO$_3^-$	mmol/L	11	Cl$^-$	mmol/L	99
Glucose	mg/dL (mmol/L)	180 (10)	Albumin	g/dL (g/L)	4.5 (45)
Creatinine	mg/dL (µmol/L)	1.8 (160)	BUN (Urea)	mg/dL (mmol/L)	8.4 (3.0)
Calcium (total)	mg/dL (mmol/L)	10 (2.5)	L-lactate	mmol/L	2.0

Questions (see margin notes for hints)

Judging from the time frame, which acid has accumulated?
Why did his blood pressure fall so precipitously?
Why did he have an elevated P_K?
Why did the intravenous calcium cause the rapid recovery?

"FAST" METABOLIC ACIDOSIS
H$^+$ are produced at a very rapid rate from endogenous sources only during tissue hypoxia; the acid produced is L-lactic acid (see the discussion of Question 6-2, page 189).

CASE 6-2: METABOLIC ACIDOSIS DUE TO DIARRHEA

(Case discussed on page 188)

One week ago, this 40-year-old man began to have several bouts of diarrhea during a trip abroad. He was treated with an antimotility drug and an antibiotic. In the past 24 hours, however, his diarrhea has increased. His only intake has been popsicles to satisfy his desire for cold liquids. On physical examination, he appeared very ill and was confused. He had poor balance and an ataxic gait. He did not have signs of a significant decrease in his effective arterial blood volume.

DANGER CAUSED BY THE NEW ANIONS
Anions of the added acids may have properties that pose threats to the patient.

His abdomen was distended and bowel sounds were scanty. There were no masses or enlarged organs. Acetone was not detected on his breath, and the urine test for ketones was negative. His arterial blood gas revealed a pH of 7.22 and a P_{CO_2} of 27 mm Hg. His P_{HCO3} was 11 mmol/L. Other data are provided in this table.

		PLASMA			PLASMA
Na	mmol/L	138	K	mmol/L	3.8
Cl	mmol/L	101	Glucose	mg/dL (mmol/L)	108 (6)
Albumin	g/dL (g/L)	3.8 (38)	Osmolality	mOsm/L	289
BUN	mg/dL	14	Creatinine	mg/dL	1.2
Urea	mmol/L	5.0	Creatinine	μmol/L	103

Question

What is the basis for metabolic acidosis?

PART A
GENERAL CONSIDERATIONS

MAJOR THREATS IN THE PATIENT WITH METABOLIC ACIDOSIS

• The threats to the patient depend on the basis of the metabolic acidosis. Therefore, emphasis in therapy is to deal with the underlying cause of the metabolic acidosis rather than focusing only on the H^+ load.

There are a number of threats for the patient with metabolic acidosis due to added acids (Table 6-1; *see margin note*). For example, although L-lactic acid may be produced at an extremely rapid rate during hypoxia, failure to regenerate ATP at a sufficiently rapid rate in vital organs, rather than the metabolic acidosis, is the most important danger for the patient. A deficiency of certain B vitamins leads to the accumulation of L-lactic acid; the most important one is vitamin B_1 (thiamin), which could cause serious problems because thiamin is

CAUTION
• It is important to recognize that the term *metabolic acidosis* is not a specific diagnosis—rather it represents common laboratory findings in a number of different disorders.
• Hence, one cannot "treat metabolic acidosis." Rather, one must decide what is the basis for metabolic acidosis in an individual patient, as this defines the actual diagnosis, which has specific implications for the care of your patient.
• Even in a diagnostic category such as L-lactic acidosis or pyroglutamic acidosis, the diagnosis has not yet been defined, as there are different mechanisms at play to explain why each of these acids has accumulated and what is the danger for an individual patient.

TABLE 6-1 **THREATS TO LIFE ASSOCIATED WITH THE CAUSE OF THE ADDITION OF ACIDS**

Although other emergencies may be present, only those that are specific to the cause of metabolic acidosis are included in this table.

ADDED ACID	MAJOR THREAT
• L-Lactic acidosis due to hypoxia	• Inadequate delivery of O_2 to vital organs, causing ATP depletion
• Diabetic ketoacidosis in children	• Cerebral edema
• Alcoholic ketoacidosis with thiamin deficiency	• Wernicke's encephalopathy
• Toxin-induced metabolic acidosis (e.g., methanol)	• Toxic aldehyde metabolites (e.g., formaldehyde)
• Metabolic acidosis with a high P_K (e.g., renal failure)	• Cardiac arrhythmia
• Metabolic acidosis with a low P_K (e.g., glue sniffing)	• Cardiac arrhythmia, respiratory failure
• Pyroglutamic acidosis	• Accumulation of reactive oxygen species

required for aerobic production of ATP in brain cells during glucose oxidation. In other causes of metabolic acidosis due to added acids, such as in the patient with methanol or ethylene glycol intoxication, the toxic aldehydes formed during acid metabolism pose the major danger because they may cause blindness in the former and be associated with acute renal failure in the latter.

There are also less well-appreciated causes of metabolic acidosis in which there is a danger for the patient that must be recognized promptly. For example, in patients with pyroglutamic acidosis, the danger results from the accumulation of reactive oxygen species (ROS), whereas in patients with D-lactic acidosis, a number of compounds produced by intestinal bacteria can cause cerebral dysfunction. In yet other causes of metabolic acidosis, the major threat may be an associated abnormality in the P_K.

BUFFERING OF H⁺ IN A PATIENT WITH METABOLIC ACIDOSIS

- The most important principle is that H^+ should be prevented from binding to proteins in brain cells. To achieve this, these H^+ should be forced to react with HCO_3^-.

When H^+ bind to proteins in cells, this alters their charge and perhaps their shape and functions; this is particularly detrimental if it occurs in vital organs (e.g., brain and heart). To prevent this "bad" form of buffering, H^+ must be "forced" to bind to HCO_3^- in the extracellular fluid (ECF) and intracellular fluid (ICF) compartments of skeletal muscle, as this is where the bulk of this H^+ removal exists. For this to occur, the P_{CO_2} in capillary blood delivered to skeletal muscle must be low. Two steps are needed to achieve this objective: an appropriate fall in the arterial P_{CO_2} and a high enough blood flow to skeletal muscle relative to the rate of production of CO_2. If this fails, the blood pH falls and more H^+ are forced to bind to all buffers in the brain, including its intracellular proteins (see Fig. 1-8, page 14). Therefore, an important aim in therapy in patients with metabolic acidosis is to improve ventilation *and* to restore blood flow to skeletal muscles to lower their capillary (as reflected by the venous) P_{CO_2}.

ISSUES IN DIAGNOSIS

- The clue that raises suspicion that metabolic acidosis is caused by an added acid is an increase in the $P_{Anion\ gap}$ (see page 47).

One must always be aware of the fact that hypoalbuminemia or another cause for a spurious reduction in the $P_{Anion\ gap}$ (e.g., cationic proteins in a patient with multiple myeloma or lithium intoxication) might lower the baseline value of the $P_{Anion\ gap}$ (see page 47).

Metabolic acidosis due to added acids is often associated with a significant decrease in the effective arterial blood volume. If not, suspect a toxin-induced form of metabolic acidosis (methanol or ethylene glycol), renal failure, or L-lactic acidosis due to slow removal of L-lactic acid.

PART B
INDIVIDUAL DISORDERS
L-LACTIC ACIDOSIS

Biochemical principles

There are several principles of metabolic control that provide the background information to develop a classification of the different types of L-lactic acidosis.

Kinetics of enzymatic reactions

A rise in the concentration of L-lactate⁻ and H⁺ can be caused by an increased rate of production and/or a decreased rate of removal of L-lactic acid. Although both of these pathways are involved in most cases, usually one predominates (Fig. 6-1). To understand how a significant degree of L-lactic acidosis may develop, the kinetics of the production of L-lactic acid and the removal of L-lactic acid should be examined. There are two major ways to increase the rate of a reaction: Either raise the concentration of its substrate as long as the enzyme that catalyzes this reaction is not saturated with that substrate, or increase the activity of the enzyme (Fig. 6-2).

Substrate concentration. In simplest terms, the rate (velocity) of that process increases when the concentration of its substrates rises until that enzyme becomes saturated with its substrates. Once saturated, the velocity of that reaction is its maximum velocity (V_{max}).

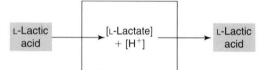

FIGURE 6-1 H⁺ balance in steady state. The *rectangle* represents L-lactic acid in the body, with its production shown *on the left* and its removal pathways *on the right*. To understand how balance is achieved, a quantitative analysis of rates of both the input and output of L-lactic acid is required.

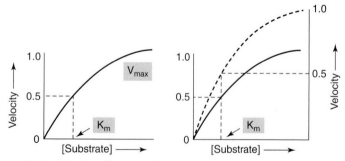

FIGURE 6-2 Kinetic of enzymatic reactions. The substrate concentration is depicted along the x-axis, and the velocity of the reaction is shown on the y-axis. In the *left portion*, the substrate concentration that causes a velocity that is one half the V_{max} is the K_m. When the substrate concentration increases, the velocity of the reaction rises until the enzyme becomes saturated (i.e., the V_{max} is achieved). In the *right portion*, the V_{max} is higher (*dashed line*) when the amount of active enzyme is increased. Notice that the K_m did not change when the V_{max} rose.

ABBREVIATIONS
V_{max}, maximum velocity
K_m, the substrate concentration for a reaction that permits its rate to be half the V_{max}

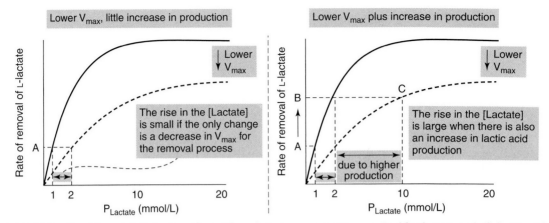

FIGURE 6-3 Two-hit model of L-lactic acidosis. The substrate concentration required for the removal of L-lactic acid ($P_{L\text{-}lactate}$) is depicted on the x-axis, and the velocity of all reactions that remove L-lactic acid is shown on the y-axis (the highest velocity of removal is called the V_{max}). When there is damage to the liver, for example, the total enzyme activity to remove L-lactic acid is lower (i.e., the V_{max} is lower, depicted by the *dashed curve*). In the *left portion of the figure*, there is only a decrease in the V_{max} of the removal of L-lactic acid. Since the removal pathways are not saturated with their substrate, a somewhat higher $P_{L\text{-}lactate}$ is needed to remove the usual production of L-lactic acid. As shown in the *right portion of the figure*, there is an initial increase in the rate of production of L-lactic acid (i.e., from its rate of production [A] to its current rate of production [B] on the y-axis); all the extra L-lactic acid is removed in steady state. When the V_{max} is lower (*dashed curve*), a much larger rise in the $P_{L\text{-}lactate}$ is needed to remove all of the L-lactic acid that is produced (*site C*).

The substrate concentration that permits a velocity of a reaction to be equal to one half the V_{max} is called the K_m.

Enzyme activity. If the concentration of substrate is not rate limiting, the V_{max} of a reaction depends on how much enzyme is present in active form. If the amount of the active form of the enzyme increases twofold, the V_{max} of that reaction doubles; the converse is also true.

Based on this analysis of the kinetics of enzymatic reactions, one can deduce three circumstances for the development of a marked degree of L-lactic acidosis (Fig. 6-3). First, there is a marked increase in the rate of production of L-lactic acid that exceeds the V_{max} for its rate of removal. Second, there is a marked decrease in the V_{max} of L-lactic acid removal without an appreciable increase in its production. Third, a combination of a small decrease in the rate of L-lactic acid removal along with a small increase in its rate of production can lead to a marked increase in its degree of L-lactic acidosis—this is likely the scenario in most cases of chronic L-lactic acidosis, in which the liver can still remove all the L-lactic acid that is produced but a higher $P_{L\text{-}lactate}$ is required.

ADP is also a substrate for glycolysis

- In virtually every example of an increased production of L-lactic acid from glucose, the cause is a rise in the concentration of ADP in cells as the result of increased conversion of ATP to ADP and inorganic phosphate.

There are four facts to appreciate. First, a low availability of ADP in cells limits the conversion of glucose to pyruvic or L-lactic acid because ADP is a *substrate* for this pathway. Second, when work is being performed, ATP is hydrolyzed and the product is ADP (Fig. 6-4). Third, in this setting, if there is a problem converting ADP to ATP in mitochondria (e.g., hypoxia, uncoupling of oxidative phosphorylation, inhibition of electron transport), a high ADP concentration in the cytosol drives the glycolytic pathway, which regenerates ATP and

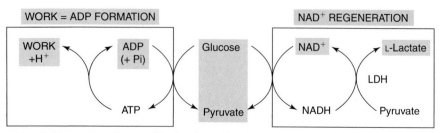

FIGURE 6-4 Metabolic process of anaerobic glycolysis. The glycolytic pathway (glucose to pyruvate) is shown in *the shaded area in the central portion.* There are two other substrates involved, ADP and NAD⁺. As shown to *the left*, the metabolic process begins with work, which stimulates glycolysis by supplying its limiting cofactor, ADP. As shown to *the right*, as soon as the concentrations of pyruvate and NADH rise, this pyruvate is converted to the "carbon end product" L-lactate, plus NAD⁺, thereby restoring this other substrate so that glycolysis can continue. Hence, control is clearly by the rate of work, which leads to the formation of ADP. LDH, lactate dehydrogenase.

HYPOXIA

Be careful when this term is used, as it can have several different meanings.

- In energy metabolism, it reflects a demand for O_2 that exceeds the delivery of O_2 to support a given rate of ATP regeneration in an organ.
- In other circumstances, it implies that the concentration of O_2 is low enough to minimize the binding of O_2 to transcription factors regulated by oxygen tension, hypoxia-inducable factor [HIF − 1 α + β], but not necessarily low enough to compromise the regeneration of ATP.

ABBREVIATIONS

NAD⁺ and NADH: the oxidized and reduced forms of the cofactor nicotinamide adenine dinucleotide, respectively (see Chapter 5, page 144 for more discussion of their role in metabolism).

NAD⁺ AND ADP ARE INTERRELATED

In glycolysis, NAD⁺ is consumed and NADH is produced. This NADH is oxidized in the mitochondrial electron transport system. In this process, ADP is consumed and ATP plus NAD⁺ are formed (see Fig. 5-12, page 145).

rapidly produces a large quantity of L-lactic acid. Fourth, because there is such a tiny concentration of ADP in cells, it takes only a 1% conversion of ATP to ADP to double the concentration of free ADP and thus double the glycolytic rate.

Metabolic processes involved in the production of L-lactic acid during ethanol oxidation

- When ethanol is oxidized in the liver, NADH is formed.
- If pyruvate can be formed *without* NADH (e.g., during the metabolism of certain amino acids), there is an increased production of L-lactic acid without a need for ADP production.

During the metabolism of alcohols such as ethanol in the liver, the concentration of NADH rises, and this causes an increase in the conversion of pyruvate to L-lactate and thus a higher concentration of L-lactic acid (Fig. 6-5). Notwithstanding, the precursor of pyruvate must *not* be glucose, because the pathway must produce pyruvate *without* NADH; otherwise the pyruvate + NADH would already have been converted to L-lactate (see Fig. 6-4). This source of pyruvate is most likely the conversion of amino acids (e.g., alanine) to pyruvate. It is also important to notice that although NAD⁺ is a substrate for both glycolysis and ethanol metabolism, it is the availability of NAD⁺ and not ADP that limits the oxidation of ethanol in a direct sense. The concentrations of ADP and NAD⁺ are, however, interrelated (*see margin note*).

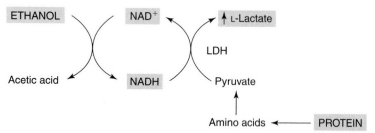

FIGURE 6-5 Production of L-lactic acid during ethanol metabolism. The substrates of this metabolic process are shown in uppercase letters in the *green rectangles.* When ethanol is oxidized in the liver, the control of acetic acid production is not via work (ADP); rather it is via the availability of NAD⁺, and the accumulation of NADH (as shown in the *green rectangle*) drives the production of L-lactate. If a supply of pyruvate is present, it is converted to L-lactate via lactate dehydrogenase (LDH).

Rate of anaerobic glycolysis

- This pathway produces ATP at a much faster rate than in the aerobic oxidation of glucose, even though it yields only 2 molecules of ATP per glucose, whereas the complete oxidation of glucose yields 38 molecules of ATP per glucose consumed (*see margin note*).

Because the rate of glycolysis can greatly exceed the rate of oxidation of pyruvate in mitochondria, L-lactic acid can accumulate very quickly when the concentration of ADP rises in cells (e.g., L-lactic acid is produced in increased amounts when the body must regenerate ATP without oxygen). The bottom line is that 1 H$^+$ plus 1 L-lactate anion are produced per ATP regenerated from glucose (*see margin note*).

Although it seems "obvious" that H$^+$ are produced during flux through the glycolytic pathway (the second step in the equations at the end of this paragraph), H$^+$ are actually formed during the hydrolysis of ATP when work is performed (the initial step that generates ADP and augments the rate of glycolysis). This misunderstanding is clarified when one includes the formation and hydrolysis of ATP and the valences of ADP, ATP, and inorganic phosphate in the overall process.

$$2\ ATP^{4-} \rightarrow 2\ (ADP + Pi)^{5-} + 2\ H^+ + \text{biologic work}$$

$$\text{Glucose} + 2\ (ADP + Pi)^{5-} \rightarrow 2\ \text{L-lactate}^- + 2\ ATP^{4-}$$

$$\text{Sum: Glucose} \rightarrow \text{biologic work} + 2\ H^+ + 2\ \text{L-lactate}^-$$

In a patient with acute L-lactic acidosis due to a low availability of oxygen, there is suddenly a very rapid rate of production of this acid because ADP must be converted to ATP rapidly enough to match the conversion of ATP to ADP when work is performed. This imbalance is short-lived because the marked rise in the concentration of H$^+$ causes one of the key enzymes in glycolysis to lose all of its activity (see equation). Although this minimizes the drop in intracellular pH, there is a huge price to pay because this may lead to an "energy crisis," especially in cells of vital organs (e.g., brain).

$$\text{PFK} - 1\ (\text{active form}) + H^+ \rightarrow \text{PFK} - 1\ (\text{inactive form})$$
(tetramer) (4 monomers)
$$\text{PFK} = \text{phosphofructokinase}$$

A high rate of glycolysis may occur in the presence of an adequate supply of oxygen if there is a defect in the electron transport system or if there is a very high rate of uncoupling of oxidative phosphorylation because in these conditions, ADP cannot be converted back to ATP quickly enough (causes are listed in Table 6-2).

Rate of removal of L-lactic acid

There are two major ways to remove L-lactic acid—first, oxidation where the critical enzyme is pyruvate dehydrogenase (PDH); and second, conversion to glucose in the liver and the kidney where the critical enzymes are pyruvate carboxylase (PC) and phosphoenolpyruvate carboxykinase (PEPCK; Fig. 6-6).

Oxidation of L-lactic acid. To oxidize 1 mmol of L-lactic acid, 3 mmol of oxygen must be consumed (18 mmol of ATP must be

---

ATP IS REGENERATED AT A FASTER RATE DURING ANAEROBIC GLYCOLYSIS THAN AEROBIC METABOLISM
To illustrate the validity of this statement, think about the facts that during a sprint ATP is generated anaerobically and that the sprinter starts from a complete stop and runs faster than the 1500-meter runner.

RATE OF PRODUCTION OF L-LACTIC ACID DURING ANOXIA
- In an adult at rest, 72 mmol/min ATP are regenerated from ADP during aerobic metabolism. If all these ATP molecules are regenerated during anoxia, there would be a net production of 72 mmol of H$^+$ per minute.
- To place this number in perspective, the entire ECF HCO$_3^-$ pool size is 375 mmol. Hence, this amount of HCO$_3^-$ would be used in close to 5 minutes of anoxia.

TABLE 6-2 **CLASSIFICATION OF L-LACTIC ACIDOSIS**

Although most patients have elements of both overproduction and reduced removal of L-lactic acidosis, one of these elements is the predominant cause of the metabolic acidosis.

A. Due predominantly to overproduction of L-lactic acid

- **Inadequate delivery of O_2**
  - Low cardiac output
  - Shunting of blood past organs (e.g., sepsis)
- **Excessive demand for oxygen**
  - Major seizure
  - Mini-seizures (e.g., isoniazid causing vitamin B_6 deficiency)
- **Increased production of L-lactic acid in absence of hypoxia**
  - Ongoing production of NADH in the liver (e.g., metabolism of ethanol)
  - Decreased pyruvate dehydrogenase activity (e.g., thiamin deficiency, inborn errors of metabolism)
  - Compromised mitochondrial electron transport system (e.g., cyanide, riboflavin deficiency, inborn errors affecting the electron transport system)
  - Excessive degree of uncoupling of oxidative phosphorylation (e.g., phenformin)

B. Due predominantly to reduced removal of L-lactate

- Liver failure (e.g., severe acute viral hepatitis, shock liver, drugs)

C. Due to a combination of reduced removal and overproduction of L-lactic acid

- Antiretroviral drugs (inhibition of mitochondrial electron transport plus hepatic steatosis)
- Metastatic tumors (especially large tumors with hypoxic areas plus liver involvement)

ATP REGENERATION DURING OXIDATION OF LACTATE
- 3 mmol ATP are formed per atom of oxygen consumed. Therefore, 6 mmol of ATP are formed per mmol O_2 consumed.
- Oxidation of 1 mmol L-lactate results in the consumption of 3 mmol of O_2 (3 mmol O_2 × 6 ATP = 18 mmol of ATP formed).

formed; *see margin note*). Hence, if (theoretically) all organs could be "persuaded" to oxidize the L-lactate anions to yield 100% of their requirement to regenerate ATP, only 4 mmol of L-lactate anion could be oxidized per minute at rest (because only 72 mmol of ADP are available per minute; *see margin note on page 166*).

$$\text{L-Lactate}^- + H^+ + 3\,O_2 + 18\,(ADP + P_i) \rightarrow 18\,ATP + 3\,CO_2 + 3\,H_2O$$

Gluconeogenesis. When L-lactate is converted to glucose in the liver and in the kidney cortex, ATP is consumed. The

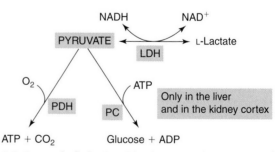

FIGURE 6-6 Removal of L-lactic acid. L-Lactate and pyruvate are linked by an enzyme-catalyzed step, L-lactate dehydrogenase (LDH), which is present in such a large amount that these two anions can be interconverted very quickly; thus, their concentrations are determined by the ratio of NADH to NAD+ in the cytosol of cells. The key compound in cells that undergoes further metabolism is pyruvate, which is shown in the *green shaded area*. There are two major fates of pyruvate; first, it can be fully oxidized in the Krebs cycle if pyruvate dehydrogenase (PDH) is active; second, it can be converted to glucose where the initial step is catalyzed by pyruvate carboxylase (PC).

maximum rate of L-lactate removal is close to 4 mmol/min in each organ. This calculation is determined by the rate at which the liver and the kidneys consume oxygen (2 mmol/min in each organ = 12 mmol ATP used per minute). This makes the assumption that all available ADP are used in gluconeogenesis and no other biologic work is performed, which is extremely unlikely.

$$L\text{-Lactate}^- + H^+ + 3\ ATP \to 0.5\ glucose$$

Clinical implications of these principles of biochemistry

1. Although both overproduction and underutilization of L-lactic acid result in L-lactic acidosis, their quantitative dimensions may differ by an order of magnitude (Fig. 6-7). The rate of production of L-lactic acid during severe hypoxia can be so high that it cannot be overcome by accelerating the rate of removal of L-lactic acid.

2. If the degree of loss of viable liver mass or the decrease in activity of the key enzymes that control the removal of pyruvate (PDH, PC, and/or PEPCK) is not very large, the presence of a significant degree of L-lactic acidosis implies that there is also a component of overproduction of this acid (see Fig. 6-3).

3. The major clinical scenario in which L-lactic acidosis is caused by an inadequate delivery of oxygen to tissues to permit a rapid enough regeneration of ATP is cardiogenic shock. This is the basis for the common clinical classification of L-lactic acidosis in which lactic acidosis is due to hypoxia, called *type A L-lactic acidosis*, while all the other causes are lumped together as *type B L-lactic acidosis*. We are not enthusiastic about this classification because cardiogenic shock is such an obvious clinical diagnosis. Furthermore, this ignores the fact that among patients in the overproduction type of L-lactic acidosis are those in which the pathophysiology also results from the accumulation of ADP in cells but for causes other than hypoxia (see Table 6-2).

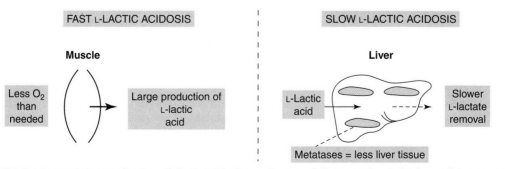

FIGURE 6-7 Fast and slow production of L-lactic acid. The production of L-lactic acid in skeletal muscle is very rapid during hypoxia, as depicted in the *left portion* (e.g., during a sprint). This rate exceeds the rate at which L-lactate can be removed in the liver as well as in the kidneys (not shown). Slower removal of L-lactic acid is depicted in the *right portion*. In this setting, a process destroys much of the liver (e.g., with hepatic metastases). Even though L-lactic acid production is not increased to a major extent, this L-lactic acid cannot be removed as fast as usual because of the reduced number of functioning liver cells. As a result, there is a slow accumulation of L-lactic acid until its removal rate equals its production rate and a steady state will be reached with a higher $P_{Lactate}$.

Clinical settings with primary overproduction of L-lactic acid

Inadequate delivery of O_2

- The most common clinical setting for rapid overproduction of L-lactic acid is a sudden, marked decrease in cardiac output.

Other examples of conditions that lead to an inadequate delivery of O_2 to tissues include acute airway obstruction, hemorrhagic shock, and carbon monoxide poisoning. In patients with sepsis, there can be circulatory disturbances that lead to tissue hypoxia in energy terms (both decreased delivery of oxygen and impaired extraction of oxygen).

When L-lactic acidosis is associated with a decreased effective arterial blood volume, in addition to an "energy crisis" due to failure to regenerate ATP, there is a "tissue form" of respiratory acidosis (see Chapter 1, page 14). As a result, the bicarbonate buffer system fails to remove enough H^+; hence, more H^+ bind to intracellular proteins in vital organs (e.g., brain cells), which may impair their functions.

Cardiogenic shock. This diagnosis is very obvious and usually results from a myocardial infarction during which the blood pressure falls markedly and the cardiac output is extremely low. This diagnosis must be made quickly because the failure to generate ATP rapidly enough in vital organs is lethal in a matter of a few minutes.

Treatment. The aim of therapy is to increase the blood flow and thereby delivery of oxygen to vital organs by whatever means needed to do so—no other therapy saves the patient if the cardiac output is not significantly improved. Therefore, the crucial issue in therapy is to improve the ability of the patient to regenerate ATP in vital organs rather than to be overly concerned with lowering the concentration of H^+ per se. Measures to improve hemodynamics to restore adequate cardiac output and tissue perfusion (e.g., ionotropic agents) are absolutely critical if there is an adequate concentration of oxygen in blood. In patients with an inadequate circulating volume, it is necessary to administer blood and/or solutions containing Na^+ and/or albumin, depending on the cause. If the problem is continuing poor myocardial contractility despite the use of ionotropic agents, one may need to use an intra-aortic balloon pump.

NaHCO$_3$ therapy in these forms of L-lactic acidosis. The use of $NaHCO_3$ during marked hypoxia is of no value because of the magnitude of the H^+ load. Nevertheless, $NaHCO_3$ may "buy a few minutes" to improve myocardial function in cases in which hypoxia is marginal and potentially reversible, but this issue remains controversial (*see margin note*). The Na^+ load accompanying the HCO_3^- poses a major limit to this type of therapy, especially in patients with cardiogenic shock and pulmonary edema. Removal of the Na^+ load by dialysis is usually not feasible because of hemodynamic instability.

ALKALI ADMINISTRATION AND REMOVAL OF INHIBITION OF PHOSPHOFRUCTOKINASE
Removal of H^+ with alkali can increase the flux in glycolysis and hence increase the rate of regeneration of ATP, providing that it leads to deinhibition of the key glycolytic enzyme phosphofructokinase-1. The "price to pay," however, is 1 mmol of H^+ per 1 mmol of ATP generated (i.e., per mmol of L-lactic acid produced). This can be of benefit only if it occurs in vital organs and if the H^+ formed are titrated by the bicarbonate buffer system and thus do not bind to intracellular proteins.

Excessive demand for oxygen

- L-Lactic acidosis due to excessive demand for oxygen occurs during seizures or extreme exercise.
- Another example is the mini-seizures that cause L-lactic acidosis in some patients given isoniazid.

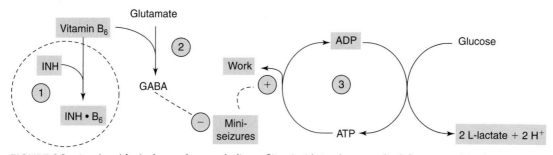

FIGURE 6-8 L-**Lactic acidosis due to the metabolism of isoniazid.** As shown in the *left portion* of the figure, the addition of isoniazid (INH) removes vitamin B_6, the necessary cofactor to synthesize GABA. Hence the major cause of L-lactic acidosis is a large increase in the production of L-lactic acid during a series of mini-seizures, owing to a deficiency of vitamin B_6.

Isoniazid. When muscle contraction is markedly increased, there can be a component of anaerobic glycolysis in which L-lactic acid is formed more rapidly than it can be removed. An example is the L-lactic acidosis seen at times in patients taking isoniazid, one of the drugs commonly used to treat tuberculosis. The mechanism of the L-lactic acidosis caused by this drug is a markedly increased muscle twitching (mini-seizures; Fig. 6-8). This may be due to the rapid development of vitamin B_6 (pyridoxine) deficiency because of the formation of an isoniazid–vitamin B_6 complex, pyridoxal-isonicotinyl-hydrazone, via a nonenzymatic reaction. This leads to a diminished rate of formation of an inhibitory neurotransmitter and increased muscle excitability (*see margin note*).

The second factor that could contribute to the degree of L-lactic acidosis in these patients is iron deficiency caused by chelation of iron by the isoniazid–vitamin B_6 complex. This could result in an electron transport defect and hence a higher production of L-lactic acid, as well as a slower rate of its removal via gluconeogenesis because of the need for iron as a cofactor in both processes.

Treatment. A deficiency of vitamin B_6 is likely to be responsible for the isoniazid-associated mini-seizure and thereby L-lactic acidosis because almost invariably there is a rapid cessation of the seizure state and recovery from L-lactic acidosis in response to a large dose of intravenous vitamin B_6.

Clinical settings with increased production of L-lactic acid in the absence of hypoxia

Ethanol

These patients usually have a mild degree of L-lactic acidosis (~5 mmol/L). This reflects the more reduced $NADH:NAD^+$ ratio because of ongoing production of NADH due to ethanol metabolism that is largely restricted to the liver (see Fig. 6-5). Other organs in the body are capable of oxidizing the L-lactate because they lack alcohol dehydrogenase and thus do not have a high $NADH:NAD^+$ ratio.

A more severe degree of L-lactic acidosis suggests that there is L-lactic acid overproduction that may be caused by hypoxia (resulting from shock due to gastrointestinal bleeding, for example), thiamin deficiency, seizures (alcohol withdrawal, delirium tremens, and/or a central nervous system lesion), and/or L-lactic acid underutilization due to severe liver disease due to acute alcoholic hepatitis that may be superimposed on chronic liver disease that is often associated with chronic alcohol use (e.g., fatty liver, cirrhosis).

VITAMIN B_6 AND SEIZURES
- Pyridoxal phosphate is a cofactor for the enzyme glutamic acid decarboxylase in which glutamate is converted to the inhibitory neurotransmitter γ-aminobutyric acid (GABA). Therefore, vitamin B_6 deficiency leads to a decrease in GABA, which could result in increased excitability and thereby to increased muscle twitching and at times seizures and the production of L-lactic acid.
- Vitamin B_6 deficiency can be suspected by finding a low activity of alanine aminotransferase in erythrocytes.
- Patients on chronic hemodialysis are at increased risk for isoniazid-induced toxicity because they tend to have lower levels of vitamin B_6 as a result of the efficient removal of this vitamin by hemodialysis.

THERAPY WITH VITAMIN B_6
The recommended dose of vitamin B_6 for treatment of isoniazid toxicity is the same gram amount as the isoniazid ingested. If the amount of isoniazid ingested is not known, the recommended approach is to give 5 grams of pyridoxine over 2 hours.

Thiamin deficiency

- L-Lactic acidosis due to thiamin deficiency occurs most often in malnourished chronic alcoholics (see Chapter 5, page 141).
- The encephalopathy in patients with thiamin deficiency has two components—depletion of ATP and binding of H^+ from the production of L-lactic acid to proteins in brain cells.
- A possible important factor in the encephalopathy is alcohol withdrawal syndrome (i.e., delirium tremens) because there is likely an increased demand for ATP regeneration, which requires an increased rate of oxidation of glucose, but it cannot be achieved after ketoacids disappear.

RATIONALE FOR THE DEVELOPMENT OF WERNICKE'S ENCEPHALOPATHY

The maximum rate of ATP regeneration suddenly becomes insufficient to meet the demand for ATP formation when pyruvate dehydrogenase has a low activity. Nevertheless, this form of encephalopathy did not develop before the episode of alcoholic ketoacidosis, although there was still a deficiency of thiamin as well as an absence of keto-acids. Accordingly, it seems that an increased demand for the regeneration of ATP is needed to explain the development of Wernicke's encephalopathy in this setting (e.g., delerium tremens due to alcohol withdrawal or uncoupling of oxidative phosphorylation by salicylate or other agents).

CHRONIC THIAMIN DEFICIENCY

In the chronic state of thiamin deficiency, hypotension, tachycardia, tachypnea, and signs of a high-output form of congestive heart failure (beri-beri heart disease) may be present.

A prolonged period of poor nutrition is needed to induce a biologically significant state of thiamin deficiency. Although L-lactic acidosis is one of the features of thiamin deficiency, damage to the brain is the major concern (discussed in Chapter 5, page 171). The brain must regenerate ATP as fast as it is being used to perform biologic work. It has the option of oxidizing two substrates—ketoacids and glucose—for this purpose. Ketoacids are the preferred fuel if they are present; they are derived from storage fat, and hence body protein is spared as a source for glucose for the brain during prolonged starvation. This fuel selection is set by an accumulation of the products of the metabolism of ketoacids, which inactivate PDH (see Fig. 5-2, page 115). In settings where the levels of ketoacids are very low (e.g., usual dietary intake of carbohydrate), ATP must be regenerated in the brain by the oxidation of glucose.

The preceding biochemistry becomes important in the clinical setting of the malnourished chronic alcoholic who presents with alcoholic ketoacidosis. After successful treatment of the disorder, ketoacids are no longer available. Thus, the brain must regenerate most of its ATP from the oxidation of glucose, but the activity of PDH may be compromised by a lack of one of its cofactors, vitamin B_1 (thiamin; Fig. 6-9). Probably of greater significance is the likelihood of an increased demand for ATP regeneration in that setting (e.g., delirium tremens or the use of salicylates that may uncouple oxidative phosphorylation in the brain; *see margin note for rationale*). Hence, the concentration of ADP rises and anaerobic glycolysis is stimulated in the brain to make ATP. As a result, there is a sudden rise in the production of H^+ (and L-lactate anions) in areas of the brain where the metabolic rate is the most rapid and/or ones that have the lowest reserve of thiamin.

The clinical manifestations include Wernicke-Korsakoff syndrome, in which the patient disguises the cerebral deficit by confabulating; hence, a high degree of suspicion is needed to make this diagnosis (*see margin note*). The background of malnutrition that leads to the thiamin deficiency might also lead to deficits of other B vitamins (e.g., riboflavin).

Treatment is obviously to administer thiamin *before* the ketoacid concentration in plasma falls to low levels (i.e., before the patient receives glucose, which stimulates the release of insulin, or has been given sufficient saline to reexpand the contracted ECF volume, which removes the α-adrenergic inhibition of the release of insulin). Thiamine should be administered intravenously to have the desired rapid onset of action.

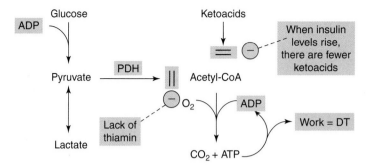

FIGURE 6-9 Regeneration of ATP during thiamin deficiency. The oxidation of glucose to yield ATP requires flux through PDH. Thiamin is a cofactor for pyruvate dehydrogenase (PDH). Hence, this flux may become too slow to meet the energy demands during thiamin deficiency. In contrast, the oxidation of ketoacids does not require flux through PDH, so it is not compromised during thiamin deficiency. Not withstanding, there must also be a demand for a higher rate of regeneration of ATP, and this may be caused by the withdrawal of alcohol (DT, delirium tremens). The accumulation of ADP drives the conversion of glucose to L-lactic acid.

Riboflavin deficiency and the use of tricyclic antidepressants

- Flavin products of vitamin B_2 metabolism (flavin mononucleotide [FMN], flavin adenine dinucleotide [FAD]) are components of the mitochondrial electron transport system that leads to the conversion of ADP to ATP.
- A lower content of these nucleotides arises when the kinase that forms them from vitamin B_2 has a reduced activity (e.g., inhibited by tricyclic antidepressants).

The active metabolites formed from vitamin B_2 (riboflavin), FMN, and FAD are components of the mitochondrial electron transport system, the principal pathway to regenerate ATP. Riboflavin must be activated via an ATP-dependent kinase to produce FMN and FAD (Fig. 6-10). Tricyclic antidepressant drugs (e.g., amitriptyline and imipramine) inhibit this kinase. The activity of this kinase is also decreased in hypothyroidism (*see margin note*).

Either a deficiency of riboflavin or inhibition of its kinase by tricyclic antidepressant drugs can lead to low levels of FMN and/or FAD and development of L-lactic acidosis. The reason why this is a chronic steady-state L-lactic acidosis is not clear but probably reflects only a partial lack of these cofactors. The diagnosis is suspected by the history suggestive of malnutrition or the intake of tricyclic antidepressant drugs and is confirmed by finding a low activity of glutathione reductase in erythrocytes (a flavoprotein-dependent enzyme). Supplementation with riboflavin may lead to a prompt reversal of the metabolic acidosis in these patients. This also is the case in patients taking tricyclic antidepressant drugs, which suggests that the defect caused by these drugs is via competitive inhibition of the kinase that can be overcome by high riboflavin levels.

METABOLIC ACIDOSIS IN PATIENTS WITH MYXEDEMA CRISIS
- L-Lactic acidosis may be seen in patients with myxedema crisis.
- Because FMN and FAD are also cofactors for the enzyme glutathione reductase (as noted in the discussion of pyroglutamic acidosis), this disorder may also be present in patients with myxedema crisis.

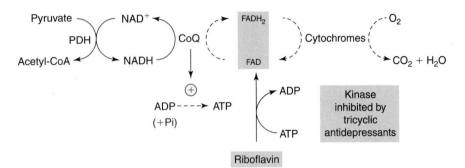

FIGURE 6-10 L-**Lactic acidosis and riboflavin deficiency.** Riboflavin (vitamin B_2) must be activated to flavin mononucleotide (FMN) or flavin adenine dinucleotide (FAD) to become a component in the electron transport system, the mitochondrial pathway to regenerate ATP. When this electron transport system goes too slowly, ADP accumulates and anaerobic glycolysis is stimulated. Either a deficiency of riboflavin or inhibition of its kinase by tricyclic antidepressant drugs can lead to low levels of FMN and/or FAD.

Uncoupling of oxidative phosphorylation

- Uncoupling of oxidative phosphorylation refers to a state in which there is consumption of oxygen without the conversion of ADP to ATP.
- Whether uncoupling of oxidative phosphorylation will cause L-lactic acidosis depends on how much ADP will accumulate.

One should think of this process as occurring in three degrees of severity. In its most severe form, there is such a rapid rate of consumption of oxygen without the ability to convert ADP back to ATP that a lethal condition is created because there is insufficient ATP available for performance of biologic work needed for survival. With a somewhat smaller degree of uncoupling of oxidative phosphorylation, ATP is still being formed at appreciable rates, but there is a somewhat higher concentration of ADP. As a result, anaerobic glycolysis is accelerated and L-lactic acid is formed faster than it can be removed (see the next paragraph). When the degree of uncoupling of oxidative phosphorylation is very modest, there is an increased rate of fuel oxidation, but ADP does not accumulate in appreciable amounts; thus, there is no overproduction of L-lactic acid.

Phenformin is a biguanide oral hypoglycemic agent that caused L-lactic acidosis, but it is no longer in use (*see margin note*). This drug has a large hydrophobic end, which enables it to cross the lipid-rich mitochondrial membrane rapidly. In so doing, H^+ are brought into the mitochondria quickly and without permitting the conversion of ADP to ATP (i.e., it uncoupled oxidative phosphorylation, see Chapter 5, page 146). As a result, ADP accumulates and anaerobic glycolysis is accelerated; thereby, a large amount of L-lactic acid is produced. Certain conditions, including renal insufficiency, reduced liver function, alcohol abuse, and heart failure, lead to higher blood levels of this drug, and hence patients with these conditions were more predisposed to a serious degree of L-lactic acidosis.

METFORMIN
- Metformin is another biguanide drug that is frequently used to treat patients with type 2 diabetes mellitus. Because it does not have a large hydrophobic tail, it is a very weak uncoupler, and therefore it causes a fall in the $P_{Glucose}$ and also in the $P_{L-Lactate}$.
- In virtually all reported cases in which metformin has been associated with L-lactic acidosis, there were other conditions that could have explained why this acid-base disturbance developed.
- If a patient is taking another uncoupler of oxidative phosphorylation (e.g., a large dose of salicylic acid), it is possible that the combined effect of the two drugs may lead to the development of L-lactic acidosis. Moreover, the concentration of metformin is much higher in portal venous blood while the drug is being absorbed, and this may cause a greater degree of uncoupling of oxidative phosphorylation in the liver.

Clinical settings with primary slow removal of L-lactic acid

- This type of L-lactic acidosis is very different from very rapid production of L-lactic acid, in which there is inadequate regeneration of ATP.
- This type of lactic acidosis is usually caused by a liver problem.

Hepatic disease

The causes for a low rate of removal of L-lactic acid are usually related to problems with the liver, due to hepatitis, replacement of normal liver cells (e.g., by tumor cells or large fat deposits), destruction of liver due to prior hypoxia (e.g., "shock liver"), or compromised activity of the enzymes responsible for conversion of pyruvate to glucose (PC or PEPCK). If the degree of loss of viable liver mass or the decrease in activity of PC and/or PEPCK is not large, the presence of a significant degree of L-lactic acidosis implies that there is also a component of overproduction of this acid (see Fig. 6-3, page 165).

For example, in patients with a malignancy and hepatic metastases, the mechanisms that contribute to the L-lactic acidosis include replacement of a sufficient number of liver cells with tumor cells to impair L-lactate removal, production of metabolites by tumor cells such as the amino acid tryptophan that may inhibit the conversion of pyruvate to glucose in the liver, and/or production of L-lactic acid by ischemic tumor cells. A chronic steady state of L-lactic acidosis often represents a modest increase in the rate of production, coupled with a decreased rate of removal of L-lactic acid (*see margin note*).

THERAPY WITH NaHCO₃
Administration of $NaHCO_3$ to patients with L-lactic acidosis due to malignancy and hepatic metastases may have detrimental long-term effects because the load of alkali might increase L-lactic acid production (from glucose) by deinhibiting an important rate-controlling enzyme in glycolysis in malignant cells (phosphofructokinase-1). When the source of pyruvate is glucose made from amino acids (gluconeogenesis), a considerable amount of lean body mass may be lost.

Antiretroviral drugs

- One older effect of these drugs is to inhibit the mitochondrial electron transport system.
- Another side-effect of these drugs is to cause replacement of normal liver tissue with storage fat.

L-Lactic acidosis has been reported in patients with human immunodeficiency virus (HIV) infection treated with various antiretroviral agents. The agent most frequently associated with L-lactic acidosis is zidovudine, but didanosine, stavudine, lamivudine, and indinavir have also been implicated. There are two possible important mechanisms whereby antiretroviral agents may cause L-lactic acidosis. First, they block the electron transport system, akin to the mechanism of action of low-dose cyanide. Hence, more ATP will be produced by anaerobic glycolysis, driven by a high availability of ADP. This may lead to mitochondrial myopathy, as manifested by ragged-red fibers and mitochondrial DNA depletion. Although this mechanism is thought to be the main cause of L-lactic acidosis, there is doubt about its validity in all patients because mild exercise does not increase the degree of acidemia. Second, these drugs may lead to hepatic parenchymal replacement with storage fat (steatosis; Fig. 6-11). This view is supported by the fact that in some of these patients a small dose of ethanol, which leads to a higher NADH concentration in hepatocytes, results in a significantly increased degree of L-lactic acidosis because it diverts pyruvate to L-lactate (see Fig. 6-5, page 165).

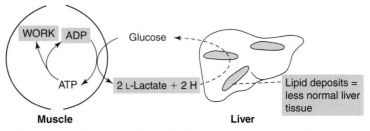

FIGURE 6-11 L-Lactic acidosis and antiretroviral drugs. The major basis for L-lactic acidosis is a problem with L-lactic acid removal by the liver. When there is a large replacement of liver parenchyma by triglycerides (hepatic steatosis, depicted by the *ovals*), a large rise in $P_{L\text{-lactate}}$ may occur because one is now operating closer to the maximum velocity of L-lactate removal in the liver (see *right portion* of Fig. 6-3, page 164). L-Lactic acidosis may also result from the effect of antiretroviral drugs causing inhibition of electron transport in muscle and hence the accumulation of ADP.

QUESTIONS

(Discussions on page 190)

6-1 *Why is the rate of production of ketoacids so much lower than that of L-lactic acid if both are regulated by the rate of turnover of ATP to yield ADP?*

6-2 *Consider the following example. An anoxic limb needs to regenerate 18 mmol/min of ATP (25% of the ATP needed in the body) via anaerobic glycolysis. If the rest of the body could be "persuaded" to oxidize L-lactate anions (+ H^+) to regenerate all needed ATP (54 mmol/min), would L-lactic acid still accumulate?*

6-3 *If a patient has hypoxia but little glycogen in the liver, does L-lactic acidosis develop? If not, what changes would you expect to find in the concentration of metabolites in blood?*

6-4 *$NaHCO_3$ was given as treatment for L-lactic acidosis, but there was no rise in the P_{HCO3}. Is it appropriate to conclude that the alkali has not been helpful?*

ORGANIC ACID LOAD FROM THE GASTROINTESTINAL TRACT (D-LACTIC ACIDOSIS)

- The importance of this diagnosis is not the acidemia, but rather that it is a sign of an overproduction of a variety of noxious compounds in the GI tract that compromise central nervous system function.
- The basis of overproduction of organic acids by the GI tract is that the usual separation of the GI bacteria and sugars (the substrates for fermentation) is not present.
- Three factors augment the formation of D-lactic acid—antibiotics that may change the intestinal bacterial flora, provision of sugars for fermentation, and a slow GI motility.

ABBREVIATION
GI, gastrointestinal

Pathophysiology

Under normal circumstances, the gut flora (mainly in the colon) do not have access to glucose because glucose is absorbed in the upper small intestine (Fig. 6-12). Disruption of this geographic separation of bacteria

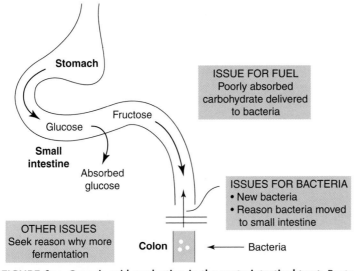

FIGURE 6-12 Organic acid production in the gastrointestinal tract. Bacteria are normally separated from dietary sugar by "GI geography." For overproduction of D-lactic acid, new bacteria need to be present (e.g., owing to intake of antibiotics). These bacteria from the lower GI tract must mix with nonabsorbed sugars. Either bacteria migrate up to and proliferate in the small intestine, where they are provided with sugar in this "friendly environment," or sugars are delivered to the colon. More D-lactic acid (and other organic acids) can be produced if bacteria and sugar coexist for longer time periods (e.g., owing to low GI motility). Of note, a variety of noxious compounds (e.g., aldehydes) are produced in the fermentation process.

and glucose is the major factor in the development of D-lactic acidosis. Altered bacterial flora (e.g., owing to antibiotic therapy) may migrate up to the small intestine and proliferate because they are provided with dietary sugar. Alternatively, certain sugars (e.g., fructose) may be delivered to the colon when their intake is high because they are poorly absorbed in the small intestine. Decreased bowel motility (from blind loops or drugs) increases the contact time for bacteria and sugar and, as a result, more organic acids may be produced. In addition, antacids or drugs that inhibit gastric H^+ secretion may lead to a higher pH that is more favorable for bacterial growth and metabolism in the intestinal tract. Organic acids, noxious alcohols, aldehydes, amines, and mercaptans produced during fermentation may lead to many of the central nervous system symptoms that are observed in this disorder.

Humans metabolize D-lactate more slowly than L-lactate. D-Lactate may also be excreted in the urine, and hence the rise in the $P_{Anion\ gap}$ may be lower than expected as judged from the fall in P_{HCO_3}, if the D-lactate anions are excreted with Na^+ and/or K^+ but not NH_4^+. In addition, if there was an appreciable loss of $NaHCO_3$ in the diarrhea fluid, the fall in P_{HCO_3} may be greater than expected from the rise in the $P_{Anion\ gap}$.

Diagnosis and treatment

- The usual laboratory test for "lactate" detects L-lactate, but not D-lactate. Hence, a specific assay for D-lactate must be performed to confirm this diagnosis.

Treatment should be directed at the GI problem. The oral intake of fructose and complex carbohydrates should be stopped. Antacids and

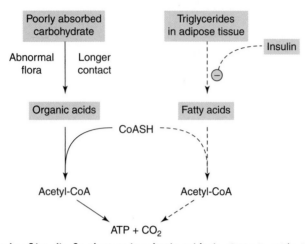

FIGURE 6-13 Possible role of insulin for therapy in D-lactic acidosis. Organic acids, including D-lactic acid at times, are produced during fermentation of poorly absorbed carbohydrate in the gastrointestinal tract (*left side*). After delivery to the liver, these organic acids are converted primarily to acetyl-CoA. To remove this H^+ load, the organic anions must be oxidized to CO_2 for the most part in the liver and skeletal muscle. This metabolic removal is slower if fatty acids are being oxidized to produce acetyl-CoA. Hence, administering insulin, which should depress the rate of oxidation of fatty acids, may permit more organic acids to be oxidized.

oral $NaHCO_3$ should be avoided because they could lead to a higher intestinal luminal pH and thereby an increased production of toxic products of fermentation. In addition, drugs that diminish GI motility should be discontinued. Intravenous $NaHCO_3$ can be given if the acidemia is severe, but this is usually not needed. Poorly absorbed antibiotics (e.g., vancomycin) could be used to change the bacterial flora. Insulin may be helpful by lowering the rate of oxidation of fatty acids and thus permitting a higher rate of oxidation of organic acids (Fig. 6-13).

QUESTION

(Discussion on page 191)

6-5 *What useful functions can be attributed to the normal production of organic acids in the colon?*

METABOLIC ACIDOSIS DUE TO TOXIC ALCOHOLS

- The major threat to patients with toxic alcohol–induced metabolic acidosis is not the acidemia; rather, it is the toxicity of the aldehyde intermediates of their metabolism (e.g., formaldehyde, glycoaldehyde).
- This diagnosis should be suspected by finding an elevated $P_{Osmolal\ gap}$ and it is confirmed by detecting methanol or ethylene glycol in the blood.
- Suspect methanol intoxication if the patient has visual disturbances and suspect ethylene glycol intoxication if there are oxalate crystals in the urine and/or acute tubular necrosis.
- The most important goal in therapy is to prevent the metabolism of the toxic alcohol; this should be followed by the removal of these alcohols by hemodialysis.

Methanol

Methanol (CH_3OH), also known as methyl alcohol, wood spirit, and wood alcohol, has a molecular weight of 32. It is used as antifreeze, an additive to gasoline, and a solvent in the manufacture of various drugs. Methanol itself is not toxic, but its metabolic product, formaldehyde, is the major cause of toxicity because it rapidly binds to tissue proteins.

Methanol is converted to formaldehyde by alcohol dehydrogenase in the liver, but a high concentration of methanol is required for rapid rates of oxidation of this alcohol. The formaldehyde formed is rapidly converted to formic acid by aldehyde dehydrogenase (Fig. 6-14). In each step, NAD^+ is converted to NADH. The latter step is much faster, which means that formaldehyde blood levels are only slightly increased, yet they are still in a toxic range.

The metabolic acidosis of methanol poisoning is associated with an increased $P_{Anion\ gap}$ due to the accumulation of formate and L-lactate anions; the L-lactate level often exceeds that of formate. The L-lactic acidosis results from inhibition of cytochrome oxidase by formate and also from the the conversion of pyruvate to lactate in the liver owing to an increased $NADH:NAD^+$ ratio caused by methanol metabolism. HCO_3^- is regenerated when formate anions are metabolized to neutral end products; folic acid is a cofactor in this metabolism. Filtered formate is reabsorbed in the proximal tubule via the formate-chloride exchanger, and thus its excretion in the urine is low.

Early on, symptoms of intoxication (e.g., inebriation, ataxia, and slurred speech) dominate the clinical picture. Later, blurred vision, blindness, abdominal pain, malaise, headache, and vomiting develop. Funduscopic examination may reveal papilledema. Visual impairment is related to metabolism of methanol to formaldehyde via an alcohol dehydrogenase in the retina (retinol dehydrogenase). Fixed and dilated pupils may result from reduced light perception caused by optic neuropathy. Abdominal pain and tenderness often result from acute pancreatitis. Overall, methanol should always be considered in the differential diagnosis of metabolic acidosis with an increased $P_{Anion\ gap}$ (*see margin note for a quantitative analysis*), particularly if the ECF volume is not contracted and renal failure is not present. This diagnosis should be suspected by finding an elevated $P_{Osmolal\ gap}$ and confirmed by a direct assay for methanol in the blood.

RATE OF PRODUCTION OF FORMIC ACID FROM METHANOL

- The molecular weight of methanol is 32. One oz (32 mL) of methanol is close to 32 g or 1000 mmol. Accordingly, 1 oz of methanol can yield 1000 mmol of formic acid.
- Hepatic alcohol dehydrogenase has a maximal activity for the metabolism of close to 7000 mmol of methanol per day, but constraints on the rate of removal of NADH cause a much lower rate of H^+ production (~1 mmol /min).

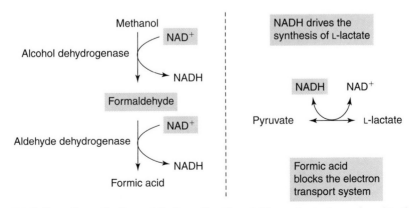

FIGURE 6-14 Metabolic pathway for the metabolism of methanol. The major toxin produced in the metabolism of methanol is formaldehyde. The metabolic conversion of methanol to formaldehyde is catalyzed by alcohol dehydrogenase. The major acid produced is formic acid, from the metabolism of formaldehyde, which is catalyzed by aldehyde dehydrogenase. Formic acid can inhibit the mitochondrial electron transport system (cytochrome c) when its concentration is very high.

Ethylene glycol (antifreeze) intoxication

> • The unique danger in ethylene glycol poisoning is acute renal failure. Therefore, do not administer too much Na^+.

Ethylene glycol ($OH-CH_2-CH_2-OH$) has a molecular weight of 62; it is a clear and colorless liquid with a sweet taste and a low vapor pressure. Ethylene glycol is widely used as an antifreeze; in hydraulic brake fluids; as a solvent in the paint and plastics industries; and in the formulation of printers' inks, stamp pad inks, and inks for ballpoint pens. The lethal dose is approximately 1.4 mL/kg body weight (about 100 mL in an average-sized adult).

Ethylene glycol is converted to glycoaldehyde by alcohol dehydrogenase in the liver (Fig. 6-15); the affinity of this enzyme to ethylene glycol is close to 100 times lower than for ethanol; thus, the rate of metabolism of ethylene glycol is rapid only when its concentration is high. Glycoaldehyde is further metabolized to glycolic acid by hepatic aldehyde dehydrogenase, which is the major acid that accumulates in ethylene glycol poisoning. One percent or less of glycolic acid is converted to oxalic acid, mainly by the action of lactate dehydrogenase. Virtually all oxalate produced is precipitated as calcium oxalate, contributing to acute renal failure and hypocalcemia. The major end product of glycolic acid metabolism is glycine in a transamination reaction with alanine that is catalyzed by the enzyme alanine glyoxylate aminotransferase; vitamin B_6 (pyridoxine) is a cofactor.

Central nervous system symptoms, such as inebriation, ataxia, and slurred speech, are the effects of ethylene glycol itself. At this stage, the $P_{Osmolal\ gap}$ is high. After a latent period of about 4 to 12 hours, patients develop nausea, vomiting, hyperventilation, elevated blood pressure, tachycardia, tetany, and convulsions. At this point, an increased $P_{Anion\ gap}$ type of metabolic acidosis is present. The tetany is most likely caused by hypocalcemia, which is postulated to be the result of deposition of calcium oxalate crystals (*see margin note*). Cranial nerve palsies may be seen; calcium oxalate deposition in the vessels and in the meninges of the brain has been noted at autopsy. Leukocytosis of an unknown mechanism is frequently observed.

BASIS FOR HYPOCALCEMIA: "IS IT THAT SIMPLE?"
- On one hand, precipitation of ionized calcium with oxalate should lower the concentration of calcium in plasma.
- On the other hand, this should just be a transient phenomenon that is corrected by the release of calcium from its bound form on albumin and an increased release of parathyroid hormone, which mobilizes calcium from bone.

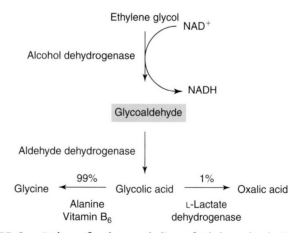

FIGURE 6-15 Pathway for the metabolism of ethylene glycol. The major toxin is glycoaldehyde, the product of alcohol dehydrogenase (*rectangle*). The major acid produced is glycolic acid, the product of aldehyde dehydrogenase.

Renal failure is common and usually develops 36 to 48 hours after the ingestion of ethylene glycol; glycoaldehyde appears to be the main toxin. It is not clear whether the deposition of calcium oxalate monohydrate crystals plays an important role in pathogenesis of renal failure in these patients. In patients who survive, calcium oxalate crystals can persist in the kidney for months (*see margin note*).

CALCIUM OXALATE CRYSTALS IN THE URINE
The crystals are usually monohydrates, which are needle shaped. Less often, there may be the envelope-shaped dihydrates.

Therapy of methanol or ethylene glycol intoxication

- The most important goal of therapy is to prevent the formation of these toxic aldehydes by giving ethanol; this should be followed by the removal of the offending alcohols by hemodialysis.

Administration of ethanol

Maintenance of a plasma ethanol level of about 20 mmol/L (100 mg/dL) nearly completely inhibits methanol and ethylene glycol tmetabolism by alcohol dehydrogenase. Because ethanol distributes throughout total body water, administer a bolus of 0.6 g of ethanol/kg of body weight (intravenously or orally) to increase its plasma level by 1 mg/mL (100 mg/dL); this amount of alcohol is contained in 4 oz of whiskey. The maintenance dose should be equal to the expected rate of metabolic removal of ethanol; at a plasma level in excess of 3 mmol/L (14 mg/dL)—the hourly amount of ethanol removal is about 0.11 g/kg of body weight. In an alcoholic patient, the amount of ethanol metabolized is expected to be about 50% higher. Hence, about 0.16 g of ethanol/kg body weight (1 oz whiskey) should be administered hourly in nondrinkers, and 0.32 g of ethanol/kg body weight (2 oz whiskey) in chronic drinkers. During hemodialysis, one can increase the rate of infusion of ethanol or add ethanol to the dialysis bath to achieve a concentration of ethanol of 20 mmol/L. It is important to ensure an optimal ethanol plasma level by measuring ethanol levels frequently and adjusting its rate of infusion.

Administration of fomepizole (4-methylpyrazole)

- Although fomepizole has few acute side effects, it is rather expensive, which limits its use.

Fomepizole is an inhibitor of alcohol dehydrogenase that has almost 8000-fold higher affinity to alcohol dehydrogenase than ethanol and is approved by the Food and Drug Administration (FDA) for the treatment of ethylene glycol intoxication. The target level of fomepizole in humans is 100 to 300 µmol/L (8.6 to 24.6 mg/dL) to ensure near-complete inhibition of hepatic alcohol dehydrogenase. Its plasma half-life varies with the dose, even in patients with normal renal function. Fomepizole distributes rapidly in total body water. With multiple doses, fomepizole augments its own metabolism by inducing the cytochrome P_{450} mixed-function oxidase system; this effect increases the elimination rate by about 50% after about 30 to 40 hours.

The side effects of fomepizole include headache, nausea, dizziness, and allergic reactions (rash and eosinophilia). Venous irritation and phlebosclerosis may occur if the drug is not diluted prior to infusion; therefore, it should be diluted with at least 100 mL of isotonic saline or D_5W.

QUESTION

(Discussion on page 192)

6-6 *If oxalic acid were the sole product formed during the metabolism of ethylene glycol, why might the degree of metabolic acidosis be less severe?*

TOXICITY CAUSED BY PROPANE 1,2-DIOL (PROPYLENE GLYCOL)

> • One of the metabolites of this compound is an aldehyde, which is oxidized quite slowly. In general, aldehydes are very toxic compounds.

This compound is a common diluent for many intravenous drug preparations (e.g., lorazepam; *see margin note*), which is commonly used in large doses as a sedative in the intensive care unit and to treat delirium tremens). When given in large quantities, this alcohol can be detected by finding a very large $P_{Osmolal\ gap}$.

Biochemistry

Propane 1,2-diol (molecular weight 76) is a 50:50 mixture of D and L isoforms (*see margin note*). Of the administered dose, 40% is excreted unchanged in the urine, and 60% is metabolized in the liver by alcohol dehydrogenase to lactaldehyde and then by aldehyde dehydrogenase to lactic acid (Fig. 6-16). D-Lactaldehyde, however, is not a good substrate for aldehyde dehydrogenase; therefore, it accumulates and leads to many of the toxic effects observed in this setting. D-Lactaldehyde can be metabolized to D-lactic acid by an alternate pathway in the liver, which uses reduced glutathione (GSH) as a cofactor. Because L-lactate is metabolized much faster than D-lactate, the acid that accumulates is principally D-lactic acid.

PROPANE 1,2-DIOL
- This solvent is used to allow elements of relatively insoluble materials (e.g., drugs, cough medicines, toothpaste) to be administered. Beware, at times, it may be present without proper labeling.
- A vial of the sedative lorazepam contains 2 mg/mL, of which 0.8 mL is propanediol. If a patient receives 10 mg/hr of lorazepam, this is 4 g/hr of propanediol, or 96 g (1300 mmol)/day of propanediol.

ASYMMETRICAL CARBON IN PROPANE 1,2-DIOL
The middle carbon of this three-carbon compound has four different chemical groups attached to it; hence, it is an asymmetrical carbon. Because it can be metabolized to lactate, both the D- and the L-forms are produced.

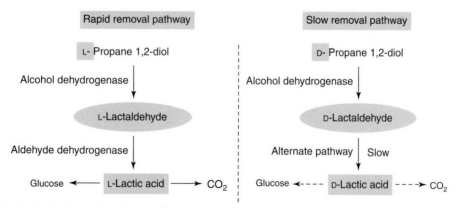

FIGURE 6-16 Metabolism of propane 1,2-diol to L- and D-lactic acid. When a large quantity of propane 1,2-diol is ingested, the body is presented with a racemic mixture; the middle carbon of this three-carbon chain has four different groups attached. Both the L-form (shown to the *left*) and the D-form (shown to the *right*) are substrates for alcohol dehydrogenase; hence, their metabolism occurs in the liver. The products are L- and D-lactaldehyde. L-Lactaldehyde is a good substrate for aldehyde dehydrogenase. The D-lactaldehyde accumulates and is responsible for most of the toxicity. When it is metabolized, the acid that accumulates is D-lactic acid, because it is metabolized much more slowly than L-lactic acid. To simplify the figure, the cofactors, NAD^+ and NADH, are not shown.

Clinical manifestations

The major findings are seizures, cardiac dysfunction, and progressive renal failure. It is likely that D-lactaldehyde is responsible for much of this toxicity. The metabolic acidosis is a sign of the metabolic abnormality rather than posing a major threat to the patient.

Treatment

Although one must stop the drug, the most important step is to stop the formation of D-lactaldehyde by giving ethanol or fomepizole. This must be followed up by removal of propane 1,2-diol by hemodialysis (*see margin note*).

DIALYSIS OF ALDEHYDES
Since the concentration of aldehydes is very low, it is unlikely that they can be removed rapidly by hemodialysis.

PYROGLUTAMIC ACIDOSIS

> • The importance of this disorder is not the acidemia but rather that it signals that there is a serious metabolic stress present owing to a high level of reactive oxygen species (ROS).

Pyroglutamic acidosis is a unique form of metabolic acidosis, which occurs most often in critically ill patients. It may not be included in the usual lists of causes of metabolic acidosis with an increased $P_{Anion\ gap}$ because it was thought to represent only rare inborn errors of metabolism in the γ-glutamyl cycle (defects in 5-oxoprolinase or in glutathione synthetase [Fig. 6-17]). It is interesting to note that the vast majority of reported cases are in women; the reason for this is not clear.

ABBREVIATIONS
GSH, reduced from of glutathione
GS-SG, oxidized from of glutathione

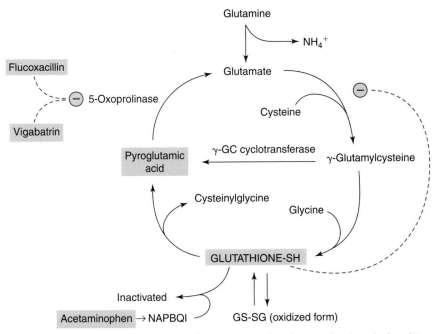

FIGURE 6-17 Production of pyroglutamic acid. When there are low levels of reduced glutathione (e.g., owing to depletion by *N*-acetyl-*p*-benzoquinonimide [NAPBQI], a highly reactive metabolite of acetaminophen), γ-glutamylcysteine synthetase is deinhibited. If the γ-glutamylcysteine accumulates, pyroglutamic acid is formed. In addition, if 5-oxyprolinase is inhibited (e.g., flucloxacillin, vigabatrin), pyroglutamic acid also accumulates. As described in the text, a diminished ability to detoxify reactive oxygen species is likely to be more dangerous than the acidosis in this setting.

GSH is made up of three amino acids: glutamate, cysteine, and glycine. It is the sulfhydryl moiety of cysteine that endows this compound with it ability to detoxify ROS. In this process, the reduced form of GSH is converted to the oxidized form of glutathione (GS-SG; see equation). Key to understanding the basis for the accumulation of pyroglutamic acid is the fact that the reduced form of GSH feeds back to inhibit the enzyme that catalyzes the first step in the cycle, γ-glutamylcysteine synthase, which converts glutamate to γ-glutamylcysteine (see Fig. 6-17). Hence, when ROS accumulate (e.g., in a patient with sepsis), the concentration of GSH declines and this results in an accelerated formation of γ-glutamylcysteine. When the concentration of γ-glutamylcysteine rises, this compound is an alternate substrate for the enzyme that produces pyroglutamic acid (see Fig. 6-17). It is important to recognize that components of the GSH cycle reside in different compartments of the cell, which adds to the complexity of understanding the regulation of this feedback system.

$$2\,GSH + ROS \rightarrow GS\text{-}SG + inactive\,ROS$$

A number of drugs have been identified as potential causes of pyroglutamic acidosis. Some, such as acetaminophen, after conversion to a metabolite, N-acetyl-p-benzoquinonimide, decrease the concentration of GSH, thereby driving the synthesis of γ-glutamylcysteine and thus the formation of pyroglutamic acid (see Fig. 6-17). Other drugs (e.g., the antibiotic flucloxacillin and the anticonvulsant vigabatrin) may inhibit 5-oxoprolinase, which converts pyroglutamic acid to glutamate. Other causes of this disorder may include drugs or inborn errors of metabolism that affect glucose 6-phosphate dehydrogenase activity, which results in a diminished concentration of NADPH, the cofactor in the reaction that reduces GS-SG to GSH (see equation) by glutathione reductase. FMN and FAD, the products of metabolism of riboflavin by its kinase (see Fig. 6-10), are cofactors for the enzyme glutathione reductase. This may explain, at least in part, why malnutrition seems to be a risk factor for the development of this type of acidosis. Severe hypothyroidism decreases the activity of riboflavin kinase and may contribute to the development of pyroglutamic acidosis (*see margin note on page 173*).

$$GS\text{-}SG + NADPH \rightarrow 2\,GSH + NADP^+$$

METABOLIC ACIDOSIS CAUSED BY THE INGESTION OF AN ACID

- Be careful; the anion accompanying H^+ may have important biologic effects.
- The acid load may lead to a very rapid rate of addition of H^+.

Patients occasionally ingest a sufficient quantity of an organic acid to cause a severe metabolic acidosis. The symptoms may be due to the acidemia or may result from a property of the anion of the acid (e.g., chelation of calcium by citrate with ingestion of citric acid, see Case 6-1). The clue for this diagnosis is that the patient presents with hyperacute metabolic acidosis with an increased $P_{\text{Anion gap}}$. L-Lactic acid is the only acid of endogenous origin that may be produced at an extremely rapid rate when the demand for O_2 outstrips its supply. Therefore, suspect the ingestion of an acid in patients with hyperacute metabolic acidosis if the plasma L-lactate level is not very high. The patient may or may not confess to

USE OF *N*-ACETYLCYSTEINE IN THE TREATMENT OF PYROGLUTAMIC ACIDOSIS

- Pyroglutamic acidosis (PGA) represents a heterogeneous group of conditions where PGA accumulates. Their important feature is that there is an impaired removal of ROS by GSH.
- *N*-acetylcysteine may be very useful to treat the subgroup of these disorders, which have a depleted GSH + GS-SG pool size (e.g., that due to large doses of acetaminophen).
- *N*-acetylcysteine should be much less effective when the GSH + GS-SG pool size is not depleted. The goal now is to convert GS-SG to GSH.

BASIS FOR THE GAIN OF H^+
H^+ accumulate only when the precursor of glutamate is glutamine and providing that the NH_4^+ so formed is metabolized to urea in the liver.

the ingestion, but he or she will have a normal $P_{Osmolal\ gap}$ unless ethanol, methanol, or ethylene glycol was also ingested.

Treatment consists of gastric suction to remove any acid that is not yet absorbed, administration of $NaHCO_3$ if the acidemia is severe, and attention to any adverse action of the anion (e.g., hypotension due to hypocalcemia caused by chelation of ionized calcium by citrate).

PART C
INTEGRATIVE PHYSIOLOGY

CASE 6-3: EXERCISE-INDUCED ACUTE RENAL FAILURE

(Case discussed on page 188)

After a 400-meter race, a 24-year-old male elite athlete felt extremely weak and experienced nausea, dizziness, and flank soreness. A few days later, he was seen in the emergency department and was diagnosed with acute renal failure based on the presence of oliguria, a BUN (P_{Urea}) of 56 mg/dL (20 mmol/L), and a $P_{Creatinine}$ of 11.5 mg/dL (1000 μmol/L). He was noted to have hyperphosphatemia and hyperuricemia, but his plasma creatinine kinase was not elevated (173 U/L). His hemoglobin was 148 g/L. His family history was noncontributory. Urine microscopy showed several red blood cells and heme-granular casts but no cellular casts. Abdominal sonography showed enlarged kidneys. Five days after hemodialysis began, renal function improved sufficiently, and hemodialysis was discontinued. His P_{Urea} and $P_{Creatinine}$ values fell to normal over a 2-week period.

His blood pressure is now 120/70 mm Hg and his effective arterial blood volume status is normal. Cardiopulmonary and neuromuscular examinations are unremarkable. On screening, all laboratory values are in the normal range except that his P_{Urate} is one tenth the lower limit of normal, but his daily excretion of urate is similar to normal subjects. Of note, however, a few hours after moderate exercise, his $P_{Creatinine}$ rose by a factor of 1.3.

Questions

Does the patient have a renal defect that causes his P_{Urate} to be so low? What is the role of the patient's low P_{Urate} in causing his exercise-induced acute renal failure?

REACTIVE OXYGEN SPECIES

Superoxide (O_2^-), the parent of many forms of ROS is formed when the concentrations of molecular oxygen (O_2) and electrons rise. An important donor of electrons is the semialdehyde form of coenzyme Q (CoQ), one of the intermediates in the electron transport system (*see margin note*). Because the reaction described in the equation does not require an enzyme for catalysis, it proceeds faster and forms more O_2^- when the P_{O_2} is high.

$$E^- (electron) + O_2 \rightarrow O_2^- (superoxide)$$

ABBREVIATIONS

$P_{Creatinine}$, concentration of creatinine in plasma

P_{Urea}, concentration of urea in plasma

P_{Urate}, concentration of urate in plasma

ETS, electron transport system in mitochondria, which is the pathway by which the energy from fuel oxidation is used to convert ADP to ATP

COENZYME Q

- Coenzyme Q (CoQ) provides the link between the first and second major steps in the mitochondrial electron transport system. This organic molecule moves in the lipid phase of the inner mitochondrial membrane and carries electrons from NADH to the flavin-containing nucleotides (FMN and FAD).
- CoQ exists in three states: an oxidized, a reduced, and a half-oxidized or semialdehyde form.
- The concentration of the semialdehyde form of CoQ rises when fuels are oxidized faster than the flux through the electron transport system can regenerate ATP (Fig. 6-18). As a result, it donates its electrons to oxygen and leads to the formation of ROS.

EXAMPLES OF BENEFICIAL EFFECTS OF REACTIVE OXYGEN SPECIES

- Low concentrations of ROS cause mild uncoupling of oxidative phosphorylation that may increase the synthesis of ketoacids in the liver during starvation (see Chapter 5, page 146).
- Activated neutrophils (e.g., during an infection) form ROS to kill bacteria that underwent phagocytosis.

EXAMPLE OF THE HARMFUL EFFECTS OF REACTIVE OXYGEN SPECIES

- *Reperfusion injury:* In the absence of hypoxia, xanthine dehydrogenase passes electrons directly to NAD^+ so there is no threat of forming O_2^-. After a sustained period of hypoxia, xanthine dehydrogenase is phosphorylated and it becomes xanthine oxidase. When blood flow is restored, this form of the enzyme donates electrons directly to oxygen. O_2^- is formed, and this may lead to tissue injury.
- *Low levels of circulating antioxidants:* An example is in the patient with a low concentration of urate in blood. For the danger to occur, ROS must be synthesized at a rapid rate (see discussion of Case 6-3, page 187).

Biologic effects of reactive oxygen species

Although low concentrations of ROS may be useful (*see margin note*), damage to tissues may occur when their concentrations rise appreciably (*see margin note*).

Methods to detoxify reactive oxygen species

There are a number of ways to detoxify ROS. The first line of defense is the catalytic destruction of O_2^- by the enzyme superoxide dismutase. Another mechanism is to convert O_2^- to peroxide (H_2O_2) and then destroy H_2O_2 using the enzyme catalase or peroxidase. Mitochondria detoxify ROS by having them react with the reduced form of GSH. The product, oxidized glutathione (GS-SG), must be converted back to GSH using NADPH generated in large part by glucose 6-phosphate dehydrogenase in the pentose-phosphate pathway. Another mechanism is to destroy O_2^- chemically in the circulation by an antioxidant, urate (see discussion of Case 6-3).

A different form of defense mechanism is to reduce the production of ROS by lowering the P_{O_2} in cells. This involves an accelerated flux in the electron transport system by increasing the rate of consumption of oxygen. There are a number of ways to accomplish this. One is to accelerate the rate of conversion of ATP to ADP by performing metabolic work, and a second is to create a futile cycle (see Fig. 5-14, page 149). On the other hand, one can induce a mild degree of uncoupling of oxidative phosphorylation, as illustrated in Figure 6-18. These uncoupler protein H^+ channels can be in an open configuration when the concentration of ROS rises *and* if fatty acids (i.e., a metabolite that is not a fuel for brain cells) are present near these mitochondria.

DISCUSSION OF CASES

CASE 6-1: PATRICK IS IN FOR A SHOCK

(Case presented on page 161)

Judging from the time frame, which acid has accumulated?

The only acid that is made endogenously at a very rapid rate is L-lactic acid during hypoxia. The concentration of L-lactate was not

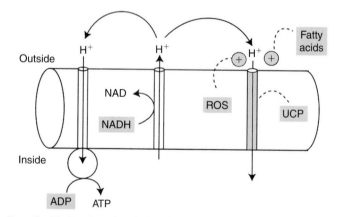

FIGURE 6-18 Uncoupling of oxidative phosphorylation decreases the production of reactive oxygen species (ROS). The *horizontal structure* represents the inner mitochondrial membrane. *On the left*, the diffusion of H^+ into mitochondria drives ATP regeneration (coupled oxidative phosphorylation). *On the right*, the uncoupler protein (UCP) is shown. When ROS rise and fatty acids are present, flux of H^+ through UCP rises, but ATP is not regenerated.

elevated in blood to a sufficient degree (only 2 mmol/L), so this is not the correct answer. Therefore, the most likely diagnosis is that he ingested an acid. Now let us see if we can deduce which acid was ingested from the properties of its anion.

Why did his blood pressure fall so precipitously?

Blood pressure is a direct function of cardiac output and peripheral vascular resistance. Cardiac output is directly related to the heart rate and stroke volume. Because his heart rate is rapid, one should look for a process that could compromise his stroke volume and/or possibly his peripheral vascular resistance. Because he has no evidence of blood loss, sepsis, or a disorder that can cause salt deficiency (e.g., a history of vomiting, diarrhea), one should suspect that there is a problem with the contractility of his heart and/or the vasoconstrictor tone of his blood vessels. The factor essential for contractility is ionized calcium. Therefore, it is possible that the new anion might have removed ionized calcium. Because citrate is a chelator of ionized calcium (e.g., this is the mechanism whereby citrate anticoagulates blood), this patient may have ingested citric acid. This was confirmed later when the composition of the ingested solution became known.

Why did he have an elevated P_K?

To shift K^+ out of cells, the resting membrane potential must become less negative. The key transporter involved in this process is the Cl^-/HCO_3^- anion exchanger, which catalyzes an electroneutral exchange of these anions. Although this is an electroneutral pathway, when activated it results in a higher concentration of intracellular Cl^-; this and the negative voltage inside the cell force Cl^- to exit cells through open Cl^- channels down the electrochemical gradient. This exit of Cl^- should diminish the degree of negative intracellular voltage so K^+ can exit from cells if K^+ channels are open (Fig. 6-19; *see margin note*).

ANION EXCHANGER
- The function of AE may not simply be limited to an acid-base issue, as it leads to the net export of K^+ and HCO_3^- from cells.
- The major physiology may be part of the response to a deficit of $KHCO_3$ (e.g., diarrhea) and for the export of $KHCO_3$ in the first phase of a sprint when cells become very alkaline due to the hydrolysis of phosphocreatine (see Chapter 1, page 32).

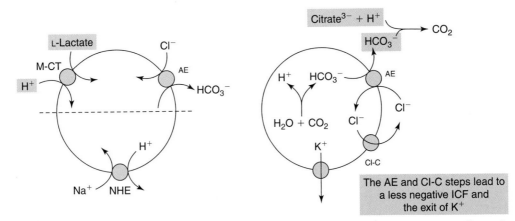

FIGURE 6-19 Role of the anion exchanger in the shift of K⁺ out of cells. The *circle* represents a cell membrane. Transporters that accelerate the movement of H⁺ and HCO₃⁻ across cell membranes are shown on the *left*. The H⁺ from citric acid cannot enter cells on any of these transporters because citrate is not a substrate for the monocarboxylic acid cotransporter (citrate is a tricarboxylic anion). As shown on the *right*, when the anion exchanger (AE) becomes active (AE is normally *inactive* in cell membrane) and citric acid lowers the P_HCO3, more HCO₃⁻ can be exported and more Cl⁻ will enter cells. The rise in intracellular Cl⁻ and the negative voltage inside the cell force Cl⁻ out of the cells down their electrochemical gradient via specific Cl⁻ channels (ClC). This exit of Cl⁻ causes the intracellular fluid (ICF) voltage to become less negative so K⁺ can exit from cells if K⁺ channels are open.

Why did the intravenous calcium cause the rapid recovery?

As part of the emergency treatment of hyperkalemia, his physician infused a calcium salt. This caused a rise in the concentration of ionized calcium in plasma, which increased myocardial contractility as well as causing vasoconstriction, which raised his blood pressure. This was another piece of the puzzle that alerted his physicians to the possibility that this patient may have ingested citric acid.

CASE 6-2: METABOLIC ACIDOSIS DUE TO DIARRHEA

(Case presented on page 161)

What is the basis for metabolic acidosis?

Metabolic acidosis in this patient is not simply the result of loss of $NaHCO_3$ in diarrhea fluid because the $P_{Anion\ gap}$ is 26 mEq/L and the $P_{Albumin}$ is not very high. L-Lactic acidosis is unlikely because there is no hemodynamic problem, liver function tests are normal, and the time period is too short for a nutritional deficiency that may cause L-lactic acidosis to develop. Moreover, he did not ingest drugs that may cause L-lactic acidosis. There is no history of diabetes or the intake of ethanol, and his blood sugar is normal. Later, L-lactic acidosis and ketoacidosis were ruled out because the concentration of each of these anions was not elevated in blood or urine. There was no history of intake of an organic acid. Toxic alcohol ingestion was not likely from the history or the laboratory data (no increase in the $P_{Osmolal\ gap}$). Renal failure was not present ($P_{Creatinine}$ is near normal). Hence, the most likely diagnosis is D-lactic acidosis (*see margin note*).

The factors that might lead to overproduction of D-lactic acid and possibly other organic acids in his GI tract include a change in his GI bacterial flora owing to the use of antibiotics, provision of substrates to these bacteria (popsicles contain sucrose and fructose; fructose is poorly absorbed in the intestinal tract), and a slower transit time owing to the drug used to decrease intestinal motility to treat his diarrhea.

CASE 6-3: EXERCISE-INDUCED ACUTE RENAL FAILURE

(Case presented on page 185)

Does the patient have a renal defect that causes his P_{Urate} to be so low?

There are three ways to have a low P_{Urate}: a decrease in its production, destruction of circulating urate, or failure to reabsorb filtered urate. Measuring the urate excretion rate distinguishes between the first two of these possibilities and a renal problem. If one of the former is the case, the rate of excretion of urate would be very low, whereas if there is a renal problem, the rate of urate excretion is the same as in other subjects. Hence, marked hypouricemia, a normal urate excretion rate, and the presence of normal urate production indicate a defect in urate reabsorption in the proximal convoluted tubule in this patient.

The usual renal handing of filtered urate is shown in Figure 6-20. The process involves two steps: a urate/organic anion exchanger (URAT-1) and a Na^+-linked reabsorption of the secreted organic anion. The binding of urate in the former step is inhibited by a number of compounds that cause hyperuricemia (e.g., L-lactate, β-hydroxybutyrate, salicylate). Molecular studies in this patient revealed a mutation in URAT-1 that diminishes its activity.

BASIS OF INCREASED $P_{Anion\ Gap}$
Of interest, part of the rise in the $P_{Anion\ gap}$ could be due to a higher $P_{Albumin}$ if his plasma volume is reduced and to a larger net negative valence on albumin in this setting. Alternatively, there may have been acids other than D-lactic acid produced by his altered GI bacterial flora.

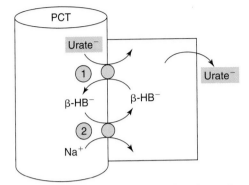

FIGURE 6-20 Proximal tubular urate transport. The traditional view on the renal transport of urate is that it is filtered and both reabsorbed and secreted. More recent data suggest that there is only filtration and reabsorption of urate. Two steps are involved in reabsorption. First, urate is reabsorbed in exchange for an organic anion via a urate-organic anion exchanger (URAT-1; *site 1*). Second, the organic anions that enter the lumen are reabsorbed using the Na^+-organic anion cotransporter (*site 2*). Compounds that interfere with URAT or this Na^+-linked organic anion cotransporter can alter the excretion of urate. Inactivating mutations in the gene that encodes URAT-1 diminish its activity, and this can lead to marked hypouricemia. β-HB, β-hydroxybutyrate anion; PCT, proximal convoluted tubule.

What is the role of the patient's low P_{Urate} in causing his exercise-induced acute renal failure?

To answer this question, we need first to examine the role of exercise in the formation of ROS. To generate more ROS, the P_{O_2} and/or the concentration of electrons (e^-) must rise. During vigorous exercise, the blood flow rate is high, but the consumption of O_2 is so large that the P_{O_2} is very low in capillaries. The concentration of e^- may also be low because of the very rapid flux through the electron transport system. Hence, the risk of forming O_2^- is low. Just after the exercise stops, however, the consumption of O_2 declines markedly while the rate of blood flow, although being lower, is less reduced than the rate of O_2 consumption. This high rate of blood flow is beneficial because it causes the P_{CO_2} to fall in muscle cells so their bicarbonate buffer system can remove the H^+ produced when phosphocreatine is formed (see Chapter 1, page 33 for more details). A "price" for maintaining this high rate of blood flow is a rise in the P_{O_2} in these cells. In addition, the slower flux of electrons in the electron transport system leads to a rise in their concentration. This together with the rise in the P_{O_2} increases the formation of O_2^-. Normally, a major route of removing O_2^- in the circulation is its reaction with urate—this cannot occur at a fast enough rate when the P_{Urate} is so low.

The question now is why the patient developed acute renal failure. Not only does the kidney receive a large proportion of the cardiac output; its proximal tubule cells are always exposed to a high P_{O_2} (*see margin note*). Therefore, it has a continuous high demand for a system to remove ROS. In fact, an almost universal symptom in patients with low P_{Urate} who develop acute renal failure shortly after exercise is bilateral flank pain due to renal parenchymal swelling, which may be the result of a sudden large rise in the concentrations of ROS and thereby, cell damage.

HIGH RENAL CORTICAL P_{O_2}
Renal cortical cells depend on having a high P_{O_2} for their ability to have a sensitive system to detect a need for the synthesis of erythropoietin (see Chapter 8, page 236 for more discussion).

USE OF DICHLOROACETATE

- Dichloroacetate is an activator of PDH, which accelerates the oxidation of L-lactic acid and thereby removes H^+, providing that oxygen is available.
- There is a minor benefit of dichloroacetate as the oxidation of pyruvate yields 6 ATP/O_2, whereas the oxidation of fatty acids yields close to 10% less ATP/O_2. Hence, in the rare case in which the degree of hypoxia is less than 10%, dichloroacetate may be useful, at least in theory, to allow more ATP to be regenerated per O_2 consumed and diminish the rate of production of lactic acid.
- Dichloroacetate is currently being tested for use in patients with cancer. The rationale is that activation of PDH will generate more of the semialdehyde form of CoQ and thereby more reactive oxygen species, which leads to tumor cell death. Some tumor cells are particularly vulnerable because PDH activity limits their rate of glucose oxidation.

6-1 *Why is the rate of production of ketoacids so much lower than that of L-lactic acid if both are regulated by the rate of turnover of ATP to yield ADP?*

The answer focuses on the restrictions set by the rate of consumption of O_2 (availability of ADP) in the major organs involved in the process and by stoichiometry.

In quantitative terms, the rate of production of ADP to form ketoacids in the liver is orders of magnitude lower than the quantity of ADP formed during vigorous muscle work.

6-2 *Consider the following example. An anoxic limb needs to regenerate 18 mmol/min of ATP (25% of the ATP needed in the body) via anaerobic glycolysis. If the rest of the body could be "persuaded" to oxidize L-lactate anions (+ H^+) to regenerate all needed ATP (54 mmol/min), would L-lactic acid still accumulate?*

The answer focuses on the stoichiometry of H^+/ATP during production and removal of L-lactic acid. For this anoxic limb to generate 18 mmol of ATP via anaerobic glycolysis, 18 mmol of L-lactic acid are formed. Examining the following equation for L-lactic acid removal reveals that oxidation of 1 mmol of L-lactic acid causes the regeneration of 18 mmol of ATP. Therefore, if the rest of the body could be "persuaded" to oxidize L-lactate anions (+ H^+) to regenerate all needed ATP (54 mmol/min), only 3 mmol of lactic acid per minute are removed (in contrast to 18 mmol/min of L-lactic acid produced). Clearly L-lactic acid will accumulate. The obvious message from this quantitative analysis is that one cannot overcome a rapid rate of production of L-lactic acid by accelerating its rate of removal. Hence, drugs such as dichloroacetate are unlikely to be of benefit during hypoxic L-lactic acidosis (*see margin note*).

$$\text{L-Lactate}^- + H^+ + 3\,O_2 + 3\,(ADP + Pi) \rightarrow 18\,ATP + 3\,CO_2 + 3\,H_2O$$

6-3 *If a patient has hypoxia but little glycogen in the liver, does L-lactic acidosis develop? If not, what changes would you expect to find in the concentration of metabolites in blood?*

Because the major substrate to make L-lactic acid during hypoxia is glucose, if there is little glucose available, one develops hypoglycemia but little L-lactic acidosis.

6-4 *$NaHCO_3$ is given as treatment for L-lactic acidosis, but there is no rise in the P_{HCO3}. Is it appropriate to conclude that the alkali has not been helpful?*

To be a successful buffer, HCO_3^- must remove H^+ bound to proteins in the ICF of vital organs (e.g., brain and heart) or accelerate the rate of production of ATP in these organs by deinhibiting phosphofructokinase (see page 166 in this chapter). In the latter case, more L-lactic acid is formed. In both cases, this disappearance of HCO_3^- could be seen as being beneficial.

In clinical medicine, the focus is on the plasma H^+ and P_{HCO3} because they are easy to measure. It actually does not matter how much the P_{HCO3} per se rises because it represents untitrated base. In patients with hypoxic L-lactic acidosis, it is really the depletion of ATP in vital organs and the binding of H^+ to proteins in cells of these organs that are detrimental rather than the concentration of H^+ in the ECF compartment. One should recognize that if HCO_3^- disappears, L-lactic acid and ATP are generated and the latter may be beneficial.

6-5 *What useful functions can be attributed to the normal production of organic acids in the colon?*

When carbohydrates that cannot be absorbed in the small intestine (some fructose, fiber) are delivered to the colon, bacteria in this location convert them to a mixture of organic acids, which are absorbed and are added to the portal venous blood. The vast majority of these organic acids are oxidized, which converts ADP to ATP. As a result, these fuels can be used to permit the performance of biologic work. As discussed in the following paragraphs, there are also specific uses for individual organic acids.

　Butyric acid: The main function of this acid is to provide much of the fuel oxidized by the colon when it regenerates its ATP. Without butyric acid, the colon may not function properly (starvation colitis), possibly due in part to a deficiency of ATP.

　Propionic acid: Although propionic acid represents only close to 20% of the total amount of organic acids produced each day in the colon, it may have an important metabolic function. In more detail, propionic acid is converted in the liver to propionyl-CoA (Fig. 6-21). There are two major fates for this compound. In the fed state, it can be converted to pyruvate, which can then be oxidized or be made into glucose. Between meals there may be a need to synthesize four-carbon catalysts for the Krebs cycle (e.g., oxaloacetate) in organs other than the liver (e.g., in the

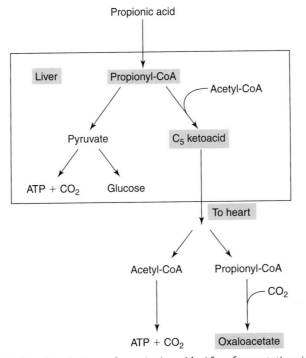

FIGURE 6-21 Metabolism of propionic acid. After fermentation in the colon to produce propionic acid, this acid is delivered to the liver (*rectangle*), where it is converted to propionyl-CoA. There are two major fates of this intermediate—conversion to pyruvate or to a C_5 ketoacid. The latter compound is released into the hepatic vein, and it can be taken up by the heart to regenerate its four-carbon tricarboxylic acid cycle intermediates.

USE OF PROPIONYL-CARNITINE
IN PATIENTS WITH HEART
FAILURE
Propionyl-carnitine has been used
to improve myocardial energetics
(ATP production) with the assumption that it is the carnitine that
provides the benefit. It is equally
possible that the supply of a precursor of oxaloacetate would be beneficial, depending on whether the
limiting factor in ATP production
is a limited supply of carnitine or
Krebs cycle intermediates in regions
of the myocardium.

OXALIC ACID
Only about 1% of gylcol acid is
metabolized to oxalic acid.

heart) if some of the four-carbon Krebs cycle catalysts are consumed during a catabolic phase of illness [*see margin note*]). To
ensure that propionic acid is not fully metabolized in the liver,
propionyl-CoA combines with a molecule of acetyl-CoA to produce a five-carbon ketoacid, which then exits the liver. When
the heart extracts this five-carbon ketoacid, the propionyl-CoA
formed could lead to improved aerobic fuel oxidation if there
were a large enough deficit of oxaloacetate.

6-6 *If oxalic acid were the sole product formed during the metabolism
of ethylene glycol, why might the degree of metabolic acidosis be less
severe?*

The unique property of oxalic acid is that it precipitates in solutions containing ionized Ca^{2+}. When ionized Ca^{2+} is precipitated in
the body as its oxalate salt, the concentration of ionized Ca^{2+} falls
and bone salts are hydrolyzed. These bone salts are alkaline, and
the anions released (PO_4^{3-} and CO_3^{2-}) remove H^+. The net result
is a diminished acidemia. Notwithstanding, there could be a major
problem of an acute fall in the concentration of ionized calcium (see
Chapter 7, page 216).

Introduction

ABBREVIATION
U$_{Cl}$, concentration of Cl$^-$ in the urine

Metabolic alkalosis is an electrolyte disorder accompanied by changes in acid-base parameters in plasma, namely an elevated concentration of HCO$_3^-$ (P$_{HCO3}$) and pH. Most patients with metabolic alkalosis have a deficit of NaCl, KCl, and/or HCl, each of which leads to a higher P$_{HCO3}$. A deficit of NaCl raises P$_{HCO3}$ primarily by lowering the extracellular fluid (ECF) volume, whereas a deficit of HCl or KCl does so by adding new HCO$_3^-$ to the body.

The most common causes of metabolic alkalosis are chronic vomiting (the initial deficit is HCl, which is transformed over time into a deficit of KCl) and the use of diuretics (the deficits are of NaCl and KCl). Measuring the concentration of electrolytes in urine is often very helpful for diagnostic purposes; the U$_{Cl}$ is particularly valuable in this regard. The major goal for therapy is to replace these deficits.

OBJECTIVES

- To illustrate that metabolic alkalosis is really an electrolyte disorder in which there are deficits of compounds that contain Cl^-, $NaCl$, KCl, and/or HCl.
- To emphasize that the deficits described may increase the HCO_3^-/ECF volume ratio by influencing its numerator and/or denominator.
- To illustrate how measuring the urine electrolytes can help reveal that there is a deficit of $NaCl$, KCl, and/or HCl; the U_{Cl} is the most helpful of these measurements.
- To emphasize that the goal for therapy should be to replace existing deficits.

CASE 7-1: A BALANCED VIEW OF "VOMITING"

(Case discussed on page 204)

(Case discussed on page 204)

REASON FOR SELECTING THIS CASE

This case was selected to illustrate the pathophysiology of metabolic alkalosis because the data needed to calculate balances were available. It differs, however, from the usual clinical presentation of protracted vomiting in that there was no significant deficit of NaCl.

BODY COMPOSITION
- Weight 70 kg, 67% water
- ICF volume: 30 L
- ECF volume: 15 L

NAMES OF PERIODS
- We have named the periods by their principal Cl compound deficits.
- Hence, the period in which the deficit is primarily HCl represents the *drainage period*.
- The period in which the deficit is primarily KCl is also called the *postdrainage period*. There is overlap in that the deficit of KCl begins during the drainage period.

A deficit of HCl is induced in a healthy human volunteer in a clinical research center by aspirating gastric contents for several days while balance data were obtained *(see margin notes)*. The drainage period and postdrainage periods are easy to define, and some of the adaptive responses to the deficit of HCl are clearly evident during the time that drainage occurred. The P_{HCO3} at the end of the drainage period was 37 mmol/L and the plasma pH was 7.47. Losses of Na^+ were replaced with nonchloride salts of Na^+ to maintain the selective deficit of HCl. Although there were no appreciable changes in plasma acid-base values in the postdrainage period, there was a progressively larger negative balance of K^+—its cumulative deficit was virtually equal to the cumulative deficit of Cl^-. Nevertheless, the story is not complete until one understands how electroneutrality has been achieved. With NaCl therapy, the P_{HCO3} fell from 37 mmol/L to 25 mmol/L. There was a large positive balance of Na^+ and Cl^-, however, enough to overexpand the ECF volume by close to 5 L.

CUMULATIVE BALANCE (mmol)

	DAYS	Na^+	K^+	Cl^-
HCl loss	0–2	−5	−10	−200
KCl deficit	3–6	−10	−190	0
Cumulative		−25	−200	−200
Cumulative balance after treatment with NaCl		+1000	−300	+700

Questions

How large was the deficit of HCl?

Why did the deficit of K^+ equal that of Cl^- at the end of the postdrainage period?

What is the therapy for metabolic alkalosis at this stage?

CASE 7-2: THIS MAN SHOULD NOT HAVE METABOLIC ALKALOSIS

(Case discussed on page 206)

(Case discussed on page 206)

After a forced 6-hour run in the desert in heat of day, an elite corps soldier was the only one in his squad who collapsed. He had perspired profusely but had free access to water and glucose-containing fluids during the exercise. He did not vomit and denied the prior intake of medications. Physical examination revealed a markedly contracted effective arterial blood volume. Initial laboratory data are provided below.

P_{Na}	mmol/L	116	pH		7.47
P_K	mmol/L	2.7	P_{HCO_3}	mmol/L	37
P_{Cl}	mmol/L	56	Arterial P_{CO_2}	mm Hg	47
Hematocrit		0.50			

Questions

What is the basis for metabolic alkalosis?

What is the therapy for metabolic alkalosis in this patient?

CASE 7-3: WHY DOES METABOLIC ALKALOSIS DEVELOP SO QUICKLY?

(Case discussed on page 207)

A 52-year-old Asian man has chronic lung disease. Prior to this admission, his arterial pH was 7.40, P_{CO_2} was 40 mm Hg, and P_{HCO_3} was 24 mmol/L. In the past 24 hours, he developed an acute attack of asthma with very prominent wheezing that was resistant to his usual medications (inhaled β-adrenergics and theophylline). In the emergency department, he received a large dose of cortisol, and this treatment was continued for the next 4 days in the hospital. On day 3, his breathing had improved markedly, and he was able to eat without difficulty. He did not vomit or use diuretics. Surprisingly, a severe degree of hypokalemia and metabolic alkalosis (arterial pH 7.47, P_{CO_2} 50 mm Hg) were present on day 4. At this time, his urine Na+, K+, and Cl− concentrations were 54 mmol/L, 23 mmol/L, and 53 mmol/L, respectively. He had a calculated creatinine clearance of 80 mL/min and a $P_{Glucose}$ of 102 mg/dL (6 mmol/L).

DAY		0	3	4
P_K	mmol/L	4.0	3.2	1.7
P_{HCO_3}	mmol/L	24	29	37

Question

Why did metabolic alkalosis develop on days 3 and 4?

ABBREVIATIONS

$P_{Glucose}$, concentration of glucose in plasma

P_K, concentration of potassium in plasma

P_{Na}, concentration of sodium in plasma

$P_{Albumin}$, concentration of albumin in plasma

$P_{Anion\ gap}$, anion gap in plasma

GFR, glomerular filtration rate

PART A
PATHOPHYSIOLOGY

OVERVIEW

- The term *Cl− depletion alkalosis* is an incomplete description of the pathophysiology of any form of metabolic alkalosis because it fails to indicate how electroneutrality was achieved.

Metabolic alkalosis is a process that leads to a rise in the P_{HCO_3} and the plasma pH. The following fundamental principles are necessary to understand why metabolic alkalosis develops. The concentration of HCO_3^- is the ratio of the content of HCO_3^- in the ECF compartment (numerator) and the ECF volume (denominator). A rise in the concentration of HCO_3^- might be due to an increase in its numerator (addition of HCO_3^-) and/or a decrease in its denominator (diminished ECF volume). A quantitative estimate of the ECF volume is critical to assess the quantity of HCO_3^- in the ECF compartment and thereby to assess the basis of the metabolic alkalosis. Because electroneutrality must be present, terms such as *Cl⁻ depletion alkalosis* are misleading; deficits must be defined as HCl, KCl, and/or NaCl. Knowing the balances for Na^+, K^+, and Cl^- allows one to decide why the P_{HCO3} has risen and what changes have occurred in the composition of the ECF and ICF compartments. Even though balance data are not available in most patients, careful attention to other available laboratory measurements such as the hematocrit helps the clinician obtain a quantitative assessment of ECF volume. Thus, it is possible to reach a reasonable conclusion about the contribution of deficits of the different Cl^--containing compounds to the development of the metabolic alkalosis (see Case 7-2 and Fig. 7-1).

Critical to the understanding of the pathophysiology of metabolic alkalosis is that there is no tubular maximum for HCO_3^- reabsorption in the kidney. Angiotensin II and the usual pH in proximal convoluted tubule cells are the two major physiologic stimuli for $NaHCO_3$ reabsorption in this nephron segment. Both of these stimuli must be removed for $NaHCO_3$ to be excreted (see Chapter 1, page 19 for more details).

Metabolic alkalosis is usually thought of as a "primary" acid-base disorder; however, this is true only in the very initial stage of HCl deficiency. In contrast, in some patients, the high P_{HCO3} is secondary to a disorder of K^+ homeostasis, causing a deficit of KCl (see the discussion of postdrainage phase of Case 7-1). In yet other

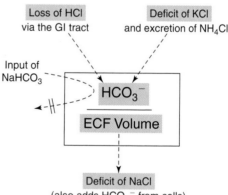

FIGURE 7-1 **Basis for a high concentration of HCO_3^- in the extracellular fluid (ECF) compartment**. The *rectangle* represents the ECF compartment. The concentration of HCO_3^- is the ratio of the content of HCO_3^- in the ECF compartment (numerator) and the ECF volume (denominator). The major causes for a rise in the content of HCO_3^- in the ECF compartment is a deficit of HCl and/or a deficit of KCl (*upper portion*). The major cause for a fall in the ECF volume is a deficit of NaCl (*see margin note*). An intake of $NaHCO_3$ is not sufficient on its own to cause a sustained increase in the content of HCO_3^- in the ECF compartment, except if there also is a marked reduction in the glomerular filtration rate or if there is another lesion that augments the usual stimuli for the reabsorption of $NaHCO_3$ in the proximal convoluted tubule (*double lines in the left portion* indicate reduced renal output of $NaHCO_3$). GI, gastrointestinal.

A DEFICIT OF NaCl MAY CAUSE A GAIN OF HCO_3^-

If a deficit of NaCl causes a severe degree of ECF volume contraction, there will be a rise in the venous Pco_2 and thereby in the cell Pco_2. As a result, HCO_3^- are formed and added to the ECF compartment (see Fig 3-1, page 66).

patients, the high P_{HCO3} is due to a deficit of NaCl that raises the P_{HCO3} owing to a contracted ECF volume (see the discussion of Case 7-2). Accordingly, we emphasize how each of these primary deficits (HCl, KCl, and NaCl) can cause the P_{HCO3} to be high in this chapter; we refer the reader to Chapter 13 for a more detailed discussion of the physiology of K^+ and to Chapter 9 for a more detailed discussion of the physiology of Na^+.

DEVELOPMENT OF METABOLIC ALKALOSIS

A deficit of HCl, KCl, and/or NaCl causes the P_{HCO3} to rise (Flow Chart 7-1). Determining whether there is a negative balance of each of these Cl^--containing compounds has implications for understanding the pathophysiology of metabolic alkalosis in a given patient and changes in the composition of the ECF and ICF compartments and in designing appropriate therapy.

Deficit of HCl

- The net result of a deficit of HCl is a gain of HCO_3^- that is equimolar to the loss of Cl^-.
- Electroneutrality is maintained because there is simply an exchange of anions in the ECF compartment.

Gain of HCO_3^-

The gain of HCO_3^- in the ECF compartment is the result of H^+ secretion into the lumen of the stomach and its loss in vomiting.

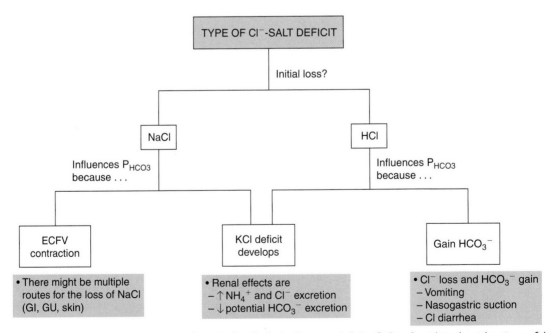

FLOW CHART 7-1 Pathophysiology of metabolic alkalosis due to a deficit of Cl^- salts. This algorithm is useful for understanding how a deficit of HCl, KCl, and/or NaCl contributes to the development of metabolic alkalosis. Later in this chapter, we address metabolic alkalosis due to a gain of $NaHCO_3$. ECFV, extracellular fluid volume; GI, gastrointestinal; GU, genitourinary.

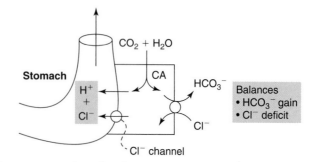

FIGURE 7-2 Secretion of HCl in the stomach. The *stylized structure* is the stomach with a parietal cell on its right border. In this cell, $CO_2 + H_2O$ are converted to H^+ and HCO_3^-, a reaction that is catalyzed by carbonic anhydrase (CA). H^+ are secreted into the lumen of the stomach by an H^+/K^+-ATPase, while K^+ recycle back into the parietal cell (not shown, for simplicity). Cl^- from the extracellular fluid compartment enter parietal cells on the HCO_3^-/Cl^- anion exchanger; Cl^- enter the lumen of the stomach via Cl^- ion channels. Overall, there is a loss of Cl^- and a gain of HCO_3^- in the body during vomiting.

Electroneutrality

The steps involved in the loss of HCl via vomiting are illustrated in Figure 7-2. The process that adds H^+ to the lumen of the stomach is electroneutral because there is an equivalent secretion of Cl^-. Within the parietal cells that secrete HCl, the immediate source of H^+ (and HCO_3^-) is carbonic acid (H_2CO_3), which is made from $CO_2 + H_2O$—the enzyme carbonic anhydrase catalyzes this reaction. The process is electroneutral because both H^+ and HCO_3^- exit from the cell. In the ECF compartment, electroneutrality is maintained because HCO_3^- exits the cell via a Cl^-/HCO_3^- anion exchanger with a 1:1 stoichiometry; hence, there is simply an exchange of Cl^- for HCO_3^- in the ECF compartment.

Balance

The net effect is a loss of Cl^- and an equivalent gain of HCO_3^- in the body.

Renal contribution to the high P_{HCO3}

- Angiotensin II and the usual pH in proximal convoluted tubule cells are the two major physiologic stimuli for $NaHCO_3$ reabsorption in the proximal convoluted tubule. To reabsorb less $NaHCO_3$, both of these stimuli must be removed.

ALKALINE TIDE
This term refers to the consequences of secreting HCl in the stomach. Although this causes a higher P_{HCO3} (the P_{HCO3} rises to ~30 mmol/L), it does not induce an appreciable rate of excretion of HCO_3^- in the urine. It is advantageous to avoid the loss of HCO_3^- because ultimately, the P_{HCO3} will decrease when $NaHCO_3$ is secreted into the duodenum.

Although some invoke a special renal action to augment the reabsorption of filtered $NaHCO_3$ to maintain metabolic alkalosis, this is not necessary. In fact, addition of HCO_3^- to the ECF compartment under physiologic conditions does not automatically cause a large excretion of this anion (e.g., the higher P_{HCO3} owing to alkaline tide following the secretion of HCl in the stomach; *see margin note*). Because angiotensin II and the usual pH in proximal convoluted tubule cells are the two major physiologic stimuli for $NaHCO_3$ reabsorption in the proximal convoluted tubule, a large input of $NaHCO_3$ is excreted because its Na^+ load expands the effective arterial blood volume, and thus results in a fall in angiotensin II levels while its HCO_3^- load causes an increase in the intracellular pH in proximal convoluted tubule cells.

Later in the course of gastric HCl loss, hypokalemia develops owing to renal loss of K^+ with an anion other than Cl^- or HCO_3^-. Hypokalemia is associated with an acidified proximal convoluted tubule cell pH, which leads to an enhanced excretion of NH_4^+ and a diminished excretion of organic anions and HCO_3^-. This continues until the P_{HCO3} rises sufficiently to return the pH in proximal convoluted tubule cells toward its normal value but at the expense of a higher P_{HCO3}.

Deficit of KCl

- A deficit of KCl results in a gain of HCO_3^- in the ECF compartment and it also ensures that the kidneys retain this extra HCO_3^-. The signal for these two processes is a lower pH in cells of the proximal convoluted tubule (*see margin note*).

METABOLIC ALKALOSIS DUE TO A DEFICIT OF KCl

- This is common in patients with chronic vomiting and/or diuretic use.
- In chronic vomiting, there is also a large deficit of HCl early in the time course and a variable deficit of NaCl.
- In patients with diuretic use, while balance data are not available, one component of the pathophysiology of metabolic alkalosis is due to a deficit of KCl (i.e., a gain of HCO_3^- in the ECF compartment plus a gain of H^+ and Na^+ in the ICF compartment).
- If Na^+ is retained in cells, there must be a reason why it was not exported on the Na-K-ATPase.
- There is also a prominent deficit of NaCl.

Gain of HCO_3^-

The gain of HCO_3^- in the ECF compartment is the result of two renal processes that are driven by a deficit of K^+. They share a common signal, an acidified proximal convoluted tubule cell pH. The first process is an enhanced excretion of NH_4^+ in the urine with Cl^-, which adds HCO_3^- to the body (Fig. 7-3). The second process is the reduced excretion of organic anions such as citrate (i.e., potential HCO_3^-) in the urine. As presented in Figure 1-5, page 10, dietary alkali load is eliminated by the excretion of organic anions (e.g., citrate)—this process is diminished when there is an acidified proximal convoluted tubule cell pH (e.g., associated with a deficit of K^+).

Electroneutrality

A deficit of KCl satisfies the need for electroneutrality in whole body terms. Nevertheless, because most of the K^+ is lost from the

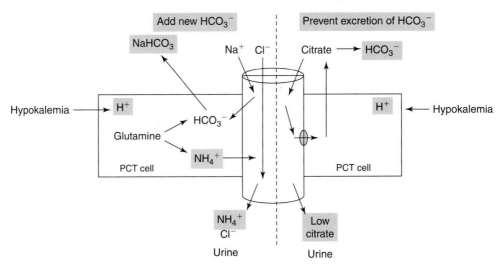

FIGURE 7-3 Retention of HCO_3^- in the body during a deficit of KCl. The *central cylindrical structure* represents the lumen of the proximal convoluted tubule (PCT) with two PCT cells. A deficit of K^+ is associated with intracellular acidosis in PCT cells. As shown to the *left of the dashed vertical line*, the production of $NH_4^+ + HCO_3^-$ is augmented. NH_4^+ is excreted in the urine with Cl^- while the new HCO_3^- is added to the body. As shown to the *right of the dashed vertical line*, intracellular acidosis augments the reabsorption of filtered organic anions (e.g., citrate), which compromises the elimination of dietary HCO_3^-.

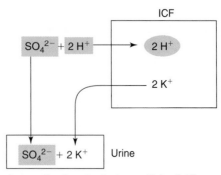

FIGURE 7-4 Balance of cations in the intracellular fluid (ICF) compartment in the postdrainage period. The *large rectangle* represents the ICF compartment, which contains the vast bulk of body K^+. Early in the drainage period of selective depletion of HCl, there is a deficit of Cl^- and a gain of HCO_3^- in the ECF compartment (see Fig. 7-2). In the postdrainage period, the balance becomes one of a KCl deficit; K^+ are excreted in the urine with an anion other than Cl^- or HCO_3^-. SO_4^{2-} anions that are produced with H^+ during the oxidation of sulfur-containing amino acids, which yields H_2SO_4. For electroneutrality in the ICF compartment, the shift of K^+ out of cells is likely to be accompanied primarily by a shift of H^+ into cells, while this exported K^+ is excreted with SO_4^{2-} anions.

ICF compartment, one needs to understand how electroneutrality is achieved in both the ECF and ICF compartments because each compartment has lost a single ion. Because electroneutrality must be present, an anion is retained in the ECF compartment (HCO_3^-) and a cation (H^+ or Na^+) is retained in the ICF compartment (Fig. 7-4). The balance data to reveal how electroneutrality is achieved in both the ECF and ICF compartments are available from the postdrainage period of the study of selective depletion of HCl. These data indicate that K^+ is lost in the urine with an anion other than Cl^- or HCO_3^-. In more detail, H^+ are produced during the oxidation of sulfur-containing amino acids to yield H_2SO_4, and K^+ is excreted with SO_4^{2-} (see Chapter 13, page 438 for a discussion of the mechanisms involved). For electroneutrality in the ICF compartment, the shift of K^+ out of cells is accompanied by a shift of H^+ into cells.

Balance

- In the postdrainage period of the selective depletion of HCl, the deficits of K^+ and Cl^- are equal. Hence, the gain of HCO_3^- in the ECF compartment is equal to the gain of H^+ in the ICF compartment, and in *total* body terms, there is a nil balance of the sum of H^+ and HCO_3^-.

The net result of this loss of KCl is a gain of HCO_3^- in and an equivalent loss of Cl^- from the ECF compartment as well as a gain of H^+ in and a loss of K^+ from the ICF compartment (Fig. 7-5; *see margin note*). Because the deficits of K^+ and Cl^- are equal, the gain of HCO_3^- in the ECF compartment is equal to the gain of H^+ in the ICF compartment.

Renal contribution to the high P_{HCO3}

Hypokalemia leads to an enhanced rate of excretion of NH_4^+ and a diminished rate of excretion of organic anions, which raise the P_{HCO3}. Once the P_{HCO3} rises sufficiently to return the ICF pH toward its

METABOLIC ALKALOSIS DUE TO KCl DEFICIT IN PATIENTS WITH PRIMARY HIGH MINERALOCORTICOID ACTIVITY

- In this setting, there is an initial surplus of NaCl owing to actions of mineralocorticoids.
- The second primary event is the excretion of K^+ along with some of the Cl^- that was retained. The resulting deficit of K^+ acidifies proximal convoluted tubule cells and thereby results in the retention of some of the dietary alkali with Na^+ and in an increased rate of excretion of NH_4^+ with Cl^-; both cause the development of metabolic alkalosis.
- In total body terms, there is a net gain of $NaHCO_3$. Balance data are not available in these patients; nevertheless, it is likely that the loss of K^+ from ICF is accompanied by a gain of H^+ and/or Na^+ in the ICF compartment. If Na^+ were retained in the ICF, there would need to be a lower activity of the Na-K-ATPase, but the mechanism for this is not clear.

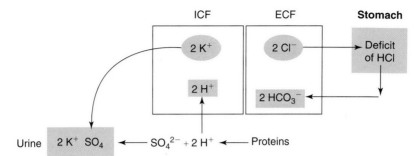

FIGURE 7-5 Balances in the extracellular fluid (ECF) and intracellular fluid (ICF) compartments in the model of selective depletion of HCl. The net balance is a deficit of K^+ and Cl^- but via different routes. Although there is metabolic alkalosis, the gain of HCO_3^- in the ECF compartment is equal to the gain of H^+ in the ICF compartment.

normal value, these patients can achieve acid-base balance by excreting the appropriate amounts of NH_4^+ and organic anions in the urine as dictated by their dietary intake, but at a higher P_{HCO3}.

Deficit of NaCl

• A deficit of NaCl results in a higher P_{HCO3} primarily because of a contracted ECF volume.

Although a deficit of NaCl leads to an increase in the HCO_3^- concentration in the ECF compartment, the content of HCO_3^- is largely unchanged. Nevertheless, a minor gain of HCO_3^- in the ECF compartment can occur if there is a high P_{CO_2} in cells owing to a very contracted effective arterial blood volume. This causes the equation for the bicarbonate buffer system to be displaced toward H^+ and HCO_3^-. The latter is added to the ECF compartment, raising the P_{HCO3} somewhat (see Fig. 3-1, page 66).

$$CO_2 + H_2O \rightleftharpoons H_2CO_3 \rightleftharpoons H^+ (\text{bind to protein}) + HCO_3^- (\text{to the ECF})$$

Electroneutrality

Electroneutrality is maintained because both Na^+ and Cl^- are lost from the ECF compartment.

Balance

There is a loss of Na^+ and Cl^- from the ECF compartment without an appreciable change in the content of HCO_3^- in this compartment.

Renal contribution to the high P_{HCO3}

When the effective arterial blood volume is contracted, renin is released and angiotensin II is formed. Angiotensin II is the most potent stimulator of the reabsorption of $NaHCO_3$ in the proximal convoluted tubule (see Chapter 1, page 17 for more discussion).

Input and retention of NaHCO$_3$

> • To understand the basis of this type of metabolic alkalosis, seek the source of NaHCO$_3$ input and also the reason why stimuli for NaHCO$_3$ reabsorption are still present.

Source of alkali

A diet that contains fruit and vegetables provides an alkali load in the form of K$^+$ salts of organic anions (potential HCO$_3^-$; see Fig. 1-5, page 10); this daily intake in a typical Western diet is 30 to 40 mEq. At times, the source of alkali is certain medications; examples include NaHCO$_3$ tablets, acetate anions (e.g., in total parental nutrition solutions), citrate anions (e.g., in K$^+$ supplements), and/or carbonate or hydroxyl anions (e.g., in certain antacid preparations).

Renal reasons for a markedly reduced rate of excretion of NaHCO$_3$

> • There are two reasons for a reduced excretion of NaHCO$_3$: (1) a marked reduction in the GFR, and/or (2) an enhanced reabsorption of HCO$_3^-$ in the proximal convoluted tubule.

The first reason for a markedly reduced rate of excretion of NaHCO$_3$ is a relatively large decrease in its filtered load owing to a significant reduction in the GFR. The second reason is the presence of the stimuli for NaHCO$_3$ reabsorption by proximal convoluted tubule cells. The latter is due to an acidified proximal convoluted tubule cell pH (usually because of hypokalemia) or a condition in which the level of angiotensin II is high despite an expanded effective arterial blood volume (e.g., renal artery stenosis or a renin-producing tumor).

Renal reabsorption of NaHCO$_3$: A more detailed analysis

The traditional view of the renal handling of HCO$_3^-$ is that there is a renal threshold and a tubular maximum for the reabsorption of HCO$_3^-$ in the proximal convoluted tubule. This conclusion is based largely on experimental studies performed by Pitts many decades ago. When examining the results of these experiments, it is important to consider some pertinent aspects of regulation of HCO$_3^-$ reabsorption by proximal convoluted tubule cells; these are summarized in the following paragraph.

Stimuli for the reabsorption of filtered NaHCO$_3$

> • The usual concentration of H$^+$ in cells of the proximal convoluted tubule and/or the usual level of angiotensin II are sufficient stimuli for the reabsorption of most of the filtered NaHCO$_3$.

H$^+$ secretion in the proximal convoluted tubule occurs largely via the Na$^+$/H$^+$ exchanger (NHE-3). The usual circulating levels of angiotensin II and the usual concentration of H$^+$ in proximal convoluted tubule cells provide sufficient stimuli to permit the reabsorption of most of the filtered NaHCO$_3$. In contrast, if a subject is given a load of NaHCO$_3$, the kidney is unable to reabsorb this extra filtered load of HCO$_3^-$ because the Na$^+$ load expands the effective arterial blood volume, which leads to suppression of the release of angiotensin II, and the load of HCO_3^- lowers the concentration of H^+ in proximal convoluted tubule cells.

Experiments carried out by Pitts

- The experimental design was to administer $NaHCO_3$ and hence the gain of HCO_3^- was *not* accompanied by a deficit of Cl^- in the ECF compartment.

The experiments were designed to define the physiologic renal response to an administered load of HCO_3^- (notice this term lacks electroneutrality) in dogs. Really, it is the renal response to a load of *NaHCO_3*, which, as mentioned previously, would diminish the stimuli for the reabsorption of $NaHCO_3$ that are normally present in the proximal convoluted tubule. Hence, the results of these experiments are predictable; all the extra $NaHCO_3$ that is filtered will be excreted in the urine. These results, however, were interpreted to indicate that there is a tubular maximum for the rate of reabsorption of $NaHCO_3$ by the kidney (Fig. 7-6).

Renal response to a physiologic load of HCO_3^-

Evidence to support the physiology of an absence of a tubular maximum for the reabsorption of HCO_3^- is that the rise in the P_{HCO3} caused by the secretion of HCl in the stomach during the daily alkaline tide does not cause appreciable bicarbonaturia. As shown in Figure 7-2, and described in electroneutral terms, a gain of HCO_3^- occurs when the stomach secretes HCl. This gain of HCO_3^- is accompanied by an equivalent deficit of Cl^- in the ECF compartment, and accordingly, there is no increase in the ECF volume with this rise in P_{HCO3}. Hence, there is no inhibition of the reabsorption of HCO_3^- by the proximal convoluted tubule, and virtually all the surplus of HCO_3^- is retained in this setting (see Fig. 7-6). If a large amount of HCO_3^- were to be excreted, a deficit of HCO_3^- would be created when $NaHCO_3$ is secreted into the duodenum at a later time to neutralize this HCl; the resultant Na^+ and Cl^- are absorbed.

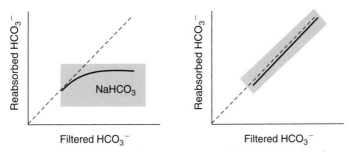

FIGURE 7-6 Control of the renal reabsorption of $NaHCO_3$. In this figure, the *horizontal axis* represents the filtered load of HCO_3^- (P_{HCO3} × GFR), and the *vertical axis* represents the amount of HCO_3^- reabsorbed. The *left* graph depicts the results of experiments when a load of $NaHCO_3$ is given, and the *right graph* depicts the results of experiments in which a rise in the P_{HCO3} was induced without ECF volume expansion. The *dashed line* represents the complete reabsorption of all of the filtered load of HCO_3^- and the *solid line* represents the data from that experiment.

To correct this deficit, new HCO_3^- would have to be generated by the kidney via increased ammoniagenesis, a process that consumes the amino acid glutamine. Furthermore, for electroneutrality, the excretion of the anion HCO_3^- obligates the excretion of a cation, Na^+ and/or K^+, that might result in deficits of these cations.

Experimental studies in animals also demonstrated the absence of a tubular maximum for HCO_3^- reabsorption when the gain of $NaHCO_3$ was matched with a loss of NaCl. In these studies, the P_{HCO3} rose to 50 mmol/L without inducing appreciable bicarbonaturia.

DISCUSSION OF CASES 7-1, 7-2, and 7-3

CASE 7-1: A BALANCED VIEW OF "VOMITING"

(Case presented on page 194)

How large was the deficit of HCl?

In electroneutral terms, the net effect of this selective deficit of HCl is a loss of Cl^- and a gain of HCO_3^- in a 1:1 stoichiometry (see Fig. 7-1). Therefore the magnitude of the HCl deficit (or the gain of HCO_3^- in the body) is equal to the negative balance for Cl^- (200 mmol). The strategies for therapy at this stage are illustrated in Figure 7-7.

Balances during the period of HCl deficit

Prior to the loss of HCl, this subject weighs 70 kg and has 45 L of total body water, with 15 L in his ECF compartment and 30 L in his ICF compartment.

Cl^- balance. Before withdrawing the HCl, he had 1545 mmol of Cl^- in his ECF compartment (P_{Cl} 103 mmol/L × 15 L). After the negative balance of 200 mmol of Cl^-, his ECF contains about 1345 mmol of Cl^- (1545 mmol – 200 mmol). If there were no change in his ECF volume (15 L) and all the Cl^- were lost from his ECF compartment, his final P_{Cl} would be about 90 mmol/L (1345 mmol/15 L).

HCO_3^- balance. His ECF compartment contained 375 mmol of HCO_3^- before the withdrawal of HCl (25 mmol/L × 15 L) and 575 mmol of HCO_3^- after the addition of 200 mmol of new HCO_3^- (375 mmol + 200 mmol). Hence his new HCO_3^- concentration would have been 39 mmol/L if none of the HCO_3^- entered cells (575 mmol/15 L). Thus a final P_{HCO3} of 37 mmol/L would imply that almost all of the HCO_3^- remained in the ECF compartment in the period when the only deficit consisted of HCl.

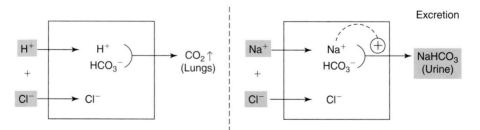

FIGURE 7-7 Therapy to replace a deficit of H^+ + Cl^-. The *rectangle* represents the body. There is gain of HCO_3^- and a loss of Cl^- of equal magnitudes. This mass balance can be corrected by giving HCl (*left portion*) or NaCl, providing that the resultant ECF volume expansion leads to the renal excretion of $NaHCO_3$ (*right portion*).

Why did the deficit of K⁺ equal that of Cl⁻ at the end of the postdrainage period?

The deficit of K^+ occurs primarily via the renal excretion of K^+. The mechanism for this renal excretion of K^+ is described on page 438 in Chapter 13.

Balances during the period of K⁺ deficit

Since there were only minor changes in the P_{Cl}, P_{HCO3}, and ECF volume (as judged from the minor negative balance for Na^+ along with little change in the hematocrit), the anion lost when the deficit of K^+ occurred was an anion other than Cl^- and HCO_3^-. Therefore, to understand how electroneutrality was maintained, two other areas must be evaluated: the ICF compartment and the urine.

Electroneutrality in the ICF compartment. The negative balance for K^+ was about 200 mmol. Since the vast majority of K^+ is located in cells, the origin of this K^+ loss is from the ICF compartment, but the exact organ involved was not defined in this experiment (it is likely that the major organ that lost this K^+ was skeletal muscle, owing to the magnitude of the K^+ deficit). As judged from the balance data, there was little excretion of HCO_3^- or Cl^- in this period (no change in the P_{Cl} or P_{HCO3}). The mechanism for the retention of HCO_3^- in the ECF compartment is likely an enhanced reabsorption of HCO_3^- (and organic anions such as citrate; *see margin note*) in the proximal convoluted tubule once the P_K fell below 3.5 mmol/L.

To maintain electroneutrality in cells when K^+ exits, there must be either a loss of anions from the ICF compartment (predominantly from organic phosphates such as RNA, DNA, phospholipids, phosphocreatine, or ATP) or a gain of a cation (Na^+ or H^+). The former is not likely since there was little negative balance for phosphate. It is also unlikely that the loss of K^+ from the ICF was accompanied by a gain of Na^+ because there was no significant change in ECF volume. Moreover, to gain Na^+ in the cells, there must be inhibition of the Na-K-ATPase. Therefore, the most likely event is a gain of H^+ as discussed in a following section.

Electroneutrality in the urine. There must be an anion in the urine to accompany K^+ and it was not Cl^- or HCO_3^- as discussed above. Therefore these "occult" urine anions must enter the body without Na^+ or K^+ (i.e., as an acid) to account for the balance data for these cations. Since H_2SO_4 is produced daily during the metabolism of dietary sulfur-containing amino acids, the excretion of 2 K^+ per SO_4^{2-} in the urine could explain the balance data and also account for the electroneutrality in the ICF compartment (gain of H^+ is largely equal to this deficit of about 200 mmol of K^+ in the urine; see Fig. 7-4).

Bottom lines

1. The balance data reveal near-equal deficits of Cl^- from the ECF compartment and K^+ from the ICF compartment (i.e., an early deficit of HCl becomes a secondary deficit of KCl).
2. The current surplus of HCO_3^- in the ECF compartment (~200 mmol) is almost perfectly matched by a surplus of H^+ (~200 mmol) in cells.
3. The entire deficit of KCl must be replaced to correct all the deficits in this patient. One cannot replace a deficit of KCl by giving *only* NaCl.

EXCRETION OF ORGANIC ANIONS IN THE URINE
- Endogenous organic anion excretion with a cation other than H^+ or NH_4^+ represents a net loss of HCO_3^- (see Chapter 1, page 9 for more discussion of base balance).
- The excretion of organic anions should be low once a degree of hypokalemia develops because of a higher [H^+] in cells of the proximal convoluted tubule.

What is the therapy for metabolic alkalosis at this stage?

It is obvious that KCl must be given to replace the deficit of KCl. When K^+ and Cl^- are retained, K^+ enters the ICF compartment in conjunction with the net transfer of H^+ to the ECF compartment. These exported H^+ react with HCO_3^- to form H_2O and CO_2. After the CO_2 is exhaled, both a higher $[H^+]$ in the ICF and ECF alkalemia are corrected. In addition, Cl^- remains in the ECF compartment, replacing its deficit, which preserves electroneutrality.

Although it is possible to lower the concentration of HCO_3^- in the ECF compartment with a large infusion of saline, this does not correct the gain of HCO_3^- in the ECF compartment or the gain of H^+ in the ICF compartment. It is obvious that NaCl cannot replace a deficit of KCl. This is yet another example of why we do not belive that the term *Cl^- depletion* is an adequate description of the process that has led to metabolic alkalosis.

QUESTIONS

(Discussions on pages 220 and 221)

7-1 *Why might a deficit of NaCl occur in patients with protracted vomiting or nasogastric suction?*

7-2 *Why is it advantageous not to have a tubular maximum for the renal reabsorption of $NaHCO_3$?*

7-3 *When HCl is secreted into the stomach during the cephalic phase of gastric secretion (before food is ingested), the P_{HCO3} rises. What is the renal response to this high P_{HCO3}?*

7-4 *Why do some infants who vomit have metabolic alkalosis, whereas others develop metabolic acidosis?*

CASE 7-2: THIS MAN SHOULD NOT HAVE METABOLIC ALKALOSIS

(Case presented on page 194)

What is the basis for metabolic alkalosis?

There is no ingestion of $NaHCO_3$ or the Na^+ salts of anions that can be metabolized to HCO_3^-. Hence, we must look for a deficit of HCl, KCl, and/or NaCl to explain why metabolic alkalosis has developed (see Flow Chart 7-1).

Deficit of HCl: There was no history of vomiting or diarrhea (*see margin note*), which means that this is a very unlikely basis for the metabolic alkalosis.

Deficit of KCl: The basis of hypokalemia could be due to a shift of K^+ into cells or a loss of KCl in the urine. To lower the P_K to 2.7 mmol/L, especially in this muscular elite solider, the loss of KCl must be very large. Moreover, it is extremely unlikely that this happened over such a short period of time. In addition, even if there was a KCl deficit, it is difficult to attribute the rise in the P_{HCO3} to the formation of new HCO_3^- owing to the renal effects of K^+ depletion because the time course is too short.

Deficit of NaCl: There is evidence on clinical examination to suspect that his effective arterial blood volume is contracted; we can use his hematocrit value of 50% to provide a quantitative assessment of his plasma volume and deduce whether his deficit of NaCl is sufficient to cause a degree of ECF volume contraction to explain why metabolic alkalosis was present.

INDIRECT LOSS OF HCl DURING DIARRHEA
When the Cl^-/HCO_3^- anion exchanger has a low activity, the diarrhea fluid may contain more Cl^- than $Na^+ + K^+$, as the H^+ secreted by NHE in the colon bind to bacterial proteins in the lumen (see Chapter 4, page 81 for more information).

LOSS OF K^+ AND Cl^- IN SWEAT IN PATIENTS WITH CYSTIC FIBROSIS
- The concentrations of Na^+ and Cl^- can be as high as 60 mmol/L in sweat in patients with cystic fibrosis as compared to <30 mmol/L in normal subjects.
- The mechanism for the loss of K^+ and Cl^- is described in the legend for the figure in the margin on page 207.
- Aldosterone is released owing to contraction of the effective arterial blood volume.
- The cystic fibrosis transmembrane regulator Cl^- channel (CFTR) is the pathway for Cl^- absorption; it is defective in patients with cystic fibrosis.

Quantitative analysis: Using his hematocrit value of 50%, one can estimate that his ECF volume has decreased from its normal value of 15 L (because his weight was 80 kg) to close to 10 L. Accordingly, he has lost 5 L of ECF.

The second calculation is to define how much this degree of ECF volume contraction would raise his P_{HCO3}. For this calculation, simply divide the normal content of HCO_3^- in his ECF compartment ($15\ L \times 25\ mmol/L = 375\ mmol$) by his new ECF volume of 10 L. The result is 37.5 mmol/L, a value that is remarkably close to the observed 37 mmol/L. Therefore, the major reason for his metabolic alkalosis is the NaCl deficit (a "contraction" form of metabolic alkalosis).

The next issue is to examine possible routes for a large loss of NaCl in such a short time period. Because both diarrhea and polyuria were not present, the only route for a large NaCl loss is via sweat. To have a high electrolyte concentration in sweat, the likely underlying lesion would be cystic fibrosis (*see margin note on page 206*). This diagnosis was confirmed later by molecular studies of the gene encoding for the cystic fibrosis transmembrane regulator Cl^- channel.

It is also possible to have a loss of KCl in sweat in patients with this disease (*see margin note*). Nevertheless, it is unlikely that this is a quantitatively important mechanism to explain why he developed metabolic alkalosis so quickly. It is more likely that the deficit of NaCl was more important as revealed in the previous calculation.

What is the therapy for metabolic alkalosis in this patient?

Knowing that the basis for the metabolic alkalosis is largely a deficit of NaCl, he needs to receive NaCl as his major treatment; the goal is to replace the deficit (*see margin note*). Nevertheless, there are several cautions to note because of associated findings:

1. *Acute hyponatremia*: Given the marked danger of brain herniation, hypertonic saline should be administered rapidly to increase the P_{Na} by close to 5 mmol/L ($5\ mmol\ NaCl \times 45\ L$ total body water = 225 mmol).
2. *Hypokalemia*: We suspect that a large β_2-adrenergic surge, the ingestion of food that caused the release of insulin, and perhaps the alkalemia may all have contributed to a shift of K^+ into cells (*see margin note*). The response to therapy with KCl will provide the answer to this uncertainty about the magnitude of the deficits of K^+ and Cl^-.

CASE 7-3: WHY DOES METABOLIC ALKALOSIS DEVELOP SO QUICKLY?

(Case presented on page 195)

Why did metabolic alkalosis develop on days 3 and 4?

The first step is to look for the common causes of metabolic alkalosis. Because there is no history of vomiting or nasogastric suction, there is no evidence for a loss of HCl. Similarly, there is no evidence of an unusually large loss of NaCl by any of the usual routes, and the absence of a rise in hematocrit provides evidence to support the impression that there is not a large deficit of NaCl. Therefore, only a KCl deficit is considered as a possible etiology for the metabolic alkalosis in this patient.

He appears to have renal K^+ wasting on day 3 because he is modestly hypokalemic (P_K 3.2 mmol/L) and his urine on the morning of day 4 contains more K^+ than expected (~4 mmol K^+/mmol creatinine, expected about 1 mmol K^+/mmol creatinine). Moreover, there is a

ION BALANCE IN SWEAT

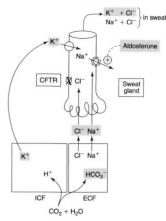

The *structure with a coil* represents the sweat gland with its channels for Na^+ (ENaC) and Cl^- (cystic fibrosis transmembrane regulator [CFTR]). Aldosterone causes ENaC to be open, and Na^+ is reabsorbed faster than Cl^- when CFTR is defective. To the extent that there are open K^+ channels in the luminal membrane of sweat ducts, some K^+ are lost with Cl^-. The *lower rectangles* represent the body with its extracellular fluid (ECF) and its intracellular fluid (ICF) compartments. Electroneutrality is achieved in each compartment when K^+ and Cl^- are lost—H^+ replace K^+ in the ICF, and HCO_3^- replace Cl^- in the ECF compartment. When Na^+ and Cl^- are lost, this represents electroneutral loss from the ECF compartment.

P_K DURING VIGOROUS EXERCISE
The P_K usually rises during vigorous exercise. What is different in this patient is the combination of a stimulus for the release of insulin (large intake of sugar), a large β_2-adrenergic surge, and the high P_{HCO3}. Some K^+ and Cl^- may be lost in sweat as well, but quantitatively this is likely a minor cause of the low P_K.

CALCULATE THE DEFICIT OF Na^+
- He lost 700 mmol of Na^+ in the 5-L loss from his ECF compartment ($5\ L \times 140\ mmol/L = 700\ mmol$).
- Each remaining liter of ECF (10 L) has a deficit of 24 mmol/L ($140 - 116\ mmol/L$). Hence the total is 240 mmol.
- The total deficit of Na^+ is 940 mmol (700 + 240 mmol).

EFFECTS OF A LARGE DOSE OF CORTISOL ON K⁺ EXCRETION

EFFECTS OF A LARGE DOSE OF CORTISOL ON K⁺ EXCRETION
- When very large amounts of cortisol are given, some of this hormone escapes destruction by the enzymes, 11β-hydroxysteroid dehydrogenase in principal cells of the cortical distal nephron (see Chapter 14, page 496 for more discussion).
- As a result, some cortisol binds to the mineralocorticoid receptor, resulting in aldosterone-like actions that promote a kaliuresis, even when aldosterone levels in plasma are very low.

possible reason for the excessive excretion of K⁺: high doses of cortisol were administered (*see margin note*).

The sudden fall in the P_K from 3.2 to 1.7 mmol/L in just 24 hours while the K⁺ excretion rate was modest suggests that there had been an acute shift of K⁺ into cells. Perhaps this is related to high insulin levels (dietary intake of carbohydrate), prolonged β₂-adrenergic actions of his medications for treatment of asthma, and perhaps the sudden rise in his P_{HCO3}.

For a rise in P_{HCO3}, he needs an input of alkali and the preservation of the stimuli for the reabsorption of $NaHCO_3$ in the proximal convoluted tubule. The input of alkali was due to his dietary intake of fruit and vegetables (but the amount needed is larger than that in the usual dietary intake). The presence of the mild degree of hypokalemia leads to an acidified proximal convoluted tubule cell pH, which promotes the reabsorption of HCO_3^- and diminishes the elimination of dietary alkali via the excretion of citrate and other organic anions (see Fig. 7-3, page 199). Of note, he did have a high urine pH on day 4 and a large excretion of $NaHCO_3$ during therapy.

Although it is difficult to determine how large a deficit of KCl was present and to what degree an acute shift of K⁺ into cells was contributing to this profound degree of hypokalemia, this will become evident from the amount of KCl that is needed to correct the hypokalemia.

PART B
CLINICAL SECTION

CASE 7-4: MILK-ALKALI SYNDROME, BUT WITHOUT MILK

(Case discussed on page 216)

A 60-year-old man complained of malaise, anorexia, and constipation over the past several weeks. He denied vomiting or the intake of diuretics. He has chewed close to 40 betel nuts on a daily basis for many years. To avoid the bitter taste of the betel nut, he adds a paste that contains $Ca(OH)_2$. On physical examination, his ECF volume was contracted and his tongue, the oral mucosa, and the angles of his mouth were stained brick red by the betel nut juice. The laboratory data are provided below. Of note, he had hypercalcemia, and the levels of both his parathyroid hormone and 1,25-dihydroxyvitamin D_3 in plasma were below the normal range (data not shown).

		PLASMA	URINE
pH		7.47	—
HCO₃⁻	mmol/L	36	—
Na⁺	mmol/L	137	21
K⁺	mmol/L	3.2	21
Cl⁻	mmol/L	91	42
Creatinine	mg/dL (µmol/L)	9.7 (844)	108 (9400)
Calcium	mg/dL (mmol/L)	12.8 (3.2)	23.4 (5.9)
Phosphate	mg/dL (mmol/L)	5.7 (1.8)	5.9 (2.1)
Albumin	g/dl (g/L)	3.9 (39)	—

Questions

What is the basis for the metabolic alkalosis?
What should the initial therapy be?

CLINICAL APPROACH

A list of causes of metabolic alkalosis is provided in Table 7-1. Four aspects of the clinical picture in a patient with metabolic alkalosis merit careful attention—these include the medical history (e.g., vomiting, diuretic use), the presence of hypertension, the effective arterial blood volume status, and the P_K.

Our clinical approach to a patient with metabolic alkalosis is outlined in Flow Chart 7-2. The first step is to rule out the common causes of metabolic alkalosis, vomiting and use of diuretics. Although this may be evident from the history, some patients may deny the intake of diuretics or inducing vomiting; examining the urine electrolytes is particularly helpful if you suspect these diagnoses (Table 7-2). An excellent initial test is to examine the concentration of Cl^- in the urine (U_{Cl}). A very low U_{Cl} is expected when there is a deficit of HCl and/or NaCl. Nevertheless, the U_{Cl} may not be low if there is a recent intake of diuretics to cause the excretion of Na^+ and Cl^-. If the U_{Cl} is not low, assessment of effective arterial blood volume and blood pressure helps separate patients with disorders of high ENaC (see Table 7-7; effective arterial blood volume is not low, presence of hypertension) from those with Bartter's or Gitelman's syndromes (effective arterial blood volume is low, absence of hypertension). Serial measurements of U_{Cl} in spot urine samples are helpful to separate patients with Bartter's or Gitelman's syndromes (persistently high U_{Cl}) from those with diuretic abuse (intermittently high U_{Cl}).

Effect of metabolic alkalosis on ventilation

Because the concentration of H^+ in plasma is a major determinant of ventilation, the alkalemia in metabolic alkalosis depresses

TABLE 7-1 **CAUSES OF METABOLIC ALKALOSIS**

Causes usually associated with a contracted effective arterial blood volume

Low U_{Cl}

- Loss of gastric secretions (e.g., vomiting, nasogastric suction)
- Remote use of diuretics
- Delivery of Na^+ to the CCD with nonreabsorbable anions plus a reason for Na^+ avidity
- Posthypercapnic states
- Loss of HCl via lower gastrointestinal tract (e.g., congenital disorder with Cl^- loss in diarrhea, acquired forms of DRA)

High U_{Cl}

- Recent diuretic use
- Endogenous diuretics (occupancy of the Ca-SR in the thick ascending limb of the loop of Henle, inborn errors affecting transporters of Na^+ and/or Cl^- in the nephron, such as Bartter's or Gitelman's syndrome)

Causes associated with an expanded extracellular volume and possibly hypertension

Disorders with primary enhanced mineralocorticoid activity causing hypokalemia

- Primary aldosteronism
- Primary hyper-reninemic hyperaldosteronism (e.g., renal artery stenosis, malignant hypertension, renin-producing tumor)
- Disorders with cortisol acting as a mineralocorticoid (e.g., apparent mineralocorticoid excess syndrome, licorice ingestion, ACTH-producing tumor)
- Disorders with constituitively active ENaC in the CCD (e.g., Liddle's syndrome)

Large reduction in glomerular filtration rate plus a source of $NaHCO_3$

ACTH, adrenocorticotropic hormone; Ca-SR, calcium-sensing receptor; CCD, cortical collecting duct; DRA, down-regulated Cl/HCO_3 exchanger in adenoma/adenocarcinoma.

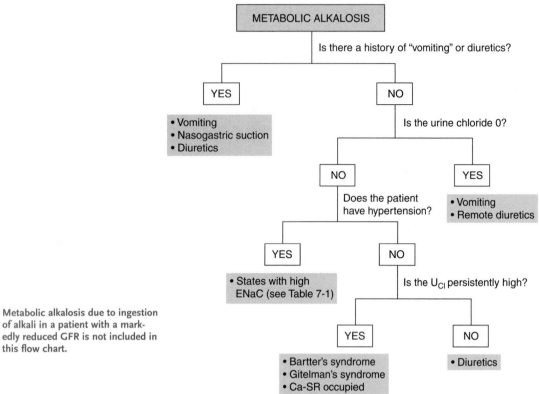

FLOW CHART 7-2 **Clinical approach to the patient with metabolic alkalosis.** The U_{Cl} should be close to nil if the cause of metabolic alkalosis is vomiting or the remote use of diuretics. If the U_{Cl} is not low, an assessment of effective arterial blood volume and blood pressure helps differentiate patients with disorders of high primary mineralocorticoid activity from those with Bartter's-like syndromes. Ca-SR, calcium sensing receptor in thick ascending limb of loop of Henle.

CAVEATS IN THE USE OF URINE ELECTROLYTES TO DETECT EFFECTIVE ARTERIAL BLOOD VOLUME CONTRACTION

- Both Na^+ and Cl^- concentrations may be high (e.g., recent intake of diuretics, acute tubular necrosis).
- Na^+ concentration may be high in a patient with recent vomiting because the excretion of the anion HCO_3^- obligates the loss of the cation, Na^+.
- Cl^- concentration in the urine may be high during diarrhea or laxative abuse, because excretion of the cation NH_4^+ obligates the excretion of the anion Cl^-.

TABLE 7-2 **URINE ELECTROLYTES IN THE DIFFERENTIAL DIAGNOSIS OF EFFECTIVE ARTERIAL BLOOD VOLUME CONTRACTION**

In this table, "high" indicates a concentration of the electrolyte in the urine that is greater than 15 mmol/L, and "low" indicates a concentration that is less than 15 mmol/L. These values are based on a urine volume of 1 L/day and therefore must be adjusted for the urine volume if polyuria is present. Note that chronic diarrhea and the abuse of laxatives are usually associated with hyperchloremic metabolic acidosis.

CONDITION	URINE ELECTROLYTE	
	Na+	*Cl-*
Vomiting		
Recent	High	Low
Remote	Low	Low
Diuretics		
Recent	High	High
Remote	Low	Low
Diarrhea or laxative abuse	Low	High
Bartter's or Gitelman's syndrome	High	High

ventilation. In fact, there is a linear relationship between the increase in the P_{HCO3} and the increase in the arterial Pco_2; the slope is approximately 0.7. Thus, when patients present with CO_2 retention and metabolic alkalosis, the metabolic alkalosis should be corrected before attributing the CO_2 retention to lung disease.

TABLE 7-3 **EFFECT OF ALKALEMIA ON PATIENTS WITH CO_2 RETENTION**

Data are derived from eight patients with chronic respiratory acidosis prior to and following therapy for metabolic alkalosis. All values reported are from measurements in arterial blood. There is a little difference in the [H^+] in plasma before and after therapy of the coexisting metabolic alkalosis in patients with chronic respiratory acidosis. After correction of these disorders, however, the arterial Pco_2 is lower and the arterial Po_2 is higher. The increase in the O_2 content of blood can be large if the changes are occurring on the steeper portion of the sigmoid shape of the O_2 saturation curve: the arterial Po_2 curve (see Chapter 8, Fig. 8-4, page 235).

METABOLIC ALKALOSIS	H^+ (nmol/L)	P_{HCO_3} (mmol/L)	Pco_2 (mm Hg)	Po_2 (mm Hg)
Before therapy	40	37	61	52
After therapy	42	28	48	69

As hypoventilation develops, it is accompanied by a somewhat lower Po_2, which may offset the degree of respiratory suppression by alkalemia and thus a rise in the arterial Pco_2 may be observed in patients receiving O_2 supplementation when hypoxia is corrected. The reduced delivery of O_2 to tissues owing to hypoxemia caused by hypoventilation in patients with metabolic alkalosis is further aggravated by the fact that alkalemia shifts the O_2-hemoglobin dissociation curve to the left; this shift increases the affinity of hemoglobin for O_2.

Because patients with chronic lung disease and chronic respiratory acidosis often take diuretics to minimize the Na^+ retention that is commonly seen in these patients, they may develop metabolic alkalosis. This may return the plasma H^+ concentration to the normal range, but their clinical condition may deteriorate when they no longer have the effects of acidemia to drive ventilation (Table 7-3).

COMMON CAUSES OF CHRONIC METABOLIC ALKALOSIS

Vomiting or nasogastric suction

• The key laboratory findings in patients with metabolic alkalosis due to vomiting or nasogastric suction are hypokalemia and the virtual absence of Cl^- in the urine.

The diagnosis is obvious if the patient has a history of prolonged vomiting or nasogastric suction (*see margin note*). The difficulty arises if the patient denies vomiting. Nevertheless, there are several helpful clues to make the diagnosis—the patient is particularly concerned with body image, has a profession where weight control is a very important factor (e.g., ballet dancer, fashion model), has an eating disorder, and/or has a psychiatric disorder that might lead to self-induced vomiting.

The physical examination may also provide some helpful clues. The effective arterial blood volume is often contracted because some NaCl is lost in the gastric fluid (see the discussion of Question 7-1, page 220). Be careful if the effective arterial blood volume is very contracted because one must look for other reasons for excessive loss of Na^+ in the urine, gastrointestinal tract, and/or sweat along with a very low intake of NaCl. Hypokalemia is always present and the deficit of KCl is a major factor in the pathophysiology of the metabolic alkalosis in

ZOLLINGER-ELLISON SYNDROME
• Metabolic alkalosis might be particularly severe when there is a gastrin-producing tumor because this hormone stimulates the secretion of HCl in the stomach.
• The most common symptoms are abdominal pain and diarrhea owing to intestinal irritation by HCl and destruction of digestive enzymes by H^+.

these patients. Alkalemia suppresses the respiratory center and this leads to hypoventilation. A primary respiratory acidosis may be present if respiratory muscle weakness occurs owing to hypokalemia. On the other hand, a primary respiratory alkalosis may be present if the patient develops aspiration pneumonia, for example.

The urine electrolytes are very helpful when this diagnosis is suspected—the key finding is an extremely low U_{Cl}. If there was recent vomiting, the U_{Na} might be high owing to bicarbonaturia (the urine pH is >7.0), obligating the excretion of Na^+.

Diuretics

- The key findings in patients with metabolic alkalosis due to the use of diuretics are a low effective arterial blood volume, hypokalemia, and intermittently high concentrations of Na^+ and Cl^- in the urine (i.e., when the diuretic acts); hypokalemia is more likely to occur in patients who have a low intake of K^+.
- Diuretics are commonly administered to treat hypertension. A large deficit of NaCl is most commonly seen in patients who also have a low intake of NaCl (e.g., in the elderly).

It is important to emphasize that the use of diuretics might be denied at times, especially in patients concerned with their body image or those seeking medical attention. To help sort out these patients from those with rare causes of hypokalemia, metabolic alkalosis, and a contracted effective arterial blood volume (e.g., Bartter's and Gitelman's syndromes), measure the urine electrolytes using multiple random urine samples (see Table 7-2). If there is doubt, an assay for diuretics in the urine may be helpful; make sure that the assay is performed in a urine sample that contains high concentrations of Na^+ and Cl^-.

At times, the loss of NaCl is due to a genetic disorder that causes inhibition of the reabsorption of Na^+ and Cl^- in one of the nephron segments or due to agents that may bind the calcium-sensing receptor in the loop of Henle (*see margin note*; see Chapter 14, pages 486–493 for more discussion of Bartter's and Gitelman's syndromes).

BARTTER'S-LIKE SYNDROME
Some cationic agents (e.g., drugs such as gentamicin or cisplatin or cationic proteins) may bind the calcium-sensing receptor in the loop of Henle function and lead to a picture that mimics Bartter's syndrome (see Chapter 14, page 493 for more discussion).

LESS COMMON CAUSES OF CHRONIC METABOLIC ALKALOSIS

Conditions with high mineralocorticoid activity

- Clinical clues to conditions with high mineralocorticoid activity as the cause of metabolic alkalosis include hypokalemia and hypertension.

The associated hypokalemia is of major importance in causing metabolic alkalosis in these patients. The specific disorders are listed in Table 7-1 and are discussed in detail in Chapter 14.

Pathophysiology

Because of the high mineralocorticoid activity or a constitutively active ENaC, principal cells of the cortical distal nephron are poised to reabsorb Na^+. Initially Na^+ and Cl^- are retained and thus the ECF volume is expanded. Subsequently, K^+ is lost in the urine with Cl^- if principal cells have open K^+ channels in their luminal membrane and if more Na^+ is reabsorbed than Cl^-. Hypokalemia leads to an acidified proximal tubule cell, which results in the excretion of more NH_4^+ with Cl^- and the retention of dietary alkali (low excretion of potential HCO_3^-, i.e., organic anions) with Na^+ (see Fig. 7-3). Overall, the body continues to have a surplus of Na^+ and HCO_3^-, but some of the retained Cl^- are excreted in the urine (with NH_4^+) and therefore Cl^- are replaced with HCO_3^-. The ICF compartment has a deficit of K^+. Since balance data are not available, the cations retained in the ICF should be H^+ and Na^+.

Metabolic alkalosis associated with milk-alkali syndrome

Although milk and absorbable alkali are not used nowadays to treat duodenal ulcers, this form of metabolic alkalosis still continues to be present, but the setting has changed. Its cardinal features are still a source of dietary alkali and absence of suppression of the stimuli for the proximal tubule to retain this alkali. Hypercalcemia is the key player in this clinical scenario that induces the high levels of angiotensin II and causes a degree of hypokalemia. The intake of calcium supplements, commonly in the form of calcium carbonate tablets, is now a common cause of hypercalcemia, particularly in elderly women (*see margin note*). Hypercalcemia develops primarily because more calcium is absorbed in the intestinal tract (especially if the intake of calcium exceeds that of dietary phosphate, see Part C for more details). When more calcium binds to its receptor in the medullary thick ascending limb of the loop of Henle, it acts as a loop diuretic that leads to an excessive excretion of NaCl and KCl. Later in the illness, the combination of a contracted effective arterial blood volume and direct effects of hypercalcemia can cause a marked reduction in the GFR, which itself further reduces the filtration and excretion of HCO_3^-. A deficit of K^+ is associated with intracellular acidosis in proximal convoluted tubule cells, which leads to the retention of ingested alkali. Therapy consists of stopping the intake of calcium and alkali, and replacing the deficits of NaCl and KCl.

Metabolic alkalosis associated with a posthypercapnic state

In the course of chronic hypercapnia, an increased P_{HCO3} results because of the high Pco_2, causing acidosis in the cells of the proximal convoluted tubule and thus an enhanced excretion of NH_4Cl in the urine. If the patient has a contracted effective arterial blood volume after the hypercapnia resolves, $NaHCO_3$ will be retained because of the high angiotensin II levels that stimulate the reabsorption of $NaHCO_3$ by proximal convoluted tubule cells. Expansion of the effective arterial blood volume lowers angiotensin II levels and causes the excretion of the excess $NaHCO_3$.

Metabolic alkalosis associated with the intake of nonreabsorbable anions

If a patient has a contracted effective arterial blood volume and takes a Na^+ salt with an anion that cannot be reabsorbed by the kidney (e.g., penicillinate$^-$), he or she may develop hypokalemia and metabolic alkalosis. Hypokalemia develops due to actions of aldosterone, which cause Na^+ to be reabsorbed in conjunction with K^+ secretion providing that the delivery of Cl^- to the cortical distal

HYPERCALCEMIA IN ELDERLY WOMEN ON CALCIUM SUPPLEMENTS

- To treat osteoporosis, these patients are given a source of oral calcium ($CaCO_3$) along with vitamin D to increase the absorption of calcium in the duodenum.
- Because of a low dietary intake of phosphate, excessive absorption of calcium may occur downstream in the intestinal tract and cause hypercalcemia (see page 219 for more discussion).
- A similar pathophysiology applies to patients with chronic renal insufficiency who are treated with $CaCO_3$ as a phosphate-binding agent and are placed on a low intake of phosphate.

nephron is low. The rise in P_{HCO3} in these patients is the result of the NaCl and the KCl deficits.

The urine provides the clues to the diagnosis. The U_{Cl} should be low. The U_{Na} varies depending on whether the load of nonreabsorbable anion is recent or remote; when the intake of nonreabsorbable anions is discontinued, the U_{Na} should be very low.

Metabolic alkalosis associated with magnesium depletion

Patients with Mg^{2+} depletion may have hypokalemia and metabolic alkalosis. The usual clinical setting for this deficiency includes malabsorption, diarrhea, or the administration of drugs that act on the loop of Henle (e.g., loop diuretics, cisplatin, or aminoglycosides). These patients must be distinguished from those with primary hyperaldosteronism as well as those with Bartter's or Gitelman's syndrome who may also have hypomagnesemia.

THERAPY FOR METABOLIC ALKALOSIS

Because metabolic alkalosis represents a number of different primary conditions, there is no single therapy for this disorder. Rather, each of the underlying causes must be treated. The following guidelines should help the clinician design a plan for therapy.

> **Guidelines for the treatment of a patient with metabolic alkalosis**
> One must recognize that there are two major groups of disorders that can cause metabolic alkalosis: those that are due to deficits of HCl, KCl, or NaCl and those that are due to the retention of an input of $NaHCO_3$. In the former, one must replace the appropriate deficit, whereas in the latter group, one must induce a loss of $NaHCO_3$ by treating the underlying disorder.

Patients with metabolic alkalosis due to deficits of Cl⁻ salts

THERAPY FOR A DEFICIT OF K⁺ IN THE ICF
- If the deficit of K⁺ in cells was accompanied by a gain of H⁺, giving KCl will cause K⁺ to enter cells and H⁺ to exit; these H⁺ will remove the extra HCO_3^- in the ECF while retained Cl⁻ replaces the deficit of Cl⁻ in the ECF.
- If the deficit of K⁺ in cells was accompanied by a gain of Na⁺, giving KCl will cause the exit of Na⁺ from cells and this extra NaCl will be excreted if there is not a deficit of NaCl.

Although a deficit of more than one Cl⁻-containing compound—HCl, NaCl, or KCl—may be present in a single patient, the presentation is different when a particular deficit dominates the clinical picture. Some authorities use NaCl as the main therapy for what they call "saline-responsive metabolic alkalosis," but NaCl will *not* replace a deficit of KCl. Although one can lower the P_{HCO3} by overexpanding the ECF volume (see discussion of Case 7-1, page 204), clearly this does *not* return balances and the composition of the ECF and ICF compartments to normal when there is a deficit of KCl. The ECF still has its gain of HCO_3^-, whereas the ICF still has its deficit of K⁺ and surplus of H⁺. Nevertheless, if a patient with a deficit of KCl consumes a diet that contains K⁺ salts, there can be a gain of K⁺ over time that corrects the K⁺ deficit providing that HCO_3^- or organic anions are excreted while Cl⁻ are retained.

Deficit of HCl

This is present in the first few days of vomiting or nasogastric suction. At this stage, there are no major threats to life directly related to the metabolic alkalosis per se. The issues related to the correction of the deficit of HCl is provided in the discussion of Case 7-1, page 204.

Deficit of NaCl

If there is hemodynamic instability, one must administer an isotonic Na^+-containing solution quickly until this emergency is removed. One should use the hematocrit and/or the $P_{Albumin}$ to obtain a quantitative estimate of the deficit of NaCl. Comparing the arterial to the brachial venous P_{CO_2} provides a very useful guide to adjust the rate of infusion of saline (see Chapter 3, page 67 for more discussion). There is an extremely important caution here if the patient also has chronic hyponatremia. If that is the case, consider the administration of dDAVP at the outset to avoid a rapid water diuresis, which can cause too rapid a rise in the P_{Na} and the development of osmotic demyelination. On the other hand, if hyponatremia is acute (see discussion of Case 7-3, page 207), administer hypertonic saline to increase P_{Na} rapidly by close to 5 mmol/L.

ABBREVIATION
dDAVP, desamino, D-arginine vasopressin

Deficit of KCl

The emergencies to consider in this setting are a cardiac arrhythmia and hypoventilation because of respiratory muscle weakness. Emergency treatment of hypokalemia is discussed in Chapter 14, page 500.

One is not able to accurately quantitate the deficit of KCl even if the ECF volume is known because the vast majority of K^+ in the body resides in the ICF compartment. Furthermore, it is not possible without balance data (virtually never available) to know the quantitative importance of a shift of K^+ into cells versus a deficit of K^+ as a cause for hypokalemia. Nevertheless, the time course of the illness can be helpful; rapid and large changes in the P_K are most likely due to a shift of K^+ into the ICF compartment (see discussion of Case 7-4, page 216).

Patients with metabolic alkalosis due to retention of NaHCO₃

- In the subgroup of patients with high mineralocorticoid activity, lowering the P_{HCO3} is usually a minor component of the therapy.

The major goal of therapy is to deal with the cause of the high mineralocorticoid effects. Specific therapy for the hypokalemia depends on the underlying disease, and this is discussed in Chapter 14, page 500. Notwithstanding, there might be a large excretion of $NaHCO_3$ if enough KCl is given to correct this deficit of K^+. The carbonic anhydrase inhibitor acetazolamide is sometimes used to diminish the degree of alkalemia when there is a need to do so (e.g., when weaning the patient from a ventilator). Nevertheless, when a large load of $NaHCO_3^-$-rich fluid is delivered to the cortical distal nephron, K^+ loss can be very large. If the alkalemia is very severe, one can give H^+ in the form of HCl or NH_4Cl. If the patient has a fixed alveolar ventilation, the arterial P_{CO_2} may rise with H^+ administration (high CO_2 production); a small increase in the arterial P_{CO_2}, however, might not pose a significant risk if it is a transient phenomenon.

Therapy is more difficult in the group of patients in whom there is retention of alkali owing to a very low GFR. It is obvious that the input of alkali must be diminished (e.g., in patients on hemodialysis, lower the concentration of HCO_3^- in the bath). As a preventive measure to minimize the risk of developing metabolic alkalosis in a patient with a markedly reduced GFR, a blocker of the gastric H^+/K^+-ATPase can be administered if nasogastric suction is required.

DISCUSSION OF CASE 7-4

CASE 7-4: MILK-ALKALI SYNDROME, BUT WITHOUT MILK

(Case presented on page 208)

What is the basis for the metabolic alkalosis?

Deficit of HCl: There was no history of vomiting or nasogastric suction, which means that there was no deficit of HCl.

Deficit of NaCl: He did not take a diuretic drug, but hypercalcemia can cause inhibition of the reabsorption of Na^+ and Cl^- in the thick ascending limb of the loop of Henle. The facts that he had a contracted effective arterial blood volume and that his urine Na^+ and Cl^- concentrations were not low are consistent with this impression. The presence of a high plasma renin activity would add support to this interpretation. A contracted ECF volume owing to the deficit of NaCl is an important reason for the high P_{HCO3}.

Deficit of KCl: There was a modest degree of hypokalemia and a high rate of K^+ excretion in this setting. Thus, a deficit of KCl has also contributed to the development of his metabolic alkalosis.

Ingestion of alkaline calcium salts: There was an ingestion of alkaline calcium salts, but this would not be sufficient on its own to cause chronic metabolic alkalosis. Alkali was retained owing to the presence of angiotensin II (caused by a contracted effective arterial blood volume) and an acidified proximal convoluted tubular cell (caused by hypokalemia).

What should the initial therapy be?

The most important component of the initial therapy in this patient is the administration of intravenous isotonic saline to reexpand his effective arterial blood volume. There should be a fall in P_{HCO3} with administration of saline. His calcium concentration in plasma fell to normal levels by the end of day 1, and this was due to both a decrease in calcium input and an enhanced excretion of calcium owing to the expanded effective arterial blood volume. The metabolic alkalosis resolved completely due in large part to reexpansion of his ECF volume and to a lesser degree to bicarbonaturia. The KCl deficit was corrected with the administration of KCl, and the P_K rose to 4.0 mmol/L.

PART C
INTEGRATIVE PHYSIOLOGY

CHRONIC K+ DEFICIENCY AND HYPERTENSION

- Epidemiologic evidence suggests that there is a higher prevalence of hypertension in populations who have a low dietary K^+ intake.
- The blood pressure–lowering effect of diuretics is diminished if the patient becomes hypokalemic.

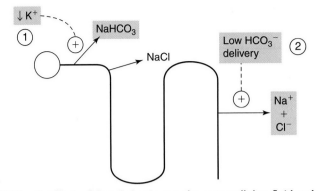

FIGURE 7-8 Effect of hypokalemia on the extracellular fluid volume.
See the text for details; *site 1* is the proximal convoluted tubule, and *site 2* is the cortical distal nephron.

It is well known that patients who have a deficit of K^+ are pre-disposed to retain dietary NaCl. Certain patients are susceptible to develop hypertension if they have an expanded effective arterial blood volume (i.e., low-renin hypertension). As to mechanism, one speculation is that the K^+ deficiency is associated with intracellular acidosis in proximal convoluted tubule cells, which augments the reabsorption of $NaHCO_3$ in this nephron segment. This raises the luminal Cl^- concentration, which drives the reabsorption of Cl^- and secondarily the reabsorption of Na^+ in the proximal convoluted tubule. A low distal delivery of HCO_3^- may enhance the reabsorption of Cl^- in the cortical distal nephron (see Chapter 13, page 444). As a result, this positive balance for NaCl in these subjects expands their effective arterial blood volume and raises their blood pressure. In studies where these subjects were given KCl, they retained the K^+ and excreted the extra Na^+ and Cl^- that was located in their ECF compartment. This was accompanied by a fall in their blood pressure (Fig. 7-8).

INTEGRATIVE PHYSIOLOGY OF CALCIUM HOMEOSTASIS

• Hypercalcemia develops when calcium input exceeds its excretion rate in steady state.

We use data from Case 7-4 to provide an understanding of some aspects of the integrative physiology of calcium homeostasis and illustrate how hypercalcemia might develop.

Input of calcium from the gastrointestinal tract

This has two aspects that need discussion, the type of calcium salt ingested and the absorption of calcium.

Type of calcium salt

The patient ingested calcium hydroxide ($Ca[OH]_2$), a sparingly soluble compound used to remove the bitter taste of the betel nut preparation (a form of local anesthetic to the taste buds). This poorly

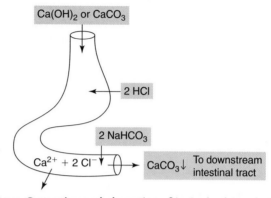

FIGURE 7-9 Generation and absorption of ionized calcium in the upper intestinal tract. Alkaline calcium salts, $Ca(OH)_2$ and $CaCO_3$, are poorly soluble in water but are converted to ionized calcium (Ca^{2+}) by gastric HCl, which can be absorbed. $NaHCO_3$ is added in the duodenum, forming insoluble $CaCO_3$.

soluble form of calcium is converted to ionized calcium in the stomach owing to HCl secretion (Fig. 7-9).

Absorption of calcium

> • Key to the process leading to absorption of calcium is the presence of more $CaCO_3$ than inorganic phosphate in the upper intestinal tract because once ionized calcium is formed, it soon precipitates as calcium phosphate.

There are two possible fates of ionized Ca^{2+} within the duodenum. First, Ca^{2+} can be absorbed once it is in its ionic form; the active form of vitamin D stimulates this process. Second, if sufficient $NaHCO_3$ is secreted into the duodenum, Ca^{2+} is precipitated as $CaCO_3$. This formation of $CaCO_3$ has two major effects. First, it stops the absorption of more calcium because this cation is no longer in its ionized form. Second, the very low level of ionized calcium permits dietary phosphate to remain as ionized inorganic phosphate once it is produced by digestion of organic phosphates. After the body absorbs the requisite amount of inorganic phosphate, $CaCO_3$ and the residual inorganic phosphate ions (HPO_4^{2-}) are delivered downstream in the intestinal tract.

The next issue to consider is the fate of $CaCO_3$ and residual HPO_4^{2-} in the lower intestinal tract (Fig. 7-10). For if the $CaCO_3$ can be redissolved, it forms a precipitate with HPO_4^{2-}. This conversion of $CaCO_3$ to ionized calcium needs a source of H^+. There is a large source of H^+ in the colon—the fermentation of carbohydrates (fiber and fructose from the diet) by colonic bacteria (in fact, twice as many H^+ are produced in the colon as are secreted by the stomach each day). Hence, a low phosphate intake, such as a diet poor in meat and fish, leaves ionized calcium in the lumen where it is reabsorbed passively at a site where its reabsorption is not regulated.

Output of calcium

> • The excretion of calcium is increased principally by decreasing its reabsorption in the nephron.

CaCO₃ TABLETS

• These are commonly used to prevent or treat osteoporosis. The use of $CaCO_3$ tablets is the third leading cause of hypercalcemia in adults, especially when there is a low intake of phosphate (e.g., the elderly and anorexic individuals who ingest calcium supplemented with vitamin D).

• When $CaCO_3$ plus the phosphate in the diet ($K^+ + H_2PO_4^-$) react, a precipitate of calcium phosphate is formed. The net reaction in acid-base terms yields CO_3^- as described in Figure 7-10.

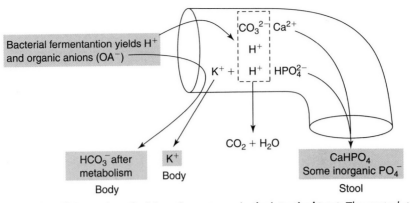

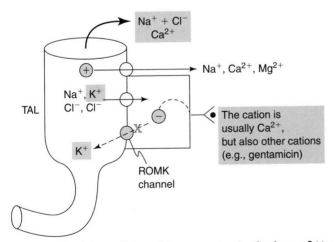

FIGURE 7-10 Prevention of absorption of calcium downstream in the intestinal tract. The *central structure* represents the colon, where calcium can be reabsorbed if it exists in an ionized form. Calcium is delivered as a precipitate of $CaCO_3$. Ionized calcium (Ca^{2+}) is formed when H^+ are produced by bacterial fermentation of dietary fiber and/or fructose and from $H_2PO_4^-$. Should the delivery of inorganic phosphate (HPO_4^{2-}) be *less* than required to precipitate all the ionized calcium as calcium phosphate, some ionized calcium could remain in the lumen and be absorbed passively. A potential bicarbonate load in the form of organic anions (OA^-) is also absorbed, representing the conversion of some of the alkali in $CaCO_3$ to HCO_3^- in the body when these organic anions are metabolized to neutral end products. The stool may contain some K^+.

Expansion of the effective arterial blood volume diminishes the reabsorption of Na^+ and Cl^- and thereby of calcium in the proximal convoluted tubule because when less Na^+ is reabsorbed, less water follows and this diminishes the rise in the luminal concentration of calcium, which decreases its reabsorption.

When the calcium-sensing receptor on the basolateral surface of the thick ascending limb of the loop of Henle is occupied by calcium (e.g., because of a high P_{Ca}), this diminishes the entry of K^+ into the lumen of this nephron segment, and hence the lumen-positive voltage is decreased (Fig. 7-11). As a result, less ionized calcium is reabsorbed in this nephron segment. The net result is a large increase in the delivery

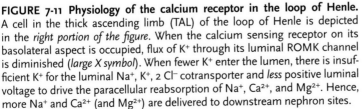

FIGURE 7-11 Physiology of the calcium receptor in the loop of Henle. A cell in the thick ascending limb (TAL) of the loop of Henle is depicted in the *right portion of the figure*. When the calcium sensing receptor on its basolateral aspect is occupied, flux of K^+ through its luminal ROMK channel is diminished (*large X symbol*). When fewer K^+ enter the lumen, there is insufficient K^+ for the luminal Na^+, K^+, 2 Cl^- cotransporter and *less* positive luminal voltage to drive the paracellular reabsorption of Na^+, Ca^{2+}, and Mg^{2+}. Hence, more Na^+ and Ca^{2+} (and Mg^{2+}) are delivered to downstream nephron sites.

of calcium to the last regulated site of its reabsorption, the connecting tubule where reabsorption of calcium should decline because parathyroid hormone secretion is suppressed by hypercalcemia. The net effect is to increase the rate of excretion of calcium in this setting.

DISCUSSION OF QUESTIONS

7-1 *Why might a deficit of NaCl occur in patients with protracted vomiting or nasogastric suction?*

To create a negative balance for NaCl, its loss must exceed intake. Because losses are small in this setting, a prerequisite for a deficit of NaCl is a low intake of this salt. There are, however, two sites of loss of NaCl in patients with vomiting or nasogastric suction.

1. *Loss in the gastric fluid:* Although there is no Na^+ to speak of in gastric fluid per se, nevertheless it might contain NaCl for two reasons. First, saliva, which contains NaCl, is swallowed and this adds some NaCl to the gastric contents. Second, in most subjects who vomit, the gastric fluid contains some $NaHCO_3^-$-rich fluid from the small intestine that enters the stomach via retrograde flux (notice the color of bile in vomited fluid). The combination of HCl and $NaHCO_3$ results in a NaCl loss plus some CO_2 formation (see following equation).

$$H^+ + Cl^- + Na^+ + HCO_3^- \rightarrow Na^+ + Cl^- + CO_2 + H_2O$$

2. *Loss in the urine:* When the urine is HCO_3^--rich, there appears to be a slower reabsorption of Cl^- in the cortical distal nephron. Should this occur, there is a loss of KCl and also of NaCl in the urine (see Chapter 13, page 441 for more discussion).

7-2 *Why is it advantageous not to have a tubular maximum for the renal reabsorption of $NaHCO_3$?*

If there were a tubular maximum of its reabsorption, $NaHCO_3$ would be lost in the urine during the daily alkaline tide. If this were to occur, the ECF volume would decrease. This would be an important problem for subjects who have little NaCl in their diet (e.g., our Paleolithic ancestors). There are other problems as well. For example, by excreting HCO_3^- in the urine, its pH could be high enough to cause calcium phosphate kidney stones. A high rate of excretion of HCO_3^- in the urine would lead to high rates of K^+ excretion and K^+ depletion. In addition, there would be a deficit of HCO_3^- when the HCl is absorbed in the duodenum (secretion of $NaHCO_3$). The resultant metabolic acidosis would require high rates of excretion of NH_4^+ to regenerate new HCO_3^- by the kidney. Were this to occur, it could cause medullary damage, and ultimately, this could lead to renal insufficiency. In summary, there are too many disadvantages in having renal loss of $NaHCO_3$. Hence, it is not surprising that there is no tubular maximum for the renal reabsorption of HCO_3^-.

7-3 *When HCl is secreted into the stomach during the cephalic phase of gastric secretion (before food is ingested), the P_{HCO3} rises. What is the renal response to this high P_{HCO3}?*

- The kidney can increase its reabsorption of filtered $NaHCO_3$ as long as there is no "message" to excrete $NaHCO_3$ (e.g., decreased level of angiotensin II or an alkaline proximal convoluted tubule cell pH).

When gastric cells secrete HCl, there is a gain of HCO_3^- in the ECF and a deficit of Cl^- in a 1:1 stoichiometry. Notice that the ECF volume should not be altered appreciably by this simple exchange of anions in the ECF compartment. Hence, without an expanded effective arterial blood volume, there is sufficient angiotensin II to reabsorb most of the filtered load of HCO_3^-. Nevertheless, if alkalemia were to occur, there might be a decrease in H^+ secretion in the distal nephron and as a result, there could be a small degree of bicarbonaturia. This represents the alkaline tide of urine pH. Hence, the renal response is to retain the extra HCO_3^- until the HCl is absorbed in the small intestine (really $NaHCO_3$ is secreted, leaving Na^+, Cl^-, CO_2, and H_2O as the products; subsequently, Na^+ and Cl^- are absorbed in the small intestine).

7-4 Why do some infants who vomit have metabolic alkalosis, whereas others develop metabolic acidosis?

The key to answering this question is whether fluid from the small intestine can enter the stomach through the pyloric sphincter. When the pylorus is blocked (congenital hypertrophic pyloric stenosis), the net result is the loss of HCl owing to vomiting and the production of metabolic alkalosis. In contrast, with a patent pylorus, the net loss is a mixture of fluid containing HCl with fluid containing $NaHCO_3$. When the amount of $NaHCO_3$ exceeds that of HCl in the stomach, metabolic acidosis develops when vomiting occurs. There are two settings for this scenario. First, normal young infants often have a less tight pyloric sphincter and lose more $NaHCO_3$ than HCl during vomiting. Second, adults with reduced secretion of HCl as part of a disease or with aging, or following the intake of drugs that inhibit the secretion of HCl (H_2-blockers or proton pump inhibitors) also have more $NaHCO_3$ than HCl in their stomach so metabolic acidosis may develop when vomiting occurs.

Respiratory Acid-Base Disturbances

Introduction

In the traditional approach to the diagnosis and management of respiratory acid-base disorders, the emphasis is on values for the *arterial* P_{CO_2} and P_{HCO_3}. In this chapter, we emphasize the importance of the P_{CO_2} *in capillaries* of individual organs because this determines whether the bicarbonate (HCO_3^-) buffer system can remove H^+ during metabolic acidosis. Since most of the bicarbonate buffer system exists in the interstitial compartment and in cells of skeletal muscle, buffering of a H^+ load by the bicarbonate buffer system is impaired if blood flow to skeletal muscle is low and/or the production of CO_2 in muscle is high, as these states are accompanied by a higher capillary and thereby higher cellular P_{CO_2}. Therefore, the degree of acidemia will be more severe and more H^+ will be delivered to and thus bind to intracellular proteins in vital organs (e.g., heart and brain). We refer to this state as a tissue form of respiratory acidosis.

OBJECTIVES

■ To emphasize that a respiratory acid-base disorder is present when the P_{CO_2} in the extracellular fluid (ECF) and/or in the intracellular fluid (ICF) compartment is higher or lower than expected.

■ To illustrate that the *arterial* P_{CO_2} reflects alveolar ventilation; nevertheless, it also sets the lower limit for the P_{CO_2} in capillary blood of all organs.

■ To illustrate that the *capillary* P_{CO_2} directly determines whether the bicarbonate buffer system is able to remove H^+ in all organs. Although the capillary P_{CO_2} cannot be measured directly, one can predict its value for an individual organ by measuring the P_{CO_2} in the vein that drains this organ.

■ Because the bulk of the bicarbonate buffer system is in skeletal muscle, impaired function of this buffer system results in a larger circulating H^+ load and thereby, more H^+ bind to proteins in brain cells.

CASE 8-1: DOES THIS PATIENT HAVE RESPIRATORY ACIDOSIS?

(Case discussed on page 239)

A 58-year-old man had a myocardial infarction and was brought to hospital with great haste. On arrival in the emergency department, he had a cardiac arrest. He was intubated, ventilated, and successfully resuscitated. Nevertheless, he continued to have a very low cardiac output. At this point, both an arterial and a venous blood were examined.

		ARTERIAL BLOOD	BRACHIAL VENOUS BLOOD
H^+	nmol/L	50	80
pH		7.30	7.10
P_{CO_2}	mm Hg	30	60
P_{HCO_3}	mmol/L	15	18
L-Lactate	mmol/L	10	12

Questions

Does the patient have respiratory acidosis of the ventilatory type?
Does the patient have respiratory acidosis of the tissue type?
Is the patient able to buffer H^+ appropriately using his bicarbonate buffer system in skeletal muscle?

PART A
REVIEW OF THE PERTINENT PHYSIOLOGY

THE BICARBONATE BUFFER SYSTEM

This topic was discussed in detail in Chapter 1, page 11; hence, we provide only a brief synopsis in this chapter. The major function of the bicarbonate buffer system is to prevent an unwanted large rise in the concentration of H^+ and thereby excessive binding of H^+ to proteins in cells, which causes their charge to become more positive (or less negative, $H \cdot PTN^+$; Fig. 8-1). To achieve this "good buffering" of H^+, there must be a low P_{CO_2} in the location where the vast majority of HCO_3^- are present (i.e., in the ICF and ECF of skeletal muscle).

Which P_{CO_2} should be used to assess buffering of H^+ by bicarbonate buffer in skeletal muscle?

Arterial P_{CO_2}

- The arterial P_{CO_2} is the lowest possible value for the P_{CO_2} in capillaries, but it does not reflect the actual value of the capillary P_{CO_2}.
- Therefore, the arterial P_{CO_2} does not provide the needed data to assess buffering of H^+ by the bicarbonate buffer systems in skeletal muscle.

The P_{CO_2} in arterial blood has the same value as the P_{CO_2} in alveolar air because there are no important diffusion barriers for CO_2 in alveoli; hence, it is valuable to assess alveolar ventilation. In acid-base terms, however, it directly influences the function of the bicarbonate buffer system only in the arterial component of the vascular volume. The P_{CO_2} in *capillaries* is the one that reflects the P_{CO_2} in *both* the interstitial fluid in the ECF compartment and in cells surrounding these capillaries. Nevertheless, the arterial P_{CO_2} is indirectly related to the P_{CO_2} in capillaries in the brain because the brain has a near-constant rate of consumption of oxygen (and thus CO_2 production) and blood flow, because the latter is autoregulated. If autoregulation

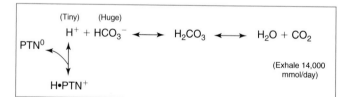

FIGURE 8-1 Bicarbonate buffer system and respiratory acid-base disorders.
Binding of H^+ to ICF proteins increases their net positive charge ($H \cdot PTN^+$) and possibly compromises their function. Thus, the key principle is that new H^+ must be removed by binding to HCO_3^- so that very few H^+ can bind to proteins (PTN^0) in cells. To force H^+ to bind to HCO_3^-, the P_{CO_2} must fall in cells despite the fact that cells produce an enormous quantity of CO_2.

of blood flow to the brain fails because of a very low effective arterial blood volume in a patient with metabolic acidosis, the P_{CO_2} rises in brain capillaries, which makes the bicarbonate buffer system ineffective and hence more of the H^+ load binds to proteins in brain cells.

Venous P_{CO_2}

- The P_{CO_2} in the venous drainage of an organ is determined by the arterial P_{CO_2} *and* the amount of O_2 extracted from each liter of blood that is supplied to that organ; the latter is influenced by the rate of blood flow to that organ; more O_2 is extracted from and more CO_2 is added to each liter of blood if blood flow to that organ declines, but its metabolic rate remains largely unchanged.
- At rest, the brachial venous P_{CO_2} is close to 6 mm Hg higher than the arterial P_{CO_2}.

The venous P_{CO_2} reflects the P_{CO_2} in capillaries and hence the P_{CO_2} in both cells and in the interstitial fluid in their venous drainage bed. CO_2 must diffuse from the cell to the capillary; therefore, the P_{CO_2} in the cell must be at least slightly higher than that in its capillary bed. Because most of the bicarbonate buffer system exists in skeletal muscles, the P_{CO_2} of brachial or femoral venous blood provides insights into how well the majority of the bicarbonate buffer system in the body is functioning (*see margin note*). If this buffer system cannot remove H^+ adequately, the concentration of H^+ rises in blood and its P_{HCO3} falls. As a result, more H^+ are delivered to vital organs (e.g., brain cells) and a larger proportion ultimately binds to their intracellular proteins.

MIXED VENOUS P_{CO_2}
The mixed venous P_{CO_2} provides an overview of buffering by the bicarbonate buffer system, but it does not indicate how this buffering was apportioned to skeletal muscles versus cells of vital organs such as the brain. Hence, it is not as valuable as the brachial or femoral P_{CO_2} to assess the likelihood of H^+ binding to proteins in the brain.

OVERVIEW OF CO₂ HOMEOSTASIS

Production of CO₂

- CO_2 is the major carbon end product of oxidative metabolism.
- More CO_2 is produced when there is increased work.

When carbohydrates are oxidized, 1 mmol of CO_2 is produced for every mmol of O_2 that is consumed (the respiratory quotient [RQ] is 1.0; *see margin note*). In contrast, less CO_2 is formed per unit of O_2 consumed when fatty acids are oxidized (RQ ~ 0.7). On a typical Western diet, the usual RQ is close to 0.8, which reflects the oxidation of the mixture of fat and carbohydrate in the diet.

RESPIRATORY QUOTIENT (RQ)
- The RQ is the quantity of CO_2 produced divided by the quantity of O_2 consumed.
- The RQ helps one deduce which type of fuel is being oxidized.

Factors that influence rate of production of CO_2 at rest

- Overall, cells consume close to 12 mmol of O_2 and produce close to 10 mmol of CO_2 per minute.

When more work is being performed, the rate of consumption of O_2 rises and more CO_2 is produced. For example, during vigorous aerobic exercise, the rate of consumption of O_2 increases close to 20-fold and more CO_2 is produced. In addition, CO_2 is also produced in this setting as a result of buffering of H^+ from L-lactic acid by HCO_3^-

TABLE 8-1 **CLINICAL SETTINGS WITH ALTERED RATES OF PRODUCTION OF CO_2**

The rate of production of CO_2 is shown as mmol/min in a 70-kg adult. These values are estimates and are for illustrative purposes only.

STATE	ORGAN	USUAL CO_2 PRODUCTION RATE	ALTERED CO_2 PRODUCTION
Coma/anesthesia	Brain	3	1.5
Low glomerular filtration rate	Kidney	2	<1
Cachexia/paralysis	Muscle	2.4	<1
Vigorous exercise	Muscle	2.4	180
Ketogenesis	Liver	2.4	0

CO_2 PRODUCTIONS DURING METABOLISM

- There are circumstances when O_2 is consumed but no CO_2 is produced (e.g., when ethanol or fatty acids are converted to keto-acids in the liver; see Table 8-2 for more discussion).
- There are also settings where CO_2 is produced, but no O_2 is consumed—examples include fatty acid synthesis with increased flux in the hexose monophosphate shunt or the pentose-phosphate pathway, or during the buffering of H+ by the bicarbonate buffer system.

during a sprint. This "acid-base" CO_2 influences only the P_{CO_2} in the venous drainage bed of the organ that performs this anaerobic work; this extra CO_2 is eliminated when blood is delivered to the lungs. A list of clinical settings with altered CO_2 production in individual organs is provided in Table 8-1.

Because arterial blood contains 8 to 9 mmol/L of O_2, close to 8 mmol of CO_2 can be added to 1 L of blood when most of its O_2 is extracted—hence, the venous P_{CO_2} is considerably higher than the arterial P_{CO_2}. There are two extremes where most of the O_2 that is delivered in a liter of blood may be consumed—a rise in the rate of metabolism without a change in the rate of O_2 delivery, and the delivery of fewer liters of blood per minute, with no change in the rate of metabolism. *Of clinical relevance, when the effective arterial blood volume is contracted and the blood flow rate falls, more oxygen is extracted from each liter of blood delivered, and hence each liter of capillary blood must carry more CO_2 to the lungs; to do this, there must be a higher P_{CO_2} in capillaries and in cells.*

The type of fuel that is being oxidized also influences the rate of production of CO_2; this can be evaluated by considering the amount of CO_2 formed per ATP regenerated from the oxidation of the different fuels (Table 8-2; *see margin note*).

Removal of CO_2

- CO_2 excretion = alveolar ventilation × P_{CO_2} in alveolar air.

All of the CO_2 produced (~10 mmol/min) enters the venous blood so that it can be transported to the lungs for elimination. Because the cardiac output is 5 L/min at rest, venous blood must carry an extra 2 mmol/L of CO_2 (10 mmol/min ÷ 5 L/min) compared with arterial

TABLE 8-2 **IMPORTANCE OF THE METABOLIC FUEL UTILIZED IN DETERMINING THE RATE OF CO_2 PRODUCTION**

The oxidation of carbohydrates produces more CO_2 than does the oxidation of fat-derived fuels when viewed in terms of the yield of ATP. No CO_2 is produced when O_2 is consumed in the liver if fatty acids or ethanol are converted to ketoacids.

FUEL	PRODUCTS	mmol CO_2/100 mmol ATP
Carbohydrate	$CO_2 + H_2O$	17
Fatty acids	$CO_2 + H_2O$	12
Fatty acids	Ketoacids	0
Ethanol	$CO_2 + H_2O$	11
Ethanol	Ketoacids	0

TABLE 8-3 **QUANTITATIVE ANALYSIS OF ALVEOLAR VENTILATION**

When the concentration of CO_2 in alveolar air is 2 mmol/L, its P_{CO_2} is 40 mm Hg. Similarly, when the concentration of CO_2 in alveolar air is 2.5 mmol/L, its P_{CO_2} is 50 mm Hg, and if this were a steady-state condition, the patient would have chronic respiratory acidosis of the ventilatory type.

	CO_2 EXCRETION	ALVEOLAR VENTILATION	$[CO_2]$ IN ALVEOLAR AIR
Normal	10 mmol/min	5 L/min	2 mmol/L
Chronic respiratory acidosis	10 mmol/min	4 L/min	2.5 mmol/L

blood. This 10 mmol of CO_2 is exhaled in 5 L of alveolar ventilation per minute (same numeric value as the cardiac output per minute). If the alveolar ventilation is doubled to 10 L/min (e.g., during metabolic acidosis or salicylate overdose) and if there is no change in the rate of production of CO_2, the P_{CO_2} of alveolar air and arterial blood falls by 50%. Conversely, as alveolar ventilation falls, the concentration of CO_2 in alveolar air must rise in steady state (as does the arterial P_{CO_2}) to remove all the CO_2 that is produced (this is akin to the concentration of creatinine in plasma and the glomerular filtration rate (GFR). When the GFR falls to half its usual value, the concentration of creatinine in plasma is double its usual value (Table 8-3).

Control of ventilation

As an overview, the concentration of O_2 (6 mmol/L) is much higher than the concentration of CO_2 (2 mmol/L) in alveolar air, and the consumption of O_2 and the production of CO_2 occur in close to a 1:1 ratio. Therefore, the supply of O_2 to the alveolus markedly exceeds demand. Accordingly, it is not surprising that the control of the rate of ventilation is to adjust the P_{CO_2} rather than the P_{O_2} in blood unless the arterial P_{O_2} is quite low (see the discussion of Question 8-2 on page 240 for more discussion).

FOCUS: SUPPLY O_2 WITH A HIGH P_{O_2} TO CELLS
(Examine the *shaded portion* of the figure.)
- When CO_2 and/or L-lactic acid is produced in cells, the concentration of H^+ rises in plasma and in red blood cells (in the *top white circle*).
- This higher concentration of H^+ increases the binding of H^+ to *oxyhemoglobin* and, as a result, O_2 is released (*lower white circle*).

PHYSIOLOGY OF CO_2 TRANSPORT

About 10 mmol of CO_2 are produced per minute, and they diffuse into red blood cells in capillary blood. The carbonic anhydrase in these cells converts CO_2 into H^+ and HCO_3^- (Fig. 8-2). This maintains a low P_{CO_2} in the red blood cells, which aids further diffusion of CO_2. The HCO_3^- formed is transported into the plasma in exchange

FOCUS: EXTRACT O_2 AND EXCRETE CO_2 IN ALVEOLAR AIR
(Begin at the *bottom far right corner* of the figure.)
- When the P_{O_2} is high in the alveoli and thus in red blood cells, this higher concentration of O_2 binds to *deoxyhemoglobin* and, as a result, H^+ are released.
- These H^+ react with HCO_3^-, forming CO_2, which is exhaled, completing the cycle.

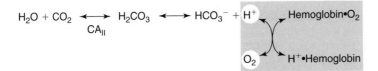

FIGURE 8-2 Carriage of CO_2 in blood. When CO_2 diffuses into red blood cells, it is converted very rapidly to H^+ plus HCO_3^- because of the high activity of carbonic anhydrase (CA_{II}). As shown in the *green shaded area*, the resulting H^+ bind to hemoglobin, which promotes the dissociation of O_2. Most of the CO_2 is carried as HCO_3^- in venous blood and delivered to the lungs. Another property of hemoglobin is that it binds CO_2 to form a carbamino compound, and this helps lower the P_{CO_2} in capillary blood (*see margin note*).

TABLE 8-4 **EXPECTED RESPONSES IN PATIENTS WITH RESPIRATORY ACID-BASE DISORDERS**

DISORDER	EXPECTED RESPONSE
Respiratory acidosis	
Acute	For every 1-mm Hg rise in the arterial P_{CO_2} from 40 mm Hg, the plasma $[H^+]$ rises by close to 0.8 nmol/L from 40 nmol/L.
Chronic	For every 1-mm Hg rise in arterial P_{CO_2} from 40 mm Hg, the P_{HCO_3} should rise by close to 0.3 mmol/L from 25 mmol/L.
Respiratory alkalosis	
Acute	For every 1-mm Hg fall in arterial P_{CO_2} from 40 mm Hg, the plasma $[H^+]$ falls by close to 0.8 nmol/L from 40 nmol/L.
Chronic	For every 1-mm Hg fall in arterial P_{CO_2} from 40 mm Hg, the P_{HCO_3} should fall by close to 0.5 mmol/L from 25 mmol/L.

for Cl^- ("chloride-shift"), and the H^+ bind to deoxyhemoglobin ($H^+ \cdot Hgb$).

In the lung, the process is reversed. This begins when the high P_{O_2} of alveolar air drives the diffusion of O_2 into blood, which raises the P_{O_2} in red blood cells and thereby promotes the binding of O_2 to hemoglobin. As a result, the H^+ that are bound to deoxyhemoglobin combine with the HCO_3^- in red blood cells to form CO_2; this new CO_2 diffuses into the alveoli. The lower concentration of HCO_3^- in red blood cells leads to the entry of HCO_3^- on the Cl^-/HCO_3^- anion exchanger in their cell membranes with the exit of Cl^-. The net result is the addition of O_2 and removal of CO_2 from capillary blood in the lungs.

RENAL RESPONSE TO A CHRONIC CHANGE IN P_{CO_2}

- The P_{HCO3} is higher than normal in chronic respiratory acidosis.

In chronic respiratory acidosis, the intracellular acidosis in proximal convoluted tubule cells leads to an increase in both HCO_3^- reabsorption and NH_4^+ production and excretion, but for only a transient period; this increase leads to a higher P_{HCO3}. Therefore, patients with chronic respiratory acidosis have a P_{HCO3} that is persistently higher than normal. The opposite occurs in chronic respiratory alkalosis. Thus, individuals with chronic respiratory acid-base disturbances have a different steady-state P_{HCO3}, and hence H^+ concentration, than those with acute respiratory acid-base disorders (Table 8-4). It is therefore important for the clinician to clarify, on clinical grounds, whether the acid-base disturbance is acute or chronic.

QUESTIONS

(Discussions on pages 239 and 240)

8-1 *Can respiratory alkalosis and respiratory acidosis occur in the same patient at the same time?*

8-2 *What allows oxygen to diffuse quickly to skeletal muscle cells during the performance of vigorous exercise despite a low P_{O_2} in capillary blood?*

PART B
RESPIRATORY ACID-BASE DISORDERS

- The traditional definition of respiratory acid-base disorders is based on changes in the arterial Pbn_2.
- The definition of respiratory acidosis should also include the "tissue" type of respiratory acidosis.

Because there is a very large flux of CO_2 relative to the P_{CO_2}, if a transient discrepancy between production and removal of CO_2 develops, the resultant change in arterial P_{CO_2} is large enough to cause a significant displacement of the bicarbonate buffer system equilibrium (see Fig. 8-1). A rise in the arterial P_{CO_2} results in an increased concentration of H^+ (respiratory acidosis), and a fall in arterial P_{CO_2} causes a fall in the concentration of H^+ (respiratory alkalosis). Notwithstanding, it is the capillary P_{CO_2} (reflected by the venous P_{CO_2}) that determines whether H^+ are buffered by the bicarbonate buffer system or bind to intracellular proteins.

RESPIRATORY ACIDOSIS

- The hallmark of respiratory acidosis is a high Pbn_2 in arterial and/or venous blood.

Respiratory acidosis can be divided into two types: respiratory acidosis of the ventilatory type and respiratory acidosis of the tissue type.

Ventilatory type

This form of respiratory acidosis occurs when ventilation transiently fails to remove all the CO_2 produced by normal metabolism. As a result, the alveolar P_{CO_2} rises, and this increases the arterial P_{CO_2}. At this new level of arterial and alveolar P_{CO_2}, all the CO_2 that is produced can now be removed despite the reduced ventilation (*see margin note*).

The clinician should establish the basis of the hypoventilation. Patients who hypoventilate can be divided into two groups—those who will not breathe (e.g., defective stimuli because of drugs that suppress the respiratory center), and those who cannot breathe (e.g., respiratory muscle weakness, pulmonary parenchymal disease, or obstructive airway disease).

Tissue type

Although this form of respiratory acidosis is less well appreciated by clinicians, it is important to recognize because of its implications for normal function of cells. The arterial P_{CO_2} might be suitably low, but the venous P_{CO_2} may still be high because either CO_2 production is increased in cells and/or the rate of blood flow to an organ is not as high as is needed to maintain a low venous P_{CO_2} (*see margin note* for a quantitative example). The venous P_{CO_2} reflects the P_{CO_2} in *capillaries* and

EXPECTED VALUE FOR THE ARTERIAL P_{CO_2}
Although the normal arterial P_{CO_2} is 40 mm Hg, its value must be evaluated in conjunction with other clinical information (e.g., in a patient with metabolic acidosis and a P_{HCO_3} of 10 mmol/L, the expected arterial P_{CO_2} should be close to 25 mm Hg).

EFFECT OF RATE OF BLOOD FLOW ON THE VENOUS P_{CO_2}
Consider an organ that extracts 6 mmol of O_2 per minute to perform its biologic work.
- If the rate of blood flow to this organ is 2 L/min, each liter of blood would lose 3 mmol of its total of 8 mmol of O_2 if the hemoglobin is fully saturated with oxygen. Now if the RQ is 1 for simple arithmetic, each liter of venous blood would have to carry an extra 3 mmol of CO_2 (largely as HCO_3^-) to the lungs, and it would have a P_{CO_2} in the mid-40 mm Hg range.
- If the blood flow rate to that organ is reduced to 1 L/min and its biologic work is unchanged, this liter of blood would lose 6 mmol of its O_2 and be forced to carry an extra 6 mmol of CO_2 to the lungs. Hence, the venous P_{CO_2} will be close to 60 mm Hg.

hence the P_{CO_2} in cells and in the interstitial fluid in this drainage area. As mentioned previously, the P_{CO_2} of brachial or femoral venous blood provides insights into how well the majority of the bicarbonate buffer system could function. If the bicarbonate buffer system in skeletal muscles (in the cells and interstitial space) does not function adequately, the pH in blood falls and more H^+ bind to intracellular proteins in vital organs, which changes their charge and may affect their shape and function.

Clinical approach

The diagnostic approach to the ventilatory type of respiratory acidosis is outlined in Flow Chart 8-1. First, decide whether the patient has chronic lung disease by the history, physical examination, and available past records. Then, compare the acid-base status with that expected for this acid-base disorder. If the expected responses are not present, the patient has a mixed acid-base disorder.

The diagnostic approach to the tissue type of respiratory acidosis is shown in Flow Chart 8-2. The key elements to analyze are reasons for a high production of CO_2 and/or a slow blood flow rate.

Permissive hypercapnia

- This name is incorrect, because the primary aim is to minimize the risk of ventilator-induced lung injury—the consequence, however, is a higher arterial P_{CO_2}.

This form of hypercapnia is not "permissive" but rather "permitted" to minimize lung trauma resulting from high pressure/volume ventilation. With the traditional way of mechanical ventilation, although one could achieve better arterial blood gases, the price to pay, especially

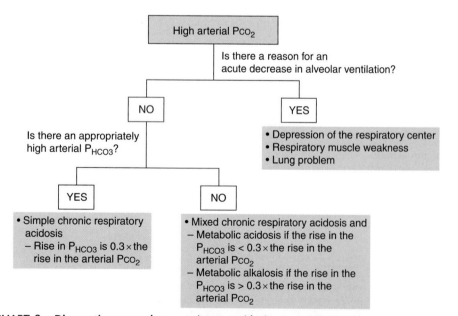

FLOW CHART 8-1 Diagnostic approach to respiratory acidosis. In a patient with an elevated arterial P_{CO_2}, determine whether the patient has acute respiratory acidosis on clinical grounds, because emergency therapy is usually needed. Conversely, if there is no evidence of an acute disorder, the patient may have chronic lung disease or a chronic central reason for hypoventilation. The causes of the acid-base disorder and the laboratory features are shown in the *green boxes*.

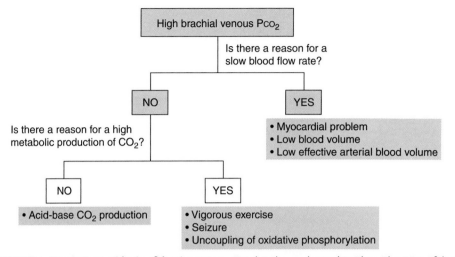

FLOW CHART 8-2 Respiratory acidosis of the tissue type. For details, see legend to Flow Chart 8-1. If the brachial venous P_{CO_2} is greater than 10 mm Hg above the arterial P_{CO_2}, determine whether the problem is a low blood flow rate and/or a high rate of production of CO_2.

in patients with high airway pressures, is the danger of causing barotrauma and/or a pneumothorax. Hence, the strategy is to deliberately ventilate these patients with a lower tidal volume and pressure. The lungs may be "saved"; however, the ability to exhale CO_2 at a low alveolar P_{CO_2} is compromised, and the result is a higher concentration of CO_2 in the alveolus and in arterial blood. In other words, hypercapnia is not the goal but rather the consequence of this therapy.

Because a high P_{CO_2} causes dilatation of cerebral arterioles, permissive hypercapnia is potentially dangerous in the patient with traumatic brain injury or cerebrovascular disease. Another concern with this mode of ventilation is in the patient with metabolic acidosis, as the high venous P_{CO_2} compromises the effectiveness of the bicarbonate buffer system in removing a H^+ load. Therefore, H^+ bind to intracellular proteins. This results in a change in their charge and perhaps shape and function, leading to possible detrimental effects on cell function, especially in vital organs (e.g., brain and heart). To date, no prospective, randomized controlled studies have unequivocally demonstrated appreciable improvements in clinical outcome when permissive hypercapnic ventilation was compared with conventional mechanical ventilation.

RESPIRATORY ALKALOSIS

Respiratory alkalosis is a common abnormality that is often ignored. In fact, the mortality rate in hospitalized patients with respiratory alkalosis is greater than that in patients with respiratory acidosis, which likely reflects the importance of the underlying disease process. Respiratory alkalosis may result from stimulation of the peripheral chemoreceptors (hypoxemia), the afferent pulmonary reflexes (intrinsic pulmonary disease), or the respiratory center in the brain (Table 8-5). An increase in ventilation may be difficult to recognize clinically, and the diagnosis of respiratory alkalosis is often made only by determination of the blood gases.

Respiratory alkalosis occurs when the removal of CO_2 via ventilation transiently exceeds its rate of production; thus, the alveolar and arterial P_{CO_2} fall. If this persists, a new steady state is achieved where the daily production of CO_2 is removed, but at a lower arterial P_{CO_2}.

TABLE 8-5 **CAUSES OF RESPIRATORY ALKALOSIS**

CONDITION	CAUSES
Hypoxia	Intrinsic pulmonary disease, high altitude, congestive heart failure, congenital heart disease (cyanotic)
Pulmonary receptor stimulation	Pneumonia, pulmonary embolism, asthma, pulmonary fibrosis, pulmonary edema
Drugs	Salicylates, alkaloids, catecholamines, theophylline, progesterone
Central nervous system disorders	Subarachnoid hemorrhage, primary hyperventilation syndrome
Miscellaneous	Psychogenic hyperventilation, liver cirrhosis, fever, gram-negative sepsis, pregnancy

A fall in the P_{CO_2} in cells lower their concentration of H^+ and thereby result in the removal of H^+ from intracellular proteins. This leads to a change in their charge, shape, and possibly function.

Clinical approach

- Chronic respiratory alkalosis is the only acid-base disorder in which the concentration of H^+ in plasma may be in the normal range (see Table 8-4 for the expected P_{HCO3} in a patient with chronic respiratory alkalosis).

The diagnostic approach to respiratory alkalosis begins by deciding on clinical grounds whether there is a disease process present that is associated with acute respiratory alkalosis; if not, the patient is presumed to have chronic respiratory alkalosis. Salicylate intoxication is the most important cause of respiratory alkalosis, and it is discussed in more detail subsequently.

Salicylate intoxication

- Respiratory alkalosis is the usual acid-base disorder that accompanies salicylate intoxication.
- The major issue is not the respiratory alkalosis but rather the toxicity of salicylate anions in cells.
- The treatment is to accelerate the removal of salicylate. If alkali is used, avoid creating a severe degree of alkalemia. If acetazolamide is used, give a small dose because it competes with salicylate for binding to albumin.

Toxicity of salicylate

The major issue with an overdose of aspirin is the toxicity related to the effect of salicylate anions in cells. This may result from direct toxic effects of salicylate on cell functions. It is also possible that this organic acid could uncouple oxidative phosphorylation, akin to dinitrophenol or metformin (see Chapter 6, page 174 for more discussion). This may lead to some of the central nervous system manifestations of salicylate intoxication. For example, if an increased consumption of O_2 and production of CO_2 occurs near the respiratory center, this could stimulate alveolar ventilation and perhaps explain the respiratory alkalosis that is commonly seen in these patients. In severe intoxications, the degree of uncoupling of oxidative phosphorylation may be excessive. If this compromises the rate of conversion of ADP to ATP, anaerobic glycolysis is stimulated and a severe degree of L-lactic acidosis develops (*see margin note*).

ABBREVIATIONS
ASA, acetylsalicylic acid
SA, salicylate anions
H•SA, nonionized salicylic acid

UNCOUPLING OF OXIDATIVE PHOSPHORYLATION BY SALICYLATE
The degree of uncoupling must be low enough to prevent an appreciable rise in the already tiny concentration of ADP, which leads very quickly to very rapid rates of glycolysis. Because the velocity of glycolysis is much greater than that of pyruvate oxidation, the net result is an acute accumulation of L-lactic acid. If the degree were to become more severe, ATP levels will fall, and this can be catastrophic.

TABLE 8-6 **EFFECT OF ACIDEMIA ON THE CONCENTRATION OF SALICYLATES IN CELLS**

In the example shown, the total salicylate concentration in the extracellular fluid (ECF) is 7 mmol/L. Because of its low pK (~3.5), only a very tiny fraction is in the undissociated form at normal blood pH values (i.e., salicylic acid [H•SA = 0.3 μmol/L]). H•SA diffuses across cell membranes and at equilibrium, its concentration is equal inside and outside cells. In the cell, the concentration of salicylate depends on the intracellular fluid (ICF) pH. Because the ICF pH is normally close to 0.3 pH units lower than the ECF pH, the intracellular salicylate will be half that in the ECF at equilibrium (3.5 mmol/L vs. 7.0 mmol/L). If the pH in ECF drops to 7.1, the concentration of H•SA will rise from 0.3 μmol/L to 0.6 μmol/L. Because H•SA diffuses across cell membranes to achieve equilibrium, the difference between the ECF and ICF pH now is small, so the intracellular salicylate concentration rises from 3.5 mmol/L to 6.0 mmol/L.

	NORMAL		ACIDEMIA	
	ECF	*ICF*	*ECF*	*ICF*
pH	7.4	7.1	7.1	7.0
H•SA (μmol/L)	0.3	0.3	0.6	0.6
Salicylate (mmol/L)	7.0	3.5	7.0	6.0

Reye's syndrome is a specific example of central nervous system toxicity of salicylate related to uncoupling of oxidative phosphorylation (*see margin note*).

The effect of acidemia on the concentration of salicylates in blood and in cells is illustrated in Table 8-6 . The key point in this table is that there is a much larger change in the pH outside as compared to inside these cells. Therefore, the concentration of salicylate rises appreciably in cells during acidemia and this should increase its toxicity. Thus, one should take measures to keep the arterial pH in the high-normal to modestly alkalemic range.

Signs and symptoms

The central nervous system manifestations of aspirin overdose include tinnitus, fever, vertigo, and nausea. The gastrointestinal manifestations include upper abdominal pain, vomiting, and diarrhea. Lung toxicity is manifested by noncardiogenic pulmonary edema. With more severe intoxication, the degree of altered mental status is more profound (e.g., coma), and this may lead, ultimately, to death.

Acid-base considerations

The most common acid-base disturbance associated with salicylate intoxication is respiratory alkalosis from central stimulation of respiration. Metabolic acidosis may be present in acute salicylate intoxication, but it is not usually an important issue (*see margin note*).

Diagnosis

The diagnosis of salicylate intoxication should be suspected on the basis of a history of ingestion or symptoms of tinnitus and lightheadedness and a severe degree of respiratory alkalosis. An unexplained ketosis, hypouricemia (high-dose salicylate has a uricosuric effect), noncardiogenic pulmonary edema, or an increased urine net charge (Na^+ and K^+ greatly exceed Cl^- when the urine does not contain HCO_3^-, as a result of the excretion of salicylate anions) should

REYE'S SYNDROME
In these patients, the activity of pyruvate dehydrogenase in the brain may be barely sufficient to regenerate the usual amount of ATP needed by that organ. In the absence of ketoacids, glucose oxidation is the only pathway of importance for ATP regeneration in the brain; hence, a small increment in the degree of uncoupling of oxidative phosphorylation may compromise brain function because of a lower rate of regeneration of ATP and also binding of H^+ to proteins in brain cells as a result of the production of L-lactic acid.

THIAMIN DEFICIENCY
Patients with thiamin deficiency also have a decreased activity of pyruvate dehydrogenase in their brain. Therefore, the intake of salicylates can lead to similar sequences in the brain as described earlier.

METABOLIC ACIDOSIS DURING SALICYLATE INTOXICATION
- Toxicity caused by the monovalent salicylate anion occurs when its concentration is 3 to 5 mmol/L. Thus, if the $P_{Anion\ gap}$ is elevated by a much greater amount, look for reasons why other anions are present (e.g., L-lactate or ketoacid anions).
- A modest degree of uncoupling of oxidative phosphorylation can increase the production of ketoacids in the liver (see Chapter 5, page 147).
- A more severe degree of uncoupling can lead to L-lactic acidosis.

raise suspicion of salicylate intoxication. The diagnosis is confirmed by measuring the concentration of salicylate in blood.

Treatment

- The focus of treatment is to avoid salicylate toxicity in cells.

Dialysis should be instituted if salicylate levels exceed 90 mg/dL (6 mmol/L). If levels of salicylate exceed 60 mg/dL (4 mmol/L), dialysis should be considered, particularly if further absorption is anticipated. In patients with an unexplained decreased level of consciousness, dialysis should be started at even lower levels of salicylate in blood because of the poor prognosis. Hemodialysis is more efficient for the removal of salicylate, but peritoneal dialysis may be considered if there will be a long delay before hemodialysis can be initiated.

In the absence of severe toxicity, the therapeutic efforts in salicylate intoxication are to decrease the concentration of salicylic acid in blood and to promote the urinary excretion of salicylate via the following two maneuvers.

Alkali therapy. This should be instituted in a patient with salicylate intoxication who has metabolic acidosis to decrease the concentration of H·SA in the blood and thus diminish its diffusion into brain cells (see Table 8-6; Fig. 8-3). Some authorities advise creating an alkaline urine pH to promote salicylate excretion. Notwithstanding, aggressive therapy with $NaHCO_3$ should be avoided because the patient may become very alkalemic due to the coexistent respiratory alkalosis.

Use of acetazolamide

- Acetazolamide, a carbonic anhydrase inhibitor, may be useful in the therapy for salicylate intoxication. Its mechanism of action is controversial.
- Avoid using large doses of acetazolamide because this drug can diminish binding of salicylate to albumin.

The traditional view is that acetazolamide increases the excretion of the salicylate by raising the pH in the lumen of the proximal convoluted tubule, thereby decreasing the concentration of the

INCREASING SALICYLATE EXCRETION WITH ACETAZOLAMIDE

- In the proximal convoluted tubule, the effect of acetazolamide is to *increase* (not decrease) the concentration of H^+ of tubular fluid via inhibition of luminal carbonic anhydrase. Hence, the likely mechanism for acetazolamide to increase the excretion of salicylate cannot be a result of lowering the H·SA concentration in luminal fluid.
- We suggest that there is a direct effect of HCO_3^- to inhibit the reabsorption of salicylate in the proximal convoluted tubule; hence, an increase in luminal HCO_3^- resulting from the effect of acetazolamide may explain its effect to increase salicylate excretion if salicylates are a substrate for a transport system.

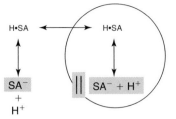

FIGURE 8-3 Nonionic diffusion of salicylic acid versus salicylate anions. The *circle* represents the cell membrane or the luminal membrane of the proximal convoluted tubule. The assumption made is that the organic acid form of salicylate (H·SA) can cross cell membranes by diffusion because it is uncharged, whereas salicylate anions cannot do so (*see double vertical lines*) unless there is a transporter that can permit transport of salicylate anion.

undissociated acid form of salicylic acid (H·SA), which can cross cell membranes by diffusion (*see margin note*). Caution is needed, however, since acetazolamide may increase the toxicity of salicylate because it competes with salicylate anions for binding to $P_{Albumin}$, which may increase the free salicylate concentration in blood. In addition, acetazolamide may induce acidemia by increasing the excretion of HCO_3^- in the urine, which may make more uncharged salicylic acid available to enter cells, and hence increase the toxicity.

There is some experimental evidence in humans, which suggests that 250 mg of acetazolamide has a tubular effect that lasts for about 16 hours. Therefore, very little drug is needed to achieve beneficial effects, and one could use a low dose instead of alkali therapy in the patient with a high blood pH (i.e., >7.5) and a modestly elevated level of salicylate.

PART C
INTEGRATIVE PHYSIOLOGY

PHYSIOLOGY OF O_2

The vast majority of O_2 in blood is bound to hemoglobin (4 mmol of O_2 per mmol of hemoglobin). Because blood contains 2 mmol/L of hemoglobin, the content of O_2 in blood is 8 mmol/L (*see margin note*). The affinity of hemoglobin for O_2 is high, but it can be reduced by elevated concentrations of H^+, CO_2, and 2,3-bis-phosphoglycerate or 2,3-dis-phosphoglycerate. All of these factors cause the S-shaped oxygen-hemoglobin dissociation curve to be shifted to the right (Fig. 8-4). Therefore, when O_2 is extracted, there is a higher P_{O_2}, which aids in diffusion of oxygen to cells (Fig. 8-5).

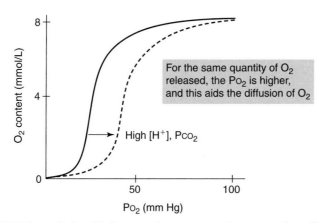

For the same quantity of O_2 released, the P_{O_2} is higher, and this aids the diffusion of O_2

High $[H^+]$, P_{CO_2}

FIGURE 8-4 Relationship between the content and concentration of O_2 in 1 liter of blood. The content of O_2 in each liter of blood (shown on the y-axis) has a sigmoid relationship to the arterial P_{O_2} (shown on x-axis). When the concentration of H^+ and/or the P_{CO_2} rises in capillaries, the S-shaped curve is shifted to the right, so the affinity of hemoglobin for O_2 is diminished and the P_{O_2} rises. Therefore, there is a higher P_{O_2}, which aids the diffusion of O_2.

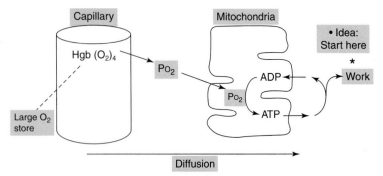

FIGURE 8-5 Delivery of O₂ to mitochondria by diffusion. *The structure on the left* is a capillary and the *structure on the right* is a mitochondrion. A large quantity of O₂ must be delivered to mitochondria in exercise to have a high rate of regeneration of ATP. Both a high Po₂ in capillaries and "stirring of the interstitial compartment" are needed for rapid rates of diffusion of O₂ to muscle cells. Nevertheless, the Po₂ in mitochondria needs to be only a few mm Hg to regenerate ATP at maximal rates. Hgb, hemoglobin.

THE ALVEOLAR-ARTERIAL Po₂ DIFFERENCE

- Calculation of the alveolar-arterial (A-a) Po₂ difference is used clinically to assess the cause of hypoxemia (*see margin note*).

The arterial Po₂ is determined by both the Po₂ of alveolar air and the ability of O₂ to diffuse across the alveolar capillary membrane. The A-a Po₂ difference is useful to estimate how much of the fall in the arterial Po₂ is the result of a change in alveolar Po₂ (ventilation) and how much is the result of reduced transfer of O₂ from alveolus to blood (intrinsic lung disease). One must, however, be able to estimate the Po₂ of the inspired air to calculate the A-a difference (*see margin note*). In the alveoli, CO₂ is part of the "non-nitrogen" gases. Therefore, as the Pco₂ of alveolar air rises, the Po₂ falls. One can calculate the alveolar Po₂ using the abbreviated alveolar gas equation (see equations).

$$\text{Alveolar air Po}_2 = \text{inspired air Po}_2 - (\text{arterial Pco}_2)/\text{RQ}$$
$$= \text{inspired air Po}_2 - (\text{arterial Pco}_2)/0.8$$

Two major types of pulmonary lesions cause the arterial Po₂ to be substantially lower than that of alveolar air. First, blood can pass from the pulmonary artery to the pulmonary vein without perfusing alveoli that have a high Po₂ (i.e., a shunt). Second, there may be a barrier to diffusion of O₂ from alveolar air to the capillaries in lungs (e.g., inflammation, pulmonary edema).

The usual value for the A-a Po₂ difference is up to 10 mm Hg, and higher values are observed with increasing age. The usual value for the A-a Po₂ difference results from mixing of a small shunt of blood with a lower oxygen content with the fully oxygenated blood leaving the lungs.

Pitfalls in the use of the alveolar-arterial difference

- The A-a difference uses the Po₂ instead of the O₂ saturation, which reflects the content of O₂.

ALVEOLAR-ARTERIAL Po₂ DIFFERENCE
The difference in Po₂ between the alveolar air and arterial blood is referred to as the A-a *gradient*. In truth, this calculation is a "difference" rather than a "gradient" because diffusion of a nonelectrolyte is involved.

ESTIMATE THE Po₂ OF INSPIRED AIR
Room air is 21% O₂, barometric pressure is 760 mm Hg, and water vapor pressure is 47 mm Hg. Therefore, the Po₂ of inspired air is 0.21 × (760 − 47), or close to 150 mm Hg.

The pitfalls are the following:

1. The same reduction in O_2 content has a different impact on the Po_2 at different sites on the oxygen-hemoglobin dissociation curve because of its sigmoid shape (see Fig. 8-4). Therefore, a disease process that causes a reduction in content of O_2 of blood from 8 mmol/L to 6 mmol/L results in a large A-a difference because it lies on the flat portion of the oxygen-hemoglobin dissociation curve. Therefore, there is a relatively large fall in its Po_2 despite a very small change in O_2 saturation or the content of oxygen. A similar decrease in its content of O_2 of blood, but from 6 mmol/L to 4 mmol/L, results in a much smaller increase in the A-a difference. As a result, a worsening pulmonary condition may not be readily detected by the A-a difference.

2. With a fixed volume of a shunt from pulmonary artery to pulmonary vein, the arterial Po_2 is strongly influenced by the content of O_2 in the blood in the pulmonary artery (*see margin note*). Therefore, nonpulmonary factors (e.g., sepsis or liver disease) can influence the magnitude of the A-a difference.

3. In the calculation of the alveolar Po_2, one must estimate the amount of O_2 removed and replaced by CO_2. To do so, one uses the arterial Pco_2 and assumes an RQ of 0.8. Notwithstanding, the RQ could be 1.0 if carbohydrate is the only type of fuel being metabolized. This will increase the A-a difference (*see margin note for an example*).

CONTROL OF THE RELEASE OF ERYTHROPOIETIN

- The central issue is that the Po_2 at the site of release of erythropoietin should be influenced *solely* by the concentration of hemoglobin in blood.

The following features make the renal cortex the ideal site for the O_2 sensor that regulates the release of erythropoietin because they allow the concentration of hemoglobin to be the only variable that influences the Po_2 at the site of the O_2 sensor (*see margin note*).

Fall in Po_2 induced by small reduction in the concentration of hemoglobin must be easily recognized

- The key to understanding this sensitivity is revealed by examining the oxygen-hemoglobin dissociation curve (compare the right and the left graphs of Fig. 8-6).

Because the kidney has a large blood flow, only a small amount of O_2 is extracted from each liter of blood. When the same amount of O_2 is extracted from blood that has a lower content of O_2 because of a lower hemoglobin concentration, the drop in Po_2 would be larger because one is still operating near the flat part of the sigmoid-shaped oxygen-hemoglobin dissociation curve (see Fig. 8-6).

Ratio of consumption of O_2 to delivery of O_2 in renal cortex must be constant to ensure that sensor for O_2 is exposed to near-constant Po_2 unless blood has lower hemoglobin concentration

- O_2 is consumed when work is performed.

LOW Po_2 IN CELLS
- One might think that a very low Po_2 in cells might limit ATP regeneration. Nevertheless, the large amount of O_2 bound to myoglobin and a high affinity of cytochrome C for O_2 avoids the difficulty of not having enough O_2 during exercise.
- Having a low Po_2 in cells at rest (due to slow diffusion owing to poor mixing) prevents the development of too high a Po_2 in cells, and thereby, an excessive formation of reactive oxygen species.

IMPACT OF THE CONTENT OF O_2 IN SHUNTED BLOOD ON THE ALVEOLAR-ARTERIAL DIFFERENCE
Assume that arterial blood has 8 mmol/L of O_2 and that 10% of the blood in the pulmonary artery bypasses aerated alveoli via a shunt into the pulmonary vein.
- In one example, assume that the content of O_2 in the blood in the pulmonary artery is 6 mmol/L. After this 10% shunt, arterial blood would contain 7.8 mmol of O_2/L (0.9 L with 8 mmol/L + 0.1 L with 6 mmol/L).
- In another example, assume that blood in the pulmonary artery contains 3 mmol/L of O_2. After the 10% shunt, the arterial blood would have 7.5 mmol/L of O_2 (0.9 L with 8 mmol/L + 0.1 L with 3 mmol/L). As a result, the new arterial Po_2 in the first instance would be 95 mm Hg and it would be 65 mm Hg in the second example. The corresponding A-a differences would be 5 and 35 mm Hg.

EFFECT OF THE RESPIRATORY QUOTIENT ON THE ALVEOLAR-ARTERIAL DIFFERENCE
- Assume an RQ of 0.8:

Alveolar O_2 = 150 − (40/0.8)
            = 100 mm Hg

- Assume an RQ of 1:

Alveolar O_2 = 150 − (40/1)
            = 110 mm Hg

Therefore, the A-a increases by 10 mm Hg.

ERYTHROPOIETIN AND THE KIDNEY
The hypothesis presented here may improve our understanding of why erythropoietin is synthesized in the renal cortex and why having both a high GFR and a very large renal blood flow rate are essential components of this efficient control system.

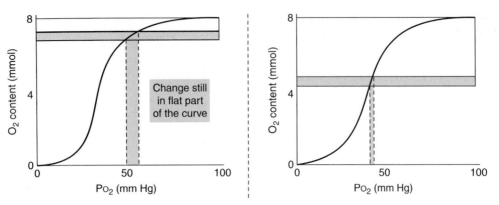

FIGURE 8-6 Importance of the renal blood flow in determining the sensitivity of the receptor for erythropoietin synthesis. The arterial Po_2 is depicted on the x-axis and the quantity of O_2 in 1 liter of blood is depicted on the y-axis. The *clear portion of the horizontal rectangle* represents the total quantity of O_2 extracted per liter of blood flow when the hemoglobin concentration in blood is in the upper normal range. In contrast, the *green rectangle* represents the extra quantity of O_2 extracted per liter of blood flow when the hemoglobin concentration in blood is in the lower normal range. The *vertical dashed lines* indicate the change in arterial Po_2 as a result of this extra extraction of O_2 per liter of blood flow. The drop in Po_2 would be larger if one is still operating near the flat part of the sigmoid-shaped oxygen-hemoglobin dissociation curve; compare the *right* with the *left portion of the figure*, where in other organs, there is more work per O_2 delivery.

NEED FOR A HIGH GFR
Because a high renal blood flow rate is needed to increase the sensitivity of the Po_2 signal for the release of erythropoietin, there is also a need for a high GFR to have enough extraction of O_2, independent of other demands of renal physiology.

FILTRATION FRACTION
To calculate the filtration fraction, the renal plasma flow is used. Conversely, the renal blood flow is substituted for the renal plasma flow for this concept because we are assessing the signal system in terms of oxygen.

Filtration fraction = GFR ÷ renal
plasma flow
(O_2 consumption ÷ O_2 delivery)

• The vast majority of renal work is to reabsorb close to 99.5% of filtered Na^+ (*see margin note*).

The amount of filtered Na^+ is the product of the GFR and the P_{Na}. Because there is little variation in the P_{Na} in healthy subjects, renal work (or O_2 consumption) is directly related to the GFR. Moreover, the *ratio* between the GFR (O_2 consumption) and renal plasma flow rate (O_2 delivery)—that is, filtration fraction—does not vary appreciably from day to day in humans (*see equation in margin note*). This is achieved because the glomerulus lies between two arterial systems, each with different modulators of vessel tone. If the filtration fraction does not vary appreciably, the sensor for O_2 should be exposed to a near-constant Po_2 unless blood has a lower hemoglobin concentration.

A high renal cortical blood flow rate speeds up the diffusion of O_2 from its capillaries to the receptor for O_2 deep in the renal cortex

The high cortical blood flow eliminates another variable, the slow speed of diffusion of O_2. This makes the signal to release erythropoietin related to only an abnormal concentration of hemoglobin in blood (see the discussion of Question 8-2).

A shift in the oxygen-hemoglobin dissociation curve must not interfere with the sensitivity of this system to release erythropoietin

If the oxygen-hemoglobin dissociation curve in capillaries of the renal cortex is always shifted to the right, the Po_2 signal is not influenced by other factors that may influence this shift. In fact, this is achieved by having a high Pco_2 in blood vessels in the renal cortex (~65 mm Hg).

QUESTIONS

(Discussions on pages 240 and 242)

8-3 *Why might sports anemia* (see margin note) *be tolerated without an apparent erythropoietin-induced drive to synthesize red blood cells to correct the anemia?*

8-4 *Why does a young patient with diabetes mellitus who has a high GFR not develop polycythemia?*

DISCUSSION OF CASE 8-1

CASE 8-1: DOES THIS PATIENT HAVE RESPIRATORY ACIDOSIS?

(Case presented on page 223)

Does the patient have respiratory acidosis of the ventilatory type?

The low blood pH (7.30) and low P_{HCO_3} (15 mmol/L) indicate that he has metabolic acidosis. Because the P_{HCO_3} has fallen 10 mmol/L, the expected arterial P_{CO_2} should be close to 30 mm Hg, and it is. Hence, he does not have respiratory acidosis of the ventilatory type.

Does the patient have respiratory acidosis of the tissue type?

Because his brachial venous P_{CO_2} is higher than expected (60 vs. close to 46 mm Hg), he does have respiratory acidosis of the tissue type. To decide why it is present (see Flow Chart 8-2), we see that he has a low cardiac output as a result of his myocardial infarction. It is also possible that he had a high production of CO_2 if L-lactate + H^+ were being released from his muscles and some of the H^+ were being titrated by his bicarbonate buffer system.

Is the patient able to buffer H^+ appropriately using his bicarbonate buffer system in skeletal muscle?

This patient's brachial venous P_{CO_2} is higher than expected; therefore, his bicarbonate buffer system is compromised in the interstitial fluid as well as in the ICF compartment of skeletal muscle. Because these sites contain the vast majority of bicarbonate buffer system, a much larger fraction of the H^+ load is presented to vital organs because of the more severe acidemia, which results from removing fewer H^+ in skeletal muscle. As a result, a much greater number of H^+ are bound to proteins in brain cells. This may have untoward effects; therefore, efforts should be made to increase the blood flow rate to skeletal muscles.

DISCUSSION OF QUESTIONS

8-1 *Can respiratory alkalosis and respiratory acidosis occur in the same patient at the same time?*

On the surface, the obvious answer is "no," because one cannot have a high and a low P_{CO_2} at the same time. Nevertheless, when considered in more depth, and defining events at the cellular level, the answer becomes "yes."

Think of ventilation controlling the arterial P_{CO_2} in a patient with diabetic ketoacidosis who is hyperventilating excessively because of aspiration pneumonitis (respiratory alkalosis is present). Because of the low ECF volume, the cardiac output is very low. Now the venous P_{CO_2} is high and therefore the tissue P_{CO_2} is high, so the patient has respiratory acidosis at the cellular level (tissue form of respiratory acidosis is present). This is not just a play on words, because the emergency therapy is to allow buffering of H^+ by the bicarbonate buffer system in skeletal muscles (increase their blood flow rate). As a result of reexpansion of the effective arterial blood volume, the P_{CO_2} in brachial and femoral venous blood will fall. This permits more H^+ removal by the bicarbonate buffer system in skeletal muscles, which in turn diminishes the binding of H^+ to intracellular proteins in vital organs (e.g., in brain cells).

8-2 *What allows oxygen to diffuse quickly to skeletal muscle cells during the performance of vigorous exercise despite a low P_{O_2} in capillary blood?*

Because O_2 is poorly soluble in water, virtually 100% of O_2 is transported in blood bound to hemoglobin in red blood cells. It is important to ensure that the P_{O_2} is high in capillary blood so that the diffusion of O_2 into mitochondria can proceed at a sufficiently rapid rate (see Fig. 8-5). There are three issues to consider.

1. *Raise the P_{O_2} in capillaries during vigorous exercise*: To have O_2 delivery at a *high* P_{O_2} (O_2 concentration), the kinetics of O_2 binding to hemoglobin must have special properties. Hence, the shape of the curve relating the content of O_2 in 1 liter of blood to its P_{O_2} is S-shaped (see Fig. 8-4). When the objective is to have a large off-loading of O_2 from hemoglobin at the highest P_{O_2}, this curve must be shifted to the right. The most likely set of signals for this rightward shift can be deduced from the setting where the demand for O_2 is maximal—vigorous exercise. Therefore, the signals that cause this rightward shift are the products associated with high rates of ATP turnover (CO_2, H^+, heat).

2. *"Stirring" of the interstitial compartment*: When the blood flow rate is very high, many more capillaries are open, which shortens the distance for diffusion of O_2 and accelerates the speed of the diffusion step. "Stirring" has the same result. The importance of this effect becomes evident when one notes that while the cardiac output rises four to five times during vigorous exercise,the consumption of O_2 increases by more than 20 times; virtually all of this rise in cardiac output goes to muscles and the skin for heat dissipation.

3. *Faster diffusion of oxygen through the cytoplasm of muscle*: Because the concentration of O_2 is tiny, having O_2 bind to another compound with a much higher concentration in muscle cells accelerates this diffusion step. The concentration of myoglobin is high in muscle cells, and its affinity for O_2 (a few mm Hg) is in an appropriate range to achieve this function.

8-3 *Why might sports anemia be tolerated without an apparent erythro-poietin-induced drive to synthesize red blood cells to correct the anemia?*

During training, athletes retain extra NaCl and water. Thus, they have a larger ECF volume than prior to training. This is retained as long as training persists, even though exercise is performed over perhaps less than 10% of the day. Part of this extra ECF volume is retained in the vascular bed, which lowers the hematocrit without lowering the red blood cell volume. Perhaps most of this volume is stored in the large venous capacitance vessels; if there were a lower venous tone, this would not provide a signal to excrete the extra Na^+ in the urine. In physiologic terms, there may be an advantage when exercise is performed. In this context, the adrenergic surge would cause venoconstriction to cause this "extra" blood to enter the effective vascular volume and lead to an improved cardiac output (*see margin note*). Thus, physicians may recognize this condition as sports anemia, whereas a thin runner may recognize it by weight gain during training or weight loss that occurs along with a diuresis several days after training stops.

There must also be a diminished stimulus to produce erythropoietin even though anemia is present. We speculate that there may be a lower filtration fraction resulting from less efferent arterial constriction and/or a higher renal blood flow rate, which could cause the Po_2 to be higher deep in the renal cortex. In addition, with higher renal blood flow, there is more vigorous stirring to aid diffusion of O_2 or shorten the distance for diffusion if more capillaries are open (see the discussion of Question 8-2). A new steady state could exist with a low hematocrit, a higher plasma volume, and an altered hemodynamic pattern in the kidney. Direct data are needed to test this hypothesis.

Sports anemia is an example of a change in erythrocytosis, which may occur if the ratio of O_2 consumption (GFR) to O_2 delivery (renal blood flow) is altered because the hemoglobin concentration would not be the only variable that determines the Po_2 near the sensor for the release of erythropoietin. We stress that it is *not* the GFR per se that alters the signal to cause the release of erythropoietin. Rather it is the ratio of renal O_2 consumption (GFR) to O_2 delivery plus the

ADVANTAGE OF SPORTS ANEMIA
- Blood in the vascular tree is in three locations: arteries, veins, and capillaries.
- The capacity of the capillaries to "hold" blood is enormous. Therefore, the capillary volume cannot expand appreciably, as this would cause a hemodynamic emergency.
- During vigorous exercise, there is more blood in capillaries in skeletal muscles and in the skin. This extra capillary volume cannot exceed the "extra" volume contained in the circulation (due to contraction of capacitance vessels and the decrease in capillary volume elsewhere in the body) if hemodynamics are to be preserved during vigorous exercise. Hence, having a higher blood volume is an advantage.

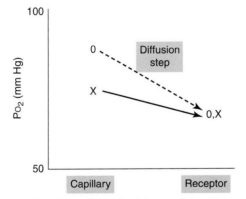

FIGURE 8-7 Possible independent role of the renal blood flow rate on the Po_2 near the receptor for O_2 deep in the renal cortex. The graph depicts the Po_2 that is likely to be present in capillary blood deep in the renal cortex (*points to the left of the line* depict diffusion) and its fall during diffusion to the site of the receptor for O_2 near the corticomedullary junction (*points to the right of the line*). The o *symbols* represent the normal control subjects and the X *symbols* represent patients with type 1 diabetes mellitus who have hyperfiltration and a higher filtration fraction. Although the capillary Po_2 is likely lower in the group with diabetes, the higher renal blood flow rate may accelerate the slow diffusion step and thereby diminish the fall in Po_2 during diffusion. As a result, the Po_2 near the receptor may not be appreciably different in these two populations.

**THERAPY FOR
ERYTHROCYTOSIS AFTER
RENAL TRANSPLANTATION**
Angiotensin-converting enzyme
inhibitors are used to diminish
the red blood cell mass in this
setting. One possible explanation
of why these drugs are effective is
that they reduce efferent arteriolar
tone; hence, they lead to a lower
GFR and thereby renal work (O_2
consumption) without influencing
the renal blood flow to a major
extent. Thus, there is a higher Po_2
in capillary blood in the renal cortex,
which diminishes the stimulus for
the release of erythropoietin.

**EARLY RENAL LESION IN
DIABETES MELLITUS**
The patients with very early
changes of diabetes mellitus are
not necessarily symptomatic. Therefore, what is called "early" is likely
to represent a somewhat later stage
of the disease.

absolute value for the renal blood flow rate that may influence the renal cortical Po_2 in steady state. When less O_2 is extracted *per liter* of renal blood flow, the Po_2 in the interstitial compartment near the O_2 sensor is higher and less erythropoietin is released. The result could be the development of chronic anemia. Perhaps, one example of this pathophysiology could be the chronic anemia associated with the use of an angiotensin-converting enzyme inhibitor. To identify which patient with chronic anemia has this functional form of erythropoietin deficiency, the GFR and renal plasma flow could be measured to reveal the low filtration fraction, and the absolute value for the renal blood flow rate should be examined as well (*see margin note*).

8-4 *Why does a young patient with diabetes mellitus who has a high GFR not develop polycythemia?*

The hyperfiltration early on in patients with diabetes mellitus does not lead to erythrocytosis despite the fact that they may have higher filtration fractions and thereby, a lower Po_2 in renal cortical *capillaries*. To explain this finding, it is noteworthy that this population, with diabetes, has higher renal plasma flow rates (*see margin note*). If a higher blood flow rate could minimize the fall in Po_2 in the slow diffusion step between capillaries and the receptor for O_2 deep in the renal cortex, there may not be a lower Po_2 near its receptor to signal the release of more erythropoietin (Fig. 8-7). Hence, one must examine both the filtration fraction and the renal blood flow rate to deduce what the Po_2 may be deep in the renal cortex.

section two
Salt and Water

Sodium and Water Physiology

Introduction

ABBREVIATIONS

P_{Na}, concentration of Na^+ in plasma

P_K, concentration of K^+ in plasma

EABV, effective arterial blood volume

AQP, aquaporin water channels

GFR, glomerular filtration rate

PCT, proximal convoluted tubule

DtL, descending thin limb of the loop of Henle

AtL, ascending thin limb of the loop of Henle

mTAL, medullary thick ascending limb of the loop of Henle

DCT, distal convoluted tubule

CCD, late distal cortical nephron including the cortical collecting duct

MCD, medullary collecting duct

NKCC-2, Na^+, K^+, 2 Cl^- cotransporter 2

ROMK, rat outer medullary K^+ channel

NCC, Na^+, Cl^- cotransporter

ENaC, epithelial Na^+ channel

It is important to understand the physiology of Na^+ and of water homeostasis to explain why the extracellular fluid (ECF) volume and/or the P_{Na} may be abnormal, to recognize how this pathophysiology may create a medical emergency, and how to plan optimal therapy to deal with these disorders.

This chapter is divided into four sections. The first section deals with the factors that determine the distribution of water between the ECF and ICF compartments as well as the distribution of saline between the vascular and interstitial subdivisions of the ECF compartment. The second section deals with how balance for Na^+ is achieved. The third section describes how balance for water is accomplished. In the final section, we provide a more in-depth look at selected aspects of integrative physiology of Na^+ and water homeostasis.

PART A
BODY FLUID COMPARTMENTS

OBJECTIVES

- To emphasize that the number of effective osmoles in the ECF and ICF compartments determines their respective volumes.
- To emphasize that the hydrostatic pressure in capillaries and the concentration of albumin in plasma ($P_{Albumin}$) are the two major factors that determine the distribution of the ECF volume between its two major subcompartments, the intravascular and the interstitial fluid volumes.
- To emphasize that P_{Na} reflects ICF volume, but in an inverse fashion.
- To point out that Na^+ and water homeostasis are regulated by different control systems.

CASE 9-1: A RISE IN THE P_{Na} AFTER A SEIZURE

(Case discussed on page 308)

A 20-year-old man experienced his first grand mal seizure one day prior to presenting to the hospital. He had no known illnesses prior to this time. The physical examination today is normal, and all the results of blood tests performed, including the P_{Na} (140 mmol/L), were in the normal range. Several hours later, he had a second grand mal seizure. A brachial venous blood was drawn immediately after the seizure; the results revealed the expected metabolic acidosis with a large increase in the $P_{Anion\ gap}$ because of accumulation of L-lactic acid, but this returned to normal in less than an hour. To everyone's surprise, however, his P_{Na} was 154 mmol/L after the seizure, but it fell over a short period of time to 140 mmol/L. There was no change in his weight and no large increase in urine output prior to the development of hypernatremia, and he did not ingest a large volume of water nor was he given hypotonic fluids after the seizure.

Question

What is the basis for the acute rise in his P_{Na}?

TOTAL BODY WATER

- Water is the most abundant constituent of the body; it accounts for approximately 60% of the body mass. Close to two thirds of this water is located inside cells.
- The percentage of body weight that is due to water content depends on the relative proportions of muscle and fat in the body.

Skeletal muscle is the largest organ in the body, which means that half of total body water is located in the ICF and ECF compartments of muscle. Because neutral fat does not dissolve in water, triglycerides are stored in fat cells without water. Accordingly, when relating total body water to body weight, one must consider the relative proportions of muscle and fat (*see margin note;* see Table 9-1). For example, females tend to a higher proportion of fat to body weight and hence a lower percentage of water than males (50% of body weight vs. 60%). Similarly, older people have less water per body weight because they often have a relatively smaller proportion of muscle. Newborn infants, on the other hand, have less adipose tissue and therefore they have a higher proportion of water per body weight (~70%).

OBESITY AND BODY WATER
- Fat stores vary considerably in individuals.
- Obese individuals have much less water per kg body weight.

Distribution of water across cell membranes

- Water crosses cell membranes until the sum of the concentrations of effective osmoles is equal on both sides of these membranes (*see margin note*).
- The number of effective osmoles in each compartment determines its volume.

OSMOTIC FORCE
The osmotic force generated by an osmotic pressure difference of 5 mOsm/kg H_2O is almost equal to the mean arterial blood pressure (1 mOsm/L = 19.3 mm Hg).

Water crosses cell membranes rapidly through AQP1 channels to achieve osmotic equilibrium. Not all materials that are dissolved in water disperse equally in the ICF and ECF compartments, however, because there are differences in permeability, transporters, and active pumps that affect the distribution of individual solutes (Table 9-2). Water distribution across cell membranes depends on the number of particles that are restricted to either the ICF or the ECF compartment (Fig. 9-1); these particles account for the effective osmolality, or the tonicity, in these compartments. The particles restricted to the ECF compartment are Na^+ and its attendant anions (Cl^- plus HCO_3^-); hence, their content in this compartment determines the ECF volume. Na^+ that enter the ICF compartment are actively exported from cells by the Na-K-ATPase, which is located in cell membranes.

TABLE 9-1 **VOLUMES AND MAJOR CATION COMPOSITION OF BODY FLUID COMPARTMENTS***

COMPARTMENT	WATER (L)	Na+ (mmol)	K+ (mmol)
ECF	15	2250	60
ICF	30	150–300	4500
Total body	45	2550	4560

*Values are approximations for a 70-kg nonobese male.
ECF, extracellular fluid; ICF, intracellular fluid.

PHOSPHATE ANIONS IN CELLS
- The majority of the anionic charge in cells is associated with organic phosphates. Because they are very large molecules, they exert little osmotic force. Hence, one should use mEq rather than mmol terms to describe their impact on balance of charges in cells. In general, these organic phosphates are monovalent in cells.
- The ICF macromolecules are largely organic phosphate esters (RNA, DNA, phospholipids, phosphocreatine, and ATP); these compounds are essential for cell function. Hence, only small changes are likely to occur in their content in normal physiology.

ORGANIC OSMOLES IN MUSCLE CELLS
- The organic solutes that have the highest concentration in skeletal muscle cells are phosphocreatine and carnosine (each is present at ~25 mmol/L; see Chapter 1, pages 32 and 36 for more discussion of their function).
- Other solutes including amino acids and their derivatives (e.g., taurine), peptides (e.g., glutathione), and sugar derivatives (e.g., myoinositol) constitute the bulk of the remaining effective intracellular osmoles. The individual compounds, however, differ from organ to organ.
- Because the vast amount of magnesium in cells is held in a bound form, magnesium does not contribute to the number of effective osmoles in cells in an important way.

TABLE 9-2 CONCENTRATION OF IONS IN THE EXTRACELLULAR FLUID AND THE INTRACELLULAR FLUID

Data are expressed as mEq/kg of water. Some water is held in "bound form," and there are regions of cytoplasm where there appears to be less "solvent water," so concentrations of ions in the ICF are not known with certainty. Moreover, these concentrations differ from organ to organ. Values provided are approximations for the ICF in skeletal muscle (*see margin note*).

	ECF	ICF
Na^+	150	10–20
K^+	4.0	120–150
Cl^-	113	~5
HCO_3^-	26	10
Phosphate	2.0 (inorganic)	130 (in macromolecules)

ECF, extracellular fluid; ICF, intracellular fluid.

Determinants of the volume of cells

- The *content* of Na^+ in the ECF compartment is the major determinant of its volume.
- The *concentration* of Na^+ in the ECF compartment is the most important factor that determines the ICF volume (except when cells or the ECF compartment have other effective osmoles).
- The major intracellular factor responsible for accumulation of water in cells is the retention of K^+ due to the presence of large macromolecular anions (organic phosphates).

Although macromolecules do not exert a large osmotic pressure (they do not represent a large *number* of particles), organic phosphates bear a large anionic net charge and as a result help retain a large number of cations (primarily K^+) to achieve electroneutrality (see Table 9-2). In addition, there are a number of organic osmoles (*see margin note*). Because particles in the ICF are relatively "fixed" in number and charge, changes in the ratio of particles to water in

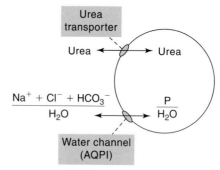

FIGURE 9-1 Factors regulating water distribution across cell membranes. The circle represents the cell membrane. Water crosses this membrane rapidly through AQP1 to achieve osmotic equilibrium. The major particles that are restricted largely to the extracellular fluid compartment are Na^+ and its attendant anions Cl^- and HCO_3^-. The major particles (P) that are restricted to the intracellular fluid compartment are predominantly K^+ and small organic compounds. Because organic phosphates and proteins are macromolecules in cells, they make only a minor direct contribution to the effective osmolality in cells. Particles such as urea cross cell membranes rapidly via urea transporters; hence, urea does *not* play a role in determining the distribution of water across cell membranes.

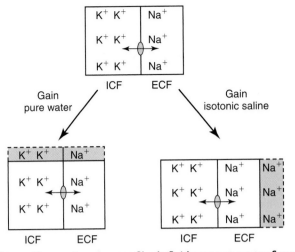

FIGURE 9-2 Changes in volumes of body fluid compartments after administering water or saline. The normal volumes of the extracellular fluid (ECF) and intracellular fluid (ICF) compartments are shown in the *top rectangle.* Water moves across cell membranes through AQP1 water channel (represented by the *oval structure*) until the tonicity is equal in both compartments. A surplus of water (*bottom left*) distributes in the ICF and ECF in proportion to their existing volumes (shown by the *horizontal green rectangle* above the normal compartment sizes); this causes hyponatremia. In contrast (*bottom right*), when there is a positive balance of isotonic saline, only the ECF volume expands (shown in the *vertical green rectangle*) and there is no change in the P_{Na} or the ICF volume in this setting.

the ICF compartment usually come about by changes in its content of water.

Particles such as urea cross cell membranes rapidly via facilitated diffusion (i.e., aided by urea transporters). Hence, the concentration of urea is equal in the ICF and the ECF compartments, and urea does *not* play a role in the distribution of water across cell membranes (i.e., urea is not an effective osmole).

Under normal conditions, it is believed that there are roughly twice as many particles in the ICF compartment as in the ECF compartment; therefore, it follows that the ICF volume is twice as large as the ECF volume (*see margin note*). The effects of administering isotonic saline or water on ECF and ICF volumes are illustrated in Figure 9-2.

Defense of cell volume

- Only brain cells maintain a near-constant volume by altering the number of their intracellular small particles.

Defense of brain cell volume is necessary because the brain is contained in a rigid box (the skull; Fig. 9-3). When brain cells swell (as occurs when the P_{Na} is low), the initial defense is to expel as much water as possible from the ventricles and out of the skull to prevent a large rise in intracranial pressure. If brain cells continue to swell, the intracranial pressure will eventually rise (see Fig. 10-2, page 319). When the intracranial pressure rises, the cerebral cortex is pushed down, which compresses veins against the bony margin of the foramen magnum, and venous outflow declines. Since the arterial pressure is high enough to permit the inflow of

ACTUAL EXTRACELLUALR FLUID AND INTRACELLULAR FLUID VOLUMES
The volume of the ICF compartment is said to be double that of the ECF compartment, but the data that support this are not robust and differ based on the method used to measure the ECF volume. It is equally possible that slightly more than half of body water (55%) is in the ICF compartment and 45% is in the ECF compartment.

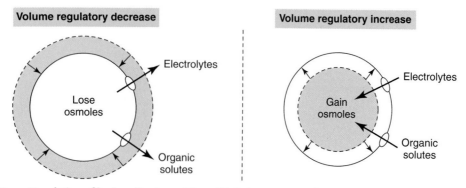

FIGURE 9-3 Regulation of brain cell volume. The *solid circle* represents the normal volume of a brain cell. In the *left portion*, brain cells have increased in size (*dashed circle*) in acute hyponatremia. To return their volume toward normal (*solid circle*), these cells export effective osmoles, K^+ with an anion (other than organic phosphate), and organic osmoles. In the *right portion*, brain cells have decreased in size (*dashed circle*) in acute hypernatremia. To return their volume toward normal (*solid circle*), these cells must import effective osmoles, $Na^+ + K^+ + Cl^-$, and some organic osmoles.

blood to continue, the intracranial pressure rises abruptly because there is a positive balance of water in the skull. This may lead to serious symptoms (seizures, coma) and herniation of the brain through the foramen magnum, causing irreversible brain damage and death.

In contrast, excessive shrinkage of brain cell volume—as occurs when the P_{Na} is high—stretches the vascular connections from the skull. This may lead to an intracranial hemorrhage (see Fig. 11-4, page 375). Because the large intracellular macromolecular anions are essential compounds for cell structure and function, defense of brain cell volume requires that small ions or nonelectrolyte osmoles be imported into shrunken brain cells to increase their size.

Regulatory decrease in brain cell volume

> • The primary mechanism to return swollen brain cells toward their original volume is to decrease their number of effective osmoles; close to half of this decrease is the result of exporting K^+.

CONCENTRATION OF Cl⁻ IN BRAIN CELLS

• Astrocytes are abundant cells in the brain. One of their major functions is to ensure a constant composition of the intracerebral ECF compartment (e.g., they keep the concentration of K^+ in the ECF of the brain from varying appreciably after neurons fire). We are not certain what the concentration of Cl⁻ is in these cells.

• Of note, the concentration of Cl⁻ in the ICF in other organs varies widely between 3 mmol/L in skeletal muscle cells to 70 mmol/L in red blood cells.

Because electroneutrality must be maintained when K^+ are exported out of cells, an anion (other than organic phosphate) must be lost as well. One of these anions could be Cl⁻, but this is not likely, however, because the concentration of Cl⁻ is low. Notwithstanding, the concentration of Cl⁻ may be higher in non-neuronal brain cells (*see margin note*). It is also unlikely that this volume defense mechanism involves the export of HCO_3^- because changes in its concentration alter the pH in cells and thereby the net charge on intracellular proteins (see Fig. 1-6, page 12).

Another mechanism to cause water to exit from cells is to have some intracellular effective ions "disappear" and thereby lower the osmolality in this compartment. This could occur if ions were to become bound and hence "osmotically inactive"; this, however, is not known to occur in brain cells. Organic solutes, if present in high enough concentrations, may be extruded from cells as part of the regulatory decrease in volume. The major organic osmoles lost from brain cells are amino acids, taurine, and myoinositol.

Regulatory increase in brain cell volume

Typically, return of shrunken cells toward their original volume begins with an influx of Na^+ and Cl^- (*see margin note*; see Fig. 9-3), which usually occurs via the furosemide-sensitive Na^+, K^+, 2 Cl^- cotransporter (NKCC-1), but it is also possible that this may be achieved by parallel flux through the Na^+/H^+ exchanger and the Cl^-/HCO_3^- anion exchanger. A change in the number of organic compounds in brain cells (e.g., amino acids, taurine, and myoinositol) seems to account for close to half of the increase in the number of effective osmoles in this adaptive process. Because it is difficult to determine all the osmoles that are responsible for the regulation of cell volume, the term *idiogenic osmoles* has been used to describe these missing osmoles (*see margin note*).

Distribution of water in the extracellular fluid compartment

- There are two subdivisions of the ECF compartment, the plasma volume and the interstitial fluid volume.
- Movement of an ultrafiltrate of plasma across capillary membranes does not cause water to shift between the ECF and ICF compartments because there is no change in the P_{Na}.
- The hydrostatic pressure and the oncotic pressure across the capillary membrane are the major forces that determine the distribution of the ECF volume between its intravascular and interstitial spaces.

The ECF compartment consists of the plasma fluid volume (~4% of body weight) and the interstitial fluid volume (i.e., fluid in tissues between the cells; ~16% of body weight; Table 9-3). In certain disease states, fluid accumulates in the interstitial space of the ECF compartment to an appreciable degree, causing peripheral edema, ascites, or pleural effusion (*see margin note*).

The factors controlling the movement of an ultrafiltrate across the capillary membrane are shown in Figure 9-4; the major outward driving force is the hydrostatic pressure difference. The hydrostatic pressure at the venous end of the capillary is higher under conditions that lead to venous hypertension (e.g., venous obstruction, congestive heart failure).

The major driving force for inward flow of fluid (from the interstitial space to the intravascular space) is the colloid osmotic pressure difference, which is largely the result of a higher $P_{Albumin}$ (40 g/L) compared with the concentration of albumin in the interstitial fluid (close to 10 g/L). The content of albumin in the interstitial space (10 g/L × 12 L), however, is virtually equal to that in the vascular volume (40 g/L × 3 L; *see margin note*).

TABLE 9-3 SUBDIVISIONS OF THE EXTRACELLULAR FLUID COMPARTMENT*

COMPARTMENT	WATER (L)	AMOUNT OF ALBUMIN
Total ECF volume	15	240 g
• Interstitial volume	12	~120 g (10 g/L × 12 L)
• Plasma volume	3	~120 g (40 g/L × 3 L)

*Values are approximation in a 70-kg nonobese male.
ECF, extracellular fluid.

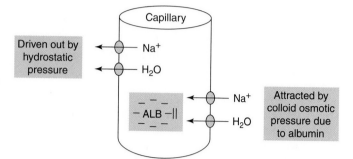

FIGURE 9-4 Factors controlling the distribution of an ultrafiltrate across the capillary membrane. There are two major forces to consider: A higher hydrostatic pressure causes fluid to leave the vascular space, and a higher colloid osmotic pressure causes fluid to enter the vascular space. ALB, albumin.

Interstitial fluid returns to the venous system via the lymphatics. Because the interstitial fluid volume is so much larger than the intravascular volume, any time expansion of the interstitial space is detected (e.g., peripheral edema), the patient always has an expanded ECF volume even if the intravascular volume is reduced (e.g., in a patient with chronic hypoalbuminemia).

Gibbs-Donnan equilibrium

The net negative valence on albumin causes ions to redistribute between the intravascular and interstitial spaces; albumin attracts cations (largely Na^+) and repels anions (largely Cl^- plus HCO_3^-) out of capillaries. In this equilibrium, the product of the concentrations of the major cations and anions in one compartment is equal to the product of their concentrations in the other compartment because these ions diffuse readily across the capillary membrane. Therefore, the intravascular space ultimately has a slightly larger total concentration of ionic species than the interstitial space. Although this difference in ion concentration is small in quantitative terms (~0.4 mmol/L), it is appreciable relative to the concentration of albumin in plasma (0.6 mmol/L; *see margin note*); hence, it makes it a significant contribution to the colloid osmotic pressure.

COLLOID OSMOTIC PRESSURE IN CAPILLARIES
The capillary colloid osmotic pressure (COP) is close to 24 mm Hg. Because the molecular weight of albumin is close to 70,000 and the $P_{Albumin}$ is 40 g/L, there is 0.6 mmol of albumin per liter of plasma. This would generate an osmotic pressure of close to 13 mm Hg. The bulk of the other 11 mm Hg of capillary COP is caused by the effect of the anionic charge on albumin, which results in a slightly higher total concentration of ionic species in the intravascular space (Gibbs-Donnan effect).

QUESTIONS

(*Discussions on pages 308 and 309*)

9-1 *Hypertonic saline is the treatment of choice to shrink brain cell size in a patient with acute hyponatremia. What is the major effect of hypertonic saline to reduce the risk of brain herniation?*

9-2 *What would happen acutely to the ICF volume if the permeability of capillary membranes to albumin were to increase?*

9-3 *What is the volume of distribution if 1 L of each of the following intravenous fluids was retained in the body: isotonic saline, half-isotonic saline, 300 mmol of NaCl/L, or 1 L of D_5W? What would the change in the P_{Na} be in a normal 50-kg subject who has 30 L of total body water before the infusion?*

PART B
PHYSIOLOGY OF SODIUM

OBJECTIVES

■ To emphasize that the content of Na^+ in the ECF compartment is regulated by modulation of the rate of the reabsorption of Na^+ by the kidneys.
■ To emphasize that the signals for regulation of the ECF volume are related to *pressure* rather than to the *volume* in large blood vessels; hence, the term *effective arterial blood volume* is used. When the effective arterial blood volume rises, the excretion of Na^+ is enhanced; this phenomenon is called a *pressure natriuresis*.

OVERVIEW

Although there is some evidence for stimulation of Na^+ intake in humans when the ECF volume is low (salt craving), this is not an important element in the control of Na^+ homeostasis. Rather, balance for Na^+ is regulated primarily by adjusting the rate of excretion of Na^+ because of signals related to the degree of expansion of the effective arterial blood volume. In more detail, the typical Western diet provides an input of close to 150 mmol of NaCl each day; hence, 150 mmol of NaCl must be excreted daily to achieve balance. For this to occur, the control system that maintains Na^+ balance must sense this extra NaCl (i.e., an expanded effective arterial blood volume) and send messages to the kidney so that this extra NaCl can be excreted (with or without water depending on the independent controls of water balance).

Work performed in the kidney

- The major renal work that requires energy expenditure is the reabsorption of filtered Na^+.
- This reabsorption of Na^+ is linked to many other functions of the kidney, depending on how this reabsorption actually occurs.

The kidneys use a large amount of fuel to provide the ATP needed to reabsorb more than 99% of the enormous filtered load of Na^+ (27,000 mmol/day). Depending on the properties of the nephron site where this reabsorption of Na^+ occurs, it could "help" the kidney reabsorb valuable compounds or ions (e.g., glucose in the proximal convoluted tubule) or secrete others (e.g., K^+ in the late cortical distal nephron). Nevertheless, filtering and reabsorbing such a large quantity of Na^+ may be thought of as a "waste of energy" at first glance. Filtering this large amount of Na^+ is dictated by the high GFR. While there are several hypotheses to explain why there is such a high GFR, the one favored by the authors is to think of the high GFR in energy or O_2 consumption terms. As discussed in Chapter 8,

ANOTHER BENEFIT FOR THE HIGH GFR
- Having a high GFR permits more fuel oxidation, as there is more work being done.
- During metabolic acidosis, the fuel consumed to provide the energy to reabsorb Na^+ is primarily glutamine. Thus, the kidneys can have a higher rate of production of NH_4^+ (and HCO_3^-; discussed in Chapter 1, page 20).

NEED FOR AN EXPANDED EFFECTIVE ARTERIAL BLOOD VOLUME WHEN THERE IS A LARGE INTAKE OF NaCl
- Control mechanisms were developed in Paleolithic times; there are no survival-related pressures in modern times that have enough control strength to negate this regulation.
- Because the diet in modern times contains more NaCl than in Paleolithic times, when little NaCl was ingested, it is "physiologically not correct" to think of our ECF volume as being "normal."
- In fact, an expanded ECF volume (actually an expanded effective arterial blood volume) is needed to provide the kidney with a message to prevent it from reabsorbing virtually all the filtered Na^+.

RETENTION OF Na^+ AND Cl^- IN TRAINED ATHLETES
- Athletes retain extra Na^+ and Cl^-. As a result, they have an expanded plasma and ECF volume as evidenced by the fact that they have a low hematocrit with a normal red blood cell mass (called sports anemia, discussed in Chapter 8, page 240).
- Although the ECF volume is expanded, the extra Na^+ and Cl^- are retained, probably because of dilatation of venous capacitance vessels, and hence the effective arterial blood volume is not expanded.
- This serves a physiologic function because the adrenergic surge during exercise causes a shift of blood from the venous capacitance vessels to the heart, which increases the cardiac output.
- It is not clear what causes dilatation of the venous capacitance vessels in this setting. Furthermore, it is not clear why this extra Na^+ load is retained even though exercise occurs during only part of the day.

page 238, having both a high rate of delivery of O_2 to the kidney (high blood flow rate per mass) and the utilization of a *constant* proportion of this O_2 (~20%) for the reabsorption of filtered Na^+, the kidneys become the ideal site for the production of erythropoietin (*see margin note*).

CONTROL SYSTEM FOR Na^+ BALANCE

"Normal" extracellular fluid volume
- Control mechanisms are set to defend the effective arterial blood volume rather than the ECF volume.
- What is considered as a "normal" effective arterial blood volume in modern times is in fact an "expanded" one compared with what this volume was in Paleolithic times (*see margin note*).
- The tone in venous capacitance vessels determines the volume of blood in the venous portion of the circulation.

What is a "normal" extracellular fluid volume?

A "normal" ECF volume may be defined based on measurements in a representative population of subjects consuming a typical Western diet in which the intake of NaCl is close to 150 mmol/day. This does not represent a "normal" value for the ECF volume; rather, it represents an expanded volume to provide a stimulus for the excretion of this large daily intake of NaCl (*see margin note*).

From a physiologic perspective, a "normal" ECF volume should be defined based on measurements in subjects with a low intake of NaCl, because this represents the conditions in Paleolithic times, when important control mechanisms developed. Hence, our Paleolithic ancestors had a "nonexpanded" ECF volume.

The most important component of the ECF compartment is the effective arterial blood volume; thus, there is a need to define this latter term. It is important to recognize that the signals for regulation of the ECF volume are related in fact to *pressure* rather than to the *volume* in large blood vessels. For example, if the tone of the venous capacitance vessels decreases, the central venous pressure and the filling pressure in the right atrium of the heart falls. This, in turn, initiates signals to retain Na^+ and Cl^- even though the ECF volume is unchanged. This may be why, for example, we excrete *so much less Na^+ and Cl^- overnight* than during the day (the rate of excretion of Na^+ and Cl^- is typically close to one third of their median 24-hour rate of excretion in young healthy subjects) despite the fact that blood has moved from the legs into the trunk when a person lies down. There is a lower adrenergic stimulation that results in decreased tone of the venous capacitance vessels while sleeping—this illustrates the dissociation between volume and pressure. In contrast, when the sympathetic tone rises during the day, these venous capacitance vessels constrict, which causes the central pressure to rise and thereby, the rate of excretion of Na^+ to increase (called a *pressure natriuresis*). Another example of this physiology is discussed in the *margin note*.

Consider two persons who consume a constant amount of NaCl; one has a disorder that results in an increased ability and the other has a disorder that causes a decreased ability to excrete Na^+

and Cl⁻. Independent of the usual control system for achieving an "ideal" ECF volume, balance for Na⁺ and Cl⁻ will be achieved in steady state, but with a different degree of expansion of the ECF volume.

1. If the disorder enhances the ability of the kidneys to reabsorb Na⁺ and Cl⁻ in the absence of a low effective arterial blood volume (e.g., chronic low intake of K⁺ (*see margin note*) or possibly a high carbohydrate intake, which causes high levels of insulin [see Chapter 16, page 565]), a significantly larger positive balance for Na⁺ and Cl⁻ will be required in steady state to provide the signal to excrete the entire daily intake of NaCl. Excessive expansion of the ECF volume may lead to edema and/or hypertension.

2. If the disorder diminishes the ability of the kidneys to reabsorb Na⁺ and Cl⁻ (e.g., the intake of a natriuretic agent such as thiazide diuretics or an inborn error such as Gitelman's syndrome; see Chapter 14, page 490 for more discussion), a much smaller positive balance for Na⁺ and Cl⁻ will be required to provide the signal to excrete the entire daily intake of NaCl. As a result, the ECF and effective arterial blood volumes will be expanded to a lesser degree in steady state and this person could be less likely to have high blood pressure.

Experimental study to illustrate the physiology of the control of Na⁺ homeostasis

A very careful investigator, R. A. McCance, reported a very interesting observation in experiments he performed on himself and his colleagues in 1936. He consumed very little salt and created a deficit of close to half of the content of NaCl in his ECF compartment by sitting in a "sweat box." Surprisingly, he did not suffer from circulatory collapse; rather, his blood pressure was somewhat low and his pulse rate was modestly elevated; in fact, he was able to continue cycling to work in this state. Hence, he had a somewhat low, but not a *very* low, effective arterial blood volume despite the large deficit of NaCl.

In contrast, McCance observed that patients with adrenal insufficiency have a much poorer hemodynamic state, even though their degree of ECF volume contraction was much less severe than his own. Perhaps these patients lack the usual constrictor tone of their venous capacitance vessels because of their very low levels of glucocorticoids, and therefore they may have a much lower effective arterial blood volume (see the discussion of Case 3-1, page 70).

Sequestration of Na⁺ in an osmotically inactive form

There are data that appear to be consistent with "osmotic inactivation" of Na⁺ (i.e., Na⁺ is held in a bound form, and it is no longer dissolved in body water). Because this process must obey the law of electroneutrality, an anion (Cl⁻ or HCO_3^-) must be removed as well. We speculate that this process is likely to represent "osmotic inactivation" of $NaHCO_3$. From a Paleolithic perspective, this process served the purpose of temporarily "hiding" the $NaHCO_3$ load that resulted from a shift of some of the K⁺ into cells in exchange of Na⁺ because K⁺ were accompanied by organic anions (HCO_3^- precursors; *see margin note*). A more detailed analysis of this topic is provided in the discussion of Questions 9-4 through 9-6 and in Chapter 13, page 436.

RETENTION OF NaCl IN K⁺-DEPLETED PATIENTS
- A low intake of K⁺ may be an important risk factor for the retention of Na⁺ and Cl⁻ and thereby the development of hypertension in certain patients.
- A supplement of KCl may have more therapeutic leverage in lowering the blood pressure than decreasing the intake of NaCl.
- Beware—the usual advice to increase the intake of K⁺ is by consuming more fruit (e.g., bananas); this may lead to a large increase in caloric intake over time and contribute to the development of obesity.

$KHCO_3$ LOAD FROM INTAKE OF FRUIT AND BERRIES
- When fruit is ingested, there is an input of K⁺ and organic anions (e.g., citrate).
- Because citrate chelates ionized calcium, it is removed on a single pass by intestinal cells and the liver—the product of citrate metabolism is HCO_3^-. Hence, K⁺ and HCO_3^- are added to the body.
- If some of this K⁺ shifts into cells in exchange for Na⁺, there is a temporary net gain of $NaHCO_3$ in the ECF compartment.

QUESTIONS

(Discussions on page 310)

9-4 *A person normally eats very little NaCl. When an extra 50 mmol of NaCl were added to the diet, this added Na$^+$ was not excreted and there was a gain of weight of 0.6 lb (0.3 kg). Does this represent osmotic inactivation of Na$^+$?*

9-5 *A patient retained ingested NaCl; the Na$^+$ entered cells while K$^+$ exited to achieve electroneutrality. The K$^+$ that shifted out of cells and the extra Cl$^-$ in the ECF compartment were excreted in the urine. Would this represent osmotic inactivation of Na$^+$?*

9-6 *When a normal volunteer increased his intake of NaCl from 200 mmol/day to 600 mmol/day for a number of days, there was a large positive balance of Na$^+$ but there was no change in weight or in the P_{Na}. Might this represent osmotic inactivation of Na$^+$?*

Sensor

- The majority of the sensors for the regulation of the effective arterial blood volume are located in the large arterial blood vessels (the carotid sinus and the aortic arch), the afferent glomerular arterioles, and the large central veins.
- These are baroreceptors or stretch receptors that recognize the pressure inside or the "filling" of these vessels.

Once the rise in the effective arterial blood volume is recognized, these sensors send messages to the kidney to promote the excretion of NaCl by decreasing their reabsorption. Because it is so important to defend the effective arterial blood volume, there are many mediators of regulation of the reabsorption of Na$^+$ that act in concert to achieve this task. The pathways to deliver the needed messages include changes in renal sympathetic stimulation and hormone levels (e.g., angiotensin II and aldosterone); these may act directly on the renal tubules, or they may act via modulation of renal hemodynamics.

Control of the excretion of Na$^+$

- The reabsorption of NaCl and water are regulated in an independent fashion.

The regulation of Na$^+$ excretion is the most important factor that maintains our effective arterial blood volume. In an adult who consumes a typical Western diet that contains 150 mmol NaCl, only 150 mmol of Na$^+$ and Cl$^-$ need to be excreted to achieve balance for these electrolytes. Thus, 99.5% of filtered Na$^+$ must be reabsorbed. In fact, filtration and reabsorption of Na$^+$ are linked so that the right amount of Na$^+$ is excreted within a relatively large range of GFR (called *glomerular tubular balance*).

Before dealing with Na$^+$ reabsorption in individual nephron segments, the overall strategy for the reabsorption of Na$^+$ will be considered. There are two elements: a driving force (a low concentration of Na$^+$ in tubular cells and a negative intracellular voltage) and a means (transporters or channels) to permit Na$^+$ to cross the luminal membrane in each nephron site.

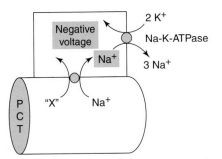

FIGURE 9-5 Overview of the mechanism of Na⁺ reabsorption in the nephron. The Na-K-ATPase causes the concentration of Na⁺ to be low inside cells; it also generates an inside-negative electrical voltage directly, because it pumps three Na⁺ out while importing two K⁺ into cells, and indirectly when K⁺ diffuse out of cells through basolateral membrane K⁺ ion channels. The mechanism for the entry of Na⁺ is different in individual nephron segments; the example shown in this figure is the cotransport of Na⁺ and other ligands indicated by *X* (e.g., glucose, amino acids, inorganic phosphate) in the proximal convoluted tubule (PCT) via a sodium-linked cotransporter.

GENERAL RULES
- The reabsorption of Na⁺ in downstream nephron sites will be upregulated when Na⁺ reabsorption is inhibited in a proximal nephron site.
- Because the mechanisms to reabsorb Na⁺ in downstream nephron sites are different, other effects may be observed. For example, if Na⁺ reabsorption is inhibited in the early distal convoluted tubule, there may be increased electrogenic reabsorption of Na⁺ in the late cortical distal nephron, which may lead to a higher rate of secretion of K⁺ in these nephron segments.

Driving force

The creation of a low concentration of Na⁺ and a negative voltage in renal tubular cells is achieved by electrogenic pumping of Na⁺ out of cells by the Na-K-ATPase in their basolateral membranes. This ion pump exports 3 Na⁺ while importing 2 K⁺; hence, it also helps create a net negative voltage inside cells (Fig. 9-5; *see margin note*).

MAGNITUDE OF THE DRIVING FORCE
The concentration difference for Na⁺ and the electrical driving force are each close to an order of magnitude. Hence this force is approximately 100-fold.

Transport mechanism

The Na-K-ATPase generates an electrochemical gradient that favors the absorption of Na⁺, but cell membranes are *not* permeable to Na⁺. Therefore, specific transporters (cotransporters or antiporters) that bind Na⁺ and another ligand or a specific Na⁺ ion channel in the luminal membrane of cells are required for the transport of Na⁺ in different nephron segments.

Tubular reabsorption of Na⁺; general principles

- The major function of the initial functional nephron unit is to reabsorb most of the filtered Na⁺ in order to deliver a small quantity of Na⁺ to downstream sites; these latter sites can adjust their reabsorption of Na⁺ to achieve daily balance for this cation in steady state.
- We shall divide the nephron into three *functional* regions, based on their permeability to water (i.e., the presence or absence of AQP).
- It is important to integrate the renal handling of ionized calcium with that of Na⁺ to gain insights into regulation of the renal reabsorption of Na⁺.

Rationale for dividing the nephron into functional units

Background. A recent important observation is that AQP1 water channels are not present in the majority of descending thin limbs of the loop of Henle. The critical implication of this finding is that, in contradiction to the traditional view, the majority of the descending

FUNCTIONAL ANALYSIS OF Na⁺ REABSORPTION
A similar approach was utilized to understand the physiology of the role of the kidney in acid-base balance. As discussed in Chapter 1, page 15, since the kidneys filter 20-fold more HCO_3^- each day than is present in the ECF compartment, the proximal nephron must reabsorb almost all of the filtered HCO_3^- before distal segments fine-tune the addition of new HCO_3^- to the body (i.e., excrete NH_4^+).

thin limbs of the loop of Henle are *impermeable* to water. This, therefore, makes the entire loop of Henle of the majorty of the nephrons impermeable to water (Fig. 9-6). Based on this observation, we define three functional units of the nephron (*see margin note*).

1. *AQP1 are constituitively present in the initial functional unit.* Hence, when Na⁺ and Cl⁻ are reabsorbed, water follows. Accordingly, the fluid reabsorbed is isotonic to plasma. The initial functional unit consists of the proximal convoluted tubule, including its pars recta.

2. *All AQP are absent in the middle functional unit.* Hence, this unit is *always* impermeable to water. Accordingly, when Na⁺ is reabsorbed, there is no reabsorption of water and therefore luminal fluid becomes hypotonic while the peritubular fluid becomes hypertonic. The middle functional unit consists of the entire loop of Henle including its cortical thick ascending limb and the early distal convoluted tubule.

3. *AQP2 can be inserted into the luminal membrane in the final functional unit, but only when there is a need to conserve water (see Fig. 9-6).* This insertion of AQP2 is under the influence of the hormone vasopressin. This final unit consists of the late portion of the distal convoluted tubule, the connecting segment, the cortical collecting duct, and the medullary collecting duct.

Importance of considering regulation of calcium reabsorption in the analysis of the control of Na⁺ reabsorption

- The control of the reabsorption of calcium is intimately linked to control of the reabsorption of Na⁺ in the initial and middle functional units of the nephron.

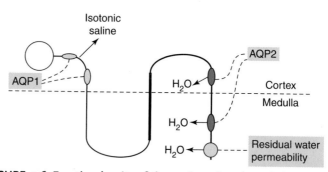

FIGURE 9-6 Functional units of the nephron based on their content of AQP1 and AQP2. The *stylized structure* represents a nephron; AQP1 is represented as an oval with *light green shading,* and AQP2 is represented as an oval with *darker green shading.* In the initial functional nephron unit with AQP1, the reabsorption of Na⁺ is accompanied by water and thus isotonic saline is reabsorbed. The middle functional nephron unit lacks AQP1 and AQP2, so in its segments where Na⁺ are reabsorbed, water is not, their luminal fluid becomes hypotonic, and the interstitial compartment becomes hypertonic. In the final functional nephron unit, AQP2 may or may not inserted. When they are present in the late cortical distal nephron, there is a rapid reabsorption of a large volume (~21 L/day) of osmole-free water in the cortex as soon as the hypotonic filtrate arrives at this site. The inner medullary collecting duct is always somewhat permeable to water, even in the absence of vasopressin actions (called *residual water permeability; see margin note*).

RESIDUAL WATER PERMEABILITY
The reabsorption of water by residual water permeability is only important during a water diuresis (i.e., when there is no AQP2 in the luminal membrane of the inner medullary collecting duct; this is discussed on page 277).

One major risk for the kidney is the formation of precipitates of calcium salts in the renal medulla (i.e., nephrocalcinosis) or in the final luminal fluid (i.e., kidney stones). Hence, it is important to integrate the renal handling of calcium in the first two functional units of the nephron to understand the physiology of the renal regulation of the reabsorption of Na^+ and water.

Initial functional unit of the nephron; the proximal convoluted tubule

- *Na^+ and water*: Since this site contains AQP1, it must reabsorb a solution that is isotonic to plasma when Na^+ and Cl^- are reabsorbed.
- *Calcium*: The guiding principle is to reabsorb as much Ca^{2+} as possible in the proximal convoluted tubule to limit its delivery to the medullary thick ascending limb of the loop of Henle.

The mechanism for the reabsorption of Na^+ in the proximal convoluted tubule is active and is driven by its basolateral Na-K-ATPase. Virtually all the valuable water-soluble compounds and some ions (e.g., glucose, amino acids, HCO_3^-) that are filtered have transport systems that are linked directly to the reabsorption of Na^+.

Quantitative analysis. When considering Na^+ reabsorption in the proximal convoluted tubule, it is important to reexamine the experimental data used to infer how much Na^+ is reabsorbed in this location. These data were derived from experiments in the *fed* rat using the micropuncture technique, in which a thin, sharp micropipette is inserted under direct vision into the proximal convoluted tubule. Of note, the experimenter is obligated to insert the pipette into the last accessible portion of the proximal convoluted tubule that is at the *surface* of the kidney. The data obtained by this technique suggested that two thirds of the water is reabsorbed at this site, as reflected by the $(TF/P)_{Inulin}$ (*see margin note*). Of great importance, this site is *not* the end of the proximal convoluted tubule. Hence, the traditional estimates of the amount of Na^+ and Cl^- and the volume of filtrate reabsorbed in the proximal convoluted tubule, which uses data gathered from this site, are in fact too low. In support of this view, the descending thin limbs of the loop of Henle in superficial nephrons lack AQP1, and they are very likely to be impermeable to water. Since all subsequent nephron sites in these nephrons prior to the early distal convoluted tubule are impermeable to water, the $(TF/P)_{Inulin}$ in this latter nephron site actually provides the best information to deduce the volume of filtrate delivered to the loop of Henle. The lowest $(TF/P)_{Inulin}$ at this site is about 6, which suggests that close to five sixths of the filtrate was reabsorbed prior to the loop of Henle. This is the basis for our reinterpretation of the data concerning the volume of filtrate and the amount of Na^+ and Cl^- reabsorbed in the proximal convoluted tubule in the fed rat is more likely to be about 80% rather than about 67% (*see margin notes*).

Reabsorption of calcium in the proximal convoluted tubule

- The mechanism for the reabsorption of Ca^{2+} in the proximal convoluted tubule is passive.

When isotonic saline is reabsorbed in this nephron segment, the concentration of Ca^{2+} in the luminal fluid rises. Hence, calcium

$(TF/P)_{Inulin}$
- Inulin is freely filtered and not reabsorbed or secreted by the tubules.
- The $(TF/P)_{Inulin}$ is the ratio of the concentrations of inulin in tubular fluid (TF) to that in plasma (P). Thus, this ratio reveals the volume of filtrate that was reabsorbed between the glomerulus and the site of micropuncture.

DATA IN HUMANS
- The reabsorption of lithium probably reflects the reabsorption of Na^+ in the PCT.
- In quantitative terms, 80% of filtered lithium is reabsorbed in humans, which supports the speculation that 80% of filtered Na^+ is reabsorbed in the PCT.

CAVEAT IN EXTRAPOLATING DATA FROM THE FED RAT TO HUMANS
- One must appreciate that fed rats consume four times more NaCl and 10-fold more K^+ per kg body weight than do humans.
- Hence, fed rats should have an expanded effective arterial blood volume and, accordingly, reabsorb a smaller proportion of Na^+ and Cl^- in their proximal convoluted tubules.

TABLE 9-4 **REVISED ESTIMATES OF VOLUME OF FILTRATE AND AMOUNT OF Na⁺ REABSORBED IN THE PROXIMAL CONVOLUTED TUBULE**

The traditional interpretation is based on the assumption that the last part of the proximal convoluted tubule that is accessible to micropuncture is the end of this nephron segment. Our reinterpretation is based on the fact that there is an additional portion of the proximal nephron prior to the delivery of fluid to the loop of Henle, and the majority of the thin descending limbs of the loop of Henle are impermeable to water. Hence the $(TF/P)_{Inulin}$ in early distal tubule reflects the volume of filtrate reabsorbed in the entire proximal convoluted tubule.

	TRADITIONAL VIEW	REVISED ESTIMATES
GFR (L/day)	180	180
Filtered Na⁺ (mmol/day)	27,000	27,000
Proximal convoluted tubule reabsorption		
Water (L/day)	120	150
Na⁺ (mmol/day)	18,000	22,500
Exit from the proximal convoluted tubule		
Water	60	30
Na⁺	9000	4500

can diffuse between cells into the interstitial compartment down its concentration difference. Therefore, since a much larger volume of filtrate is reabsorbed in the proximal convoluted tubule than previously thought, more ionized calcium is reabsorbed here and thus less is delivered to the loop of Henle (Table 9-4).

Process

- Na⁺ is reabsorbed in the proximal convoluted tubule using different types of processes.
- A Na⁺/H⁺ exchanger is the primary mechanism to reabsorb Na⁺ and HCO₃⁻.
- Na⁺ reabsorption also occurs via Na⁺-linked ligand transporters (e.g., for glucose, amino acids, phosphate).
- The reabsorption of Na⁺ and Cl⁻ in this nephron segment is carried out largely by passive mechanisms using the chemical driving force for Cl⁻.

An electrochemical gradient for Na⁺ provides the driving force for the reabsorption of Na⁺ with glucose or other filtered solutes (e.g., amino acids, phosphate, and organic anions; i.e., these are Na⁺-dependent transporters). The reabsorption of filtered glucose is considered in more detail in Chapter 16, page 551. In contrast, Na⁺ can be reabsorbed in exchange for H⁺ in cells of the proximal convoluted tubule via the Na⁺/H⁺ exchanger (NHE-3; discussed in Chapter 1, page 16). The reabsorption of Na⁺ and HCO₃⁻ in the early proximal tubule results in the transport of water and thereby causes a rise in the concentration of Cl⁻ in the remaining tubular fluid. This Cl⁻ concentration difference is sufficient to drive a considerable amount of passive proximal Cl⁻ reabsorption, probably via the paracellular pathway.

OTHER MECHANISMS FOR Cl⁻ REABSORPTION
Cl⁻ reabsorption may occur via an anion exchanger in the luminal membrane, which exchanges luminal Cl⁻ for anions in cells such as formate. In addition, a Na⁺-linked formate cotransporter is needed to recycle formate back into the cell.

QUESTION

(*Discussion on page 311*)

9-7 *What might the significance be of having the reabsorption of NaHCO₃ as the first form of Na⁺ reabsorption in the proximal convoluted tubule?*

Effect of hormones. A low effective arterial blood volume results in increased proximal reabsorption of filtered Na⁺. A fall in the renal perfusion pressure and a rise in the levels of β_1-adrenergic agonists cause the release of renin from cells of the juxtaglomerular apparatus. This in turn increases the production of angiotensin II, which stimulates the reabsorption of $NaHCO_3$ in the proximal convoluted tubule (the effects of this hormone are discussed in Chapter 7, page 202, in the context of metabolic alkalosis, and in Chapter 13, page 441, in the context of renal K⁺ excretion; *see margin note*).

Angiotensin II is also a potent vasoconstrictor, especially of renal efferent arterioles (and to a lesser degree, the afferent arterioles). Efferent arteriolar constriction increases the GFR and thereby the filtration fraction (see Part D, Chapter 8, page 237 for more discussion of this issue as it relates to control of the release of erythropoietin) and hence the peritubular capillary oncotic pressure. The latter promotes the uptake of fluid into capillaries, and as a result, an increase in the net proximal reabsorption of Na⁺, Cl⁻, and water.

Inhibitors. Dopamine (derived from the circulation or formed locally) inhibits the reabsorption of Na⁺, Cl⁻, and water in the proximal convoluted tubule (*see margin note*). The only important pharmacologic diuretic that acts on the proximal convoluted tubule is acetazolamide, which inhibits carbonic anhydrase IV, and hence diminishes the reabsorption of $NaHCO_3$ and thus NaCl.

Disorders involving the proximal convoluted tubule. The presence of excessive excretion of glucose, phosphate, organic anions, HCO_3^-, and/or urate (i.e., in the presence of low values for their concentrations in plasma) indicates a defect in proximal convoluted tubule function (*see margin note*). These defects may occur in isolation or as part of generalized proximal tubular dysfunction (Fanconi syndrome). The clinical diagnosis of proximal renal tubular acidosis can be confirmed by detecting a high fractional excretion of HCO_3^- during $NaHCO_3$ loading and the presence of a high rate of excretion of citrate in the presence of metabolic acidosis (see Chapter 4, page 88 for more discussion).

Middle functional unit of the nephron. Much of this functional unit exists in the renal medulla, and the remainder is in the cortex. All segments of this unit are impermeable to water (*see margin note*); hence, absorbed Na⁺ are added to the interstitial compartment without water, which makes the luminal fluid hypotonic. In this section, the major events in each of the components of this functional unit will be described for segments in the renal medulla and segments in the renal cortex.

Nephron segments in the renal medulla

Events in the descending thin limb of the loop of Henle

- The handling of Na⁺ and water in this nephron segment differs markedly depending on whether one incorporates an important new finding concerning the lack of AQP1 in the majority of descending thin limbs of the loop of Henle.

In the traditional view of the physiology of this nephron segment, it has AQP1 and is hence *permeable* to water. This means that when the interstitial osmolality doubles, for example, half of the volume of water reaching the descending thin limb is reabsorbed in this

CONTROL OF Na⁺ REABSORPTION IN THE PCT
- Precise control of the excretion of Na⁺ *cannot* be exerted in the proximal convoluted tubule because 27,000 mmol of Na⁺ are filtered and ~22,500 mmol are reabsorbed in this location. Hence, it is extremely unlikely that the PCT could adjust its reabsorption by ± 100 mmol/day.
- This does not mean that there is no regulation of Na⁺ reabsorption in the PCT but rather that it is not the primary mechanism to adjust the quantity of Na⁺ excreted in absolute terms.

MECHANISMS OF ACTION OF DOPAMINE IN THE PROXIMAL CONVOLUTED TUBULE
- Dopamine increases cyclic AMP, which decreases the activity of the NHE in the luminal membrane.
- Dopamine also inhibits the Na-K-ATPase pump in the basolateral membrane.

CLINICAL RELEVANCE
More calcium is reabsorbed in the proximal convoluted tubule and thereby the delivery of calcium to downstream nephron sites falls when the effective arterial blood volume declines; this may be why thiazide diuretics are useful to prevent the recurrence of calcium stones in patients with idiopathic hypercalciuria.

MINOR EXCEPTION
The descending thin limbs of loops of Henle of juxtamedullary nephrons enter the inner medulla. They account for 15% of the total nephrons, and all of them have AQP1 in their luminal membranes.

TABLE 9-5 **CHANGES IN COMPOSITION IN LUMINAL FLUID TRAVERSING THE LOOP OF HENLE**

Our reinterpretation is based on the following fact. If both the descending thin limb of the loop of Henle of superficial nephrons and their mTAL are impermeable to water, then micropuncture data obtained from early distal convoluted tubules reveal the volume of filtrate delivered to their loops of Henle. In addition, since the nephrons that enter the inner medulla are permeable to water, as they have AQP1 throughout their descending thin limbs, 3 L of water are reabsorbed from these nephrons in the outer medulla.

	TRADITIONAL VIEW	REVISED ESTIMATES
Fluid entering the loop of Henle from the proximal convoluted tubule		
Water (L/day)	60	30
Na$^+$ (mmol/day)	9000	4500
Changes in composition at the end of the descending thin limb		
Water (reabsorbed L/day)	40	3
Na$^+$ (added mmol/day)	0	~1600
Reabsorption in the medullary thick ascending limb		
Water (L/day)	0	0
Na$^+$ (mmol/day)	6000	~2500

location. On the other hand, if there truly are no AQP1 in the majority of descending thin limbs, this implies that there is little, if any, water reabsorbed in this nephron segment. The quantitative implications of these two views are provided in Table 9-5.

Necessity for a high Na$^+$ and Cl$^-$ concentration in the luminal fluid at the bend of the loop of Henle. Although the following will be discussed in more detail subsequently in Part D, page 295, it is mentioned briefly here to provide the rationale to understand why the concentration of Na$^+$ must rise in the luminal fluid in the descending thin limb of the loop of Henle. The reabsorption of Na$^+$ in the medullary thick ascending limb of the loop of Henle occurs by two different routes—each of which reabsorbs 50% of Na$^+$, and both are dependent on the entry of K$^+$ via luminal membrane K$^+$ channels. This entry of K$^+$ adds a necessary substrate for the first route, the Na$^+$, K$^+$, 2 Cl$^-$ cotransporter-2 (NKCC-2) in the luminal membrane. In addition, K$^+$ entry creates a lumen-positive voltage to drive the second half of Na$^+$ reabsorption via the paracellular pathway, which is permeable to Na$^+$.

Since 1 K$^+$ must enter the lumen of the medullary thick ascending limb of the loop of Henle to drive 1 Na$^+$ out by the passive pathway, it follows that there must *not* be a concentration difference for Na$^+$ or a voltage difference between the luminal and interstitial compartments at the bend of the loop of Henle to ensure that there is no movement of Na$^+$ into or out of the luminal fluid in the medullary thick ascending limb of the loop of Henle other than that due to changes in voltage caused by the movement of K$^+$ through the luminal membrane via these K$^+$ channels.

The rise in the concentration of Na$^+$ in the lumen of the descending thin limb of the loop of Henle could occur if water were to exit (requires the presence of AQP1) or if Na$^+$ (via Na$^+$ channels) and Cl$^-$ (via Cl$^-$ channels) were to enter. In the absence of AQP1 (see Fig. 9-6), it is unlikely that the majority of the descending thin limbs of the loop of Henle will have sufficient water permeability to have the former option for raising the luminal Na$^+$ concentration. Accordingly, it is more likely that entry of Na$^+$ and Cl$^-$ is responsible for the bulk of this rise in the luminal Na$^+$ and Cl$^-$ concentrations.

Na⁺ reabsorption in the medullary thick ascending limbs of the loop of Henle

> - Water reabsorption from the medullary collecting duct and from the descending thin limbs of the loop of Henle of juxtamedullary nephrons provides the signal to stimulate the reabsorption of Na^+ and Cl^- without water in the medullary thick ascending limb of the loop of Henle, which maintains a high osmolality in the medullary interstitial compartment.
> - Regulation is likely to be by dilution of an inhibitor (e.g., ionized calcium) in the medullary interstitial compartment, which causes ROMK to be open. This provides the impetus for the transcellular and the paracellular reabsorption of Na^+ in this nephron segment (*see margin note*).

There are five important facts to bear in mind to understand how much Na^+ is reabsorbed in the loop of Henle. First, the delivery of fluid to the loop of Henle is close to one sixth of its filtered load ($\frac{1}{6} \times 180$ L/day = 30 L/day). Second, because the concentration of Na^+ in the fluid delivered to the loop of Henle is similar to the arterial P_{Na}, approximately 4500 mmol of Na^+ are delivered to the loop of Henle each day (150 mmol/L × 30 L/day). Third, because the thin descending limbs of the loop of Henle of superficial nephrons in humans (~85% of nephrons) *lack AQP1* water channels, this suggests that water is *not* reabsorbed in these structures. Fourth, the concentration of Na^+ in the lumen of the descending thin limbs of the loop of Henle must rise as they descend deeper into the renal medulla; therefore, a considerable quantity of Na^+ must *diffuse into* their lumen (this nephron segment is permeable to Na^+ and Cl^- as a result of the presence of ion channels; Fig. 9-7). Fifth, the concentration of Na^+ in fluid exiting the medulla in the medullary thick ascending limb of the loop of Henle is distinctly hypotonic and the volume is close to 27 L/day (*see margin note*) because this is a water-impermeable nephron site (see Fig. 9-6). The following description of Na^+ reabsorption reflects this new interpretation.

There are two functions of Na^+ and Cl^- reabsorption into the medullary thick ascending limbs of the loop of Henle.

1. *Replace Na^+ that entered the descending thin limbs of the loop of Henle of superficial nephrons from the medullary interstitial compartment.* This represents close to 60% of the Na^+ reabsorbed in this nephron segment. In overall terms, this component of Na^+ reabsorption simply restores the interstitial concentration of Na^+ to its original hypertonic value. While a considerable quantity of Na^+ was reabsorbed, there was no net reabsorption of filtered Na^+ (i.e., this is merely recycling of Na^+).

2. *Na^+ that are added into the medullary interstitial compartment in response to water reabsorption from water-permeable nephron segments.* This represents close to 40% of the Na^+ that is reabsorbed in the medullary thick ascending limbs of the loop of Henle (*see margin note*; see Part D, page 304 for a quantitative analysis). It is this component of Na^+ reabsorption that maintains the high interstitial Na^+ and Cl^- concentrations so that water can be reabsorbed from these water-permeable nephron sites. Since every liter of this water must exit the renal medulla in the ascending vasa recta, it must have the same $Na^+:H_2O$ ratio as in plasma in the descending vasa recta

ABBREVIATION
ROMK, rat outer medullary K^+ channel

SPECULATION
- It is possible that the primary regulation is to prevent a rise in the ionized calcium concentration in the medullary interstitial compartment.
- This form of regulation will also result in a high interstitial osmolality (see Part D, page 295 for more discussion of this topic).

ESTIMATE OF THE VOLUME OF FILTRATE DELIVERED TO THE LOOP OF HENLE
- Five sixths of the GFR is reabsorbed in the PCT (150 of the filtered 180 L/day). Hence 30 L/day are delivered to the loop of Henle.
- The juxtamedullary nephrons (15% of the total number) enter the inner medulla. Since they have AQP1, their luminal Na^+ concentration rises by water abstraction (4.5 L/day enter from the PCT, and 3 L/day are reabsorbed in the descending thin limbs; see page 306 for a more detailed calculation).
- Hence, 27 L/day (30 L/day – 3 L/day) enter the bends of the loop of Henle.

ESTIMATE OF THE FALL IN THE [Na⁺] IN THE LUMEN OF THE mTAL
- Only the reabsorption of Na^+ that is needed to abstract water (4 L/day from the medullary collecting duct and 3 L/day from the descending thin limbs of the loop of Henle of juxtamedullary nephrons [those with AQP1]) in the outer medulla leads to a fall of the luminal [Na^+] into the hypotonic range.
- Since 8.5 L/day must exit the medulla via the vasa recta with a [Na^+] of 150 mmol/L, there is a need to reabsorb 1275 mmol of Na^+ (8.5 L/day × 150 mmol/L).
- The amount of Na^+ remaining is 3225 mmol (4500 mmol – 1275 mmol) in 27 L (i.e., the concentration of Na^+ is ~120 mmol/L).

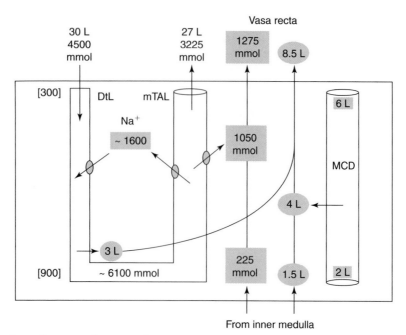

FIGURE 9-7 Balance for Na⁺ and water in the renal outer medulla. The *large rectangle* represents the renal outer medulla, and it contains the loop of Henle with its descending thin limb (DtL) and the medullary thick ascending limb (mTAL) and the medullary collecting duct (MCD). For simplicity, those DtL that enter the inner medulla are not shown. The addition of water to the outer medullary interstitial compartment is shown in the *green shaded ovals* whereas the Na⁺ added to the interstitial compartment is shown in the *green shaded rectangle*. The 3 L of water reabsorbed in the DtL are from the juxtamedullary nephrons. There is also water and Na⁺ added from the inner medulla. All of this added water and Na⁺ exit the medulla as isotonic saline via the ascending vasa recta. Na⁺ balance has two components. First, about 1600 mmol of Na⁺ diffuses into the DtL of superficial nephrons (~85% of all nephrons) each day. Therefore, these Na⁺ are replaced when Na⁺ is reabsorbed in the mTAL. Second, 1050 mmol of Na⁺ are reabsorbed from the mTAL to accompany the 8.5 L of water reabsorbed from the water-permeable MCD and DtL of juxtaglomerular nephrons with a concentration of Na⁺ that is 150 mmol/L. Hypotonic fluid exits via the mTAL (the concentration of Na⁺ is ~120 mmol/L).

(~150 mmol/kg H_2O). It is only this component of Na⁺ reabsorption that reclaims filtered Na⁺.

Process. In response to a low concentration of Na⁺ in cells of the mTAL because of the action of Na-K-ATPase at the basolateral membrane, Na⁺ enters these cells passively from the lumen on the electroneutral NKCC-2. This transporter is limited by the quantity of K⁺ in the lumen of this nephron segment. Hence, K⁺ must enter the lumen via an ROMK channel. This entry of K⁺ into the lumen generates a lumen-positive voltage (Fig. 9-8), which drives the electrogenic reabsorption of the second half of the quantity of Na⁺ reabsorbed, as well as the reabsorption of calcium and magnesium ions through the paracellular pathway.

Control

- Because regulation is most likely to be by inhibitory controls, this process is not likely to be regulated by activators of NKCC-2 or the quantity of NKCC-2 in the luminal membrane.

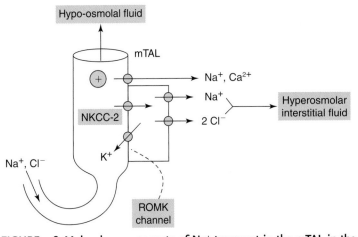

FIGURE 9-8 Molecular components of Na⁺ transport in the mTAL in the loop of Henle. The medullary thick ascending limb of the loop of Henle (mTAL) is not permeable to water. The major form of ion entry into cells of the mTAL of the loop of Henle is via the reabsorption of 1 Na⁺, 1 K⁺, and 2 Cl⁻ on the Na⁺, K⁺, 2 Cl⁻ cotransporter (NKCC-2) in their luminal membrane. K⁺ must enter the lumen via ROMK to supply the needed K⁺ for the continued operation of this transporter. This also generates a positive voltage in the lumen that "pushes" Na⁺ (and Ca²⁺ + Mg²⁺, which, for simplicity, are not shown) between cells of the mTAL of the loop of Henle; this accounts for the other half of the of Na⁺ reabsorbed in this nephron segment. The driving force for NKCC-2 is the low concentration of Na⁺ in mTAL cells, which is the result of active export of Na⁺ by the Na-K-ATPase in its basolateral membranes. Cl⁻ exit the cell via Cl⁻ channels in the basolateral membrane.

The signal to increase the reabsorption of Na⁺ in the medullary thick ascending limb of the loop of Henle is likely to be mediated by a fall in the concentration of an inhibitor in the medullary interstitial compartment. This fall in concentration of the inhibitor may begin with the addition of water that is reabsorbed from the water-permeable nephron segments that traverse the medullary interstitial compartment. One possible candidate that has ideal properties for this function is the activity of ionized calcium in the medullary interstitial compartment. In more detail, when this concentration rises, it binds to the calcium-sensing receptor at the basolateral membrane of cells of the medullary thick ascending limb of the loop of Henle, which generates a signal that leads to inhibition of ROMK (*see margin note*). This latter step supplies the K⁺ for NKCC-2 and generates the positive luminal voltage for the passive reabsorption of the other half of the Na⁺ (Fig. 9-9; see page 281, where the process of concentrating the urine is discussed).

Role of hormones. Several compounds can increase the number of NKCC-2 in the luminal membrane of cells of the medullary thick limb of the loop of Henle (e.g., WNK kinase 3, vasopressin, and possibly other hormones in some species). These likely act to facilitate faster rates of transport once the interstitial concentration of the inhibitor of ROMK in the luminal membrane has decreased.

Inhibitors. Loop diuretics (furosemide, bumetanide, ethacrynic acid) inhibit the reabsorption of Na⁺ and Cl⁻ in the thick ascending limb of the loop of Henle by competing with luminal Cl⁻ for binding to NKCC-2.

ROMK AND THE REABSORPTION OF Na⁺ IN THE MEDULLARY THICK ASCENDING LIMB OF LOOP OF HENLE
- Active reabsorption of Na⁺ on NKCC-2 requires a luminal source of K⁺, which is supplied via ROMK in the luminal membrane.
- Paracellular reabsorption of Na⁺ requires a positive lumen voltage, which is also dependent on K⁺ entry via ROMK.

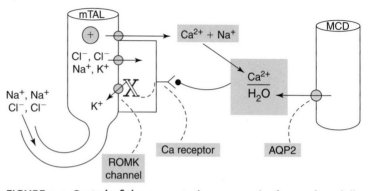

FIGURE 9-9 Control of the concentrating process in the renal medulla by interstitial ionized calcium. To reabsorb Na^+ and Cl^- in the medullary thick ascending limb (mTAL) of the loop of Henle, K^+ must be secreted via ROMK. This raises the lumen-positive voltage to drive the reabsorption of more Na^+ and also Ca^{2+} in the mTAL of the loop of Henle. Once the activity of Ca^{2+} rises sufficiently in the medullary interstitial compartment, a signal is generated to inhibit flux of K^+ through luminal ROMK and hence further reabsorption of $Na^+ + Cl^-$ in the mTAL of the loop of Henle. When more water is reabsorbed from the medullary collecting duct (MCD), the concentration of ionized Ca^{2+} in the medullary interstitium falls, allowing more Na^+ and Cl^- (and also Ca^{2+}) to be reabsorbed in this nephron segment, reestablishing this inhibitory control. DtL, descending thin limb (of the loop of Henle).

BARTTER'S SYNDROME
This inherited disorder results from mutations in one of the genes encoding for one of the transporters or channels involved in the process of Na^+ reabsorption in the thick ascending limb of the loop of Henle.

Disorders involving this nephron segment. Inhibition of NaCl reabsorption in the thick ascending limb of the loop of Henle leads to a clinical picture resembling Bartter's syndrome (*see margin note*) with wasting of Na^+, K^+, and Cl^-; a contracted effective arterial blood volume; hypokalemia; metabolic alkalosis; a renal concentrating defect; hypercalciuria; and less commonly, renal magnesium wasting (for more discussion, see Chapter 14, page 486).

Nephron segments in the cortex. There are two nephron segments in this portion of the middle functional unit of the nephron: the cortical thick ascending limb of the loop of Henle and the early distal convoluted tubule.

*Na^+ reabsorption in the cortical thick ascending limb
of the loop of Henle*

- This nephron segment has the same major transporters for Na^+ and Cl^- as the medullary thick ascending limb of the loop of Henle (luminal NKCC-2 and ROMK; basolateral Na-K-ATPase, Cl^- channels, K^+ channel; Na^+ and Ca^{2+} permeability between cells).
- The function of this nephron segment is to reabsorb a large proportion of the Na^+ that is delivered from the medullary thick ascending limb of the loop of Henle. Therefore, there is a major difference in regulation of Na^+ reabsorption, as the interstitial ionized calcium concentration is always close to its concentration in plasma owing to the very high blood flow rate.

Process. This nephron segment needs a larger lumen-positive voltage to reabsorb a bigger proportion of the Na^+ that is delivered

TABLE 9-6 **REABSORPTION OF Na$^+$ IN THE CORTICAL DISTAL NEPHRON SEGMENTS**

The volume of and the Na$^+$ concentration in the fluid that exits the medullary thick ascending limb of the loop of Henle were defined earlier. The early cortical distal nephron is always impermeable to water. The volume of water and the quantity of Na$^+$ reabsorbed are estimates. At the bottom of this table, we added data for the first portion of the third functional nephron unit, which is permeable to water when vasopressin acts, to illustrate that the net fluid reabsorbed is somewhat hypotonic saline (i.e., 3225 mmol Na$^+$ in the cortical distal nephron segments divided by 21 L is ~143 mmol/L).

NEPHRON SEGMENTS	Na$^+$			Na$^+$ (mmol/L)	
	ENTER	REABSORBED	EXIT	ENTER	EXIT
Medullary thick ascending limb of the loop of Henle					
Na$^+$ (mmol/L)	4500	1275	3225	150	120
Water (L/day)	30	3	27		
Cortical distal nephron				~120	~37.5
Na$^+$ (mmol/L)	~3225	~3000	~225		
Water (L/day)	27	21	6		

from the medullary thick ascending limb of the loop of Henle and have such a low concentration of Na$^+$ in the luminal fluid at its end (i.e., final concentration of Na$^+$ in the lumen is three- to fourfold lower than in the interstitial compartment; Table 9-6). This higher lumen-positive voltage will, however, cause the reabsorption of a large amount of ionized calcium. Notwithstanding, since the cortical plasma flow rate is large (~900 L/day) this will cause only a tiny rise in the interstitial concentration of calcium.

Control. The major difference between the cortical and medullary thick ascending limbs is the relative lack of an inhibitory effect of the activity of interstitial ionized calcium on the reabsorption of Na$^+$ and Cl$^-$ because of the enormous renal blood flow rate in the cortex. Accordingly, the limit for the reabsorption of Na$^+$ and Cl$^-$ in this nephron segment could be set either by the maximum lumen-positive voltage or by the affinity of its NKCC-2 for the concentration of Cl$^-$ in the lumen (K$_m$ ~40 mmol/L). Hence, there is a large quantity of Na$^+$ and Cl$^-$ reabsorbed each day in this nephron segment.

Na$^+$ and Cl$^-$ reabsorption in the early distal convoluted tubule

- The major property of this nephron segment is that Na$^+$ and Cl$^-$ are reabsorbed in an electroneutral fashion (i.e., via a Na$^+$ and Cl$^-$ cotransporter [NCC]).
- Regulation of Na$^+$ and Cl$^-$ reabsorption in this nephron segment must allow for a large enough delivery of Na$^+$ and Cl$^-$ (~400 mmol/day) to the late cortical distal nephron to permit the secretion of sufficient K$^+$ to excrete the large K$^+$ load of Paleolithic times.
- The major regulation of NCC is via aldosterone released in response to the current effective arterial blood volume.

Because this nephron segment has low luminal concentrations of Na$^+$ and Cl$^-$, only a small quantity of Na$^+$ and Cl$^-$ can be reabsorbed; the reabsorption of these ions must stop when their concentrations are equal in the lumen and in their cells. Since the intracellular concentration of Na$^+$ is 15 to 20 mmol/L, enough Na$^+$ (27 L/day × 15 to 20 mmol/L) will remain in the lumen to be delivered

RENAL CORTICAL PLASMA FLOW RATE
The renal plasma flow rate is close to 900L/day (i.e., GFR of 180 L/day × 5, as one fifth of the renal plasma flow is filtered [that is, the filtration fraction is ~20%]).

to the late cortical distal nephron, which is advantageous to permit maximal rates of K^+ excretion (~400 mmol/day) when needed.

Process. Because of the action of Na-K-ATPase in the basolateral membrane, the concentration of Na^+ in cells of the distal convoluted tubule is 15 to 20 mmol/L; hence, there is a chemical driving force for the entry of Na^+ and Cl^- into these cells, which is mediated by an electroneutral NCC. The intracellular concentration of Na^+ sets the lower limit for the Na^+ concentration in the lumen of the distal convoluted tubule.

Role of hormones. Aldosterone causes an increase in the number of NCC units in the luminal membranes of the distal convoluted tubule cells and the abundance of the Na-K-ATPase in their basolateral membranes.

Regulation

Function. The reabsorption of Na^+ and Cl^- is increased when there is a larger delivery of these electrolytes. Nevertheless, there must be a limit to this reabsorption so that enough Na^+ and Cl^- can be delivered distally to promote the excretion of K^+.

Control. The reabsorption of Na^+ and Cl^- is increased when the effective arterial blood volume is decreased. The mechanism begins with the release of aldosterone, which increases the activity of the Na-K-ATPase and thereby causes a fall in the intracellular Na^+ concentration, and hence this enhances the reabsorption of Na^+ via NCC. There is also an important control system to adjust the number of NCC units in the luminal membranes of the distal convoluted tubule. Actions of the WNK kinase system are critical for this form of regulation (*see margin note*).

Inhibitors. Thiazide diuretics inhibit NCC by competing with Cl^- for its binding site on NCC. Hence, the natriuretic effect of these diuretics is diminished when the effective arterial blood volume is low, as there is more avid reabsorption of Na^+ and Cl^- in upstream nephron sites. The reabsorption of Na^+ and Cl^- in this nephron segment helps desalinate the luminal fluid, and this may contribute to the development of hyponatremia in certain patients taking this class of drugs (see Chapter 10, page 357 for more discussion of this topic).

Disorders involving NCC. There is a decreased activity of this cotransporter in patients with Gitelman's syndrome (see Chapter 14, page 490) and an increase in its activity in patients with Gordon's syndrome (see Chapter 15, page 526).

Synopsis of the reabsorption of Na+ in the middle functional nephron unit

The three major features that regulate Na^+ reabsorption in these nephron segments are summarized below.

1. This is an important site to reabsorb a large proportion of the filtered load of Na^+ that escaped reabsorption in the proximal convoluted tubule.
2. During a water diuresis, there must be a stimulus for reabsorption of Na^+ and Cl^- to ensure that water can be excreted with as little Na^+ as possible (see page 276 for a more detailed discussion of water diuresis).
3. The last segment, the early distal convoluted tubule, must have a limit to its reabsorption of Na^+ and Cl^- so that enough Na^+ can be delivered to the late cortical distal nephron, which permits it to secrete a large load of K^+.

Na⁺ handling in the final functional unit of the nephron

- This functional unit is permeable to water when vasopressin causes the insertion of AQP2 into luminal membranes of its principal cells. This results in the addition of a large volume of water into the interstitial compartment of the renal cortex.
- The nephron segments of this functional unit do some of the fine-tuning so that the balance for Na⁺ can be achieved.
- A major function for Na⁺ reabsorption in the cortical portion of this unit is to permit an increase in the excretion of K⁺.

The nephron segments that make up this functional unit are the late distal convoluted tubule, the connecting tubule, the cortical collecting duct, and the medullary collecting duct. Earlier nephron segments reabsorb the vast majority of filtered Na⁺ and Cl⁻ so that fine-tuning of the excretion of these ions can be achieved in these nephron segments. Urea is an important constituent of the luminal fluid; it aids the secretion of K⁺ when Na⁺ is reabsorbed (*see margin note*). The quantitative issues are illustrated in Table 9-6.

We begin with a summary figure to illustrate how the luminal fluid composition will change as soon as hypotonic fluid is delivered to the third functional nephron unit (Fig. 9-10).

UREA AND THE EXCRETION OF K⁺
- The concentration of urea rises from 50 mmol/L to greater than 200 mmol/L secondary to the reabsorption of water in the CCD.
- Because urea is not reabsorbed in the cortical distal nephron, it is an effective osmole, which ensures that a larger volume of water remains in the lumen of these cortical nephron segments. This permits the excretion of a large amount of K⁺ without requiring a very large lumen-negative voltage in these nephron sites.

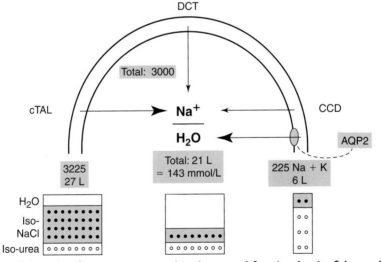

FIGURE 9-10 Fate of electrolyte-free water generated in the second functional unit of the nephron. In the *top portion of the figure*, the major point is that electrolyte-free water was generated in the cortical thick ascending limb of the loop of Henle (cTAL) and the early distal convoluted tubule (DCT). If vasopressin acts and AQP2 are inserted in the luminal membrane of the late cortical distal nephron (CCD), there will be a rapid reabsorption of about 21 L of electrolyte-free water, which must not cause hemolysis. In the *bottom portion of the figure*, the composition of the luminal fluid in each region is illustrated (i.e., the cTAL in the *far left*, the end of the early DCT in the *middle*, and the CCD after water was reabsorbed in the *far right*). The width of the rectangles represents the volume of fluid. To illustrate the difference in the composition of luminal fluid between these segments, we have divided the rectangles into an imaginary volume of isotonic saline (*middle green shaded portion with solid dots representing Na⁺*), electrolyte- and urea-free water (*clear region*), and an isotonic solution of urea (*bottom clear area with open dots representing urea*). After the reabsorption of the osmole-free water in the late cortical distal nephron, the fluid reaching the terminal CCD has an osmolality equal to plasma, but urea is the major effective osmole.

ALDOSTERONE PARADOX
- On the one hand, aldosterone acts as a NaCl-retaining hormone in response to a low effective arterial blood volume. In this setting, the release of aldosterone is stimulated by high levels of angiotensin II. On the other hand, aldosterone acts as a kaliuretic hormone in response to a large K$^+$ load. In this setting, the release of aldosterone is stimulated by a high P$_K$.
- One possible mechanism for the two different responses in the aldosterone paradox may be due to the different effects of the secretagogues for this hormone on the delivery of HCO$_3^-$ to the CCD and the effect this may have on the apparent permeability for Cl$^-$ in CCD. In more detail, high angiotensin II levels lead to a decreased delivery of HCO$_3^-$ to the CCD, whereas a high P$_K$ leads to an increased delivery of HCO$_3^-$ to the CCD (see Chapter 13, page 444 for more discussion of this topic).
- It is also possible that the mechanism for the aldosterone paradox involves changes induced by the WNK kinases.

Na$^+$ reabsorption in the late distal convoluted tubule, the connecting tubule, and the cortical collecting duct

- The pathway for the reabsorption of Na$^+$ is an epithelial Na$^+$ channel (ENaC), which can lead to the reabsorption of Na$^+$ and Cl$^-$, or the secretion of K$^+$ if Cl$^-$ is not reabsorbed (*see margin note*).
- Aldosterone is the major regulator of the number of open ENaC units in the luminal membrane of principal cells in these nephron segments.

Na$^+$ is reabsorbed in the connecting segment and the cortical collecting duct via ENaC. When there is a fall in the effective arterial blood volume, Na$^+$ is reabsorbed with equal amounts of Cl$^-$ (electroneutral reabsorption of Na$^+$). In contrast, when there is a need to secrete K$^+$, Na$^+$ is reabsorbed faster than Cl$^-$ and this creates the needed lumen-negative electrical driving force (electrogenic reabsorption of Na$^+$; see Chapter 13, page 441 for more discussion).

Process. The entry of Na$^+$ is via ENaC.

Role of hormones. Aldosterone plays a central role in Na$^+$ transport, primarily by increasing the number of open ENaC in the apical membrane of principal cells in these nephron segments. More detailed information about the mechanism of action of aldosterone can be found in Chapter 13, page 444, where we discuss what we call the "aldosterone paradox" (*see margin note*).

Inhibitors. The K$^+$-sparing diuretics, amiloride and triamterene, and the antibiotic trimethoprim, in its cationic form, block ENaC. The concentration of these inhibitors in the luminal fluid is critical for their ability to inhibit ENaC (see Chapter 15, page 530 for more discussion). In contrast, spironolactone competes with aldosterone for binding to its receptor in principal cells.

Disorders involving the epithelial Na$^+$ channel, causing its inhibition. In addition to renal salt wasting, hyperkalemia with a low rate of excretion of K$^+$ in the urine should be present if the activity of ENaC is diminished in the luminal membrane of principal cells or if ENaC is blocked (e.g., by amiloride or trimethoprim). The diagnostic approach in these patients is discussed in Chapter 15, page 530.

Na$^+$ reabsorption in the medullary collecting duct

- The medullary collecting duct is the site where final decisions are made about the excretion of NaCl, but little Na$^+$ is reabsorbed deep in the medulla owing to its poor supply of oxygen.
- When the right atrium is stretched, atrial natriuretic hormone is released, and it inhibits Na$^+$ reabsorption in this nephron segment.

The medullary collecting duct will reabsorb all the Na$^+$ that is delivered unless it receives a message to inhibit this reabsorptive process. Therefore, when the right atrial volume is low (i.e., the effective arterial blood volume is contracted), there is no inhibitor present, and virtually all the Na$^+$ delivered to this site is reabsorbed. In contrast, if the right atrial volume is high (i.e., the effective arterial blood volume is expanded or there is cardiac failure), atrial natriuretic factor is released. As a result, Na$^+$ reabsorption is inhibited in this nephron segment, which leads to a higher rate of excretion of Na$^+$.

Role of hormones. Atrial natriuretic peptide is primarily released from the right atrium of the heart in response to stretch caused by a high central venous volume. Atrial natriuretic peptide is both a peripheral vasodilator, which may lower the systemic blood pressure, and a natriuretic hormone. This latter effect is mediated by increasing the GFR and decreasing Na$^+$ reabsorption in the medullary collecting duct. Atrial natriuretic peptide increases the GFR without raising the renal blood flow, suggesting that it causes efferent arteriolar constriction.

Inhibitors. Atrial natriuretic peptide directly inhibits sodium reabsorption in the medullary collecting duct via activation of cyclic GMP.

Integrative physiology of Na$^+$; cerebral salt wasting

- There are two major requirements for the diagnosis of cerebral salt wasting, a cerebral lesion and salt wasting; of the two, salt wasting is the one that is difficult to establish.

This is a clinical diagnosis that is usually based on a triad of a cerebral lesion, salt wasting, and hyponatremia. Each of these components is considered below.

Cerebral lesion

Although obviously a cerebral lesion must be present, this alone is not sufficient to establish a diagnosis of cerebral salt wasting even if salt wasting is present, because salt wasting may have another cause.

Salt wasting

- For salt wasting to be present, patients must excrete salt while their effective arterial blood volume is contracted.

There are several ways one may be misled with respect to establishing a diagnosis of salt wasting.

1. The physical examination is not sensitive enough to provide reliable information about the effective arterial blood volume unless this volume is very significantly contracted.
2. Salt wasting is present when Na$^+$ and Cl$^-$ are excreted while the effective arterial blood volume is definitely low. In more detail, subjects who consume a typical Western diet must have an expanded effective arterial blood volume to provide the stimulus to inhibit the reabsorption of Na$^+$ and Cl$^-$ in the nephron. Accordingly, they can excrete their daily intake of NaCl. Hence, to diagnose salt wasting, the negative balance for Na$^+$ must be large enough to ensure that a normal kidney would have retained virtually all of the filtered Na$^+$ (usually >2 mmol/kg body weight in an adult; *see margin note*).
3. Patients who are under marked stress may have a high adrenergic tone, which leads to constriction of the venous capacitance vessels and/or increased myocardial contractility. Hence, these patients may have an expanded effective arterial blood volume with an increased central venous pressure, and thereby increased arterial blood pressure, which causes a pressure natriuresis even though there is a negative balance for Na$^+$ (Fig. 9-11).
4. When a patient receives a large volume of isotonic saline over a period of many days (e.g., to diminish spasm of cerebral arteries in a patient with a subarachnoid hemorrhage), a sustained stimulus to excrete Na$^+$ develops. In more detail, this expanded effective arterial blood volume for a prolonged period of time causes transporters

CLINICAL PEARL
When calculating the balance for Na$^+$, one must consider *all* the Na$^+$ administered in the ambulance, in the emergency department, in the operating room, and on the ward. It is an error to restrict the examination to shorter time periods, because this does not reflect the overall balance of Na$^+$.

IV SALINE
The large infusion of saline raises the effective arterial blood volume and augments the natriuresis caused by the adrenergic surge.

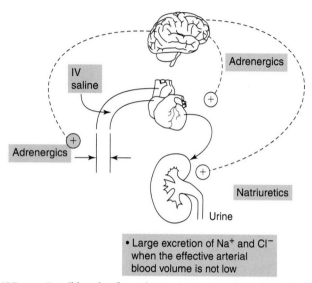

• Large excretion of Na⁺ and Cl⁻ when the effective arterial blood volume is not low

FIGURE 9-11 Possible role of an adrenergic surge in the natriuresis. Three major actions of adrenaline (*dashed lines*) can lead to a natriuresis. First, contraction of the venous capacitance vessels can lead to a rise in central venous pressure and thereby diastolic filling of the heart. Second, there may be an ionotropic action of this hormone on the heart that can lead to a higher effective arterial blood volume. Third, they can lead to the release of a renal vasodilator such as dopamine.

to be removed from the membranes of cells of individual nephron segments, and they become less able to reabsorb filtered Na⁺ (Fig. 9-12). Should there be a decrease in the rate of infusion of saline in this setting, the patient will continue to excrete Na⁺ rapidly; this excessive natriuresis continues until the transporters for Na⁺ can be reinserted into the membranes of the cells of the nephron. Therefore, a form of secondary renal salt wasting develops, but this is not cerebral salt wasting (at least the patient's cerebral lesion is not directly involved). Thus, one should *not* make a diagnosis of cerebral salt wasting in this setting. A list of other possible causes of renal salt wasting is provided in Table 9-7.

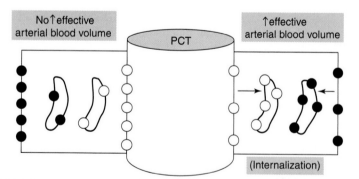

FIGURE 9-12 Development of a salt-wasting state by prior chronic expansion of the effective arterial blood volume. The *left portion* represents the normal state with luminal Na⁺ transport systems (*white circles*) and basolateral Na-K-ATPase (*black circles*) that are the components of the overall process to reabsorb filtered Na⁺ in the proximal convoluted tubule (PCT). The *right portion* shows the response to chronic expansion of the effective arterial blood volume. Elements for Na⁺ reabsorption are transferred to the intracellular compartment where they reside in vesicles inside PCT cells (internalization).

TABLE 9-7 FACTORS TO RULE OUT BEFORE MAKING A DIAGNOSIS OF CEREBRAL SALT WASTING

Because this is a diagnosis of exclusion, one must be confident that the effective arterial blood volume is low before confirming that salt wasting is present.

Ensure that there is not a renal cause for excessive excretion of Na^+
- Lack of a stimulator of the reabsorption of Na^+ (e.g., aldosterone)
- Presence of an inhibitor of the renal reabsorption of Na^+
  - Osmotic or pharmacologic diuretic
  - High concentration of a ligand for the calcium-sensing receptor (e.g., hypercalcemia, aminoglycoside antibiotic)
  - A high arterial effective blood volume despite a contracted ECF volume (e.g., a high adrenergic surge that constricts venous capacitance vessels and/or increases myocardial contractility)
- Tubular damage (e.g., obstructive nephropathy, interstitial nephritis, acute tubular necrosis)
- Inborn error (e.g., Bartter's or Gitelman's syndrome)
- A prolonged period of positive Na^+ balance that expanded the effective arterial blood volume and led to down-regulation of Na^+ transporters in the nephron

5. Although a brain-derived natriuretic peptide and/or a digitalis-like compound levels were found to be elevated in some patients with this diagnosis of cerebral salt wasting, this is not true in others. Furthermore, it is not clear that the criteria to establish the presence of negative salt balance were present in these patients with high levels of these hormones.

Presence of hyponatremia

Although almost every patient with this syndrome has hyponatremia, this electrolyte disorder represents a "physician error" in the selection of intravenous fluids rather than being a component of cerebral salt wasting. In more detail, vasopressin is released as a result of pain, drugs, and so on, in this setting. Therefore, in a patient who has a normal renal concentrating ability, the concentration of Na^+ in the urine should rise to close to 300 mmol/L. If the patient is given a large volume of isotonic saline (150 mmol/L), hyponatremia develops; its basis is illustrated in the tonicity balance in Figure 9-13. In the upper part of Figure 9-13,

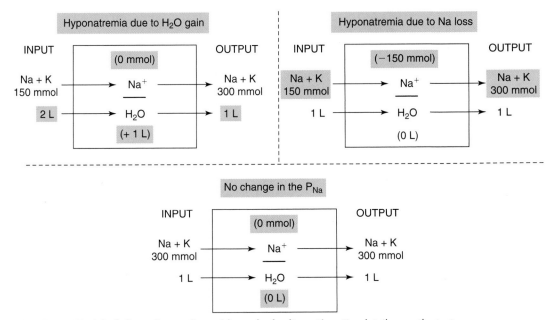

FIGURE 9-13 Tonicity balance in a patient with cerebral salt wasting. For details, see the text.

electrolyte-free water is generated when the intravenous volume is twice the urine output to achieve balance for Na^+ or when the volume of isotonic saline infused was equal to the urine volume, and hence there is a negative balance of Na^+. If the infusate has the same concentration of Na^+ as in the urine and if the volume infused were equal to the urine output, hyponatremia would not develop, although the patient may still have cerebral salt wasting (*bottom portion of the figure*).

PART C
PHYSIOLOGY OF WATER

OBJECTIVES
To emphasize that: ■ The contents of Na^+ and H_2O in the body are regulated by independent mechanisms. ■ A change of tonicity of body fluid compartments is usually synonymous with a change in the P_{Na}. ■ Water balance is primarily the result of the interplay of thirst and renal actions of vasopressin. ■ The upper limit on the rate of excretion of water is set by the distal delivery of filtrate when actions of vasopressin are absent in the distal nephron. ■ When vasopressin acts, the volume of urine is dependent on the rate of excretion of effective urine osmoles and the effective osmolality in the papillary interstitial compartment.

ANTIDIURETIC HORMONE
- This is another name for vasopressin.
- This hormone is synthesized in the paraventricular and supraoptic cells in the hypothalamus.
- Secretory granules containing vasopressin travel in neuronal axons to the posterior pituitary gland, where vasopressin is stored prior to its release in response to a rise in P_{Na}.

TERMS TO DESCRIBE THE EXCRETION OF WATER
Osmole-free water excretion
- The volume of water that is excreted in the urine without solutes is called the *osmole-free water excretion*.
- This term does not reveal the influence of urinary loss on water distribution in the body because urea is not an effective osmole in the body and hence does not affect the distribution of water across cell membranes.
Electrolyte-free water
- This term describes the imaginary volume of water in a solution that would be present if all of the Na^+ plus K^+ salts were separated into a solution of isotonic saline. If the solution is hypotonic, the residual water is called *electrolyte-free water*. If the solution is hypertonic, the volume of water that is needed for the residual $Na^+ + K^+$ salts to form an isotonic solution is called *"negative" electrolyte-free water*.
- As we shall discuss in Chapter 11, page 381, the calculation of electrolyte-free water balance predicts the change in P_{Na}, but is *not* useful to determine its basis or what is needed to restore the tonicity and volume of both ECF and ICF compartments.

OVERVIEW

Regulation of water balance has an input arm and an output arm. The input of water is stimulated by thirst. When enough water is ingested to cause a fall in the P_{Na} and swelling of cells of the osmostat (tonicity receptor), there is a decrease in thirst and inhibition of the release of vasopressin, which leads to the excretion of dilute urine.

The output arm for water balance has two components—the volume of distal delivery of filtrate and the absence of actions of vasopressin; the latter leads to removal of AQP2 from the luminal membranes of the late cortical and the medullary collecting ducts. Conversely, when there is a deficit of water and thereby a high P_{Na}, which causes thirst and stimulates vasopressin release to augment water reabsorption until the osmolalities are equal in the lumen of the late distal nephron segments and in the interstitial compartments. This results in the excretion of a small volume of concentrated urine (*see margin note*).

CONTROL OF WATER BALANCE

When 1 L of water is ingested and absorbed, it mixes with all the water in the body; hence, the P_{Na} falls. To excrete *only* this 1 L of water without electrolytes, this fall in the P_{Na} must be sensed.

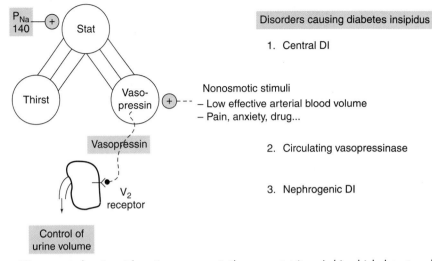

FIGURE 9-14 Water control system. The primary sensor is the osmostat (*top circle*), which detects a change in P_{Na} via an effect on its cell volume. The osmostat is linked to the thirst center (*lower left circle*) and to the vasopressin release center (*lower right circle*). Nonosmotic stimuli (e.g., nausea, pain, anxiety) also influence the release of vasopressin. Vasopressin release is also stimulated when there is a large decrease in the effective arterial blood volume; a lower P_{Na} is needed to suppress the release of vasopressin in this setting. When vasopressin acts, the urine flow rate depends on the number of effective osmoles to be excreted and the effective osmolality in the inner medullary interstitial compartment. The clinical disorders associated with a large excretion of electrolyte-free water (e.g., diabetes insipidus [DI]) and the sites of these lesions are listed on the *right*.

A message must be sent to the kidney to segregate this 1 L of water from Na^+ that it was filtered with so that only this excess water can be excreted in maximally dilute form (i.e., without obligating the excretion of electrolytes; *see margin note*).

The components of the control system for water balance are shown in Figure 9-14. The goal of this system is to return the P_{Na} to 140 mmol/L.

Sensor

> • Addition of water to the ECF compartment causes its P_{Na} to fall, which leads to swelling of all cells, including those in the osmostat.

The sensor (the osmostat or tonicity receptor) is located in the hypothalamus and is linked to both the thirst center and the vasopressin release center via nerve connections. Particles such as urea are not effective osmoles because they have similar concentrations in the ICF and ECF compartments, and hence the hypothalamic tonicity receptor does not sense them. Glucose is also not an effective osmole for the cells of the osmostat, and hence hyperglycemia does not stimulate thirst or the release of vasopressin directly (*see margin notes*).

Thirst is stimulated by an increase in the tonicity of plasma (high P_{Na}). Contraction of the effective arterial blood volume is a weak stimulus of thirst; an elevated level of angiotensin II may mediate this effect. Other factors unrelated to a need for a positive water balance may lead to a higher intake of water (e.g., dryness of the mouth, habit, culture, psychological conditions).

U_{Osm} IN THE ABSENCE OF ACTIONS OF VASOPRESSIN
The U_{Osm} in subjects consuming a typical Western diet is usually close to 60 mOsm/kg H_2O. Nevertheless, the U_{Osm} may be higher if there is a need to excrete a larger number of osmoles (Na^+, K^+, urea, ethanol). Therefore, to assess the ability of the kidney to excrete water, the primary focus should be on the *volume* of dilute urine rather than only on the U_{Osm}.

EFFECT OF HYPERGLYCEMIA
Stimulation of thirst and the release of vasopressin in patients with severe hyperglycemia are likely related to a low effective arterial blood volume secondary to the osmotic diuresis rather than a direct effect of hyperglycemia on the osmostat.

EFFECT OF ETHANOL
Although it is said that ethanol inhibits the release of vasopressin, a direct effect of ethanol to inhibit the release of vasopressin to cause a water diuresis occurs only with an extremely high blood ethanol level (>100 mmol/L [460 mg/dL]).

Messages

When cells in the tonicity receptor swell appreciably in response to a low P_{Na}, a message is sent to the thirst center to diminish the intake of water. A second message is sent to the vasopressin release center to suppress the release of vasopressin and thus to permit the excretion of the maximum volume of dilute urine to return P_{Na} to normal. The converse occurs with shrinkage of tonicity receptor cells in response to a high P_{Na}.

Pathways for the reabsorption of water

In the kidney, saline is filtered, and some of the Na^+ and Cl^- are reabsorbed without water in the thick ascending limbs of the loop of Henle; this causes the luminal fluid to become dilute (have an osmolality of close to 150 mOsm/kg H_2O; *see margin note*). Reabsorption of Na^+ and Cl^- without water in the distal nephron increases the volume of electrolyte-free water that can be excreted. The water remaining in the lumen of the distal nephron can be excreted if the luminal membranes of distal nephron segments have a low permeability to water (i.e., absence of AQP2 water channels in their luminal membranes because vasopressin is not acting). When vasopressin is not present, there is some water reabsorption in the inner medullary collecting duct because this nephron region has a modest permeability to water (called *residual water permeability*) and there is a large osmotic driving force due to the very low luminal osmolality (see page 277 for more discussion).

Excretion of a large volume of dilute urine

There are three steps to excrete a large volume of water with a low concentration of electrolytes, as shown in the following box:

- Delivery of a large volume of filtrate to the distal nephron.
- Vasopressin must be absent to prevent the insertion of AQP2 into the luminal membranes of the late distal nephron.
- Na^+ and Cl^- must be reabsorbed from water-impermeable distal nephron sites.

Distal delivery of filtrate

Distal delivery of filtrate is equal to the GFR minus the volume of water reabsorbed in the proximal convoluted tubule because virtually all subsequent nephron segments are impermeable to water when vasopressin fails to act. The major exception is the descending thin limbs of loop of Henle of nephrons that enter the inner medulla (~15% of the nephrons) because this nephron segment has AQP1.

The major factor responsible for a large distal delivery of filtrate is the avidity for reabsorption of Na^+ and secondarily water in the proximal convoluted tubule. Hence, the absence of a contracted effective arterial blood volume is needed for maximal excretion of water. Conversely, when there is both a low GFR and an enhanced proximal reabsorption, distal delivery may be very low. If the volume of distal delivery of filtrate does not exceed the volume of water that is absorbed via residual water permeability, chronic hyponatremia may

OSMOLALITY OF FLUID OBTAINED FROM THE EARLY DISTAL CONVOLUTED TUBULE
Fluid obtained during micropuncture of the early distal convoluted tubule has an osmolality of close to 150 mOsm/kg:
- Urea: 50 mmol/L
- Na^+: 50 mmol/L
- Cl^-: 50 mmol/L

develop, even with a modest water load and the absence of actions of vasopressin. (see Case 12-1, page 404, and the section on syndrome of inappropriate antidiuresis in Chapter 10, page 333).

Absence of actions of vasopressin

Because the distal nephron is impermeable to water when vasopressin fails to act, almost all the water delivered past the end of the pars recta of the proximal convoluted tubule is excreted in the urine. Therefore, there must be a low P_{Na} and the absence of nonosmotic stimuli for the release of vasopressin for a water diuresis to occur.

Reabsorption of Na^+ and Cl^- in nephron segments that are impermeable to water during a water diuresis

- Na^+ and Cl^- are *always* reabsorbed without water in the middle functional unit of the nephron.
- Na^+ and Cl^- are reabsorbed without water in the final functional nephron unit when the actions of vasopressin to insert AQP2 are not present.
- During a water diuresis, there is a need to reabsorb more Na^+ and Cl^- in the middle and final functional nephron units to avoid large losses of these ions in the urine, as there is typically a very large delivery of Na^+ and Cl^- to these nephron segments. These mechanisms are initiated by the high flow rate and are independent of the effective arterial blood volume status.

The requirement to reabsorb much of the Na^+ that remains in the lumen of diluting sites becomes obvious when the quantity of Na^+ that normally exits the medullary thick ascending limb of the loop of Henle (~3300 mmol/day) is considered. In quantitative terms, this amount of Na^+ is larger than the amount of Na^+ that is present in the entire ECF compartment in a 70-kg adult (2250 mmol, or 15 L × 150 mmol of Na^+ per L of ECF). Therefore, there must be powerful signals delivered to the second and third functional nephron units to stimulate Na^+ reabsorption in this setting. *The following discussion emphasizes the fact that a high flow rate and a low luminal osmolality provide the signals for this to be achieved.*

Desalination of luminal fluid in the medullary thick ascending limb of the loop of Henle during a water diuresis

- Residual water permeability and a low luminal osmolality permit the reabsorption of enough water from the medullary collecting duct to "de-inhibit" (i.e., activate) the reabsorption of Na^+ and Cl^- in the medullary thick ascending limb of the loop of Henle.

To reabsorb the same amount of or somewhat more Na^+ and Cl^- in this nephron segment, the inhibitory effect exerted by the interstitial concentration of ionized calcium must be diminished. This can be achieved if water is reabsorbed from the inner medullary collecting duct via its residual water permeability, as this lowers the interstitial concentration of ionized calcium.

TABLE 9-8 **DRIVING FORCE FOR WATER REABSORPTION VIA RESIDUAL WATER PERMEABILITY IN THE INNER MEDULLARY COLLECTING DUCT DURING A WATER DIURESIS**

The major factors that influence the reabsorption of water are the small degree of permeability of the inner medullary collecting duct to water and the large osmotic driving force to draw water from its lumen (i.e., the difference in osmolality between the interstitial compartment and the lumen of the inner medullary collecting duct multiplied by 19.3, the number of mm Hg per mOsm/L). Note that the osmotic driving force is huge (shown in bold).

CONDITION	INTERSTITIAL OSMOLALITY (mOsm/L)	LUMEN OSMOLALITY (mOsm/L)	DRIVING FORCE (mm Hg)
Vasopressin is acting	900	900	0
No vasopressin actions	450	50	**~8000**

RESIDUAL WATER PERMEABILITY: QUANTITATIVE ASPECTS

- The distal delivery of filtrate is ~27 L/day.
- The maximum urine flow rate during a water diuresis is close to 15 mL/min (extrapolates to 22 L/day).
- Accordingly, 27 L/day – 22 L/day or ~5 L/day appear to be reabsorbed via residual water permeability during a maximum water diuresis.
- The paradox is that reabsorption of water via residual water permeability initiates the excretion of a larger volume of electrolyte-free water during a water diuresis because it removes the inhibition exerted on reabsorption of Na⁺ in the mTAL by the concentration of ionized calcium in the medullary interstital compartment.
- During a large water diuresis, the flow rate through the inner medullary collecting duct is too fast to permit water to move to osmotic equilibrium via residual water permeability. Notwithstanding, with each renal pelvic contraction, a small volume of fluid moves in a retrograde fashion up the medullary collecting duct, while most of the urine in the pelvis descends in the bladder. Perhaps the small volume of refluxed urine may approach osmotic equilibrium, but this is obscured when examining the large volume of very dilute urine in the urinary bladder.

Importance of residual water permeability in the inner medullary collecting duct

During a water diuresis, water is reabsorbed from the inner medullary collecting duct because it is constituitively somewhat permeable to water (see Fig. 9-6). The driving force for this reabsorption of water is due to the large difference in osmolality between the interstitial compartment (higher) and the fluid in its lumen (very low; Table 9-8). In fact, it is the very low luminal osmolality that is paramount for this osmotic driving force, and it is only present when there is no AQP2 in the luminal membrane of upstream nephron sites. This reabsorption of water will lead to dilution of the medullary interstitial compartment and thereby to a fall in the concentration of ionized calcium in the outer medullary interstitial compartment (*see margin note* for quantitative aspects). As a result, the reabsorption of Na⁺ and Cl⁻ in the medullary thick ascending limb of the loop of Henle is "de-inhibited," which leads to continued reabsorption of Na⁺ and Cl⁻ and thereby to "desalination" of the luminal fluid that will be delivered to the cortical thick ascending limb of the loop of Henle during a maximum water diuresis (Fig. 9-15).

Desalination of luminal fluid in the third functional nephron unit of the nephron during a water diuresis

- A high flow rate increases the reabsorption of Na⁺ via ENaC.

There is one major diluting site in the third functional nephron unit that contributes to the excretion of the maximum volume of electrolyte-poor urine mainly by enhancing the reabsorption of Na⁺ and Cl⁻ from its luminal fluid. There is flow activation of ENaC in these nephron segments. This means that more Na⁺ can be reabsorbed during a large water diuresis. Although most of the Na⁺ that is reabsorbed will be accompanied by Cl⁻, it is possible that there can be some secretion of K⁺.

It is unlikely that there will be an appreciable secretion of K⁺ in the CCD during a water diuresis. But should some K⁺ be secreted, much of it can be reabsorbed by the H⁺/K⁺-ATPase in the inner medullary collecting duct. If the anion accompanying K⁺ were HCO_3^-, it would be absorbed indirectly by the H⁺ secreted by the H⁺/K⁺-ATPase.

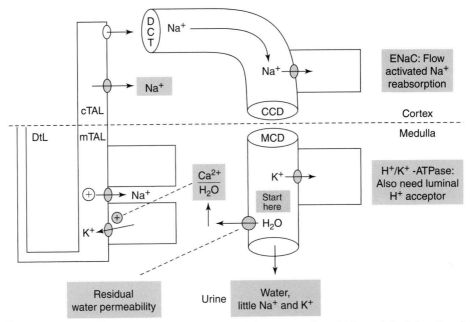

FIGURE 9-15 Removal of Na⁺ and Cl⁻ from luminal fluid that enters the middle and final functional units of the nephron during a maximum water diuresis. When more Na⁺ and Cl⁻ are reabsorbed in the middle and final functional units of the nephron, water with fewer electrolytes will be excreted. The stimulus begins with a high flow rate in the inner medullary collecting duct (MCD), which leads to more water reabsorption via residual water permeability (*green shaded circle near the "Start here" message*). As a result, there is a signal (lower concentration of ionized calcium in the outer medullary interstitial compartment), which increases the reabsorption of Na⁺ and Cl⁻ in the medullary thick ascending limb of the loop of Henle (mTAL) to begin the desalination process. In the late cortical distal nephron (CCD), flow activation of the epithelial Na⁺ channel (ENaC) accelerates Na⁺ reabsorption (and perhaps the secretion of a small quantity of K⁺). In the inner MCD, the luminal H⁺/K⁺-ATPase reabsorbs some of the K⁺ that are delivered. If the anions accompanying K⁺ were HCO_3^-, the latter would be removed as well. If the anions were Cl⁻, enhanced entry of NH_3 should result in the replacement of luminal K⁺ with NH_4^+. cTAL, cortical thick ascending limb of the loop of Henle.

Conversely, if the anion were Cl⁻, the most likely mechanism for H⁺ removal would involve enhanced entry of NH_3 and the excretion of NH_4^+ with Cl⁻.

Retain "nondangerous" water for future sweat

- In the absence of a water load, vasopressin is released on a continuous basis.
- To retain a moderate volume of water (~1 L in an adult) for future loss as sweat for heat dissipation, vasopressin must continue to be released despite a fall in the P_{Na} toward 136 mmol/L.

The retention of close to 1 L of water for future sweat will result in a fall in the P_{Na} (*see margin note*). The question is, "Why does this fall in the P_{Na} not inhibit the release of vasopressin?" The answer to this question has several parts.
   1. Brain cells swell when the P_{Na} in *arterial* plasma falls. Notwithstanding, the arterial P_{Na} may be appreciably different from the P_{Na} in venous blood early after the ingestion of a large water load (Fig. 9-16).

EVAPORATIVE WATER LOSS: A QUANTITATIVE ANALYSIS
- Heat loss (2500 kcal of heat per day) occurs by multiple mechanisms: convection, conduction, radiation, and evaporation.
- When 1 L of water evaporates on the skin surface, 500 to 600 kcal are lost.
- Any sweat that drops to the ground does not cause heat loss.

SIPPING OF WATER
- While not shown in this figure, when the same volume of water was sipped slowly, there were near-equal P_{Na} values in the arterial and venous blood.
- Vasopressin continues to act despite the same fall in the P_{Na} at the 60-minutes time.

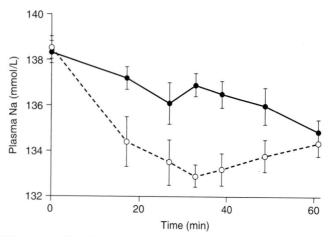

FIGURE 9-16 **Fall in the P_{Na} in arterial and venous plasma during a water load of 20 mL/kg.** The time in minutes after beginning to ingest the water, which takes about 15 minutes, is shown on the x-axis and the P_{Na} in mmol/L is shown on the y-axis. The *dashed line* depicts the arterial P_{Na} and the *solid line* depicts the P_{Na} in the brachial vein. All arterial P_{Na} values, except the zero time and the 60-minute time, are significantly lower than the venous P_{Na} values.

2. The brain must recognize when a water load may become dangerous (i.e., more brain cell swelling) and initiate a large water diuresis before the danger is serious.
3. Ingested water "dilutes" the arterial P_{Na}, but clinicians may not recognize this danger if they rely solely on the initial P_{Na} in brachial venous blood; the large muscles "suck up" water quickly, causing the venous P_{Na} to rise, which obscures the danger of brain cell swelling.
4. There are three factors that contribute to the retention of this 1 L of water. First, the electrolyte-free water load must be ingested slowly, because this prevents a large fall in the arterial P_{Na}. Second, some of this water load must be stored temporarily in the stomach and released slowly into the intestine to avoid a sudden and large fall in the arterial P_{Na}. Third, if the ingested water contains an osmole that is absorbed slowly in the intestinal tract, this delays its absorption and diminishes the fall in the arterial P_{Na} (e.g., the intake of fruit with a high content of fructose, which is poorly absorbed in the small intestine [discussed in Part D, page 293]).

ARTERIAL P_{Na} AND THE
RELEASE OF VASOPRESSIN
- Brain cells "see" the P_{Na} in arterial blood and *not* the P_{Na} in brachial venous blood.
- The fall in the arterial P_{Na} from 140 mmol/L that is needed to inhibit the release of vasopressin is appreciably larger than the rise in the arterial P_{Na} needed to stimulate the release of this hormone.
- Since the presence of nonosmotic stimuli for the release of vasopressin is variable, one cannot define an absolute value for P_{Na} that will inhibit or stimulate the release of vasopressin.

Mechanism to explain why dangerous water is excreted rapidly

Immediately following the rapid ingestion and absorption of water, the P_{Na} falls in portal venous blood and hypotonic plasma is delivered to the heart via the arterial blood. Because the brain receives such a large portion of the cardiac output (~20%) and its weight is relatively small, brain cells swell more quickly than other cells. For example, the bulk of water in the body is in skeletal muscle cells, which receive blood at one twentieth the rate of the brain on a per-kg basis (Fig. 9-17). Therefore, the release of vasopressin is suppressed and the excretion of a dangerous water load starts before enough water is retained to lower the P_{Na} in venous blood to reflect the danger of brain cell swelling (*see margin note*).

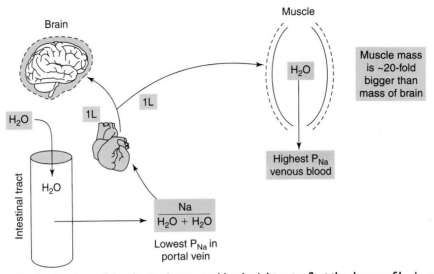

FIGURE 9-17 Mechanism to explain why P_{Na} in venous blood might not reflect the degree of brain cell swelling shortly after "gulping" water. When water is ingested rapidly (*green box on the left*), it will be absorbed from the intestinal tract and enter the portal vein. If the volume is large and the rate of stomach emptying is rapid, there will be a large fall in the arterial P_{Na}. When arterial blood is delivered to the brain and skeletal muscle cells, the initial swelling in individual brain cells is much greater than in individual muscle cells because the mass (water content) of muscle is much larger than that of the brain and their blood flow rates are similar at rest (~1 L/min). As a result, the P_{Na} in venous blood draining muscle cells will be much higher before equilibrium is reached and the impending danger of brain swelling may be underestimated.

Messages

1. *The traditional description of the physiologic response to a water load must be revised.* Ingested water, if it is not excessive, will be retained for future heat dissipation. In contrast, if a larger water load is ingested, it may lead to a rise in intracranial pressure, and if it is perceived as being dangerous, the water load will be excreted rapidly. To do so, the release of vasopressin must be suppressed.

2. *When a large volume of water is ingested and stomach emptying is rapid, the venous P_{Na} will not reveal whether the arterial P_{Na} is low enough to inhibit the release of vasopressin.* A high degree of suspicion is needed to prevent the danger of brain cell swelling and a rise in intracranial pressure.

Excretion of concentrated urine

- There are two functions of the urinary concentrating mechanism:
  - Excrete the minimum volume of water when there is a water deficit.
  - Excrete urine with the highest possible concentration of electrolytes when there is an intake of a large hypertonic salt load.

Conserve water when there is a deficit of water

The usual description of the renal concentrating process focuses primarily on conservation of water when there is a deficit of water. The first step in the overall process is to sense a deficit of water, which is recognized when the P_{Na} is close to 140 mmol/L. This stimulates the release of vasopressin, which causes the insertion of AQP2 water channels into the luminal membranes of principal cells in the third

RENAL RESPONSES TO A HYPERTONIC LOAD OF NaCl
- Vasopressin is released because of a higher P_{Na}.
- An expanded effective arterial blood volume leads to inhibition of the reabsorption of Na^+, Cl^-, and water in the PCT. Therefore, more osmoles (Na^+ and Cl^-) are delivered to the terminal cortical collecting duct and hence a larger volume of filtrate with an osmolality of ~300 mOsm/L (= P_{Osm}) will be delivered to the medullary collecting duct.
- When this filtrate reaches the 600 mOsm/kg H_2O level in the renal medulla, half of its water will be reabsorbed, but this is half of a larger volume. Accordingly, there will be a greater degree of dilution of an inhibitor in the medullary interstitial compartment. This in turn will lead to a stronger signal for the mTAL to reabsorb more Na^+ and Cl^- and thereby raise the osmolality of this interstitial compartment back to its original value.
- The urine will have the highest effective osmolality, but its volume will not be very low owing to a higher rate of excretion of effective osmoles.

RATIONALE FOR THIS QUESTION
This question was added to illustrate how a modest decline in concentrating ability poses a large threat if a person were to have both a high intake of NaCl and a limited access to water.

RECEPTORS FOR VASOPRESSIN
There are two major vasopressin receptors:
- V1 receptors are present in vascular endothelial cells, where they mediate the effect of vasopressin to cause vasoconstriction.
- V2 receptors are present in the late distal nephron, where they mediate the effect of vasopressin to increase the permeability for water (insert AQP2) and urea (insert urea transporters in the inner medullary collecting duct).

functional unit of the nephron. As soon as luminal fluid reaches the nephron segments that have AQP2 in their luminal membrane, all of the hypotonic portion of the luminal fluid will be reabsorbed and the osmolality in the luminal fluid rises until it is equal to that in the interstitial compartment surrounding these nephron segments. The net result is the excretion of a small volume of urine that has a high osmolality.

Excrete a large hypertonic load of Na^+ and Cl^-

When there is a large intake of salt with little water, this salt load must be excreted in the smallest possible volume of urine. The urine volume, however, will *not* be as low as in the setting above, as there will be a large natriuresis and thereby a salt-induced osmotic diuresis. The basis for the natriuresis is an expanded effective arterial blood volume due to the positive balance for Na^+ and Cl^- (*see margin note*). If this load of electrolytes could not be excreted with the highest possible concentration of Na^+ and Cl^- in the urine, hypernatremia would develop, and thirst would be stimulated, and the subject would drink more water. This can create a problem as illustrated in the discussion of Question 9-8.

QUESTION

(Discussion on page 311)
9-8 *Consider the following thought experiment: A man in steady state consumes and excretes 300 mosmol of electrolytes (150 mmol Na^+ + 150 mmol Cl^-) and 1 L of water. If he were to ingest an extra 300 mosmol of electrolytes without additional water, and if this extra 300 mosmol of electrolytes were excreted and his body tonicity did not change, it must be excreted in a hypertonic form. What would the change be in his body composition if his maximum urine osmolality due to electrolytes was 600 mOsm/L on one day and 400 mOsm/L on another day (see margin note)?*

Overview of the renal concentrating process

Three major effects permit the kidney to conserve water and/or excrete Na^+ and Cl^- in a hypertonic form.
1. *The presence of a unique blood supply, the vasa recta, which function as a countercurrent exchanger, will minimize the washout of osmoles from the medullary interstitial compartment.*
2. *Insertion of AQP2 water channels into the luminal membranes of the entire final functional unit of the nephron; this is the result of actions of vasopressin (see margin note).*
3. *Generation of a high medullary interstitial osmolality. This occurs when Na^+ and Cl^- are reabsorbed without water from the medullary thick ascending limb of the loop of Henle.*

The vasa recta function as a countercurrent exchanger to minimize the washout of osmoles from the renal medullary interstitial compartment

- There is a progressive rise in the concentration of solutes in the interstitial compartment as one descends into the medulla from its junction with the renal cortex to the papillary tip.

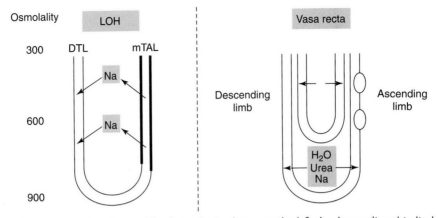

FIGURE 9-18 Countercurrent exchanger blood supply. As shown on the *left,* the descending thin limbs (DtLs) of the loop of Henle (LOH) are permeable to Na$^+$ and not water. As shown on the *right,* the thin-walled vasa recta run downward in the medulla from the corticomedullary junction (descending vasa recta), make a hairpin bend, and then run up (ascending vasa recta) in close proximity to the descending limb. Solutes (e.g., urea and Na$^+$) and water diffuse readily across at every level, and this maintains equal osmolalities at every horizontal plane. Individual vasa recta have their bend at different depths in the renal medulla. The fenestra in the ascending vasa recta permit calcium carbonate precipitates to exit from the medulla.

- There is minimal washout of solutes from the renal medullary interstitial compartment because solutes diffuse between the ascending and the descending limbs of the vasa recta.

The unique blood supply to this area avoids "washing" solutes out of the medullary interstitial compartment (Fig. 9-18). In addition to a slow rate of blood flow, its architecture is such that it functions as a *countercurrent exchanger* because the vessels that run down to the medullary tip (descending limbs) bend back and travel upward (ascending limbs). These blood vessels are very permeable to electrolytes and urea (they have a urea transporter in their luminal membranes). Moreover, water diffuses readily between the ascending limbs and the descending limbs. In fact, there are twice as many ascending as compared to descending limbs of the vasa recta, and the ascending limbs have large holes (called *fenestra*) to accelerate this diffusion process.

The ascending vasa recta carry all the water and solutes that were reabsorbed from medullary nephron segments—hence, they have a higher flow rate than in the descending vasa recta. Some vasa recta vessels bend at more superficial levels while others bend deeper in the medulla. In addition, the concentration of solutes becomes progressively lower in the lumen of both vasa recta limbs as well as in the interstitial fluid compartment as one proceeds from the papillary tip to the junction of the renal medulla with the renal cortex.

Insertion of AQP2 and the reabsorption of water when vasopressin acts

The major stimulus for the release of vasopressin is an arterial P_{Na} that is greater than 136 mmol/L (the exact threshold will vary depending on the presence of nonosmotic stimuli for the release of vasopressin). Vasopressin binds to its V_2 receptors on the basolateral membrane of principal cells of the final functional unit of the nephron (Fig. 9-19). As a result, the enzyme adenylate cyclase is activated and cyclic AMP (cAMP) is generated. This second messenger phosphorylates and hence activates cAMP-dependent protein kinase A, which leads to the insertion of AQP2 into the luminal membrane of these

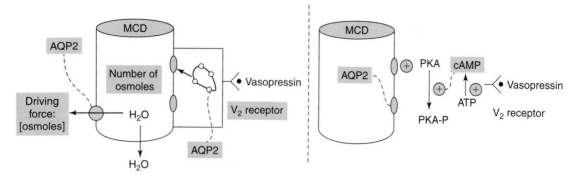

FIGURE 9-19 Vasopressin actions on the distal nephron. The *dark line with small open circles* in cells in the *left portion of the figure* represents stored AQP2 in vesicles. The insertion of AQP2 into the luminal membrane of medullary collecting duct (MCD) cells when vasopressin acts is shown to the *left of the dashed vertical line*, and the more detailed mechanisms are shown to the *right of the dashed line*. In the inner MCD, vasopressin causes the insertion of urea transporters to permit urea to diffuse across the luminal membrane and achieve equal concentrations in the lumen and in the medullary interstitial compartment (not shown). PKA, protein kinase A; PKA-P, phosphorylated protein kinase A.

VASOPRESSIN ACTS THROUGHOUT THIS DAY
This appears to be the case in most individuals who eat a typical Western diet.
- If the 24-hour urine volume is close to 1.5 L, the urine flow rate is ~1 mL/min, as there are 1440 min/day.
- If vasopressin fails to act, the urine flow rate will be 10–15 mL/min.
- Hence, there could not be many minutes in the day when vasopressin fails to act to have an average urine flow rate of 1 mL/min.

OSMOTIC FORCE FOR WATER REABSORPTION IN THE CORTEX
- Each mosmol/L exerts an osmotic pressure of 19.3 mm Hg (20 mm Hg for easy arithmetic).
- In the cortex, the interstitial osmolality is similar to the P_{Osm} (~300 mOsm/L for easy arithmetic) and the osmolality in luminal fluid that arrives here is ~150 mOsm/L. Multiplying the difference between interstitial and luminal osmolalities (150 mOsm/L) by 20 mm Hg per mosmol/L reveals that the pressure exerted is ~3000 mm Hg, a value that is equivalent to the mean arterial blood pressure (i.e., 100 mm Hg) of 30 beating hearts.
- *Overall*: Water reabsorption is very rapid in the cortex.

cells (acute effect) and the synthesis of more AQP2 (chronic effect). Of note, the duration of action of vasopressin is short; hence, there is a need for its continuous release to have the lowest possible urine flow rate (depends on the maximum interstitial osmolality and the number of effective osmoles that are being excreted; *see margin note*).

The fluid delivered to the final functional unit of the nephron always has a low osmolality. Hence, one can make an imaginary division of this volume into a component that has an osmolality equal to that in plasma and a second component, which is osmole-free water.

Reabsorption of osmole-free water

Events in the cortex. Although the difference in osmolality between the luminal and the interstitial compartments is relatively small, there is a *very large osmotic driving force* to reabsorb osmole-free water in this region (*see margin note*). While 21 L of water are reabsorbed here each day from the final functional unit when vasopressin acts and they are added rapidly to the cortical interstitial compartment, this does not pose a danger for two reasons. First, Na^+ *without* water are reabsorbed in the water-impermeable middle functional unit, which makes this net addition virtually isotonic as shown in Figure 9-10. Second, the plasma flow rate in the cortex is enormous (Fig. 9-20).

Events in the medulla. The interstitial osmolality is much higher in the renal medulla than in the cortex (Table 9-9). Nevertheless, the majority of water that is reabsorbed in the final functional unit of the nephron occurs in the cortex even though the rise in the osmolality is two- to threefold in the cortex and fourfold in the renal medulla.

Reabsorption of water and electrolytes

- When Na^+ and Cl^- are reabsorbed in a nephron segment that is permeable to water, the solution added is isotonic to the surrounding interstitial compartment.

In the renal cortex, the solution that is reabsorbed is close to isotonic saline. In the medullary collecting duct, the fluid that leaves the lumen is isotonic to the medullary interstitial compartment at that horizontal plane. Notwithstanding, this hypertonic saline will exit the

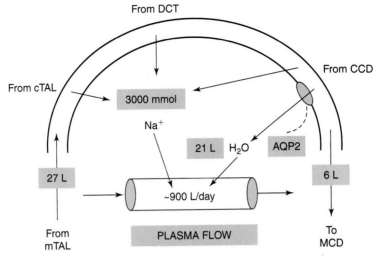

FIGURE 9-20 Reabsorption of water in the cortex. The *stylized structure* represents the entire cortical distal nephron, which has components from the middle and final functional units. Although 21 L of water are added rapidly to the cortical interstitial compartment from the final functional unit, this does not pose a risk because enough Na+ *without* water is reabsorbed in the water-impermeable middle functional unit, which makes this net addition virtually isotonic. In addition, the plasma flow rate in the cortex is enormous (~900 L/day).

medulla in the ascending vasa recta with a concentration of Na+ plus K+ that is close to isotonic saline (P_{Na} 150 mmol/kg H_2O; discussed in more detail in the following section).

Generation of a high medullary interstitial osmolality in the outer medulla

The rise in this interstitial osmolality occurs when Na+ and Cl− are reabsorbed actively *without water from the water-impermeable* medullary thick ascending limb of the loop of Henle (Fig. 9-21). While the traditional view makes this the initial step to "suck" water out of the medullary collecting duct when this nephron segment is permeable to water (i.e., when vasopressin acts), we favor an alternative definition of the first step. In our view, the first step is the reabsorption of water from the medullary collecting duct, which generates signals to

TABLE 9-9 **EFFECT OF WATER REABSORPTION IN THE FINAL FUNCTIONAL UNIT OF THE NEPHRON ON THE VOLUME AND EFFECTIVE OSMOLALITY OF THE URINE**

Approximately 27 L of hypotonic fluid is delivered to the distal nephron. Vasopressin makes the late nephron segments permeable to water. Most of the water delivered to the distal nephron is reabsorbed in the cortex so that solutes in the hypertonic medulla are not diluted by this large volume of hypotonic fluid (*see margin note*).

NEPHRON SITE	VOLUME EXITING (L)	VOLUME REABSORBED (L)	OSMOLALITY (mOsm/kg H_2O)	RISE IN OSMOLALITY
End—loop of Henle	27	—	150	—
End—cortical collecting duct	6	21	300	Factor of 2
End—medullary collecting duct	0.75	5.25	1200	Factor of 4

UREA IN THE MAJORITY OF THE FINAL FUNCTIONAL UNIT OF THE NEPHRON
It is important to remember that urea is an effective osmole until it reaches the inner MCD. Therefore, the total and effective osmolalities are the same prior to the inner MCD.

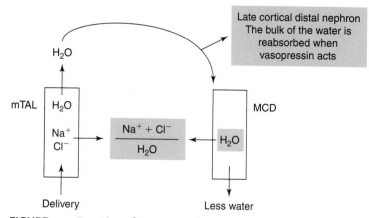

FIGURE 9-21 Excretion of concentrated urine. The *left rectangle* represents the medullary thick ascending limb of the loop of Henle (mTAL), where there is active reabsorption of Na^+ and Cl^- without water. This addition of solutes without water raises the osmolality in the medullary interstitial compartment. When vasopressin acts, the late cortical distal nephron becomes permeable to water; this is the site where much of this water is reabsorbed. The water that remains in the lumen at the end of the cortical collecting duct will be delivered to the medullary collecting duct, where most of it will be drawn out of this nephron segment by the high medullary interstitial osmolality. The intent of this figure is to illustrate the process without an emphasis on its regulation.

REGULATION OF THE REABSORPTION OF NaCl IN THE mTAL
Think about how the mTAL could know how much Na^+ and Cl^- it must reabsorb to keep the osmolality in the medullary interstitial compartment in a narrow, but high, range.

REGULATION OF Na^+ REABSORPTION IN THE LOOP OF HENLE BY IONIZED CALCIUM
• The primary control may be to decrease the likelihood of producing a high interstitial concentration of ionized calcium and thereby to minimize the risk of nephrocalcinosis.
• This regulation operates via signals elicited by binding of calcium to the calcium-sensing receptor on the basolateral aspect of cells of the medullary thick ascending limbs of the loop of Henle, which inhibits ROMK and hence voltage-driven reabsorption of calcium in the medullary thick ascending limb of the loop of Henle.
• This regulation by calcium has a secondary effect; it also controls the reabsorption of Na^+ and Cl^- in the medullary thick ascending limbs of the loop of Henle and thereby the medullary interstitial osmolality.

augment the reabsorption of Na^+ and Cl^- from the medullary thick ascending limb of the loop of Henle (see page 268 for more discussion of regulation).

Regulation of the urine concentrating process in the outer medulla. There are two possible generic mechanisms for control of the concentrating process in the renal medulla.

• *Substrate-driven control:* The primary event is accelerated reabsorption of Na^+ and Cl^- in the medullary thick ascending limb, which raises medullary interstitial osmolality to drive the reabsorption of water from the medullary collecting duct. It is not clear how this is regulated (*see margin note*).
• *Inhibitory control:* The addition of water from the medullary collecting duct lowers the concentration of an inhibitor of the reabsorption of Na^+ and Cl^- in the medullary thick ascending limb of the loop of Henle (*see margin note*).

Substrate-driven control

In this model (Fig. 9-22), which is the most popular interpretation of the control of the medullary concentrating mechanism, primary regulation is in the mTAL of the loop of Henle. This nephron segment must reabsorb just enough Na^+ and Cl^- to determine the volume of water to reabsorb from the medullary collecting duct. This raises a disquieting question, "*How can the mTAL of the loop of Henle 'know' just how much Na^+ and Cl^- to reabsorb at any one moment in time?*" For example, if too much Na^+ and Cl^- are reabsorbed from the mTAL, too much water will

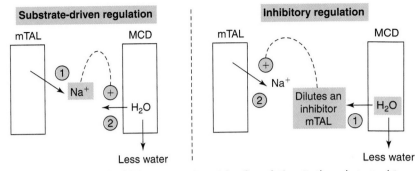

FIGURE 9-22 Substrate-driven and inhibitory control models of regulation. In the substrate-driven model shown on the *left*, the major control is exerted in the medullary thick ascending limb (mTAL) of the loop of Henle, which must reabsorb just enough Na⁺ and Cl⁻ to determine the volume of water to reabsorb from the medullary collecting duct (MCD). In contrast, in the inhibitory regulation model shown on the *right*, the major control (and "single effect") is exerted by the amount of water reabsorbed in the MCD, which dilutes an inhibitor (perhaps ionized calcium—not shown), and this permits the reabsorption of Na⁺ and Cl⁻ in the mTAL to increase by an appropriate amount (*see margin note on page 286*).

be reabsorbed from the medullary collecting duct, the urine volume will be too low, and precipitates (and eventually stones) may form.

Inhibitory control

In this model, the volume of water reabsorbed from the medullary collecting duct must signal the loop of Henle to reabsorb the correct amount of Na⁺ and Cl⁻ to maintain a steady state. To achieve this goal, there must be an inhibitor of the reabsorption of Na⁺ and Cl⁻ in the mTAL of the loop of Henle located in the medullary interstitial compartment—its concentration will fall when more water is added to the interstitial compartment, which then removes the inhibition of Na⁺ and Cl⁻ reabsorption in this nephron segment. A possible candidate is ionized calcium (Ca^{2+}) because cells of the mTAL of the loop of Henle have a receptor for Ca^{2+} on their basolateral membrane (see Fig. 9-8; *see margin note*). In addition, when Ca^{2+} binds to its receptor, a signal is generated that causes inhibition of ROMK and thereby, inhibition of the reabsorption of Na⁺ and Cl⁻ in the mTAL of the loop of Henle via both NKCC-2 and the paracellular route. When the concentration of Ca^{2+} falls, more Na⁺ and Cl⁻ are reabsorbed from the mTAL of the loop of Henle.

A critique of the two models of control

For illustrative purposes, consider heating a house in a Canadian winter (Fig. 9-23). The fuel in an oil tank represents the mTAL of the loop of Henle, the house represents the medullary interstitial compartment, and a furnace in which heat is generated represents the medullary interstitial osmolality.

Control by substrate supply. In this model, adding more oil to the tank leads to generation of extra heat, but the house may become too hot (i.e., the medullary osmolality could rise to dangerous levels and predispose to oliguria and the risk of forming kidney stones; *see margin note*).

Control by "inhibitory" signals. In this model, the house also has a thermostat; it does not overheat because when the temperature

SIGNAL RELATED TO IONIZED CALCIUM

- Although it is common to say that receptors "see" the concentration of ligands that bind to them, this is not technically true for the calcium-sensing receptor. Rather than concentration, one must think of *activity* when ions are concerned, and this is especially true for divalent ions such as Ca^{2+}.
- In the renal medullary interstitial compartment, the high concentration of electrolytes increases the ionic strength, which lowers the activity of ionized calcium at any given concentration of this electrolyte.

CONTROL BY SUBSTRATE SUPPLY

A substrate-driven control would be desired only if the goal were to remove oil rather than to achieve the desired temperature in the house.

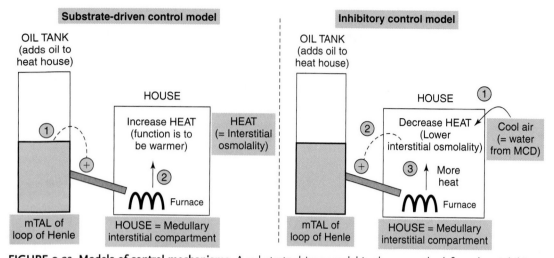

FIGURE 9-23 Models of control mechanisms. A substrate-driven model is shown on the *left*, and an inhibitory control model is shown on the *right*. The oil tank represents the medullary thick ascending limb (mTAL) of the loop of Henle, the house represents the medullary interstitial compartment, and the rise in temperature represents an increase in osmolality in the medullary interstitial compartment. In the inhibitory control model, the thermostat detects the temperature of the house (which represents the osmolality in the medullary interstitial compartment). If the temperature rises, a message is sent to stop the inflow of oil from the oil tank to the furnace. This message should persist as long as the temperature of the house is at or above the desired level. It is also noteworthy that the "single effect" in the renal medulla is to dilute the medullary interstitial compartment, and the response is to restore its composition to the original value very quickly by releasing the inhibition exerted on the mTAL of the loop of Henle. MCD, medullary collecting duct.

reaches a selected level, inhibitory controls stop the input of oil. That is, the mTAL of the loop of Henle reabsorbs Na^+ and Cl^- only *after* water is reabsorbed from the medullary collecting duct, and this reabsorption stops when the concentration of inhibitor returns to its original value.

Conclusions. If one adopts the inhibitory regulation model of control of the events in the renal medulla, two conclusions follow:

1. The new "single effect" is the reabsorption of water from the medullary collecting duct, which "dilutes" an inhibitor in the interstitial compartment, and this provides the signal to the mTAL of the loop of Henle to reabsorb the correct amount of Na^+ and Cl^- to raise the interstitial osmolality to its original value.
2. The loop of Henle does not function as a countercurrent multiplier (see Part D, page 308).

Regulation of the urine concentrating process in the inner medulla

The major functions of the inner medulla are:

- *Excrete urea without obligating the excretion of extra water.* For this to occur, urea must be an *ineffective* osmole in the luminal fluid in the inner medullary collecting duct.
- *Ensure that the urine volume is large enough when the urine contains few electrolytes.* To have a larger urine flow rate in this setting, urea must be an *effective* urine osmole.

Urea and the conservation of water

For urea to be an ineffective osmole in the urine, the concentration of urea must become equal in the inner medullary interstitial compartment and in the lumen of the inner medullary duct. This occurs when vasopressin causes the insertion of urea transporters into the luminal membrane of the inner medullary collecting duct. In addition, these transporters must permit urea to diffuse quickly enough to achieve equal concentrations in the luminal and interstitial compartments in the inner medulla when the urine has a sufficiently high concentration of electrolytes (Fig. 9-24). Also, a mechanism is needed to minimize the fall in the effective osmolality in the medullary interstitial compartment when urea and water are absorbed from the inner medullary collecting duct (discussed in the following paragraph).

Add Na⁺ and Cl⁻ to the inner medullary interstitial compartment to minimize the fall in its effective osmolality

- The "single effect" in the inner medulla is the absorption of urea *with water* from the inner medullary collecting duct; this reduces the concentration of Na⁺ and Cl⁻ as it adds water without electrolytes to the interstitium of the inner medulla.

Because the inner medullary collecting duct has *both* AQP2 and urea transporters in its luminal membrane when vasopressin acts, this nephron segment should be permeable to both water and urea if these channels are present and open. Therefore, the interstitial osmolality in this region *cannot* rise directly by reabsorbing urea from this nephron segment, because it is reabsorbed as an *iso-osmotic solution* (Fig. 9-25). Accordingly, the first step in this

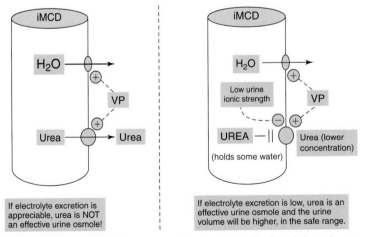

If electrolyte excretion is appreciable, urea is NOT an effective urine osmole!

If electrolyte excretion is low, urea is an effective urine osmole and the urine volume will be higher, in the safe range.

FIGURE 9-24 Urea and the conservation of water. The *barrel-shaped structure* represents the inner medullary collecting duct (iMCD). AQP2 are shown as a *green oval*, and the urea transporters are shown as a *green circle*. On the *left*, urea is an *ineffective* osmole in the inner medulla, and hence it does not obligate the excretion of water. On the *right*, urea may become an effective urine osmole when there is a low electrolyte concentration in luminal fluid (i.e., a low ionic strength; *see margin note*). VP, vasopressin.

UREA AS AN EFFECTIVE URINE OSMOLE
Urea can become an effective urine osmole if the maximum velocity for its reabsorption is exceeded by having a very large delivery of urea and/or if the urine is electrolyte poor; the latter diminishes the apparent permeability of the inner medullary collecting duct for urea even though vasopressin is present.

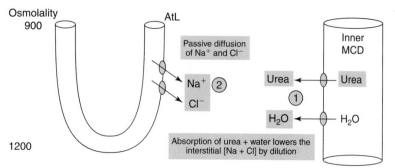

FIGURE 9-25 Events in the inner medulla. The *U-shaped structure* represents the thin limbs of the loop of Henle with its water-*permeable* descending thin limb (it has aquaporin 1 [AQP1]) and its water-*impermeable* ascending thin limb (AtL; it lacks AQP1) in the inner medulla. This latter limb has ion channels for Na^+ and Cl^- (*green ovals*). The driving force for the reabsorption of these ions is created by the fall in the interstitial concentration of Na^+ and Cl^- by dilution when an iso-osmolal urea solution (i.e., without Na^+ and Cl^- [*site 1*]) is reabsorbed from the inner medullary collecting duct (inner MCD; *large cylinder*). The addition of Na^+ and Cl^- *without* water to the interstitial compartment (*site 2*) raises its osmolality and electrolyte concentrations.

REABSORPTION OF Na^+ AND Cl^- IN THE ASCENDING THIN LIMBS OF THE LOH

- Since the luminal membrane of this nephron segment has channels for Na^+ and Cl^-, these ions will be absorbed passively when there is a favorable concentration difference (i.e., higher in the luminal fluid and/or lower in the interstitial compartment).

- A rise in the interstitial osmolality will cause water to be reabsorbed from the water-permeable descending thin limbs of the loop of Henle in the inner medulla, as they have AQP1. This results in higher luminal concentrations of Na^+ and Cl^-, which will facilitate the diffusion of these electrolytes into the medullary interstitial compartment.

process is a fall in the effective or non-urea osmolality in the inner medullary interstitial compartment by *"dilution" without a decrease in the interstitial total osmolality.* These lower interstitial concentrations of Na^+ and Cl^- create the driving force for the addition of Na^+ and Cl^- into this compartment from the water-impermeable ascending thin limb of the loop of Henle, as it is permeable to both Na^+ and Cl^-. After Na^+ and Cl^- diffuse from this nephron segment into the medullary interstitial compartment, this raises the interstitial total and its effective osmolality (*see margin note*). This is the *"passive single effect"* that raises the osmolality in the inner medullary interstitial compartment (see page 296 for more discussion of its impact on the deeper region of the outer medulla). Nevertheless, the concentrations of Na^+ and Cl^- must now be somewhat lower in both the ascending thin limb of the loop of Henle and the interstitial compartment after urea and water are reabsorbed.

Avoiding oliguria when the urine is electrolyte poor

- In this setting, urea must now be an effective osmole despite the presence of a urea transporter in the luminal membrane of the inner medullary collecting duct.

In this setting, the aim is to conserve water but also to ensure that the urine volume is not too low (see Fig. 9-24). Therefore, urea must become an effective urine osmole (i.e., have a higher concentration in the luminal fluid in the inner medullary collecting duct than in the renal medullary interstitial compartment). This must occur if this nephron segment is permeable to water (vasopressin acts) *and* if the osmolality resulting from electrolytes is higher in the interstitial compartment because the luminal fluid does not contain an appreciable quantity of electrolytes. Thus, the concentration of electrolytes and/or the ionic strength in the luminal fluid in the inner medullary ducts may lead to a signal that affects gating and/or adjust the number of active urea transport units in the luminal membrane.

Urea recycling in the nephron

- This is a critically important component to the function of the inner medulla to allow urea to be excreted without obligating the excretion of water.
- A reasonable estimate of the amount of urea that recycles each day is 900 mmol (i.e., equal to the filtered load of urea per day).

This process begins with the reabsorption of urea in the inner medullary collecting duct. For this to occur, there must be a high concentration of urea in the lumen of the inner medullary collecting duct and luminal transporters. The former is the result of a large delivery of urea to the distal nephron and the abstraction of water but not urea in upstream distal nephron segments prior to arriving at the inner medullary collecting duct when vasopressin acts (Fig. 9-26). Virtually all urea leaves the inner medulla via the ascending vasa recta, because little urea enters the descending thin limb and the ascending thin limb of the loop of Henle (*see margin note*).

Once in the outer medulla, urea enters the luminal compartment of the *lower one third* of the descending thin limbs of the loop of Henle of superficial nephrons, because this is the only nephron segment that has the urea transporter to permit the requisite high delivery of urea to the distal convoluted tubule. Of great importance, the site where urea enters the descending thin limbs of the loop of Henle is *deeper* in the outer medulla relative to the site where the bulk of water is added to this interstitial compartment (most of the water reabsorbed from the water-permeable nephron sites occurs

QUANTITATIVE ANALYSIS OF UREA RECYCLING
- Since the concentration of urea in the lumen of the early distal convoluted tubule of fed rats is ~50 mmol/L and the estimated daily volume delivered here in humans is 27 L/day, 1350 mmol of urea will be delivered to this nephron site (50 mmol/L x 27 L/day), if data from the rat can be extrapolated to humans.
- When eating a typical Western diet, human adults excrete 450 mmol of urea per day.
- Overall, urea recycling = delivery to the early DCT (1350 mmol/day) minus urea excretion (450 mmol/day) or 900 mmol/day.

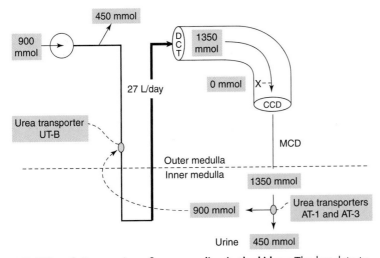

FIGURE 9-26 An overview of urea recycling in the kidney. The key data to assess this delivery of urea are derived from micropuncture experiments in fed rats in which the early distal convoluted tubule was sampled. There are two key measurements: First, the (TF/P)$_{Inulin}$ provided information to estimate the volume of filtrate delivered here (extrapolated to 27 L/day in a human adult); second, the content of urea in this fluid indicates that despite a large reabsorption of urea in the proximal convoluted tubule, more urea is delivered to this distal site than is filtered—this reflects entry of urea into the water-impermeable descending thin limbs of the loop of Henle of superficial nephrons with bends deep in the medulla (i.e., below the 600 mOsm/kg H$_2$O level).

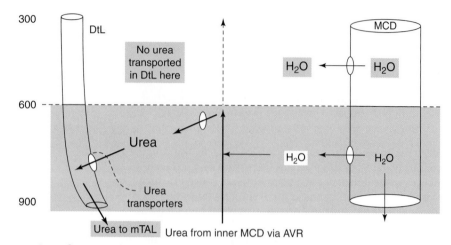

FIGURE 9-27 Sites of water reabsorption and urea recycling in the outer medulla. The descending thin limb (DtL) of the loop of Henle is the *thinner structure on the left*, the ascending vasa recta (AVR) is depicted in the *center*, and the medullary collecting duct (MCD) is the *cylinder on the right*. The *dashed line* represents a medullary osmolality of 600 mOsm/kg, and the *green shaded* area represents the site where most of the urea enters the DtL. In contrast, most of the water is reabsorbed in a more superficial area. Hence, this water does not wash most of the urea out of the interstitial compartment.

between interstitial osmolalities of 300 and 600 mOsm/kg H_2O), which markedly improves the efficiency of recycling of urea, as this minimizes the washout of urea from the medulla (Fig. 9-27). This would not be possible if the thin descending limbs had AQP1 and therefore a large amount of water was reabsorbed.

Integrative aspects

On one hand, the urine volume must be small to achieve water balance when there is a deficit of water. On the other hand, the urine volume must be high enough to decrease the risk of precipitation of poorly soluble constituents in the urine and thereby the formation of kidney stones (Table 9-10). To have a large enough volume of urine when vasopressin acts, the number of effective osmoles must increase in the urine. There are two major strategies that permit this to occur, and each depends on the setting.

Consumption of protein with little intake of water or salt. In this setting, urea is excreted, but the urine does not contain its usual content of effective osmoles (Na^+ and K^+ salts). Without another

SAFE MINIMUM URINE VOLUME

- A glance at Table 9-10 reveals that if the urine flow rate were 0.6 mL/min instead of 0.3 mL/min, the risk of forming precipitates in the urine would be markedly reduced. This strategy requires that there be a higher rate of excretion of effective osmoles when vasopressin acts.
- In this illustrative example, we did not take into account that when there is a decrease in the rate of excretion of Na^+ (e.g., a low salt intake or excessive loss of Na^+ in sweat, or during the overnight period), the rate of excretion of calcium may decline. Since there is only a modest decrease in the rate of excretion of citrate in the overnight period, the concentration of ionized calcium is significantly lower in the urine.

TABLE 9-10 EFFECT OF THE URINE FLOW RATE ON THE LIKELIHOOD OF PRECIPITATION CALCIUM OXALATE

For ease of illustration, the concentrations of Ca^{2+} and oxalate are assigned values of X and Y mmol/L, respectively, at a urine flow rate of 1.2 mL/min. Their ion product rises 4- and 16-fold when the urine flow rate halves to 0.6 mL/min and halves again to 0.3 mL/min despite the fact that the excretion rates for these ions are constant.

FLOW RATE (mL/min)	Ca^{2+} (mmol/L)	OXALATE (mmol/L)	Ca^{2+} × OXALATE
1.2	X	Y	XY
0.6	2 X	2 Y	4 XY
0.3	4 X	4 Y	16 XY

adaptation, the urine volume would be very small indeed if urea continues to be permeable (i.e., if urea remains as an ineffective osmole). In fact, experimental data in rats show that the inner medulla is not sufficiently permeable to urea when few electrolytes are being excreted and vasopressin acts (see Fig. 9-24, page 289). Hence, urea becomes an effective osmole in the urine in this setting and obligates the excretion of enough water to minimize the likelihood of precipitate formation.

Prolonged starvation. In this setting, the urine does not contain its usual effective osmoles (Na^+ and K^+ salts), and it contains little urea. Therefore, there is a need to generate new effective osmoles in the urine when there is little intake of water. This is accomplished by excreting NH_4^+ and β-hydroxybutyrate, which are effective osmoles in the urine. Because each mmol of urea has two nitrogens, and the excretion of 2 mmol of NH_4^+ is accompanied by the excretion of 2 mmol of β-hydroxybutyrate$^-$, excreting nitrogen wastes as NH_4^+ salts adds four osmoles instead of one if the nitrogen had been excreted as urea.

QUESTION

(Discussion on page 311)

9-9 *Two patients have a maximum U_{Osm} of 600 mOsm/kg H_2O when vasopressin acts. One of them has sickle cell anemia and papillary necrosis, whereas the other has a lesion that affects his outer medulla, but he has an intact papilla. Both patients eat the same diet and excrete 900 mosmol/day (urine osmoles are half urea and half electrolytes). Why do they not have the same minimum urine flow rate?*

PART D
INTEGRATIVE PHYSIOLOGY

RETENTION OF INGESTED WATER

Water intake is needed primarily to permit evaporative heat loss during periods of exercise. Because exercise and drinking water are not synchronous events, one must be able to store the ingested water for future sweat during exercise in a hot environment. There are two ways to retain ingested water.

1. Drink it slowly.
2. Drink it along with a large amount of a substance that is poorly absorbed in the small intestine, so water will be absorbed slowly, even if it was ingested rapidly. Therefore, this does not lower the P_{Na} sufficiently in the portal venous system (and hence the arterial P_{Na}) and thus it does not inhibit the release of vasopressin.

In this regard, the Paleolithic diet might have helped our primitive ancestors retain valuable water for future sweat loss because it consisted largely of fruit and berries. Hence, it was rich in the sugar fructose (fruit sugar). In the following section, we review the biochemistry of fructose.

A succinct review of the biochemistry of fructose

> • It is a great surprise that fructose, which constituted a large proportion of the calories consumed by our Paleolithic ancestors, is poorly absorbed in the intestinal tract. Therefore, it is likely that there are advantages for this physiology.

The possible benefits of having a slow absorption of fructose in the intestinal tract are discussed subsequently.

Production of valuable organic acids during fermentation of fructose in the colon

This topic was discussed in detail in Chapter 6, page 191. Butyric acid, for example, is an important fuel for the colon throughout the 24-hour period. Propionic acid is a potential source of the tricarboxylic acid cycle intermediate oxaolacetate in the heart when there is a low intake of carbohydrates. The most abundant of these organic acids is acetic acid; the advantages of its formation are discussed below.

Do not "flood" the liver with a load of glucose that is larger than this organ can remove in a single pass

ABBREVIATION
$P_{Glucose}$, concentration of glucose in plasma

The liver must be supplied with glucose at a rate that it can metabolize completely in a single pass; this keeps the $P_{Glucose}$ in arterial blood low enough to avoid glucosuria and thereby the loss of valuable Na^+ in an osmotic diuresis (as the Paleolithic diet had little NaCl). In this context, glucose that enters the portal vein is not diluted by the bulk of the ECF compartment before it is delivered to the kidney, where it is filtered. Furthermore, as discussed in Chapter 8, page 237, it is necessary to have a high GFR for the control system for the release of erythropoietin to function optimally. Hence, it is important to avoid having a $P_{Glucose}$ higher than 180 mg/dL (10 mmol/L) after meals to avoid glucosuria (*see margin note*).

Several strategies prevent an unwanted large rise in the $P_{Glucose}$ in arterial blood.

TUBULAR MAXIMUM FOR THE REABSORPTION OF GLUCOSE
The maximum amount of glucose absorbed in the proximal convoluted tubule is ~1.8 g (10 mmol) glucose per liter GFR.

1. When the $P_{Glucose}$ rises, a signal is sent to the stomach to slow gastric emptying (see Chapter 16, page 562 for more discussion).
2. Fructose represents half of the monosaccharide load in sucrose (the most common dietary disaccharide). Having a large proportion of the sugar load in the form of fructose rather than glucose avoids the delivery of more glucose to the liver than this organ can remove by metabolism in a single pass and hence this minimizes the rise in the $P_{Glucose}$ in arterial blood.
3. To have a rapid rate of removal of glucose, the controls that operate on the conversion of glucose to pyruvate in the liver must be bypassed. This is achieved when fructose is converted to acetic acid by fermentation in the colon. Metabolism of the short-chain fatty acids in the liver produces acetyl-CoA.
4. Pyruvate dehydrogenase is a key enzyme that limits the metabolism of pyruvate to its two major fates, the regeneration of ATP and the synthesis of storage fat (see Fig. 5-2, page 116). Bypassing this step by supplying acetic acid permits a slow and consistent input of substrate to make storage fat in the fed state and a brain fuel (ketoacids) early in fasting (see Chapter 5, page 117 for more discussion of this topic).

Increase the ability to retain ingested water

Because fructose is *poorly* absorbed in the intestinal tract, it causes water to be retained in the lumen of the intestine as a result of the higher luminal osmolality. This ensures that some of the ingested water is absorbed slowly. In addition, compounds in the diet that slow stomach emptying (e.g., lipids) will also convert rapidly ingested water into slowly absorbed water, increasing the likelihood that this water will be retained for future sweat and thereby be useful for heat dissipation.

INTEGRATIVE PHYSIOLOGY OF THE RENAL MEDULLA

- Our understanding of the physiology of both concentration and dilution of the urine must be revised owing to the following:
  - A reexamination of the original micropuncture data
  - The finding that AQP1 are not present in the majority of thin descending limbs of the loop of Henle.

Revised interpretation of micropuncture data

- We suggest that 150 L/day rather than 120 L/day are reabsorbed in the entire proximal tubule. Thus, 30 L/day rather than 60 L/day are delivered to the loop of Henle.
- This lack of AQ1 implies that the descending thin limbs of the loop of Henle of superficial nephrons are likely to be impermeable to water.

Two points must be kept in mind when interpreting micropuncture data. First, in the micropuncture procedure, fluid is withdrawn from nephron segments that are accessible on the renal cortical surface. Therefore, the last site that can be micropunctured in the proximal convoluted tubule is not the end of this nephron segment. In addition, this technique cannot obtain samples from deep nephrons. Second, isotonic saline is infused into anesthetized rats to maintain their blood pressure during these experiments (*see margin notes*).

The majority of the descending thin limbs of the loop of Henle lack AQP1

It has recently been identified that the descending thin limbs of the loop of Henle of those nephrons that do not enter the inner medulla (~85% of all nephrons) lack AQP1. Accordingly, the entire loop of Henle lacks AQP1 and is likely to be impermeable to water. Thus, the $(TF/P)_{Inulin}$ in luminal fluid in the early distal convoluted tubule, which is also impermeable to water, will reveal the volume of filtrate delivered to their loop of Henle. Because this value is close to 6, about five sixths of the GFR was reabsorbed in the *entire* proximal convoluted tubule (*see margin note*).

EXPANSION OF THE ECF VOLUME DURING MICROPUNCTURE EXPERIMENTS
Because anesthesia decreases the tone in venous capacitance vessels, it lowers the effective arterial blood volume. To overcome this problem, isotonic saline is infused, but the investigator does not know how much to infuse to avoid overexpansion of the effective arterial blood volume, which could induce changes in the renal handling of Na^+.

USE OF THE $(TF/P)_{Inulin}$
- Inulin is freely filtered and not reabsorbed or secreted by renal tubules. Thus, if the concentration of inulin is higher in tubular fluid than in plasma, this rise in concentration is due to the reabsorption of water between the glomerulus and the micropuncture site.
- Since the concentration of inulin at the site of micropuncture in the early distal convoluted tubule is sixfold higher than in plasma, only one sixth of the filtered water remains at this site of sampling. Hence, five sixths of the filtered water was reabsorbed up to here. Since the entire loop of Henle lacks AQP1, water cannot be absorbed between the end of the proximal and the beginning of the distal convoluted tubules. Therefore, five sixths of the filtrate is absorbed by the end of the proximal convoluted tubule (note that this micropuncture site is not the end of the proximal convoluted tubule).

Physiologic implications

1. *A smaller volume of filtrate is delivered to the loop of Henle than previously believed.* Therefore, there is a much smaller delivery of ionized calcium to the loop of Henle. This will be important when the risks for deposition of calcium salts in the renal medullary interstitial compartment (nephrocalcinosis) and the initiation of calcium-containing kidney stone formation are considered.

2. *During water deprivation, the inhibitory signals that modulate the reabsorption of Na^+ and Cl^- in the medullary thick ascending limb of the loop of Henle can only be influenced by the volume of water that is reabsorbed from the medullary collecting duct.* Therefore, signals in response to water reabsorption from the medullary collecting duct are not obscured by reabsorbing an order of magnitude more water from the descending thin limb of the loop of Henle. During a water diuresis, this same inhibitory control can be diminished by water that is reabsorbed from the medullary collecting duct via its residual water permeability; this can help desalinate the final urine.

3. *The rise in the concentrations of Na^+ and Cl^- in the descending thin limb of the loop of Henle in superficial nephrons is via addition of Na^+ and Cl^-.* This has both an advantage and a disadvantage.

   Advantage: This leads to a high concentration of Na^+ in the bend of the loop of Henle, which is required for the renal concentrating process to operate.

   Disadvantage: This addition of Na^+ requires an increased reabsorption of Na^+ from the medullary thick ascending loop of Henle. This seems to be a problem because it occurs in a region of the kidney with a low blood flow and a low hematocrit and hence an area that has a precarious delivery of oxygen. Nevertheless, this can be overcome, as we shall see in the following section.

A more detailed analysis of the concentrating process

- In the traditional analysis of the renal concentrating process, the focus is entirely on its ability to conserve water. In contrast, our emphasis includes a focus on the prevention of medullary damage due to hypoxia and by the precipitation of calcium salts.
- These two views can be thought of as opposite sides of the same coin because ionized calcium plays a central role in each of them.

Our first objective is to place the urine concentrating process in perspective by emphasizing that it has two major components: One is the ability to excrete urine with the highest osmolality (U_{Osm}) and the other is the ability to decrease the number of effective osmoles in the urine when vasopressin acts. This analysis must also be performed in quantitative terms.

1. *Deficit of water*: In human adults who consume a typical Western diet, if the urine total U_{Osm} were to decline by 50% (i.e., be 600 mOsm/kg H_2O instead of the usual 1200 mOsm/kg H_2O), the net result would be to excrete an extra 0.75 L of water per day (*see margin note*).

QUANTITATIVE PERSPECTIVE OF THE IMPORTANCE OF MAXIMAL WATER CONSERVATION

- Consider a human adult who has 37.5 L of water in his body. He remains in steady state by ingesting enough water to have a daily urine volume of 0.75 L/day because he excretes 900 mosmol/day and his maximum U_{Osm} is 1200 mOsm/kg H_2O. Hence his minimum daily urine volume is 0.75 L (i.e., 900 mosmol/1200 mOsm/L).
- If his medullary osmolality were to decline to 600 mOsm/kg H_2O, the U_{Osm} will also be 600 mOsm/kg H_2O and the urine volume will be 1.5 L/day (i.e., 900 mosmol/600 mOsm/L) when vasopressin acts.
- While having the same diet, water intake, and nonrenal losses, he would have a daily water deficit of 0.75 L. If this continues for 5 days, he would have a 10% deficit of water (5 days × 0.75 L/day = 3.75 L).
- Since there would be enough time for adaptations in brain cell volume, the impact on the degree of brain cell shrinkage will be much smaller.
- Therefore, although this ability to maximally conserve water is necessary in the long term, it is far less important in the short term.

2. *A decrease in the number of effective osmoles in the urine*: Urea becomes an ineffective osmole in the urine when vasopressin causes the insertion of urea transporters (act as urea channels) in the inner medullary collecting duct and when the urine contains the usual quantity of electrolytes. Said another way, the concentrations of urea in the urine and in the inner medullary interstitial compartment become virtually equal. Since urea accounts for half of the urine osmoles excreted each day, the urine volume is decreased by 50% due to urea becoming an ineffective osmole. This illustrates the importance of urea recycling in water conservation, but this is only one of the important contributions of urea recycling to the physiology of the renal medulla, as we shall stress later in this section.

While the stoichiometry; the presence of cotransporters, ion exchangers, ion pumps, and water; urea; and ion channels in all of the nephron segments in the renal medulla, as well as the unique countercurrent exchange blood supply, are all well known, it is still a mystery how this area is regulated in vivo. Moreover, all the models to predict how the outer and inner medullary areas carry out all of their functions have not been completely successful. Because of these problems, we provide a different view for regulation of urine concentrating mechanism. This view is based on a combination of a different emphasis on mechanism of regulation, the new findings concerning the absence of AQP1 in thin descending limbs of the loop of Henle, a reinterpretation of prior micropuncture data, and a central role for ionized calcium in the overall process. We emphasize that the concentrating process must be accomplished while preserving the integrity of the kidney (avoid anerobic metabolism, nephrocalcinosis, and luminal precipitation of calcium salts [*see margin note*]). Said another way, the conservation of water when there is a water deficit must be accomplished without creating a danger for the host or the kidneys.

Major dangers for the renal medulla

There are two important potential dangers for the renal medulla. First, there is a risk of forming precipitate of calcium salts in the lumen of the nephron and in the interstitial compartment; second, there is a risk of developing hypoxia in the deeper areas of the outer medulla, as this region has a marginal delivery of oxygen. Our hypothesis is that the inner medulla and the deep region of the outer medulla function as a coordinated unit to minimize these dangers.

Events in the inner medulla

There is one obvious difference between juxtamedullary nephrons (15% of the total nephrons), which descend into the inner medulla, and the superficial nephrons (85%), which do not enter the inner medulla—the descending thin limbs of the loop of Henle of juxtamedullary nephrons have AQP1 in their luminal membranes. Therefore, there is a rise in their luminal Na$^+$ (and calcium) concentrations due to water abstraction as one moves deeper into the renal medulla. In contrast, the descending thin limbs of the loop of Henle of superficial nephrons lack AQP1 in their luminal membranes; hence, the rise in their luminal Na$^+$ concentration as one descends deeper into the renal medulla is due to the addition of Na$^+$ and Cl$^-$. Thus, the juxtamedullary nephrons may have other unique properties that help them carry out their functions.

PRECIPITATION OF CALCIUM SALTS IN THE MEDULLARY INTERSTITIUM

- *Nephrocalcinosis*: This is the deposition of multiple small precipitates of calcium salts throughout the renal medullary interstitial compartment.
- *Deposition of apatite in the inner medulla*: The initial nidus for the formation of calcium oxalate stones in patients with idiopathic hypercalciuria is a precipitate of ionized calcium and trivalent phosphate on the basolateral membrane of the ascending thin limb of the loop of Henle in the inner medulla.

Central to the discussion to follow is the handling of HCO_3^- and the divalent cations, calcium, and magnesium in juxtamedullary nephrons. Nevertheless, since the proximal convoluted tubules of the juxtamedullary nephrons do not reach the surface of the kidney cortex, the composition of their luminal fluid cannot be measured using the micropuncture technique. Hence, there are no data that can be used to infer how much of the filtered water and ions are reabsorbed in this nephron site in the rat and in human subjects. Thus, deductive reasoning is required to obtain quantitative information about their functions.

Prevent the precipitation of calcium salts deeper in the renal medulla

- Two anions are most likely to form a precipitate with ionized calcium: divalent phosphate (HPO_4^{2-}) and carbonate (CO_3^{2-}); their concentrations rise when the pH of a solution becomes more alkaline. The important pH range for HPO_4^{2-} is close to its pK (~6.8) whereas even higher pH and HCO_3^- concentrations are needed to raise the concentration of CO_3^{2-} sufficiently to form a precipitate with ionized calcium.
- The pH of a solution of given volume and P_{CO_2} will be higher when it contains more HCO_3^-.
- The concentrations of all solutes in a solution rise when water is removed. Hence, the ion product of ionized calcium and HPO_4^{2-} or CO_3^{2-} may exceed their K_{sp} and thus form a precipitate in the luminal fluid in the deepest part in the renal medulla.

ABBREVIATION
K_{sp}: This is the solubility product constant for the activity of ions in a solution. When it is exceeded, a precipitate may form.

PERCENTAGE OF HCO_3^- REABSORBED IN THE PROXIMAL TUBULE OF SUPERFICIAL NEPHRONS
Filtered HCO_3^-: With a total GFR of 180 L/day and superficial nephrons representing 85% of the total nephrons, their GFR is 153 L/day (180 L/day × 0.85). With a P_{HCO_3} of 25 mmol/L, the filtered load of HCO_3^- in superficial nephrons is 3825 mmol/day.
HCO_3^- remaining at the end of the proximal tubules of superficial nephrons: Since the volume of filtrate delivered to the loop of Henle of these nephrons is 25.5 L/day (⅙ × 153 L/day) and if the concentration of HCO_3^- was ~12 mmol/L, the delivery of HCO_3^- to the loops of Henle of superficial nephrons would be close to 300 mmol/day.
% HCO_3^- reabsorbed in the proximal tubules of superficial nephrons: The value is 92% of the filtered load (100 × [3825 mmol/day − 300 mmol/day]/3825 mmol/day).

To understand the dangers in the renal medulla, we shall focus initially on the region that is at greatest risk—the bend of the loop of Henle near the renal papilla (i.e., at the 1200 mOsm/kg H_2O level in human subjects) in a setting where water must be conserved. Therefore, our first question is, "What are reasonable values for the composition of luminal fluid in those nephrons at the bend of the loop of Henle at the 1200 mOsm/kg H_2O level?"

If the composition of the fluid delivered to the loop of Henle was identical in both superficial nephrons and juxtamedullary nephrons, there will be a major danger of forming luminal precipitates of calcium phosphate ($CaHPO_4$) and calcium carbonate ($CaCO_3$) in the juxtamedullary nephrons.

Conundrum 1. A high luminal pH is a major risk factor for the formation of each of these precipitates. There is a major risk of forming luminal precipitates of $CaHPO_4$ and $CaCO_3$ in the juxtamedullary nephrons if the percent of $NaHCO_3$ reabsorbed in the proximal convoluted tubules of these nephrons is similar to that in the proximal convoluted tubules of superficial nephrons.

Reabsorption of $NaHCO_3$ in proximal tubules of superficial nephrons. In micropuncture studies in the fed rat, the pH of luminal fluid was considerably less than 7.4. For example, if this pH were 7.1 at the end of the proximal convoluted tubule, the concentration of HCO_3^- in luminal fluid would be approximately 12 mmol/L. Since only one sixth of the GFR of superficial nephrons reaches their loops of Henle, more than 90% of filtered HCO_3^- must be reabsorbed for the concentration of HCO_3^- in luminal fluid to be approximately 12 mmol/L (*see margin note*).

*Reabsorption of NaHCO₃ in proximal tubules
of the juxtamedullary nephrons*

> • If only 92% of filtered HCO_3^- were reabsorbed in the proximal
> tubules of the juxtamedullary nephrons, the pH of the luminal
> fluid in their loops of Henle at the 1200 mOsm/kg H_2O level
> would be ~7.7, and therefore there would be a very high risk of
> forming precipitates of $CaHPO_4$ and of $CaCO_3$.

The descending thin limbs of the loop of Henle of juxtamedullary
nephrons have AQP1 in their luminal membranes and thus water is
reabsorbed while they traverse the hyperosmolar medullary interstitial compartment. In quantitative terms, if the interstitial osmolality
rises from 300 mOsm/kg H_2O to 1200 mOsm/kg H_2O, three fourths
of the filtrate will be reabsorbed once the filtrate reaches the 1200
mOsm/kg H_2O level. Therefore, the concentration of HCO_3^- in this
fluid will be fourfold higher (i.e., it will be 48 mmol/L) and the pH
will be 7.7 if the interstitial P_{CO_2} is similar to that in the cortex. At
this high pH, the activities of HPO_4^{2-} and CO_3^{2-} along with that of
ionized calcium will exceed the K_{sp} for $CaHPO_4$ and for $CaCO_3$.

Resolution. Since appreciable precipitation of these calcium salts
must not occur, it is likely that more HCO_3^- is reabsorbed proximally
of juxtamedullary nephrons. In quantitative terms, to have a luminal
fluid pH of 7.1 in the descending thin limbs of the loops of Henle of
juxtamedullary nephrons at the 1200 mOsm/kg H_2O level, the quantity of HCO_3^- in the luminal fluid of these nephrons must be fourfold
lower than that in the superficial nephrons because of the fourfold
decrease in luminal fluid volume in the descending thin limbs of the
loops of Henle of juxtamedullary nephrons at this level in the inner
medulla. Therefore, about 98% of filtered HCO_3^- must be reabsorbed
in their proximal convoluted tubules.

**Another potential advantage of a large % reabsorption of HCO₃⁻ in
the proximal tubule.** In addition to avoiding a high pH in luminal
fluid in the descending thin limbs of the loops of Henle; there could
also be a decrease in the quantity of ionized calcium in the luminal
fluid at the bend of these loops of Henle. In more detail, when Na^+
and HCO_3^- are reabsorbed in the proximal convoluted tubules, water
follows and thus the volume of filtrate declines. As a result, the concentration of Cl^- rises in its luminal fluid, which provides a larger driving
force for its reabsorption, leaving the lumen with a small positive voltage. This in turn should increase the reabsorption of ionized calcium
and thereby lower the quantity of this divalent cation that is delivered
to the descending thin limbs of the loops of Henle of these nephrons.

Conundrum 2. The activity of ionized calcium and of HPO_4^{2-} in
the luminal fluid at the 1200 mOsm/kg H_2O level could be high
enough that, without another defense mechanism, $CaHPO_4$ would
precipitate in this location.

Resolution. A compound or ion should be present in luminal fluid
at the 1200 mOsm/kg H_2O level in the inner medulla to minimize
the risk of $CaHPO_4$ precipitate formation. We shall speculate that
the differential renal handling of ionized calcium and magnesium in
the proximal convoluted tubule and in the medullary thick ascending
limb of the loop of Henle may be important with respect to minimizing the risk of formation of potentially dangerous precipitates of
$CaHPO_4$ and $CaCO_3$ in the lumen and in the medullary interstitial
compartment at the 1200 mOsm/kg H_2O level.

Minimizing the precipitation of calcium salts; role of magnesium

> • The vast majority of ionized calcium is reabsorbed in the proximal convoluted tubule, whereas much less magnesium is reabsorbed in this nephron segment.
> • The major driving force to reabsorb ionized calcium in the proximal convoluted tubule is a higher luminal concentration secondary to the reabsorption of Na^+ and water. In contrast, the major driving force to reabsorb ionized calcium in the medullary thick ascending limb of the loop of Henle is a lumen-positive voltage. The reabsorption of ionized calcium is passive in both locations.
> • Magnesium may minimize the risk of formation of $CaHPO_4$ and $CaCO_3$ in the lumen of the loop of Henle in the inner medulla and of nephrocalcinosis deep in the outer medulla.

As background, the concentration of ionized calcium in plasma is more than twofold higher than that of ionized magnesium (1.25 mmol/L and ~0.5 mmol/L, respectively), as part of the total content of magnesium in 1 L of plasma is also bound to albumin. Nevertheless, by the time luminal fluid in the loop of Henle reaches the inner medulla, the concentration of magnesium becomes higher than that of ionized calcium, as most of the ionized calcium, but only a small proportion of filtered magnesium, is reabsorbed in the proximal convoluted tubule. As described earlier, even more ionized calcium may be reabsorbed in the proximal convoluted tubule of juxtamedullary nephrons owing to their small lumen-positive voltage.

Based on the increased product of the activities of ionized calcium with HPO_4^{2-} or CO_3^{2-} in the luminal fluid at the 1200 mOsm/kg H_2O level, it would be advantageous to have an inhibitor of these precipitation reactions in the luminal fluid in the inner medulla. Since magnesium forms ion complexes with both HPO_4^{2-} and CO_3^{2-} that have a K_{sp} that is at least three orders of magnitude higher than for their respective calcium salts, magnesium could diminish the risk of formation of these precipitates.

There is another benefit for the preferential reabsorption of magnesium in deep regions of the outer medulla. In more detail, HCO_3^- is added to this interstitial fluid secondary to the reabsorption of K^+ by the H^+/K^+-ATPase in the medullary collecting duct deeper in the medulla, and this will lead to a higher concentration of CO_3^{2-} in this location. Hence, the presence of a high concentration of magnesium in the interstitial compartment will decrease the likelihood of precipitation of $CaCO_3$ in the medullary interstitial compartment when ionized calcium is also reabsorbed in the medullary thick ascending limb of the loop of Henle. Preventing the precipitation of $CaHPO_4$ in the luminal fluid after much magnesium is reabsorbed in the medullary thick ascending limb of the loop of Henle becomes the task of Tamm Horsfall proteins that are secreted in this nephron segment (*see margin note*).

Nephron distribution in the deep region of the outer medulla. As background, very few thin limbs of loops of Henle of superficial nephrons descend into the medulla to the 900 mOsm/kg H_2O level, whereas those of all of the juxtamedullary nephrons descend into this region and into the inner medulla. Moreover, the ascending thin limbs of these nephrons do not lead directly into medullary thick ascending limbs as soon as they enter the outer medulla.

TAMM HORSFALL PROTEINS
• While Tamm Horsfall proteins permit concentrations of calcium salts that exceed their K_{sp} to remain in solution (i.e., not form precipitates), this protein is synthesized uniquely in the medullary thick ascending limb of the loop of Henle.
• Hence, a different factor is needed at the bend of the loop of Henle to minimize the formation of $CaHPO_4$ and $CaCO_3$.
• It will also be important to understand why Tamm Horsfall proteins are added after the site where it seems they were most needed.

With respect to the concentration of ions in the luminal fluid in the ascending thin limbs of the juxtamedullary nephrons, there is close to fourfold higher luminal calcium and magnesium concentrations because water was reabsorbed in their descending thin limbs throughout the medulla. Moreover, when the lumen-positive voltage develops in their medullary thick ascending limbs in the renal medulla, a relatively large amount of ionized calcium and magnesium could be added to a small volume of interstitial fluid deep in the outer medulla, which could lead to nephrocalcinosis if it occurred very quickly. Therefore, it is likely more than a coincidence that the ascending thin limbs of many of these nephrons do not lead directly into thick ascending limbs as soon as they enter the outer medulla. This extended length of ascending thin limbs will delay the addition of ionized calcium to the interstitial compartment to a level where more water is added from water-permeable nephron segments (Fig. 9-28).

Mechanisms to minimize work in the deep part of the outer medulla

- When there is an inadequate supply of oxygen, expect to find alternate ways to perform essential work (i.e., deliver more oxygen and/or regenerate ATP anerobically).

The rate of blood flow to the deeper region of the outer medulla should be high enough to deliver sufficient oxygen to permit the required rate of active transport of electrolytes (primarily Na^+ and Cl^-); nevertheless, it should be low enough to retain the high concentration of absorbed osmoles in the medullary interstitial compartment and to minimize the risk of formation of reactive oxygen species if there were a high local P_{O_2}. Blood delivered to the medulla has a low hematocrit. While this improves the blood flow rate owing to a reduction in viscosity, there may still be a low delivery of oxygen to deeper areas in the outer medulla. There is another limiting factor for the delivery of oxygen to these deeper areas: the shunting of oxygen from descending vasa recta to their ascending limbs in more superficial regions of the medulla, owing to its countercurrent exchange property.

Conundrum 3. There may not be enough oxygen delivered deep in the outer medulla to permit active reabsorption of the requisite quantity of Na^+ and Cl^-. Although anaerobic glycolysis permits ATP to be regenerated without the consumption of oxygen, it is unlikely to be a useful strategy for two reasons—first, there is also a low rate of delivery of glucose and second, one product of anaerobic glycolysis—H^+—may cause extensive local damage.

Resolution

- Passive reabsorption of Na^+ and Cl^- in inner medulla will replace the requirement for active reabsorption of Na^+ and Cl^- in the medullary thick ascending limbs of the loop of Henle deep in the renal outer medulla.
- A concentration difference for Na^+ and Cl^- is needed for passive reabsorption.

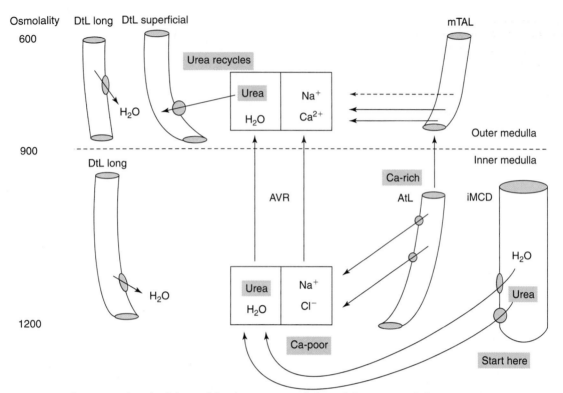

FIGURE 9-28 **Integrative physiology of the deep outer medulla and the inner medulla.** The analysis begins in the inner medulla (*below the horizontal dashed line*) in the lumen of the inner medullary collecting duct (iMCD), where urea (*circle*) and water (AQP2, *oval*) will be reabsorbed as an iso-osmotic solution; this will diminish the concentration of Na^+ and Cl^- in the medullary interstitial compartment and create the driving force for the entry of these electrolytes from the water-impermeable ascending thin limb of the loop of Henle (AtL) into the inner medullary interstitial compartment. All of the absorbed water from the iMCD and the descending thin limbs (DtL) of juxtamedullary nephrons along with the Na^+ and Cl^- reabsorbed from the AtL enter the ascending vasa recta (*arrow*) and are delivered to the deeper region of the outer medulla. Of great importance, this solution has a low ionized calcium concentration. Once in the deep outer medulla, the urea diffuses into the DtL of superficial nephrons as they have urea transporters and a low luminal urea concentration (shown to the *left*). Because of dilution of the interstitial ionized calcium activity, the reabsorption of luminal fluid in the medullary thick ascending limbs of the loop of Henle (mTAL) is stimulated (shown to the *right*). As a result, the luminal voltage becomes positive, which causes primarily the reabsorption of ionized calcium (and magnesium, not shown), as its luminal fluid has a particularly high concentration of these divalent cations (*solid arrows*). The net result is a diminished active reabsorption of Na^+ and Cl^- in this oxygen-poor region of the deep outer medulla (*dashed arrow*).

UREA RECYCLING
- It is arbitrary where to begin this description, because this is a cycle.
- Work is needed to achieve a high concentration of urea in the inner medulla to permit passive reabsorption of Na^+ and Cl^- in the inner medulla.
- This work is performed in the cortex and outer medulla, where there is an abundant supply of oxygen.

A lower concentration of Na^+ and Cl^- in the compartment where these ions will enter can be created by having fewer Na^+ and Cl^- or by the addition of a solution that does not contain Na^+ and Cl^-. In the latter case, this solution will have a high content of urea to prevent a fall in osmolality (see Fig. 9-28; *see margin note*).

Urea recycling has benefits other than conserving water in both the inner medulla and in the deeper regions of the outer medulla. First, it contributes to a diminished need for oxygen consumption deep in the renal outer medulla, as the large passive reabsorption of Na^+ and Cl^- in the inner medulla will replace the need for active reabsorption of Na^+ and Cl^- in the medullary thick ascending limbs of the loop of Henle deep in the outer medulla (*see margin notes on page 303 for a quantitative analysis*). The work needed to achieve a high concentration of urea in the inner medulla is the active reabsorption of

Na$^+$ and Cl$^-$ and thereby of water in the renal cortex and in the renal medulla near the cortex; the work occurs, however, in areas where there is an abundant supply of oxygen. Second, by virtue of reabsorbing a calcium-poor solution in the inner medulla, this process will diminish the concentration of ionized calcium in the interstitial compartment and thereby reduce the likelihood of developing nephrocalcinosis deeper in the outer medulla.

Events in the outer medulla

Minimize the work performed deep in the outer medulla, as there is a low delivery of oxygen to this region

Issues. Since there is a relatively small delivery of oxygen to deeper regions in the outer medulla, there is a need to minimize the work performed in this area.

Conundrum. A high activity of the inhibitor of active reabsorption of Na$^+$ and Cl$^-$ in the interstitial compartment is required; this inhibitor is likely to be ionized calcium. On the other hand, the fluid delivered to the interstitial compartment from the inner medulla and from the water-permeable descending limbs of the loop of Henle and the medullary collecting ducts is calcium poor, and this should stimulate the active reabsorption of Na$^+$ and Cl$^-$ in this region. There is one other contributor to this conundrum: There is a high concentration of ionized calcium in the luminal fluid of water-permeable juxtamedullary nephrons because water but not calcium was reabsorbed during their descent through the outer and inner medulla.

Resolution. The objective is to have a large input of ionized calcium to inhibit active reabsorption of Na$^+$ and Cl$^-$ in the medullary thick ascending limb of the loop of Henle in this oxygen-poor area. Notwithstanding, the mechanism to reabsorb ionized calcium is linked directly to the active reabsorption of Na$^+$ and Cl$^-$. Hence, there is a need to alter the stoichiometry of these events in the medullary thick ascending limb of the loop of Henle. Said another way, ionized calcium must be added with little active reabsorption of Na$^+$ and Cl$^-$. *This is why it is crucial to have high luminal concentrations of calcium and magnesium in the lumen of juxtamedullary nephrons.* In more detail, when the activity of ionized calcium in the interstitial compartment deep in the outer medulla falls due to the addition of water without calcium, the medullary thick ascending limb of the loop of Henle is stimulated, which increases its lumen-positive voltage. As a result, a much larger effect is exerted on the paracellular reabsorption of divalent as compared to monovalent cations because of the uniquely high luminal levels of ionized calcium and magnesium in juxtamedullary nephrons. Therefore, enough ionized calcium and magnesium will be reabsorbed to raise their activities in the medullary interstitial compartment sufficiently to induce a rapid inhibition of this active transport process in the medullary thick ascending limb of the loop of Henle. The net result is to limit the active reabsorption of Na$^+$ in this oxygen-poor region *(see margin note).*

Mechanisms to minimize the risk of precipitation of calcium salts in the outer part of the outer medulla

- The reabsorption of calcium should always follow the addition of water to the interstitial compartment to diminish the risk of developing nephrocalcinosis.

STEPS IN THE RECYCLING OF UREA

- *Add urea without water into the lumen of the descending thin limbs of the loop of Henle of superficial nephrons deep in the outer medulla:* The driving force is the high medullary interstitial urea concentration due to its reabsorption in the inner medullary collecting duct.
- *Raise the luminal concentration of urea in the final functional nephron unit:* The mechanism is to reabsorb water but not urea (AQP2 are present in their luminal membranes).
- *Reabsorb an electrolyte-free, iso-osmotic urea solution in the inner medullary collecting duct:* When this solution is added into the interstitial compartment in the inner medulla, there is a fall in the interstitial concentrations of Na$^+$ and Cl$^-$, which creates the driving force for their passive reabsorption from the ascending thin limbs of the loops of Henle in the inner medulla.
- *The reabsorbed fluid leaves the inner medulla in the ascending vasa recta:* Water, urea, Na$^+$, and Cl$^-$ are delivered to the deepest area of the outer medulla with a high concentration of urea and a low concentration of calcium.

QUANTITATIVE ANALYSIS OF EVENTS IN THE INNER MEDULLA

- *Urea:* Approximately 900 mmol of urea enter the inner medullary interstitial compartment in 1.5 L of water each day.
- *Water:* 1 L of water is reabsorbed from the inner medullary collecting duct, as most of the urea is reabsorbed close to the 900 mOsm/kg H$_2$O level. In addition, ~0.25 L of water is reabsorbed from the descending thin limbs of loops of Henle, and ~0.25 L of water is reabsorbed from the inner medullary collecting duct owing to the rise in osmolality from 900 mOsm/kg H$_2$O to 1200 mOsm/kg H$_2$O.

IONIC STRENGTH AND ION ACTIVITY
- When the concentration of all the electrolytes (ionic strength) is higher, the activity coefficient for all of the ions in a solution will be lower.
- Binding to receptors or the likelihood of forming precipitates depends on the activity rather than on the concentration of ions in a solution.
- This reduction in the activity coefficient is much more pronounced for divalent ions (e.g., calcium), as compared to monovalent ions (e.g., Na^+ or Cl^-).

ADDITION OF Na^+ AND Cl^- FROM THE INNER MEDULLA
- *Na^+*: 225 mmol of Na^+ and 225 mmol of Cl^- are reabsorbed passively from the ascending thin limbs of the loop of Henle in the inner medulla *without the need for the consumption of oxygen.*
- The final composition of the fluid that enters the outer medulla from the inner medulla via the ascending vasa recta is 1.5 L of water, 600 mmol of urea/L, 225 mmol of Na^+/L, and 225 mmol of Cl^-/L.

Issue. Mechanisms are needed to minimize the risk of precipitation of calcium salts in the outer medulla. A different strategy is required to minimize the risk of nephrocalcinosis in the more superficial area as compared to the one described above for the deeper region of the outer medulla.

Conundrum. There is a larger reabsorption of Na^+, Cl^-, and ionized calcium in the more superficial than in the deeper regions of the outer medulla. Hence, this addition of ionized calcium could increase the risk for nephrocalcinosis. In addition, when fluid with a high ionic strength and high calcium concentration is delivered from the deeper to the more superficial regions of the outer medulla via the ascending vasa recta, it is diluted with the large volume of water that is added from both the descending thin limbs of the juxtamedullary nephrons and from the medullary collecting ducts. This reduction in the ionic strength should increase the interstitial ionized calcium activity (*see margin note*).

Resolution. The first mechanism to decrease the ionized calcium activity is the large addition of water without ionized calcium to the medullary interstitial compartment. A quantitative analysis is provided in the *margin note.*

A second mechanism to diminish the risk of developing nephrocalcinosis is to reabsorb as little ionized calcium (and Na^+ with Cl^-) as possible from *individual* nephrons in this location. This will occur for two reasons: First, the lumen-positive voltage in each thick ascending limb of the loop of Henle is smaller; second, there are more nephrons above as compared to below the 600 mOsm/kg H_2O level (Fig. 9-29).

Quantitative analysis of Na^+ reabsorption in the renal outer medulla. The reabsorption of Na^+ in the outer medulla has two components: One is to replace the Na^+ and Cl^- that recycled into the descending thin limbs of the loop of Henle of superficial nephrons and the second is to add enough Na^+ and Cl^- into the medullary interstitial compartment to permit the water drawn from the descending thin limbs of the juxtamedullary nephrons and from the medullary collecting ducts to exit the renal medulla via the ascending vasa recta with a concentration of Na^+ equal to that in plasma.

Recycling of Na^+ and Cl^- in the renal outer medulla. As shown in Table 9-11, about 1400 mmol of Na^+ recycle per day in the outer medullary interstitial compartment nearer the renal cortex when the medullary interstitial osmolality rises progressively from its 300 mOsm/kg H_2O to its 600 mOsm/kg H_2O level. Owing to both fewer nephrons in the region below the 600 mOsm/kg H_2O level and the high interstitial urea concentration, much less Na^+ recycles in the deeper region of the outer medulla (~160 mmol/day). The assumptions to make this calculation are shown in the *margin note on page 305* and the rationale for quantitation of the role of urea is provided in the following paragraph.

As described previously, our best guess is that 1.5 L of water containing 900 mmol urea, 225 mmol of Na^+, and 225 mmol of Cl^- are transported from the inner medulla into the deep region of the outer medulla via the ascending vasa recta. In addition, we have assumed that the concentration of urea will be 100 mmol/L at the 750 mOsm/kg H_2O region (*see margin note*).

Reabsorption of Na^+ in the loop of Henle needed to convert the water reabsorbed in the medulla into isotonic saline. The statements in this shaded box are important in our calculations.

- The total volume of water reabsorbed in both the outer and inner medulla will enter the renal cortex as a solution that is isotonic to arterial plasma (150 mmol Na^+/L).

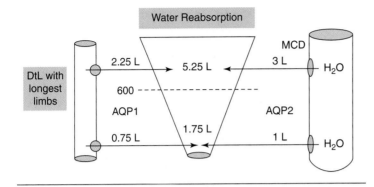

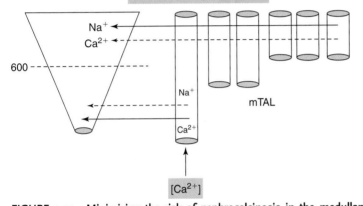

FIGURE 9-29 Minimizing the risk of nephrocalcinosis in the medullary interstitial compartment nearest the cortex. The *upper portion of the figure* depicts the reabsorption of water (volume is represented as a *triangular shape* because more water is reabsorbed above the *solid horizontal line*, which depicts the interstitial osmolality of 600 mOsm/kg H₂O). There is also an addition of 1.5 L of calcium-poor fluid that contains urea, Na⁺, and Cl⁻ from the inner medulla (not shown). The *lower portion of the figure* depicts the reabsorption of Na⁺, Cl⁻, and Ca²⁺ in the medullary thick ascending limb of the loop of Henle (mTAL). In the deeper region of the outer medulla, there is a small increase in reabsorption of Na⁺ and Cl⁻ (*dashed line*) and a relatively larger rise in the reabsorption of Ca²⁺ (*solid line*), as the mTAL units are largely from juxtamedullary nephrons, which have a three- to fourfold higher luminal concentration of ionized calcium.

TABLE 9-11 QUANTITATIVE ESTIMATE OF THE RECYCLING OF Na⁺ AND Cl⁻ IN THE RENAL OUTER MEDULLA

The assumptions made in these calculations were presented in the text. With a total GFR of 153 L/day in the superficial nephrons and five sixths of this volume reabsorbed in the entire proximal convoluted tubule, 25.5 L of the filtrate enter the loops of Henle. For the values provided, we assume that one fourth of the total number of superficial nephrons reach the 750 mOsm/kg H₂O level (*see margin note*).

LEVEL IN THE OUTER MEDULLA	VOLUME DELIVERED	↑ CONCENTRATION OF Na⁺	Na⁺ RECYCLED
450 mOsm/kg H₂O	19 L/day	75 mmol/L	~1430
750 mOsm/kg H₂O	6.4 L/day	25 mmol/L	160

- Focus on how much Na⁺ is added between the 600 mOsm/kg H₂O and 900 mOsm/kg H₂O levels in the outer medulla, bearing in mind that this is the area with the lowest supply of oxygen.
- Recognize how much Na⁺ is added to the region with the precarious supply of oxygen that was the result of passive reabsorption of Na⁺ in the inner medulla.

ASSUMPTIONS TO CALCULATE THE RECYCLING OF Na⁺ IN THE RENAL MEDULLA IN QUANTITATIVE TERMS

- If diffusion equilibrium were achieved for Na⁺ and Cl⁻, the concentration of each of these ions should rise in the luminal fluid until it is half of the osmolality at each horizontal plane.
- The quantity of Na⁺ and Cl⁻ that diffuses into an individual descending thin limb of a superficial nephron before it reaches its bend would be the same, independent of whether the rise in the concentration of Na⁺ is from 150 mmol/L to 165 mmol/L or from 250 mmol/L to 265 mmol/L.
- The interstitial concentration of urea is high, between the 600 mOsm/kg H₂O and the 900 mOsm/kg H₂O levels (the site where there are urea transporters in the descending thin limbs of the loop of Henle in superficial nephrons; this will influence the amount of recycling of Na⁺ in this region).
- If the interstitial concentration of urea were 100 mmol/L at the 750 mOsm/kg H₂O level in the outer medulla, the concentration of Na⁺ in this location would be half of the nonurea osmolality (650 mOsm/L), or 325 mmol/L.
- We assumed that all the recycling of Na⁺ in superficial nephrons between the 300 mOsm/kg H₂O and 600 mOsm/kg H₂O levels occurs at the 450 mOsm/kg H₂O level owing to the progressive decline in nephrons remaining as one proceeds deeper into the outer medulla.
- Similarly, we used the 750 mOsm/kg H₂O to calculate the amount of Na⁺ recycling between the 600 mOsm/kg H₂O and the 900 mOsm/kg H₂O levels (note that the concentration of Na⁺ is ~325 mmol/L at this point, as we assume that the concentration of urea at this level is 100 mmol/L).

Quantity of Na⁺ needed to make reabsorbed water into iso-osmotic saline throughout the renal medulla. A total of 8.5 L of water are added daily in the renal medulla (see Fig. 9-29). Hence, the total amount of Na^+ that must be added daily for this volume of water to exit the medulla in isotonic form is 1275 mmol/day (8.5 L/day $\times$ 150 mmol/L). In the sections to follow, the quantities of Na^+ added to the interstitial compartment of the outer medulla will be described, beginning with its deepest region.

Quantity of Na⁺ added between the 600 mOsm/kg H₂O and 900 mOsm/kg H₂O levels in the outer medulla. For simplicity, we performed this calculation at its midpoint (i.e., at the 750 mOsm/kg H_2O level). As discussed in the *margin note on page 305*, the concentration of Na^+ is 325 mmol/L at this level if the concentration of urea in the interstitial fluid is 100 mmol/L. Since 3.25 L/day of water enter this region (1.75 L/day + 1.5 L/day; see Fig. 9-29), close to 1050 mmol of Na^+ must be added to achieve the desired Na^+ concentration (325 mmol/L $\times$ 3.25 L/day). There are two sources of this added Na^+. First, 225 mmol of Na^+ were added via this passive route. Second, 825 mmol of Na^+ would need to be reabsorbed actively in the medullary thick ascending limb of the loop of Henle in this region (i.e., 1050 mmol/day – 225 mmol/day).

Quantity of Na⁺ added between the 300 mOsm/kg H₂O and the 600 mOsm/kg H₂O levels. Since the total amount of Na^+ that must be added is 1275 mmol/day, and since 1050 mmol of Na^+ were added daily below the 600 mOsm/kg H_2O level, 225 mmol of Na^+ must be reabsorbed actively between the 300 mOsm/kg H_2O and 600 mOsm/kg H_2O levels each day.

Total active reabsorption of Na⁺ in the renal medulla

1. *Recycling of Na⁺*: As shown in Table 9-11, the total amount of Na^+ recycling is about 1600 mmol/day; the vast majority of recycling occurs above the 600 mOsm/kg H_2O level.
2. *Conversion of added water into isotonic saline:* Overall, close to 1275 mmol of Na^+ must be added per day for this purpose, but 225 mmol of this addition of Na^+ occurs by passive reabsorption in the inner medulla. Therefore, 1050 mmol of Na^+ are added daily by active reabsorption in the entire outer medulla.
3. *Component of Na⁺ added deep in the outer medulla by active transport*: The majority of this transport is needed to convert added water into a solution with a concentration of Na^+ close to 325 mmol/L (825 mmol/day between 600 mOsm/kg H_2O and 900 mOsm/kg H_2O). In fact, most of this total reabsorbtion occurs closer to the 600 mOsm/kg H_2O level. Notwithstanding, in the deepest region, the addition of 255 mmol of Na^+ daily by passive reabsorption in the inner medulla decreases a large proportion of the work in an area with the most precarious supply of oxygen.

Clinical implications. When the amount of oxygen delivered to the renal medulla declines, the maximum urine osmolality falls appreciably. This is *initially* due to diminished recycling of Na^+, which is a way to diminish work in the medulla and prolong survival of cells of the medullary thick ascending limb of the loop of Henle, but it only has a modest effect deep in the renal outer medulla. Notwithstanding, when the medullary interstitial osmolality falls, less water is reabsorbed in medullary nephron segments that possess aquaporins. Hence, the amount of Na^+ reabsorption that is needed for water to exit the medulla in isotonic form is also reduced. In fact it is this second type of Na^+ reabsorption that is *quantitatively* more important to reduce active transport in the deepest region of the outer medulla, as discussed in the preceding paragraphs.

Based on the above, if one were to monitor the urine osmolality closely, a recent fall in this parameter may be a useful test to suggest that hypoxic injury to the renal medulla may be imminent. This may also be the time to administer an agent that will diminish Na^+ and Cl^- reabsorption in this nephron segment and/or a drug that selectively increases the blood flow rate to the medullary interstitial compartment. Moreover, these strategies may not be effective after the injury is established.

Concluding remarks

If one did not consider all of the components of the descriptions in the preceding sections, one might easily overlook its beauty. Perhaps the most important step is to avoid a linear analysis of the nephron (i.e., beginning at the glomerulus)—rather, we began our analysis with the area that is most vulnerable: the deepest regions in the renal outer medulla.

We emphasized how the deeper outer and inner medullary regions operate as a single functional unit, primarily to minimize the dangers related to the low delivery of oxygen. It is particularly important to include the passive reabsorption of Na^+ and Cl^- from the thin ascending limb in the inner medulla in this context.

Another major point in the analysis was to minimize the risks for nephrocalcinosis—its main tenet is to reabsorb water before ionized calcium is added to the medullary interstitial compartment. To minimize the likelihood of forming luminal precipitates of calcium salts in the deepest region of the inner medulla, the rate of reabsorption of filtered ionized calcium in the proximal convoluted tubule should be as high as possible, whereas the rate of reabsorption of filtered magnesium should be relatively low in this nephron segment. In addition, urea recycling and the absence of AQP1 were very important in this integrative analysis deep in the medulla so that all the parts can act in concert to accomplish an integrated function.

A CRITIQUE OF THE COUNTERCURRENT MULTIPLIER HYPOTHESIS

Traditional view

The basic tenet of the countercurrent multiplier hypothesis is that each medullary thick ascending limb of the loop of Henle at each horizontal plane in the outer medulla reabsorbs a relatively constant amount of Na^+. This implies that each nephron has a limited capacity to reabsorb Na^+ and Cl^-, which is set by an undefined mechanism.

Critique of the countercurrent multiplier model

As discussed in detail in the previous section on the integrative analysis of events in the inner and outer medulla, there is not a constant fixed quantity of Na^+ reabsorption in the medullary thick ascending limb of the loop of Henle at each horizontal plane. Moreover, calling this a countercurrent multiplier does not advance our understanding of the physiology of the concentrating mechanism. Thinking in terms of an inhibitory control system with a signal system that responds to the rate of reabsorption of water provides a better insight into this integrative system in the opinion of the authors.

DISCUSSION OF CASE 9-1

CASE 9-1: A RISE IN THE P_{Na} AFTER A SEIZURE

(Case presented on page 246)

What is the basis for the acute rise in his P_{Na}?

Because the gain of Na^+ is not of sufficient magnitude to explain this rise in P_{Na}, its basis is a loss of water from the ECF compartment. Nevertheless, there is no site for water loss, and hypernatremia resolved without administration of water. Therefore, the most likely explanation for this water loss from the ECF compartment is a shift of water into cells or into the lumen of the intestinal tract. Because of the history of a very recent seizure, the most likely site of water shift is into skeletal muscle cells (see Fig. 10-3, page 323). The driving force for this shift is a rise in the number of effective osmoles in skeletal muscle cells. Quantitatively, the breakdown of phosphocreatine to creatine and inorganic phosphate provides most of these osmoles. In addition, the breakdown of the macromolecule, glycogen, into many small molecules of L-lactic acid will also generate new osmoles, but only if their H^+ do not react with HCO_3^-, as there is no gain of osmoles (L-lactate anions replace intracellular HCO_3^-). Conversely, if some of the H^+ bind to proteins in these cells, there is an increase in the number of osmoles in the form of L-lactate anions in muscle cells. Because there is vigorous muscle activity (large production of CO_2) and a low blood supply during a seizure, there is a high tissue P_{CO_2}, and this promotes H^+ binding to proteins rather than reacting with HCO_3^- (Fig. 9-30).

There is an additional issue here. The P_{Na} in blood drawn from the brachial vein is much higher than in the rest of the body before a

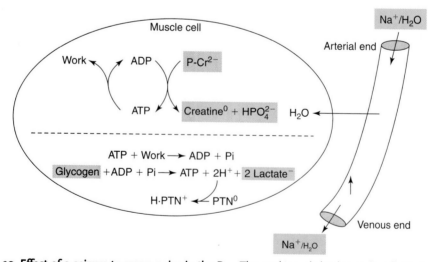

FIGURE 9-30 Effect of a seizure to cause a rise in the P_{Na}. The *oval* is a skeletal muscle cell. During a seizure, phosphocreatine is converted to creatine plus inorganic phosphate (*above the dashed horizontal line*) and glycogen is converted to many molecules of L-lactic acid as a result of the high concentration of ADP. In each of these processes, there are more molecules of the products than of the substrates. With regard to L-lactic acid, since there is a high production of CO_2 and a relatively low blood flow rate the tissue P_{CO_2} is high, many of the H^+ formed bind to proteins instead of titrating intracellular HCO_3, and there is a net rise in the number of new osmoles (L-lactate$^-$ anions) that can accumulate in these cells, as their H^+ are bound to proteins. This causes water to be drawn into cells from their capillary blood, which raises the capillary P_{Na} and thereby the venous P_{Na}.

steady state occurs. Hence, one would need to know the arterial P_{Na} to assess the impact of this hypernatremia on brain cell volume.

DISCUSSION OF QUESTIONS

9-1 *Hypertonic saline is the treatment of choice to shrink brain cell size in a patient with acute hyponatremia. What is the major effect of hypertonic saline to reduce the risk of brain herniation?*

When the P_{Na} is low, brain cells have an increased volume. Because brain cells occupy two thirds of the volume in the skull and there is a small volume of fluid to squeeze out (most of this volume of fluid is in ventricles of the brain), a point comes when intracranial pressure must rise. Hence, therapy must be directed at removing water out of the skull (not just shifting water from the ICF to the ECF compartment of the brain). Because the capillaries of the brain form tight junctions (called the *blood-brain barrier*), hypertonic saline acts like albumin when infused rapidly, and therefore water moves faster than Na^+ across the barrier. After this emergency therapy with the administration of a bolus of hypertonic saline, measures must be taken to prevent water from reentering brain cells (i.e., give more hypertonic saline or create a negative water balance).

9-2 *What would happen acutely to the ICF volume if the permeability of capillary membranes to albumin were to increase?*

There will be no change in the ICF volume because there is no change in the P_{Na}. Rather there will be a large fall in the intravascular volume and a relatively small rise in the interstitial fluid volume.

9-3 *What is the volume of distribution if 1 L of each of the following intravenous fluids is retained in the body: isotonic saline, half-isotonic saline, 300 mmol of NaCl/L, or 1 L of D_5W? What would the change in the P_{Na} be in a normal 50-kg subject who has 30 L of total body water before the infusion?*

The volumes of distribution are shown in the table below. The first step in this calculation is to assign the quantity of electrolytes into a solution of isotonic saline. The second step is to determine whether there is extra water or extra Na^+. If there is residual water, it will distribute in the body in proportion to the original compartment volumes. On the other hand, if there is residual Na^+, it will be retained in the ECF compartment and one must obtain a volume of water from the ICF compartment to make it become an isotonic solution. The glucose infused is assumed to be metabolized into $CO_2 + H_2O$ or be converted into storage compounds. In either case, the infused water that remains after the metabolism of glucose distributes in body compartments based on their original volumes (*see margin note for sample calculation for the addition of 300 mmol NaCl without water*).

SAMPLE CALCULATION: ADDITION OF 300 mmol NaCl AND 0 L OF WATER TO A 50-kg PERSON

- This person has 10 L of ECF and 20 L of ICF before these infusions.
- The quantity of osmoles added to the body is 600 mosmol (2 × 300 mmol NaCl per liter).
- The total number of effective osmoles in the body is equal to 2 P_{Na} + $P_{Glucose}$ in mmol/L terms (285 mOsm/L) × total body water (30 L) = 8550 mosmol, because the osmolality is equal in the ICF and ECF compartments.
- After adding 600 mosmol, the new osmolality in the body is (8550 + 600) ÷ 30 L = 305 mOsm/L.
- The number of osmoles in the ICF compartment does not change (20 L × 285 mOsm/L = 5700 mosmol). Hence, the new ICF volume is 5700 mosmol ÷ 305 mOsm/L = 18.7 L. The new ECF volume is its original volume (10 L) + 1.3 L that shifted from the ICF = 11.3 L. The new P_{Na} = the original quantity of Na^+ in the ECF compartment (1400 mmol; 10 L × 140 mmol/L) + 300 mmol Na^+ added = 1700 mmol ÷ 11.3 L = 150 mmol/L.

SOLUTION (1 L)	ECF VOLUME CHANGE	ICF VOLUME CHANGE	NEW P_{Na}
Isotonic NaCl	+ 1.0 L	0 L	140
Half-isotonic NaCl	+ 0.67 L	+ 0.33 L	138
300 mmol NaCl	+ 1.30 L	− 1.30 L	150
D_5W	+ 0.33 L	+ 0.67 L	136

9-4 *A person normally eats very little NaCl. When an extra 50 mmol of NaCl were added to the diet, this added Na⁺ was not excreted and there was a gain of weight of 0.6 lb (0.3 kg). Does this represent osmotic inactivation of Na⁺?*

No, if the Na^+ and Cl^- were retained with water, this is not osmotic inactivation of Na^+. In more detail, the gain of weight resulted from retention of water in the ECF compartment because there was no change in his P_{Na}. Therefore, his ECF volume is mildly expanded. In other words, this is a renal mechanism that permitted our Paleolithic ancestors to retain extra dietary Na^+ when there was an episodic intake of NaCl. They saved it for periods when they might develop a deficit of Na^+ because of their low intake of NaCl (i.e., minimize the danger of developing a low effective arterial blood volume).

9-5 *A patient retained ingested NaCl; Na⁺ entered cells while K⁺ exited to achieve electroneutrality. The K⁺ that shifted out of cells and the extra Cl⁻ in the ECF compartment were excreted in the urine. Would this represent osmotic inactivation of Na⁺?*

No, this is not osmotic inactivation of Na^+. In more detail, while intracellular K^+ are excreted with the ingested Cl^-, Na^+ is still in the body in an osmotically active form—it simply replaces K^+ in cells. Nevertheless, there is a physiologic problem with this process—there would need to be a mechanism to prevent the extra intracellular Na^+ from being pumped out of cells by the Na-K-ATPase.

9-6 *When a normal volunteer increased his intake of NaCl from 200 mmol/day to 600 mmol/day for a number of days, there was a large positive balance of Na⁺ but there was no change in weight or in the P_{Na}. Might this represent osmotic inactivation of Na⁺?*

Yes, these data do suggest osmotic inactivation of NaCl. To be sure, one would need to confirm that K^+ balance is not altered. Nevertheless, this experiment represents *pathophysiology*, so one must be cautious about extending the conclusions to normal physiology. In more detail, the response to a very large intake of NaCl is not one that developed in Paleolithic times. Therefore, it might represent the "stealing" of a component of a control mechanism that had another function.

9-7 *What might the significance be of having the reabsorption of NaHCO₃ as the first form of Na⁺ reabsorption in the proximal convoluted tubule?*

When Na^+ and HCO_3^- are reabsorbed in this water-permeable nephron segment, there is no change in the luminal concentration of Na^+ because water is also reabsorbed. Because close to 90% of filtered HCO_3^- is reabsorbed, however, there is a large fall in the concentration of HCO_3^- in luminal fluid. Moreover, the concentration of Cl^- rises in the luminal fluid as a result of the fall in its volume with no change in the content of Cl^-. This altered luminal anionic composition favors an exchange of Cl^- (exit) and HCO_3^- (entry) in the lumen, catalyzed by a luminal Cl^-/HCO_3^- exchanger. In addition, this entry of HCO_3^- now supplies the luminal H^+ acceptor for the Na^+/H^+ exchanger in the luminal membrane. The luminal carbonic anhydrase removes the H_2CO_3 that is formed to complete the cycle

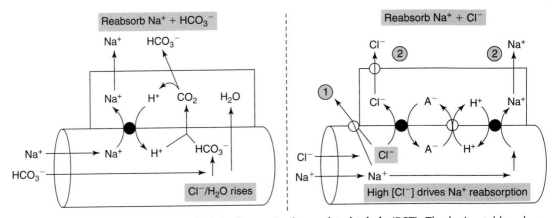

FIGURE 9-31 Reabsorption of Na$^+$ and Cl$^-$ in the proximal convoluted tubule (PCT). The *horizontal barrel* represents the PCT. The initial event is to reabsorb Na$^+$, HCO$_3^-$, and water as an iso-osmotic solution (*left*); this raises the concentration of Cl$^-$ in the lumen because the volume decreases. The higher concentration of Cl$^-$ in the luminal fluid (*rectangle*) provides the driving force to reabsorb Cl$^-$ and secondarily, Na$^+$. Two possible mechanisms are illustrated *on the right*. First, Cl$^-$ diffuses between the cells, down its concentration difference, which causes a small lumen-positive voltage to drive the passive paracellular reabsorption of Na$^+$ (*site 1*). Second, the high concentration of Cl$^-$ in the lumen drives an exchange with organic anions, including formate (A$^-$). When H$^+$ are secreted by NHE, formic acid is formed in the lumen, and this acid can enter cells of the PCT, completing a cycle that leads to the net reabsorption of Na$^+$ and Cl$^-$ (*site 2*). A similar effect will result if Cl$^-$ were exchanged with HCO$_3^-$.

(Fig. 9-31). The net result is the net reabsorption of Cl$^-$ and Na$^+$ in a 1:1 stoichiometry. There may also be an anion exchange where formate is the anion that is exchanged with Cl$^-$.

9-8 *Consider the following thought experiment: A man in steady state consumes and excretes 300 mosmol of electrolytes (150 mmol Na$^+$ + 150 mosmol Cl$^-$) and 1 L of water. If he were to ingest an extra 300 mosmol of electrolytes without additional water, and if this extra 300 mosmol of electrolytes were excreted and his body tonicity did not change, it must be excreted in a hypertonic form. What would the change be in his body composition if his maximum urine osmolality due to electrolytes was 600 mOsm/L on one day and 400 mOsm/L on another day?*

In the first setting, the extra 300 mosmol of electrolytes could be eliminated in his usual 1-L urine volume because the urine tonicity can rise from 300 to 600 mOsm/L (Fig. 9-32).

In the second setting, because the maximum urine tonicity is 400 mOsm/L, he can add only 100 mosmol of electrolytes to the original 1 L of urine. Therefore, to excrete the remaining 200 mosmol of electrolytes at a tonicity of 400 mOsm/L, *without* causing a change in body tonicity, he must excrete another 600 mosmol of electrolytes and 2 L of water (see Fig. 9-32). Therefore, this results in a loss of 2 L of ECF volume. Note that in both settings, the amount of extra electrolytes (300 mosmol) that need to be excreted in a *hypertonic form* is identical, but the urine tonicity is appreciably different (600 vs. 400 mOsm/L).

9-9 *Two patients have a maximum U$_{Osm}$ of 600 mOsm/kg H$_2$O when vasopressin acts. One of them has sickle cell anemia and papillary necrosis, whereas the other has a lesion that affects his outer*

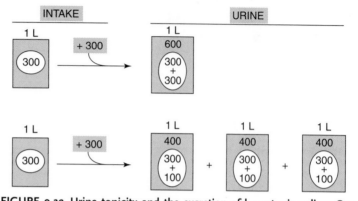

FIGURE 9-32 Urine tonicity and the excretion of hypertonic saline. One liter of urine is depicted as a *rectangle*; the osmolality due to Na⁺ salts in each liter is shown in an *oval* inside the rectangle, with its osmolality due to hypertonic Na⁺ salts written as the second line in the oval. The subject usually excretes 300 mosmol of Na⁺ salts and 1 L of water. In the first setting (*top*), the urine osmolality due to Na⁺ salts may rise to 600 mOsm/L, whereas in the second setting (*bottom*), it may rise to only 400 mmol/L. The extra 300 mosmol of electrolytes are ingested without water. Therefore, the final urine volume is 1 L in the first setting and 3 L in the second setting to excrete an extra 300 mosmol of Na⁺ salts in a hypertonic form without a change in body tonicity.

medulla, but he has an intact papilla. Both patients eat the same diet and excrete 900 mosmol/day (urine osmoles are half urea and half electrolytes). Why do they not have the same minimum urine flow rate?

There are two factors that influence the urine flow rate when vasopressin acts—the number of effective osmoles in the luminal fluid of the inner medullary collecting duct and the effective osmolality of the fluid in the medullary interstitial compartment. To illustrate the importance of each of these factors, consider the patient who has sickle cell anemia. In this disorder, there is obstruction of the blood vessels by sickled cells that descend into the inner medulla. As a result, there is necrosis of the renal papilla. Because the inner medullary collecting duct is the nephron site where vasopressin causes the insertion of urea transporters, urea cannot be reabsorbed in the inner medullary collecting duct at appreciable rates in this patient when vasopressin acts. Therefore, urea becomes an *effective* osmole in this setting and it obligates the excretion of water. In addition, if urea cannot be reabsorbed as an iso-osmotic solution in the inner medullary collecting duct, this prevents the passive reabsorption of Na⁺ and Cl⁻ from the ascending thin limb of the loop of Henle. Accordingly, the maximum medullary interstitial osmolality is likely to be close to 750 mOsm/L (*see margin note*). If this patient excreted 900 mosmol/day and all of the urine osmoles are effective, the minimum urine volume would be close to 1.2 L/day. Of greater importance, the absence of appreciable urea recycling will decrease the number of osmoles delivered to the late cortical distal nephron and thereby the volume delivered to the nephron segments that secrete K⁺. As a result, they may have a lower maximum rate of excretion of K⁺ when they ingest a large quantity of fruit and vegetables (see Chapter 13, page 446 for more details).

Contrast these numbers with the second subject who has a similar osmole excretion rate (half urea, half electrolytes) and who has a

EFFECTIVE URINE OSMOLES IN A PATIENT WITH SICKLE CELL ANEMIA

- One can easily calculate the effective osmolality due to nonurea osmoles.
- Since many of the urea transporters may have been destroyed, it is reasonable to assume that urea does not achieve diffusion equilibrium in the inner medulla and make this calculation in total osmole terms rather than effective osmole terms.

normal papilla but a maximum effective U_{Osm} that is 450 mOsm/kg H_2O. After vasopressin acts, urea transporters are present in the inner medullary collecting duct and the concentration of urea is equal in the lumen of the inner medullary collecting duct and in the papillary interstitial compartment. Since urea is not an effective urinary osmole in this setting, the rate of excretion of effective osmoles is half of 900 mosmol/day or 450 mosmol/day. Accordingly, the daily urine volume would be 1.0 L (450 effective mosmol ÷ 450 effective mOsm/L), somewhat less than in the patient with sickle cell anemia and papillary necrosis.

chapter **10**

Hyponatremia

Introduction

HYPONATREMIA
- This is a concentration term; it is the number of mmol of Na^+ per liter of ECF.
- The P_{Na}, however, reflects the ICF volume, but in an inverse fashion.

Hyponatremia is present when the P_{Na} is less than 136 mmol/L (*see margin note*). The major danger with each type of hyponatremia is a primary emphasis in this chapter.

1. *The patient with acute hyponatremia*: The danger in this setting is swelling of brain cells; this causes an increase in the intracranial pressure and may lead to herniation of the brain, which can occur abruptly. This constitutes a critical medical emergency, and

measures must be taken *immediately* to remove water from inside the cranium.

2. *The patient with chronic hyponatremia:* The danger to avoid in this setting is a large and rapid rise in the P_{Na}, which causes shrinkage of brain cells and ultimately can lead to osmotic demyelination. The major etiologic factor is a large water diuresis owing to the disappearance of actions of vasopressin and/or a large increase in the distal delivery of filtrate.

OBJECTIVES

- To emphasize that hyponatremia is a diagnostic category and *not* a single disease. Hence, treatment should be tailored to the specific pathophysiology in each patient.
- To emphasize that hyponatremia may be due to either a decrease in the content of Na^+ or the retention of water. The former is more important in patients with SIAD, whereas the latter is the major component of SIADH (*see margin note*).
- To emphasize that a low effective P_{Osm} implies that the intracellular fluid (ICF) volume is expanded. If the time course is greater than 48 hours, brain cells have had time to export enough effective osmoles to return their size toward normal.
- To emphasize that, from a clinical perspective, hyponatremia should be divided into three categories based on whether it is acute, chronic, or chronic with an acute component; this has important implications for the design of therapy.
  1. When hyponatremia is acute (i.e., <48 hours), the major risk is an increase in intracranial pressure, which may lead to brain herniation. Urgent therapy with hypertonic saline is needed to draw water out of the cranium.
  2. When hyponatremia is chronic (i.e., >48 hours) and there is no acute element, the major risk related to hyponatremia is the development of osmotic demyelination from too rapid a rise in the P_{Na}. If a water diuresis is likely to occur, consider giving dDAVP at the outset of therapy (*see margin note*).
  3. When an acute element of hyponatremia is present in a patient with chronic hyponatremia, the P_{Na} must be raised quickly to lower intracranial pressure, but this rise should not exceed the set upper limit for the rise in P_{Na} over a 24-hour period to avoid causing osmotic demyelination.

ABBREVIATIONS
P_{Na}, concentration of Na^+ in plasma
P_K, concentration of K^+ in plasma
$P_{Glucose}$, concentration of glucose in plasma
$P_{Albumin}$, concentration of albumin in plasma
P_{Osm}, osmolality in plasma
SIAD, syndrome of inappropriate antidiuresis
SIADH, syndrome of inappropriate antidiuretic hormone
AQP, aquaporin water channels
ODS, osmotic demyelination syndrome

CLASSIFICATION OF LOW EXCRETION OF WATER
SIAD: The major pathophysiology is a low distal delivery of filtrate.
SIADH: This diagnosis cannot be made if there is a low distal delivery of filtrate. In essence it is the permanent presence of AQP2 in the late distal nephron; hence, it is always permeable to water.

DESMOPRESSIN (dDAVP)
dDAVP is a chemically modified form of vasopressin in which there is a loss of the terminal NH_3 group (desamino) and a switch of L-arginine to D-arginine. These changes increase its duration of action (i.e., it acts for 6 to 36 hours).

CASE 10-1: THIS CATASTROPHE SHOULD NOT HAVE OCCURRED!

(Case discussed on page 361)

A 25-year-old woman (weight 50 kg) developed central diabetes insipidus 18 months ago—there was no obvious cause for the disorder. Treatment consisted of dDAVP to control her polyuria and maintain her P_{Na} close to 140 mmol/L. Her current problem began after she developed the "flu" one week ago; this was followed by a persistent dry cough. To alleviate her symptoms, she sipped ice-cold liquids. Because she felt progressively less well over time, she visited her physician yesterday afternoon. There was a new finding, a close to 3-kg (7-lb) weight gain. Accordingly, her P_{Na} was measured, and it was 125 mmol/L.

Although she was advised by her physician not to drink any fluids and to go to the hospital immediately, she waited until the next morning before acting on this advice. On arrival in the emergency room, she had a mild headache. There were no other new findings on physical examination, but unfortunately, her weight was not measured. Her laboratory data are summarized in the following table:

		PLASMA	URINE
Na^+	mmol/L	112	100
K^+	mmol/L	3.9	50
Cl^-	mmol/L	78	100
BUN (Urea)	mg/dL (mmol/L)	6(2.0)	120 mmol/L
Creatinine	mg/dL (μmol/L)	0.6 (50)	0.6 g/L (5 mmol/L)
Glucose	mg/dL (mmol/L)	90 (5.0)	0
Osmolality	mOsm/kg H_2O	230	420

Questions

What dangers are present on admission?

What dangers should be anticipated during therapy, and how can they be avoided?

PART A
BACKGROUND

REVIEW OF THE PERTINENT PHYSIOLOGY

The plasma Na^+ concentration

- The P_{Na} reflects the ICF volume, whereas the content of Na^+ determines the extracellular fluid (ECF) volume.

EFFECTIVE OSMOLES
Effective osmoles are those that cause water to move across cell membranes because they are largely restricted to one compartment (e.g., Na^+, glucose, or mannitol in the ECF compartment).

Although hyponatremia may result from either a negative balance for Na^+ and/or a positive balance for water, a negative balance of Na^+ is more important for patients with SIAD, whereas a positive balance of water is more important for patients with SIADH. Hyponatremia is associated with an expanded ICF volume unless its basis is a gain of effective osmoles in the ECF compartment (e.g., glucose or mannitol; Fig. 10-1; *see margin note*). The ECF volume, on the other hand,

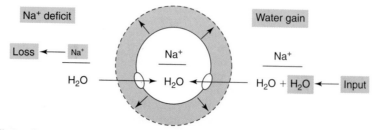

FIGURE 10-1 Cell size during hyponatremia. The *circle depicted with the solid line* represents the normal intracellular fluid (ICF) volume. Independent of whether the basis for hyponatremia is a deficit of Na^+ (*left*) or a gain of water (*right*), the ICF volume is increased (*dashed circle line, filled in green*). The *ovals* represent aquaporin 1 (APQ1) water channels in the cell membrane.

may be increased (if the basis of hyponatremia is a positive water balance) or decreased (if the basis of hyponatremia is a negative Na^+ balance).

The term *pseudohyponatremia* is used when the ratio of Na^+ to plasma water and the effective P_{Osm} are normal, but the ratio of Na^+ to the total volume of plasma is low because of an increase in the nonaqueous volume of plasma (e.g., as a result of hyperproteinemia and/or hyperlipidemia; *see margin note*).

The P_{Na} reflects the intracellular fluid volume

The physiology of the distribution of water across cell membranes is based on four facts. First, cell membranes are permeable to water because AQP1 are always present in cell membranes of most cells; accordingly, water moves rapidly to osmotic equilibrium. Second, the effective osmoles in the ECF compartment that keep water out of cells are Na^+ and its attendant anions, Cl^- and HCO_3^-. Third, the effective osmoles in the ICF compartment that keep water in cells are K^+ and a number of small organic compounds for the most part. Fourth, intracellular osmoles rarely change in amount (except in brain cells in response to an acute change in brain cell volume); accordingly, changes in the ICF volume are inversely proportional to the changes in P_{Na} in most circumstances (*see margin note*).

The content of Na^+ determines the extracellular fluid volume

Because Na^+ is an osmole that is largely restricted to the ECF compartment, it keeps water out of cells; thus the content of both Na^+ and its attending anions (Cl^- and HCO_3^-) determine the ECF volume.

Renal response to a deficit or a surplus of water

- Beware! With rapid ingestion of a large water load, the P_{Na} "seen" by the brain (the arterial P_{Na}) may be much lower than the P_{Na} in brachial venous plasma (*see margin note*).

A high P_{Na} (water deficit in cells of the osmostat) is the primary stimulus for the release of vasopressin. Another stimulus for the release of vasopressin is a low effective arterial blood volume. This volume, however, must decrease by almost 10% to cause the release of this hormone in subjects consuming a typical Western diet, as they have a high intake of NaCl and thereby have an expanded effective arterial blood volume to provide the signal to cause the excretion of this NaCl. There are also nonosmotic stimuli for the release of vasopressin (e.g., nausea, pain, anxiety).

Once a water load leads to a fall in the arterial P_{Na} and the absence of circulating vasopressin, the late distal nephron loses its luminal AQP2 channels. As a result, a large water diuresis ensues. The limiting factor for the excretion of water in this setting is the volume of filtrate delivered to the distal nephron and the amount of water reabsorbed in the inner medullary collecting duct by pathways that are independent of vasopressin (see the discussion of residual water permeability in Chapter 9, page 277). The distal delivery of filtrate may be low if there is a low glomerular filtration rate (GFR) and/or a contracted effective arterial blood volume and hence an enhanced reabsorption of Na^+ and water in the proximal

PSEUDOHYPONATREMIA
- This is present when the laboratory result for the P_{Na} is lower than the P_{Na} in the patient. In fact, it is always present when measurements are made on diluted samples of plasma because plasma has close to 7% nonaqueous volume (lipids and proteins). Hence, the true P_{Na} is 152 mmol Na^+ per liter or kg H_2O, whereas the reported value is 140 mmol/L plasma volume, which includes its nonaqueous volume.
- A greater degree of pseudohyponatremia will be observed when plasma contains more lipid and/or protein, but only if the plasma sample is diluted prior to assay.

HYPONATREMIA WITH A LOW ICF VOLUME
This may occur when hyponatremia is due to retention of effective osmoles in the ECF compartment (e.g., hyperglycemia, mannitol infusion).

ARTERIAL VERSUS VENOUS P_{Na}
- As discussed in Chapter 9, page 281, shortly after the rapid ingestion of a large water load, the arterial P_{Na} (the P_{Na} that is "seen" initially by all cells in the body) is appreciably lower than the venous P_{Na} (the P_{Na} that is measured in clinical practice).
- There will be a more severe degree of acute swelling in brain cells than in muscle cells owing to a larger blood flow per unit mass. The presence of brain cell swelling may not be suspected if one relies on only the venous P_{Na}.

U_{Osm} **DURING A WATER DIURESIS**

- Consider two subjects who excrete urine with a U_{Osm} that is much less than the P_{Osm}, indicating that vasopressin is not acting.
- Each patient excretes 600 mosmol/day. Subject 2 has a lower distal delivery of filtrate. Notice the difference in the values for their U_{Osm}.

SUBJECT	URINE VOLUME	U_{Osm}
1	10 L/day	60
2	5 L/day	120

LOSS OF INTRACELLULAR ANIONS IN THE BRAIN IN RESPONSE TO CHRONIC HYPONATREMIA

- It is not clear which anions are lost with K^+ in this process.
- Neuronal cells do not have enough Cl^- to be exported with K^+. If HCO_3^- were the anions lost with K^+, there would be serious changes in intracellular pH.
- It is possible that glial cells (which in fact constitute the bulk of cells in the brain [~80%]) do have enough Cl^- to be exported with K^+.

OSMOTIC DEMYELINATION SYNDROME

- This disorder may be observed after therapy for chronic hyponatremia, if the P_{Na} increases too rapidly.
- The process of osmotic demyelination commonly involves the base of the pons.
- Clinically, there is a wide spectrum of presentations, ranging from the absence of symptoms to a devastating disorder characterized by confusion, agitation, and, eventually, flaccid or spastic quadriparesis. This disorder may be accompanied by bulbar involvement.
- The diagnosis can be confirmed by magnetic resonance imaging, including coronal views.
- There is no known treatment, and the mortality and morbidity rates are high.

convoluted tubule (see Part D, page 350 for more discussion of this topic).

The appropriate renal response to an excess of water is to excrete the largest possible volume (~10–15 mL/min or ~16 L/day) of maximally dilute urine (~50 mOsm/kg H_2O; *see margin note*). If this response is not observed, suspect that vasopressin is acting and/or that the distal delivery of filtrate is low (see Case 12-1, page 410).

Regulation of brain volume

- Since water cannot be compressed, a positive balance of water in the skull will cause an abrupt large rise in intracranial pressure.
- Acute hyponatremia is associated with swelling of brain cells.
- When hyponatremia is present for longer than 48 hours, adaptive changes have proceeded sufficiently to shrink the volume of brain cells back toward their normal size.

The adaptive responses when brain cells swell are different in patients with acute versus chronic hyponatremia.

1. *Acute hyponatremia:* The most important issue in this setting is that there will be a gain of water in brain cells. Initially, there is a small rise in intracranial pressure, which results in the expulsion of fluid from ventricles in the brain, and this minimizes the rise in intracranial pressure. Once additional water enters brain cells due to a fall in P_{Na}, the patient is at great risk for herniation of the brain. Therefore, urgent therapy is needed.

   When brain cells swell acutely by close to 15%, these local defense mechanisms can be overcome. Therefore, a further fall in the P_{Na}, even if it is small in degree, can be very dangerous. Because of the physical restriction to swelling imposed by the rigid skull, the cerebral cortex is pushed down on the bony margin of the foramen magnum, veins become compressed, and venous outflow declines. The arterial pressure, however, is large enough to permit the continued inflow of blood, and intracranial pressure rises abruptly. This leads to serious symptoms (seizure, coma) and quickly thereafter to respiratory arrest and irreversible brain damage, unless a sufficient volume of water is removed rapidly from the skull to lower the intracranial pressure (see the section on therapy for more information, page 323).

2. *Chronic hyponatremia:* The major adaptive change to brain cell swelling in this setting is to export effective osmoles from brain cells (Fig. 10-2). Approximately half of the particles exported are electrolytes (K^+ + an anion from the ICF; *see margin note*), and the other half are organic solutes of diverse origin. When hyponatremia is present for longer than 48 hours, adaptive changes have proceeded sufficiently to shrink the volume of brain cells back toward their normal size. Therefore, if the P_{Na} rises rapidly in this setting, brain cells will shrink because water leaves the ICF compartment and this could cause osmotic demyelination (*see margin note*). To restore these essential intracellular osmoles that were exported from the ICF during volume regulation requires both time and a good dietary intake. Hence, it is not surprising that patients with chronic hyponatremia who are also malnourished and/or potassium depleted are at increased risk for osmotic demyelination if their P_{Na} rises too much and/or too rapidly. Accordingly, the

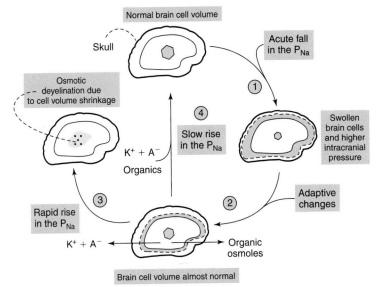

FIGURE 10-2 Changes in brain cell volume in a patient with hyponatremia. The *structure* represents the brain; its ventricles are depicted as *hexagons* and the *bold line* represents the skull, which limits expansion of the brain. When the P_{Na} falls, water enters brain cells, and there is a rise in intracranial pressure (ICP; *site 1*). This rise in ICP squeezes the ventricles and their fluid, and some of the extracellular fluid exits from the skull. As the P_{Na} approaches 120 mmol/L, the danger of herniation mounts enormously. If, however, the fall in P_{Na} has been more gradual (*site 2*), adaptive changes have time to occur (export K^+ salts and organic molecules), and brain cell size is now close to normal despite the presence of hyponatremia. If the P_{Na} rises too quickly at this stage, osmotic demyelination may develop (*site 3*; *black spots in the gray shaded area; see margin note*). If, however, the rise in the P_{Na} occurs over a much longer period, brain cells return to their normal size and composition (*site 4*).

THEORIES TO EXPLAIN THE DEVELOPMENT OF OSMOTIC DEMYELINATION

- The most common theory is that demyelination may be caused by the slow recovery of the organic osmoles such as myoinositol and taurine. This results in shrinkage of neuronal cells when the P_{Na} rises rapidly, which strips off their long myelin sheath and leads to cell damage. Oligodendrocytes are particularly vulnerable.

- Another theory is that a rapid rise in $P_{Effective\ osm}$ disrupts the blood-brain barrier, which leads to the influx of complement and other inflammatory mediators that damage cells that support the maintenance of the myelin tracts.

- Microglia may play an important role in this pathophysiology; they have been shown to accumulate in the areas of demyelination and produce inflammatory cytokines.

maximum for the allowable rate of rise of P_{Na} should be even lower in these patients (see page 347).

BASIS OF HYPONATREMIA

Although vasopressin may be present and acting, a severe degree of acute hyponatremia is not common because normal subjects will not ingest an enormous volume of water when the thirst center is intact and mental function is normal (Table 10-1). Therefore, in a patient with acute hyponatremia, one must look for a reason why so much water was ingested while there should be an aversion to drink water. In fact, most cases of acute hyponatremia occur in a hospital setting, particularly in the perioperative period, and hence this defense mechanism of aversion to drinking large amounts of water is bypassed with the intravenous administration of fluids.

In a patient with chronic hyponatremia, the major pathophysiology is a defect in the excretion of water (Table 10-2). This may be primarily due to a low distal delivery of filtrate (and, at times, the presence of vasopressin) in patients with SIAD; one usually finds an appreciable contraction of the ECF volume (*see margin note*). In the absence of a low distal delivery of filtrate, the diagnosis is SIADH.

LARGE DEFICIT OF Na⁺
In patients with a very low ECF volume (SIAD), there will be a large deficit of Na⁺ (e.g., patients with adrenal insufficiency or those consuming little NaCl while being treated with a diuretic). Hyponatremia in these patients is due primarily to a large deficit of Na⁺; the patients may also have a small positive balance for water (see Mini-Cases 10-1 and 10-2, page 361).

TABLE 10-1 CAUSES OF A LARGE INPUT OF WATER IN A PATIENT WITH HYPONATREMIA

In these patients, look for a reason why the aversion to drink water was "ignored." Also, look for a reason for a decreased rate of excretion of water (e.g., release of vasopressin [see Table 10-2] and/or a low distal delivery of filtrate).

A very large intake of water

- Aversion to water intake is suppressed by mood-altering drugs (e.g., Ecstasy)
- Drinking too much water during a marathon (e.g., owing to poor advice to avoid dehydration)
- Beer potomania
- Psychotic state (e.g., paranoid schizophrenia)

A large infusion of D_5W

- Postoperatively (especially in a young patient with a low muscle mass)

Large infusion of hypotonic lavage fluid

- Input of water and organic solutes, with little or no Na^+ (e.g., hyponatremia following transurethral resection of the prostate)

Generation and retention of electrolyte-free water ("desalination")

- Excretion of a large volume of hypertonic saline due to a very large infusion of isotonic saline or the use of a thiazide diuretic plus a stimulus to excrete Na^+ (e.g., effective arterial blood volume expansion) while vasopressin acts

TABLE 10-2 CAUSES OF A LOWER THAN EXPECTED RATE OF EXCRETION OF WATER

Lower rate of water excretion due to low distal delivery of filtrate (SIAD)

- States with a very low glomerular filtration rate
- States with enhanced reabsorption of filtrate in the proximal convoluted tuble (e.g., a low intake of salt, loss of Na^+ and Cl^- in sweat [e.g., patients with cystic fibrosis, a marathon runner], via the gastrointestinal tract [e.g., infants with diarrhea], or via the kidney [diuretics, aldosterone deficiency, renal or cerebral salt wasting])

Vasopressin release and a normal distal delivery of filtrate (SIADH)

- Nonosmotic stimuli including pain, anxiety, nausea
- Central stimulation of vasopressin release by drugs, including Ecstasy, nicotine, morphine, clofibrate, tricyclic antidepressants, antineoplastic agents such as vincristine, cyclophosphamide (probably via nausea and vomiting)
- Central nervous system or lung lesions (e.g., neoplasm, granulomatous disease such as tuberculosis)
- Exogenous administration of dDAVP (e.g., for urinary incontinence, treatment for diabetes insipidus)
- Glucocorticoid deficiency (see margin note)
- Hypothyroidism (see margin note).

BASIS FOR VASOPRESSIN RELEASE IN PATIENTS WITH:

- *Glucocorticoid deficiency:* When there is a deficit of cortisol because of an adrenal or anterior pituitary disorder, corticotropin-releasing factor is high. This hormone leads to the production of adrenocorticotropic hormone (ACTH) *and* vasopressin.
- *Hypothyroidism:* A possible mechanism is a low effective arterial blood volume resulting from decreased cardiac output, but this may not be the sole mechanism.

PART B
ACUTE HYPONATREMIA

CASE 10-2: THIS IS FAR FROM "ECSTASY"!

(Case discussed on page 361)

Amy-Sue, age 19, suffers from anorexia nervosa. She went to a "rave" party, where she took the drug Ecstasy. Following advice from others at the party, she drank a large volume of water that night to avoid "dehydration" from excessive sweating. As time progressed she began to feel unwell—her main symptoms were lassitude and an inability to concentrate. After lying down in a quiet room for 2 hours, her symptoms did not improve and she developed a headache. Accordingly, she was brought to the hospital. In the emergency department, she had a grand mal seizure. Blood was drawn immediately after the seizure and the major electrolyte abnormality was a P_{Na} of 130 mmol/L; metabolic acidosis (pH 7.20, P_{HCO3} 10 mmol/L) was also present.

Questions

Is this acute hyponatremia?
Why did she have a seizure if the P_{Na} was 130 mmol/L?
What role might anorexia nervosa play in this clinical picture?
What is your therapy for this patient?

CLINICAL APPROACH

- The clinical approach has three steps (Flow Chart 10-1):
  1. Deal with emergencies.
  2. Anticipate dangers that may develop during therapy.
  3. Proceed with diagnostic issues.

Deal with emergencies

- Beware if a patient with hyponatremia has symptoms that might be related to an increase in intracranial pressure because this is a *superacute* medical emergency demanding urgent therapy to shrink the volume inside the skull.

Is the patient symptomatic?

The symptoms that develop when brain cells swell are often very subtle in an early stage. Beware if there is a mild headache or a decrease in attention span. When the rise in intracranial pressure is somewhat greater, the patient may become drowsy and mildly confused and may

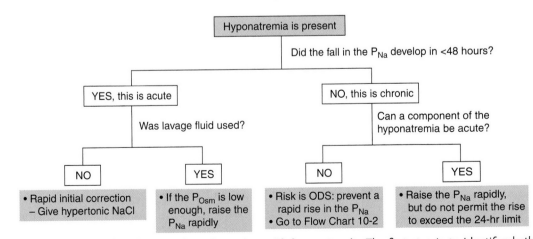

FLOW CHART 10-1 Clinical approach to the patient with hyponatremia. The first step is to identify whether hyponatremia is acute. Aggressive therapy is also needed in the patient with chronic hyponatremia if there are symptoms to suggest an acute component to the hyponatremia. ODS, osmotic demyelination syndrome.

complain of nausea. At a later stage, there may be a major degree of confusion, decreased level of consciousness, vomiting, or even coma. Notwithstanding, the time period for the transition between early mild symptoms and later severe symptoms may be very brief. Accordingly, the golden rule is, "Treat the patient with acute hyponatremia aggressively with hypertonic saline even if he or she has only mild symptoms."

Degree of acute hyponatremia

If a patient clearly has acute hyponatremia and the P_{Na} is 130 mmol/L or lower (this cutoff is an arbitrary one), we would treat this patient with hypertonic saline even if there are no symptoms for the following reasons:

1. Since it is very likely that the P_{Na} was drawn from a brachial vein, the P_{Na} in capillaries of the brain (reflected by the arterial P_{Na}) may be much lower.
2. There may be a recent, large intake of water that is currently in the stomach and may be absorbed soon and cause a major fall in the arterial P_{Na}.
3. If the patient has a small muscle mass, a smaller intake of water can create a larger fall in the arterial P_{Na} and thereby a greater degree of brain swelling, which results a large rise in intracranial pressure.
4. If a patient has a space-occupying lesion inside the skull (e.g., a tumor, infection [meningitis, encephalitis], a subarachnoid hemorrhage, or edema following recent neurosurgery), a smaller degree of brain cell swelling can lead to a dangerous rise in intracranial pressure.
5. If a patient has an underlying seizure disorder, a smaller degree of an acute fall in the P_{Na} can provoke a seizure.

Caution

In the initial phase during the use of lavage solutions, an acute and large fall in the P_{Na} may not be associated with significant brain cell swelling *providing that* the solute involved remains largely outside brain cells; this is suggested by the absence of a significant fall in the P_{Osm} (the topic of acute hyponatremia following lavage fluid retention is discussed on page 325 in this chapter).

Diagnostic issues

POSITIVE WATER BALANCE IN PATIENT WITH ACUTE HYPONATREMIA
The volume of water that must be retained to cause acute hyponatremia is large:
- A 50-kg person has 30 L of water.
- If the P_{Na} is ~120 mmol/L, there is a positive balance of 15% of body water.
- 15% of 30 L = 4.5 L

- Acute hyponatremia is almost always due to a large positive balance of water (*see margin note*).
  - The emphasis in the diagnosis is on the source of the water.
  - Look for a reason why the usual aversion to drink a large volume of water was ignored or bypassed.
  - A low rate of excretion of water must also to be present (look for a reason for the release of vasopressin and/or a low distal delivery of filtrate).

A major clue to suspect acute hyponatremia is the presence of symptoms that may be related to brain swelling (e.g., decrease in attention, confusion, lethargy, headache, nausea, seizure). Another important clue is the recent intake of a large volume of water (*see margin note*) in the presence of a setting where its excretion is diminished (see Table 10-2). Conversely, not all episodes of acute hyponatremia are associated with a dangerous rise in intracranial pressure (e.g., hyponatremia due to retained lavage fluid). The clue here is the absence of a large fall in the P_{Osm} (see page 325 for more discussion).

THERAPY OF ACUTE HYPONATREMIA

> • In a symptomatic patient with acute hyponatremia, give a bolus of hypertonic saline to raise the P_{Na} by 5 mmol/L even if the symptoms are mild (*see margin note*).

The amount of NaCl administered is calculated based on the assumption that NaCl will distribute as if it were mixing with total body water. In fact, the rise in arterial P_{Na} will be to a much greater degree in the initial period when hypertonic saline is infused rapidly, as this infusate will not yet have mixed with the total volume of body water. In the absence of obesity, the quantity of NaCl to administer is a 3 mmol/kg body weight (*see margin note*). At least one third of this dose should be given over the first 10 to 15 minutes and the remainder should be infused over the rest of the first hour. A faster rate of infusion may be needed depending on severity of symptoms. The infusion of hypertonic saline should continue at a slower rate thereafter, with a goal of raising the P_{Na} to close to the normal range in the next several hours (*see margin note*). The P_{Na} should be followed closely, as it may fall again if there is addition of water that was "hidden," for example, in the GI tract or in muscle after seizures.

Cautions

1. Another cause for the neurologic symptoms should be suspected if they persist after the P_{Na} has risen by 5 mmol/L.
2. If water was ingested and some may still be in the intestinal tract, there could be a sudden fall in the arterial P_{Na} with devastating results when that water is absorbed. Watch carefully for even a mild headache, as one cannot predict when this will occur.
3. Do not draw blood from a vein draining muscle shortly after a seizure, as this P_{Na} may not reflect the degree of brain cell swelling (Fig. 10-3).
4. One must be confident that there is no component of chronic hyponatremia to raise the P_{Na} to close to 140 mmol/L in approximately

RATIONALE FOR THE USE OF HYPERTONIC SALINE
- The immediate goal is to draw water out of the skull quickly. Therefore, the hypertonic solute must not exit from the capillaries at the blood-brain barrier at an appreciable rate (i.e., it must be given rapidly).
- Give enough solute quickly to return the P_{Na} to a level at which there are no symptoms of high intracranial pressure (raise P_{Na} by 5 mmol/L).
- After achieving this acute shift of water, continue the hypertonic infusion to prevent this water from returning back inside the skull.

CALCULATION
- Water is ~60% of body weight. Hence each kg has 600 mL of water.
- To raise the P_{Na} by 5 mmol/L in 600 mL (0.6 L), give 0.6 × 5 mmol/L or 3 mmol/kg body weight.

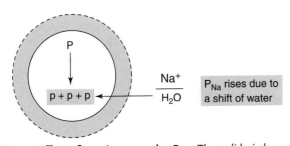

FIGURE 10-3 Effect of a seizure on the P_{Na}. The *solid circle* represents the normal muscle cell size with its complement of macromolecules (P). With vigorous exercise or a seizure, macromolecules are hydrolyzed into a greater number of smaller particles (p), and osmolality rises in the intracellular fluid compartment. This causes water to shift into muscle cells (*green area and dashed circle*), raising the P_{Na}.

24 hours. There is little if any risk of inducing osmotic demyelination if hyponatremia was present for less than 24 hours.

SPECIFIC CAUSES

Populations most at risk

- Patients who have more brain cells per volume of the skull (younger age) need a smaller decrease in their P_{Na} to have a rise in the intracranial pressure due to brain cell swelling (especially if their ECF volume within the skull is also increased).
- Patients with a smaller muscle mass develop a greater degree of hyponatremia for a given volume of retained water (*see margin note*).
- Patients with meningitis, encephalitis, or a brain tumor have less room for brain cell swelling, so they are at greater risk with acute hyponatremia.
- Patients with an epileptogenic brain lesion may be more likely to develop a seizure with a milder degree of hyponatremia.

Premenopausal women are said to be at greater risk for the development of brain cell swelling from acute hyponatremia. This is thought to be due to hormonal factors that lead to less efficient brain adaptation to changes in its cell volume. Although this may be the case, other factors including their younger age (more brain cells per volume of the skull) and smaller body size are perhaps more important. One should also note that the most common setting for the development of acute hyponatremia in adult males is the infusion of lavage fluid during a TURP. As is explained later, the hyponatremia in this setting is not usually associated with as large a degree of brain cell swelling, at least in its early phase.

Clinical settings in which acute hyponatremia develops in the hospital

Perioperative hyponatremia

- This is a common setting for the development of acute and potentially life-threatening hyponatremia.

In this setting, vasopressin is present for a number of reasons (e.g., underlying illness, anxiety, pain, nausea, and administration of drugs; see Table 10-2). These patients have two obvious sources of water. First, the most common is the intravenous administration of glucose in water (D$_5$W, virtually always a mistake; *see margin note*) or hypotonic saline (virtually always a mistake as well in the perioperative period). Second, the "kindly" provision of ice chips or sips of water (also a mistake in the perioperative period) may provide a large water load. Another source of water that may not be obvious is when isotonic saline is administered, and Na$^+$-poor water is generated and retained in the body by the excretion of urine with a very high concentration of Na$^+$. We call this process *desalination* of a saline solution (Fig. 10-4). Several liters of isotonic saline are usually administered in the perioperative period of even simple surgical procedures to maintain blood pressure and a "good" urine output. If the NaCl is excreted

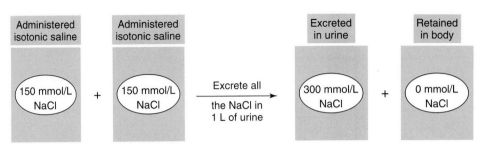

FIGURE 10-4 Desalination: Making saline into water. The *two rectangles to the left* represent two 1-L volumes of infused isotonic saline. The concentration of Na$^+$ in each liter is shown in the *ovals inside the rectangles*. The fate of the infused isotonic saline is divided into two new solutions as shown to the *right*. Because of the actions of vasopressin, all of the NaCl that was infused (300 mmol) is excreted in 1 L of urine. Therefore, 1 L of pure water is retained in the body.

(because of the expanded effective arterial blood volume) in *hypertonic* urine (as a result of presence of actions of vasopressin), water is retained in the body. Patients with small body size are particularly likely to develop a more serious degree of acute hyponatremia.

Prevention of acute hyponatremia in perioperative setting. The cautions needed to avoid perioperative hyponatremia are summarized in Table 10-3. The message concerning the input is this: *Do not give water to a patient who has a defect in water excretion.* The message concerning the output is this: *A "good" urine output is a danger sign for development of acute hyponatremia if that urine is hypertonic.*

In the circumstance in which there is a large infusion of isotonic saline (e.g., patients with a ruptured cerebral aneurysm causing a subarachnoid hemorrhage), as well as the excretion of urine with a high concentration of Na$^+$, one must prevent a fall in the P_{Na} by maintaining a tonicity balance. That is, the volume of water infused should be equal to the urine volume, and the concentration of Na$^+$ + K$^+$ in the intravenous solutions should be equal to the concentration of Na$^+$ + K$^+$ in the urine (Fig. 10-5). One may achieve this goal by decreasing the U_{Na} + U_K with the use of a loop diuretic while infusing isotonic saline at the same rate as the urine output.

Hyponatremia due to retained lavage fluid

- This type of acute hyponatremia occurs primarily in elderly males undergoing TURP. Large volumes of lavage fluid that contain organic solutes (e.g., glycine), but not Na$^+$, are used during surgery (*see margin note*).
- The clinical picture is complicated because neurologic symptoms may result from toxicity from NH$_4^+$ produced during the metabolism of glycine rather than from brain cell swelling.

USE OF LAVAGE FLUID DURING TURP
- When TURP is performed, the large venous plexus of the prostate is likely to be cut.
- Electrocoagulation is used to minimize blood loss. A large volume of lavage fluid is usually washed over the site of bleeding to permit better visualization. To make this safe, the lavage fluid must be electrolyte free (to avoid sparks when cautery is used to stop the bleeding), and therefore organic solutes are used. The lavage fluid may enter the venous blood because of the higher pressure in the urinary bladder.
- Glycine is a preferred solute because its solution is clear (nontranslucent). NH$_4^+$ may be produced at a high rate during the metabolism of glycine, with severe metabolic consequences.

TABLE 10-3 **DIAGNOSIS AND PREVENTION OF ACUTE PERIOPERATIVE HYPONATREMIA**

- Have a high index of suspicion for populations at risk.
- Even mild symptoms (nausea, headache) may be followed by a sudden and catastrophic herniation of the brain, so initiate aggressive treatment immediately.
- Do not give hypotonic fluids in the acute perioperative setting.
- Do not infuse more isotonic saline than the patient needs for hemodynamic stability.
- Be extremely cautious with the volume of fluid infused in patients with a small muscle mass.
- Be very suspicious of a "good" urine output because this may be hypertonic to the infused solutions and hence pure water will be generated and added to the body.

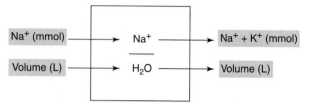

FIGURE 10-5 Maintaining a tonicity balance. To prevent a fall in the P_{Na}, a tonicity balance must be achieved. That is, the volume of water infused should be equal to the urine volume, and the concentration of $Na^+ + K^+$ in the intravenous solutions should be equal to the concentration of $Na^+ + K^+$ in the urine.

The quantitative aspects of hyponatremia that may develop in this setting and its impact on brain cell volume are illustrated in Table 10-4. The two reasons why hyponatremia develops during TURP become obvious after dividing the absorbed fluid into its two constituent parts: iso-osmolal fluid and osmole-free water.

Iso-osmolal fluid. Because glycine does not cross cell membranes at an appreciable rate in the *very* early time periods, it remains in the ECF compartment and causes water to be retained in this location and thereby leads to a severe degree of hyponatremia with a near-normal P_{Osm} (*see margin note*). These organic solutes are unmeasured osmoles in plasma; thus, the measured P_{Osm} exceeds the calculated P_{Osm} ($2 \times P_{Na} + P_{Urea} + P_{Glucose}$, all in mmol/L terms). This form of hyponatremia is not associated with brain cell swelling, and it does not pose a threat of brain herniation. Nevertheless, with subsequent metabolism of these organic solutes, there is a gain of pure water, and hence hyponatremia is now associated with an increased swelling of brain cells. A clinical clue that this may be the case is a fall in the P_{Osm} when the P_{Na} *rises*.

Osmole-free water. This is simply the remaining volume of water; it causes cells to swell. This component, however, is not the major cause for the hyponatremia following TURP (see Table 10-4).

Quantitative analysis. For simplicity, we assume that each patient in this example has 30 L of total body water and a positive balance of 3 L of fluid. When the infusate is D_5W, the distribution of the 3 L of water (after glucose is metabolized) causes 2 L of water to be located in the ICF compartment and 1 L to be located in the ECF compartment. Therefore, there is a 10% rise in the ECF volume and a fall in the P_{Na} to close to 126 mmol/L (see Table 10-4). In contrast, the 3 L of *half isotonic* lavage fluid consists of 1.5 L of osmole-free water and

TRANSLOCATION TYPE OF HYPONATREMIA

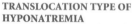

- Hyponatremia that is attributed to retained lavage fluid is often called *"translocational" hyponatremia,* which implies that there has been an addition of hyperosmolar fluid, which caused the exit of water from cells. In fact, because most lavage solutions are hypotonic, some water moves *into* cells; hence, "translocational" is the wrong term to describe the pathophysiology in this setting. The fall in P_{Na} is, in part, due to retention of water with a "Na^+-like" particle in the ECF compartment as an iso-osmolal, but Na^+-free, solution.
- A "Na^+-like" particle is one that is largely restricted to the ECF compartment (e.g., mannitol). Glycine is a "Na^+-like" particle as long as it remains in the ECF compartment (i.e., transiently before it enters cells).

TABLE 10-4 COMPARISON OF A GAIN OF WATER OR OF HALF-ISOTONIC LAVAGE SOLUTION ON THE DEGREE OF HYPONATREMIA AND ICF VOLUME

In this example, both patients have a normal total body water of 30 L, two thirds of which is in the ICF compartment. Note that although the drop in P_{Na} is larger with the retention of lavage fluid, the increase in ICF volume is smaller. Note also that because these organic solutes are not measured in plasma, the measured P_{Osm} exceeds the calculated P_{Osm}.

PARAMETER		NORMAL VALUES	D_5W GAIN 3 L	LAVAGE FLUID GAIN 3 L
Total body water	L	30	33	33
• ICF volume	L	20	**22**	**21**
• ECF volume	L	10	11	12
• P_{Osm}	mOsm/L	285	259	272
• P_{Na}	mmol/L	140	**126**	**117**
• Change in P_{Na}	mmol/L	0	**−14**	**−23**

1.5 L of iso-osmolal solution containing organic solutes. When virtually all the glycine remains in the ECF compartment, 1 L of water (two thirds of the 1.5 L gain of osmole-free water) is retained in the ICF compartment; this is only half the amount of water that is retained in the ICF compartment in the patient who gained 3 L of water with the infusion of 3 L of D_5W. The ECF compartment gains 0.5 L of water (one third of 1.5 L of osmole-free water) plus the 1.5 L of iso-osmolal glycine solution in this example (i.e., a gain of 2 L of Na^+-free water). Hence, the fall in P_{Na} is twice as much (117 mmol/L; see Table 10-4), but the increase in ICF volume is half as large compared to the retention of a similar volume of D_5W (*see margin note*).

Clinical settings for acute hyponatremia that occur outside the hospital

If acute hyponatremia develops outside the hospital, look for a reason why the normal aversion to drinking a large volume of water in the face of hyponatremia has been ignored. Examples include patients who have taken a mood-altering drug (e.g., Ecstasy), patients who have mental disturbance (e.g., schizophrenia), patients who have followed incorrect advice to drink too large a volume of water (e.g., during a marathon), or patients who have drunk a large volume of beer (e.g., beer potomania; *see margin note*; see Part C, page 336 for more discussion).

It is also important to seek a reason why vasopressin may have been released despite the absence of its usual stimulus, a high P_{Na}. The ingestion of a drug (e.g., Ecstasy) may cause the release of this hormone in the face of hyponatremia (see Table 10-2). Alternatively, a low distal delivery of filtrate may diminish the ability to excrete a large volume of water. Hence, subjects who drink a large volume of water and have a deficit of Na^+ may develop a life-threatening degree of acute hyponatremia even in the absence of vasopressin actions (see Case 12-1, page 410).

In all of the aforementioned settings, there is an additional danger if the water load is ingested over a short time period and absorbed from the intestinal tract with little delay. In more detail, a larger degree of brain swelling may develop because there is a larger decline in the arterial P_{Na} (which the brain sees); this may not be revealed by measuring the brachial venous P_{Na} because muscle cells take up a larger proportion of water as a result of their relatively larger mass per blood flow rate (see Chapter 9, Fig. 9-17, page 281).

Hyponatremia due to the intake of the drug Ecstasy

- The most important reason for the development of acute hyponatremia in this setting is a positive balance of water.
- Notwithstanding, there is also a modest deficit of Na^+ in many of these patients.

Positive balance for water. For this to occur, there must be an intake of water that is larger than its output.

Large water intake. People attending a "rave" party are usually advised to drink a large volume of water (*see margin note*). Moreover, the relaxed feeling from the drug might permit them to overcome the aversion to drink water in the presence of acute hyponatremia. It is possible that water may be stored in the lumen of the stomach and

CHANGES AFTER GLYCINE IS METABOLIZED
- At this stage, the changes in the P_{Na}, ICF and ECF volumes, and osmolalities resemble those due to a positive balance of pure water.
- If the lavage fluid contained a nonmetabolized solute (e.g., mannitol), there would be less danger, as this solute and water would be excreted in the urine.

BEER POTOMANIA
Most often, these patients have chronic hyponatremia and present with a superimposed acute hyponatremia.

ADVICE TO DRINK WATER DURING "RAVE" PARTY
Subjects attending a "rave" party are advised to drink a large volume of water. The rationale may be that they believe that they will suffer from "dehydration" because of excessive sweating or it may prevent the development of rhabdomyolysis, which has been reported predominantly in male patients.

small intestine owing to reduced gastrointestinal (GI) motility so this "occult" water is not recognized by the hypothalamic osmostat and thus the thirst center. The overzealous consumption of water, however, creates a serious problem—the development of life-threatening acute hyponatremia, especially in people with a small muscle mass (usually females).

Low output of water. There are two reasons why the excretion of water may be decreased in this setting. First, drugs such as Ecstasy lead to a nonosmotic stimulus to cause the release of vasopressin. Second, there may be a low delivery of filtrate to the distal nephron, which decreases the rate of excretion of water. In this context, it is possible that the drug decreases the constrictor tone in venous capacitance vessels and hence it could cause a decrease in the effective arterial blood volume.

Negative balance for NaCl

> • The likeliest route for NaCl loss is in sweat (the loss is hypotonic); the other route is in diffusion into the intestinal tract.
> • The deficit of NaCl is greater if there is a low intake of NaCl.

At a "rave" party, subjects have a loss of NaCl if they produce a large volume of sweat (*see margin note*). There is another possible way to lose Na^+ from the ECF compartment in this setting—Na^+ diffuses between cells of the small intestine (this area is permeable to Na^+) into its lumen, which contains water because of a large volume of ingested water (slow GI motility is also needed to "trap" this Na^+ and Cl^-; Fig. 10-6). There are also two indirect effects of this loss of Na^+ that permit hyponatremia to develop: First, the low effective arterial blood volume leads to a diminished loss of hypotonic fluid in sweat; second, there is a decreased capacity to excrete water in the urine because of a low distal delivery of filtrate coupled with residual water permeability in the terminal region of the nephron (discussed in Chapter 9, Part D, page 293).

DEFICIT OF NaCl WITH SWEATING
- The concentration of Na^+ in sweat is ~25 mmol/L.
- To develop hyponatremia, there must be a larger intake of water than the volume of sweat.
- Ecstasy may uncouple oxidative phosphorylation. If this occurs, sweat loss may increase appreciably due to excessive production of heat. Nevertheless, the data to support uncoupling of oxidative phosphorylation due to Ecstasy are not compelling.

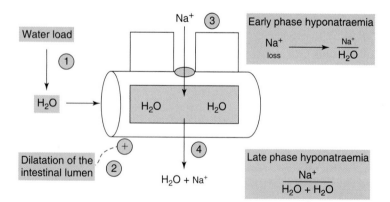

FIGURE 10-6 Role of the gastrointestinal (GI) tract in the hyponatremia due to water ingestion. The first event is water ingestion (*step 1*). An unknown volume of water remains in the lumen of a dilated GI tract (*step 2*). Na^+ diffuses from the body into the lumen of the GI tract (*step 3*). This is aided by a high local Na^+ concentration and paracellular permeability for Na^+. The P_{Na} falls and the extracellular fluid (ECF) volume is contracted at this stage. Later, when GI motility improves, the water and Na^+ in the lumen are absorbed and this causes ECF volume expansion and a low P_{Na} because of the gain of a hypotonic saline solution (*step 4*).

Hyponatremia due to diarrhea in infants and children

> • Hyponatremia in this setting usually has two components—
> Na^+ loss and water gain—its degree may be severe.

Vasopressin is released in response to both the low effective arterial blood volume (i.e., the loss of near-isotonic solutions containing Na^+ during diarrhea) and nonosmotic stimuli due to the acute illness (see Table 10-2). There is also a low distal delivery of filtrate in this setting. This leads to the retention of water if it is ingested, which is usually the case because it is common in this setting to feed these patients sugar water to "rest the GI tract" and avoid "dehydration" (*see margin note*).

Hyponatremia in a marathon runner

> • Marathon runners are often advised to drink water avidly to replace the large volume of water lost in sweat (could be as much as 2 L/hr).

A positive balance of water (reflected by weight gain; *see margin note*) is the most important factor leading to the development of acute hyponatremia. In addition, there is a deficit of Na^+ because of the large volume of sweat, which contains 15 to 30 mmol Na^+ and Cl^- per liter (see discussion of Question 11-1, page 395, for more details).

Risk factors for the development of acute hyponatremia in a marathon runner. The following conditions may contribute to the development of a severe degree of hyponatremia in a marathon runner.

- A longer duration of the race, because there is more time to drink this "extra" water. Hence, subjects who run more slowly have an increased risk.
- Runners with a smaller muscle mass (e.g., females) may have a greater risk (*see margin note on page 324*). Therefore, the amount of water intake should be adjusted per kg of lean body mass.
- Women may be at a greater risk because they are more likely to follow advice than men and hence may have a larger intake of water.
- Runners who, near the end of the race, mistakenly believe that they have a deficit of water, may *gulp* a large volume of water. The reason this is dangerous is that rapid absorption of a large volume of water causes a large decline in the arterial P_{Na} to which the brain is exposed, and hence it leads to a greater transient degree of acute swelling of brain cells (see the discussion of Case 11-3, page 399).

Risk factors after the race
- If water was retained in the stomach and/or the intestinal tract, this water may be absorbed later, causing a further fall in the P_{Na}.
- The measured brachial venous P_{Na} may not reflect this "hidden" danger, because the water that is absorbed rapidly from the intestinal tract causes a much larger fall in the arterial P_{Na} and this is the P_{Na} that causes brain cells to swell. Moreover, even if water is not absorbed because of low intestinal motility, Na^+ and Cl^- may diffuse into this luminal fluid, causing a further fall in the P_{Na} (see Fig. 10-6, page 328).
- If a runner is given a rapid infusion of isotonic saline because of suspected contraction of the ECF volume or to treat hyperthermia,

"DEHYDRATION"
- The authors avoid using this term because it is ambiguous. To some, it means a lack of water, but to others, it means a decreased ECF volume.
- In a patient with acute hyponatremia, the ICF compartment is "overhydrated" rather than dehydrated. Therefore, using this term ignores the actual danger to the patient in this setting.

WEIGHT GAIN IN MARATHON RUNNERS AND RISK OF HYPONATREMIA
Weight gain may underestimate the actual water gain in these subjects for the following reasons:
- Fuels, including glycogen in muscle, are oxidized and this could account for a weight loss of close to 0.5 kg (1 lb).
- Each gram of glycogen is stored with 2 to 3 grams of "bound" (or structural) water. Therefore, the "addition" of this water is not reflected as a gain of weight.

REEXPANSION OF THE EXTRACELLULAR FLUID VOLUME IN A PATIENT WITH A SERIOUS DEGREE OF ACUTE HYPONATREMIA

• To reexpand a contracted ECF volume in a patient with acute hyponatremia, hypertonic saline should be given if the patient has even mild symptoms of central nervous system origin.

• This caution is particularly important if there has been a large recent intake of water, which is retained in the lumen of the intestinal tract, because this may be absorbed soon and thus increase the risk of additional brain cell swelling.

this bolus of saline may alter Starling forces across capillary membranes, including those in the blood-brain barrier. As a result, the volume of the interstitial compartment of the brain increases. Recall that any further gain of volume inside the skull may raise the intracranial pressure to a dangerous level once brain cells are swollen by an appreciable degree (*see margin note*).

QUESTIONS

(Discussions on pages 363 and 364)

10-1 *Some authorities determine the basis for the change in the P_{Na} using an analysis based on electrolyte-free water balance. Does this provide different information compared with an analysis based on tonicity balance?*

10-2 *Does hypertonic saline reduce the intracranial pressure simply because it draws water out of brain cells?*

10-3 *A young woman with low muscle mass is asked to drink a standard water load (20 mL/kg) in an experimental study designed to examine the ability to excrete water; her P_{Na} prior to ingesting this water load was 140 mmol/L. Thirty minutes later, she complains of a headache, which is very unusual for her. Is therapy required at this time?*

PART C
CHRONIC HYPONATREMIA

OVERVIEW

CHRONIC CONDITIONS

• If a patient has chronic hyponatremia, the input and output of water and Na+ should be equal if this is the only disorder (i.e., there is a steady state as defined on page 341).

• Hyponatremia is ultimately the result of an altered ability to adjust the composition of the urine to match the intake of water and Na+ (i.e., the ability to excrete the appropriate volume of electrolyte-free water is decreased).

• Chronic hyponatremia ($P_{Na} < 136$ mmol/L; duration > 48 hours) is the most common electrolyte abnormality in hospitalized patients (*see margin note*).

Patients with chronic hyponatremia usually do not have specific symptoms related to this electrolyte disorder, but most suffer from a lack of energy, fatigue, and an impaired performance on both attention and tandem gait, which improve when hyponatremia is corrected. Although the presence of hyponatremia can sometimes be anticipated from other information in the history (e.g., the use of diuretics) or from findings on the physical examination (e.g., low effective arterial blood volume), hyponatremia is commonly recognized for the first time after routine measurement of electrolytes in plasma in many patients.

IMPORTANT FACTS

1. *Hyponatremia is a diagnostic category rather than a specific disease entity.* Hence, a unique design treatment will be required for each patient with this electrolyte disorder.

2. *In every patient with chronic hyponatremia, the central pathophysiology is an inability to excrete water appropriately; most of the retained water is located in cells.* In some patients, this is due to the presence of vasopressin. In others, the major defect is a low distal delivery of filtrate. To emphasize this issue, we use the term *syndrome of inappropriate antidiuresis* (SIAD).

TABLE 10-5 **SETTINGS WHERE ACTIONS OF VASOPRESSIN MAY DISAPPEAR**

- Reexpansion of a contracted effective arterial blood volume
- Decreased production of vasopressin when cortisol is administered to a patient with a deficiency of cortisol
- Disappearance of a nonosmotic stimulus for the release of vasopressin (e.g., decrease in anxiety, nausea, phobia, or discontinuation of certain drugs)
- Stopping the administration of dDAVP in patients who have been on it for a period of time (e.g., children with enuresis, the elderly with urinary incontinence, patients with central diabetes insipidus [see discussion of Case 10-1])

3. *A water diuresis may ensue if actions of vasopressin disappear (Table 10-5) and/or if the distal delivery of filtrate is increased.* Examples include reexpansion of a very low effective arterial blood volume (i.e., infuse saline in a patient with a major deficit of Na^+). Osmotic demyelination may develop unless this water diuresis falls sufficiently to prevent a rise in the P_{Na} (i.e., give dDAVP).

4. *Patients with chronic hyponatremia may also have an element of acute hyponatremia.* In a patient with chronic hyponatremia who may also have a component of acute hyponatremia, the P_{Na} must be raised quickly to lower intracranial pressure; the rise in the P_{Na} should not, however, exceed the upper limit set for 24-hour period to avoid causing osmotic demyelination.

5. *Osmotic demyelination is the major danger in patients with chronic hyponatremia, which, when very severe, can lead to quadriplegia, coma, and/or death.* Its major risk factor is a rapid and large rise in the P_{Na}. This is usually the result of a large water diuresis, which occurs if the distal delivery of filtrate is increased in a patient with SIAD or the actions of vasopressin disappear in a patient with SIADH. Patients who are malnourished and/or who are K^+ depleted are at higher risk for the development of this devastating complication. In most patients, the rise in P_{Na} should be less than 8 mmol/L/day, but in patients who suffer from malnutrition and/or K^+ depletion, the rise in the P_{Na} should be less than 4 mmol/L/day. If a water diuresis were to begin and there is a risk that P_{Na} may exceed the predefined upper limit, give dDAVP and withhold water to minimize the risk of developing this complication. Perhaps smaller rises in the P_{Na} may also lead to subclinical CNS damage. Therefore, these limits for the rise in P_{Na} should be viewed as maximums not to be exceeded rather than targets to achieve.

CLINICAL APPROACH

- The initial steps are the same as with all electrolyte disorders.
  - Identify and deal with emergencies.
  - Anticipate and prevent dangers that may occur with therapy.
- The presence of significant central nervous system symptoms or the history of a large recent intake of water suggests that an element of acute hyponatremia may be present.

Identify emergencies on admission

There are no dangers on admission that are specifically related to chronic hyponatremia. Nevertheless, there could be dangers if there are symptoms suggestive of a component of acute hyponatremia causing brain cell swelling or if there is a hemodynamic emergency when there is a large deficit of NaCl (see Flow Chart 10-1).

Anticipate risks during therapy

- Osmotic demyelination may develop during therapy if the actions of vasopressin disappear and/or distal delivery of filtrate increases, because this leads to a large water diuresis and a rapid rise in the P_{Na}.

Determine why vasopressin is released, because the reason for its release may disappear (see Table 10-5). Should this and/or an increase in the distal delivery of filtrate be anticipated, consider administering dDAVP to prevent a water diuresis, particularly in patients who are at high risk for demyelination. One must also restrict water intake at this time.

Determine why the excretion of water is too low

- There are two causes for a low excretion of water: a low distal delivery of filtrate and/or the presence of actions of vasopressin.

The next step is to determine why there is a reduced capability to excrete water; accordingly, we follow the steps outlined in Flow Chart 10-2. The issues to resolve include determining why there may be a diminished distal delivery of filtrate and/or why vasopressin may be present.

CLASSIFICATION

- The classification of patients with chronic hyponatremia should be based on why the patient has a defect in the excretion of water.

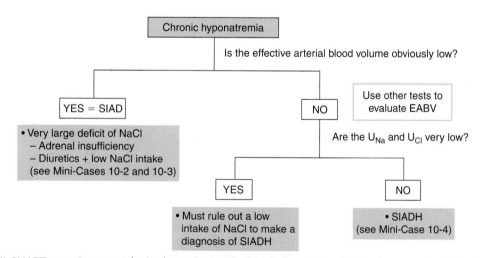

FLOW CHART 10-2 Steps to take in the patient with chronic hyponatremia. As shown on the *left*, when the effective arterial blood volume (EABV) is contracted, there is a decreased delivery of filtrate (i.e., SIAD is present). If the glomerular filtration rate is also quite low, there is a much larger decrease in the distal delivery of filtrate, and vasopression may also be present. Conversely, chronic hyponatremia may develop if there is a modest reduction in distal delivery of filtrate along with a large intake of water. When the EABV is not low, the diagnosis is usually SIADH, but if urine has low concentrations of Na^+ and Cl^-, an infusion of saline is needed to confirm that SIADH plus a low salt intake is the correct diagnosis.

Traditional approach

A common way to classify patients with chronic hyponatremia is to divide them into two groups, those with the "depletional" (Na^+ deficit) type and others with the "dilutional" (water excess) type. Although this is simple, almost every patient has both of these elements. Moreover, it is difficult to be confident about the degree of contraction of the effective arterial blood volume based on the physical examination.

Preferred classification

There are two groups in this classification (Table 10-6). The first group has SIAD, in which the major pathophysiology is a decrease in the distal delivery of filtrate ($\pm$ reabsorption of water in the inner medullary collecting duct via residual water permeability). The second group has SIADH, in which the major problem is the presence of AQP2 water channels in the luminal membrane of principal cells of the later segments of the distal nephron because of the presence of vasopressin without a physiologic stimulus for its release (i.e., the P_{Na} is distinctly < 136 mmol/L). We emphasize that a diagnosis of SIADH cannot be made if the patient has a low distal delivery of filtrate (see page 335 for more discussion). The importance of thinking in this way is that the risks associated with therapy differ in each subgroup.

Low distal delivery of filtrate

- Distal delivery of filtrate = GFR − proximal reabsorption of filtrate.
- Reabsorption of Na^+ in the proximal convoluted tubule is enhanced when the effective arterial blood volume is contracted.
- With a larger decrease in the effective arterial blood volume, the GFR falls, and this results in an even lower distal delivery of filtrate.

TABLE 10-6 **CLASSIFICATION OF PATIENTS WITH CHRONIC HYPONATREMIA**

The distal delivery of filtrate (really water) must be assessed in conjunction with the volume of water ingested. In certain settings, both low distal delivery and high levels of vasopressin may be present. To establish a diagnosis of SIADH, a low distal delivery of filtrate must be ruled out.

SIAD: Low distal delivery of filtrate for the most part

- Enhanced reabsorption of Na^+ and Cl^- in the proximal convoluted tubule due to a low effective arterial blood volume (deficit of NaCl for a variety of causes: edema states, congestive heart failure, low $P_{Albumin}$, low venous capacitance vessel constrictor tone, such as with low glucocorticoids)
- Low GFR (usually not a sole cause of chronic hyponatremia)

SIADH: High vasopressin actions

- Endocrine causes (e.g., low glucocorticoids, low thyroid hormone)
- Induced by nausea, anxiety, drugs (see Table 10-2 for a list)
- Lesions in the lungs or central nervous system
- Release of vasopressin from malignant cells (*see margin note*)
- Metabolic causes (e.g., porphyria)
- Activating mutation of the V_2 receptor (*see margin note*)

HIGH LEVELS OF VASOPRESSIN IN PATIENTS WITH A MALIGNANCY
There are often multiple reasons for the presence of vasopressin. Causes include chemotherapy (e.g., nausea), metastases in the adrenal gland (e.g., cortisol deficiency, aldosterone deficiency), and tumors in the lungs or central nervous system (may provide afferent input to suppress the release of vasopressin, or the tumor itself may release vasopressin).

ACTIVATING MUTATION OF THE V_2 RECEPTOR
In this rare disorder, there is chronic hyponatremia, vasopressin levels are very low in plasma, and a low distal delivery of filtrate is not present.

There are two reasons for a low distal delivery of filtrate: an enhanced proximal reabsorption of water and a very low GFR. Renal excretion of water will be even lower despite the absence of actions of vasopressin as a result of reabsorption of water in the inner medullary collecting duct via its residual water permeability (discussion to follow). Later in the course of the illness, when the deficit of Na^+ and Cl^- becomes quite large, vasopressin may be released in response to hemodynamic stimuli.

Enhanced reabsorption of filtrate in the proximal convoluted tubule

LOSS OF Na^+ DURING A WATER DIURESIS
- Each liter a water diuresis has 5 to 10 mmol of Na^+.
- If the water diuresis is 10 L/day, the loss of Na^+ can easily exceed 50 mmol/day.
- If there is little intake of NaCl, a deficit of Na^+ (and Cl^-) will develop over many days.

This can result from a deficit of Na^+ or a disorder that causes a low cardiac output. Because there is an obligatory minimal loss of Na^+ in each liter of urine during a large water diuresis, a deficit of Na^+ can develop during the polyuria induced by a large intake of water in a subject who consumes little NaCl for a prolonged period (*see margin note*). Assess both the intake of NaCl and the routes for its potential loss via urine, the GI tract, and/or the skin. The magnitude of the deficit of NaCl rises progressively if the reasons for negative balance of NaCl are not reversed. This will result in a progressive decline in the distal delivery of filtrate. The pathophysiology of the chronic hyponatremia in this setting, its diagnostic features, and dangers to anticipate depend on the severity of the decrease in distal delivery of filtrate (Table 10-7).

Once a given degree of chronic hyponatremia develops in this setting, it is unlikely that a true steady state will be reached, because it depends on maintaining a persistently high water intake and a constant deficit of Na^+ (*see margin note*). Therefore, the P_{Na} is likely to fluctuate in the hyponatremic range depending on the absolute intakes and losses of NaCl and water.

RELEASE OF VASOPRESSIN IN PATIENTS WITH SIAD
- Vasopressin may be present at any stage due to nonosmotic stimuli (e.g., pain or nausea due to gastritis in a patient with beer potomania). The effective arterial blood volume may not be low enough to cause the release of vasopressin; nevertheless, there is a danger of a large water diuresis if the patient consumes or is given a load of NaCl that is large enough to increase the distal delivery of filtrate.

In the next stage, the pathophysiology includes a much lower GFR, and therefore there is an even lower distal delivery of filtrate. In this stage, the P_{Na} falls to very low values if the intake of water does not decrease. Ultimately, vasopressin is released when the degree of contraction of the effective arterial blood volume is large enough (>7% to 10%), leading to a further reduction in the excretion of water.

Possible role for residual water permeability

- Residual water permeability seems to play an important role in limiting the rate of excretion of water when vasopressin does not act (see Chapter 9, page 277 for more information).

TABLE 10-7 PATHOPHYSIOLOGY OF HYPONATREMIA DUE TO A LOW DISTAL DELIVERY OF FILTRATE

The key feature is an inability to excrete all the water ingested until chronic hyponatremia develops.

STAGES	PATHOPHYSIOLOGY	DIAGNOSTIC FEATURES	DANGERS
• Modest decrease in the distal delivery of filtrate	• Modest deficit of NaCl • Large water intake	• Urine flow rate not low • ↓ Osmole excretion rate • $U_{Osm} < P_{Osm}$	• Rapid ↓ P_{Na} if ↑ water input or if sudden ↓ in water loss
• Severe decrease in distal delivery of filtrate	• Larger deficit of NaCl • Larger fall in GFR • Vasopressin may be released	• Low EABV • ↓ Osmole excretion rate • U_{Osm} may be > P_{Osm}	• Rapid ↑ P_{Na} if distal delivery of filtrate rises. • Acute hyponatremia if large intake of water (e.g., beer).

EABV, effective arterial blood volume; GFR, glomerular filtration rate.

TABLE 10-8 **WATER REABSORPTION DUE TO RESIDUAL WATER PERMEABILITY**

For water to be reabsorbed by residual water permeability (RWP), AQP2 must not be present in the luminal membrane of the inner medullary collecting duct (if vasopressin is acting, there will be no driving force to reabsorb water via RWP as depicted in the top line in this table). When there is a water diuresis (no AQP2), there is a large difference in osmolality between the inner medullary interstitial compartment and the lumen of the inner medullary collecting duct, which creates the driving force to reabsorb water (bottom line in the table). Now the contact time determines how much water is reabsorbed by RWP (*see margin note*).

VASOPRESSIN PRESENT	OSMOLE EXCRETION (mOsm/day)	INTERSTITIAL OSMOLALITY (mOsm/L)	URINE OSMOLALITY (mOsm/L)	DRIVING FORCE (mm Hg)
Yes	900	900	900	0
No	900	450	50	~8000

The following features must be appreciated to understand the contribution of residual water permeability to the pathophysiology of chronic hyponatremia in a setting of a low distal delivery of filtrate.

1. *The inner medullary collecting duct has a constitutive permeability to water.* In addition, there is an enormous driving force for water reabsorption, but only when vasopressin is absent because the osmolality in the renal medullary interstitial compartment is close to 300 mOsm/L greater than the luminal osmolality.

2. *When vasopressin acts and an abundant number of AQP2 are present in the luminal membrane of the late distal nephron, there is no function for residual water permeability.* That is, there is no driving force for water reabsorption via residual water permeability because the osmolalities are virtually identical in the lumen and in the medullary interstitial compartment.

3. *Two major factors affect the volume of fluid reabsorbed via residual water permeability during a water diuresis.* When few osmoles are being excreted, there is somewhat more water reabsorption due to a larger osmotic driving force (Table 10-8). A prolonged contact time increases the proportion of water reabsorbed by residual water permeability (*see margin note*).

QUESTION

(*Discussion on page 364*)

10-4 *What may limit the ability of water to achieve diffusion equilibrium in the inner medullary collecting duct via residual water permeability during a large water diuresis?*

Tools to detect a contracted effective arterial blood volume

A difficulty with the classification of syndrome of inappropriate antidiuresis is that many of these patients may have a modest degree of effective arterial blood volume contraction, but this cannot always be detected by the physical examination (see Chapter 9, page 276). The following laboratory tests may provide helpful clues in this context.

Concentrations of Na⁺ and Cl⁻ in the urine

- Assessment of the U_{Na} and U_{Cl} is very helpful to detect the presence of a low effective arterial blood volume, and it may also provide clues about its cause.
- These concentrations should be interpreted in conjunction with the urine flow rate, because the excretion rates are important to diagnose a low distal delivery of filtrate.

FACTORS THAT AFFECT THE URINE VOLUME DURING A WATER DIURESIS

- The two major factors are volume of fluid delivered distally and the volume of fluid reabsorbed via residual water permeability.
- Despite the large osmotic driving force, water does not move to osmotic equilibrium between the lumen of the inner medullary collecting duct and the medullary interstitium because there is insufficient time to permit the diffusion process for water to be complete.
- Contraction of the renal pelvis raises pressure and forces some urine to enter the medullary collecting duct until the pressure rises sufficiently to stop this retrograde flow. At this point, all of the remaining volume in the pelvis is forced down the ureters into the bladder. Therefore, when a large volume is in the pelvis, only a small proportion of this volume will travel by this retrograde pathway, and thus there is a small overall effect of this residual water permeability on the urine flow rate.

USE OF LABORATORY TESTS
TO ASSESS THE EFFECTIVE
ARTERIAL BLOOD VOLUME

- Patients who have a low NaCl intake can have low U_{Na} and U_{Cl} without a significant degree of contraction of their effective arterial blood volume (it is really less expanded rather than contracted).
- A low P_K, a rise in the $P_{Creatinine}$, and a high P_{HCO_3} may suggest that the effective arterial blood volume is low.
- Because the reabsorption of urea is strongly influenced by the effective arterial blood volume whereas that of creatinine is not, the rise in the P_{Urea} is more pronounced than the rise in $P_{Creatinine}$ in patients with a low effective arterial blood volume. Therefore, the ratio of urea to creatinine in plasma is likely to be high in patients with hyponatremia as a result of a deficit of Na^+ that causes a low distal delivery of filtrate. This, however, may not be the case if protein intake is low. The urea-to-creatinine ratio in plasma is likely to be low in patients with SIADH.
- Be sure to consider the muscle mass of the patient when evaluating the $P_{Creatinine}$.

BASIS FOR HYPONATREMIA

- Although a positive balance of water *in cells* is a critical component of the pathophysiology of chronic hyponatremia, in all three mini-cases presented here, the decreased water excretion is due to a low distal delivery of filtrate as a result of an appreciable deficit of Na^+ and Cl^-.
- While beer potomania is not a common clinical presentation, it is discussed in detail because it provides an excellent example of the pathophysiology involved in SIAD, a disorder caused by a low distal delivery of filtrate.

The expected renal response when the effective arterial blood volume is contracted is the excretion of urine with a very low U_{Na} and/or U_{Cl} (i.e., <15 mmol/L or <1.5 mmol Na^+/mmol $U_{Creatinine}$ [<15 mmol Na^+/g $U_{Creatinine}$]). Much lower concentrations, however, should be expected during a water diuresis. If the cause of the low effective arterial blood volume is the use of an exogenous diuretic, the excretion of Na^+ and Cl^- might be intermittently high; hence, multiple spot urine electrolyte measurements are very helpful if the patient denies taking diuretics. There are conditions, however, in which the U_{Na} is high despite the presence of a low effective arterial blood volume due to the presence of an anion in the urine that obligates the excretion of Na^+ (e.g., organic anions and/or HCO_3^- in a patient with recent vomiting). In other conditions, the U_{Cl} is high despite the presence of a low effective arterial blood volume if there is a cation in the urine that obligates the excretion of Cl^- (e.g., NH_4^+ in a patient with metabolic acidosis due to the loss of $NaHCO_3$ in diarrhea fluid).

Concentrations of urea and urate in plasma

- Patients with a low effective arterial blood volume tend to have a high P_{Urea} and P_{Urate}, because reabsorption of urea and urate is increased in the proximal tubule. The converse is also true in patients with chronic hyponatremia due to SIADH, so this subgroup has an expanded effective arterial blood volume.

The excretion rates of urea and urate are equal to their production rates in steady state; therefore, it is useful to examine their fractional excretions because this "adjusts" their excretion rates to their filtered loads. The fractional excretions of urea and urate are lower than normal when the effective arterial blood volume is contracted. For example, more urea is reabsorbed passively in the proximal convoluted tubule when its concentration is higher in the lumen owing to more fluid reabsorption. Information from other laboratory tests that may be used to assess the effective arterial blood volume is summarized in the *margin notes*.

MINI-CASE 10-1: A PROLONGED DRINKING SPREE

A 43-year-old man drinks a very large quantity of beer every day; this is virtually his only intake. Hence, he has a very low intake of NaCl. For the past several weeks, he has had a very large urine output. His urine volume has declined in the past several days; nevertheless, it is still close to 5 L/day.

When he first came to medical attention, there was no evidence of a contracted effective arterial blood volume. On laboratory testing, the P_{Na} was 126 mmol/L, $P_{Creatinine}$ was 0.7 mg/dL (60 μmol/L), the BUN was 7 mg/dL (P_{Urea} 2.5 mmol/L), and the U_{Osm} was 80 mOsm/kg H_2O. One week later, he returned to the emergency department because he was feeling unwell, but he did not have specific complaints. He had obvious evidence of a contracted effective arterial blood volume, his P_{Na} was 112 mmol/L, his P_K was 2.1 mmol/L, his $P_{Creatinine}$ was 1.5 mg/dL (130 μmol/L), and his urine volume was only 1.0 L/day, with a U_{Osm} of 350 mOsm/kg H_2O.

Questions

Why did a deficit of Na^+ develop in this patient?

Focusing on hyponatremia, were there dangers prior to admission?

Why did chronic hyponatremia develop in this patient?
Are there emergencies on admission?
Are there new dangers to anticipate with therapy on admission?
What are the options for therapy during each admission?

Discussion of Mini-Case 10-1

The P_{Na} and the composition of the urine depend on the stage of
the beer potomania. In its early stage, the picture is dominated by a
large water intake, which leads to a very large water diuresis. When
the intake of water declines, the P_{Na} rises from about 136 mmol/L to
140 mmol/L. The pathphysiology, however, begins once the patient
decreases his intake of NaCl because, in a water diuresis, the urine has
a low Na^+ concentration. For example, if the urine volume is 10 L/day
and the U_{Na} is 10 mmol/L, the excretion of Na^+ is 100 mmol/day.
Hence, a deficit of Na^+ will develop over days if the daily intake of
NaCl is significantly less than 100 mmol. Once the deficit of Na^+ is
severe enough, there is a diminished distal delivery of filtrate and a
decreased rate of excretion of water.

The stages of development of low distal delivery are clearly illustrated in this patient. The pathophysiology has several steps that
diminish the distal delivery of filtrate in a setting where residual water
permeability is important. Ultimately, the GFR falls and this leads to
an even larger reduction in the distal delivery of filtrate and hence a
lower ability to excrete water.

Why did a deficit of NaCl develop in this patient?

The deficit of Na^+ and Cl^- first developed in the polyuric phase of the
disorder after the patient decreased his intake of NaCl, and he had an
appreciable excretion of Na^+ because his urine volume was *very* large.

*Focusing on hyponatremia, were there dangers
prior to admission?*

The major danger is acute hyponatremia. For example, if this
patient were to have a nonosmotic stimulus for the release of vasopressin (e.g., alcohol-induced gastritis with pain and nausea), this
could cause a sudden and large positive water balance if his large
water intake were to continue. A second setting for acute hyponatremia would occur if he were to drink a larger volume of water or
beer while he is consuming little NaCl, which led to a significant
degree of contraction of his effective arterial blood volume. Owing
to enhanced reabsorption of Na^+, Cl^-, and water proximally, his
distal delivery of filtrate will be low, and hence some of the ingested
water would be retained and acute hyponatremia could be the result.
Notwithstanding, this water intake need not be much higher than that
in the early stage, but the main difference is the low rate of excretion
of water. Of note, the acute fall in the P_{Na} would be more dangerous
when there are more brain cells per unit volume in the skull (i.e.,
in younger patients who do not have a large reduction in brain cell
number).

Why did chronic hyponatremia develop in this patient?

Chronic hyponatremia is usually seen after the patient develops
a negative balance for Na^+. In this setting, there are two reasons
for the diminished ability to excrete water: a low distal delivery of

THE U_{Osm} AND THE URINE
VOLUME IN EARLY STAGE OF
BEER POTOMANIA
- The degree of decrease in the
  effective arterial blood volume
  is not large enough to cause the
  release of vasopressin. Hence
  the U_{osm} is low; hyponatremia
  develops despite the low U_{Osm}
  because water intake exceeds
  water excretion.
- Conversely, vasopressin may
  be released due to nonosmotic
  stimuli (e.g., pain, nausea). If this
  occurs, the U_{Osm} will be higher
  than the P_{Osm} and the urine volume will be markedly diminished.
  In this setting, the polydipsia will
  increase the risk of developing
  acute hyponatremia and, thereby,
  brain herniation.

filtrate and the presence of residual water permeability. The effect
of residual water permeability is even larger in this patient because
of the very low osmole excretion rate as a result of the poor dietary
intake of protein and salt. This leads to a lower urine osmolality
and thereby a larger osmotic driving force for water reabsorption
(see Table 10-8, page 335).

In the later stage of beer potomania, there is a much greater
reduction in the capacity to excrete water owing to a larger decrease
in the distal delivery of filtrate, the reabsorption of more water
in the inner medullary collecting duct by the residual water permeability pathway, and possibly a low GFR. Vasopressin may be
present when the degree of contraction of the ECF volume exceeds
10%. When this occurs, the urine volume should be very low
indeed. Parenthetically, the urine osmolality may be higher than
the plasma osmolality despite the fact that vasopressin is absent (*see
margin note*). We emphasize that this patient is not in a steady state
because water intake is not constant throughout the day or from
day to day. Hence, several blood tests must be performed to make
this assessment.

Usually the P_{Na} falls progressively in these patients. In more detail,
as the deficit of Na^+ increases, distal delivery of filtrate becomes much
lower and the GFR falls as well. As a result, the urine output declines
and the U_{Osm} is even greater than the P_{Osm} despite the fact that vasopressin is absent because the flow rate is slower and there is more
time for the diffusion of water via the residual water permeability
(*see margin note on page 335*). In addition, perhaps vasopressin may
be released intermittently as a result of the presence of nonosmotic
stimuli (*see margin note above*).

Are there emergencies on admission?

- There are obvious emergencies if the patient has significant
  symptoms that could be associated with an acute component
  of hyponatremia.
  - A smaller fall in the P_{Na} may cause a larger than expected
    rise in intracranial pressure if there is a space-occupying
    lesion in the skull (e.g., subdural hematoma).
  - Water may be "hidden" in the stomach and this may cause
    an acute fall in the P_{Na} when it is absorbed later.
- An emergency due to hypokalemia may develop during therapy. Hypokalemia may not be evident early on if α-adrenergic
  release inhibits the release of insulin and causes a shift of K^+
  out of cells.

There may be a medical emergency if the patient has ingested
a large volume of water recently and some of it is retained in his
stomach. When this water is absorbed quickly, there is an "acute
infusion" of "electrolyte-free water." Hence, he should be monitored very closely. Hypertonic saline should be given if there are
symptoms suggestive of acute hyponatremia. We would also give
hypertonic saline if the P_{Na} is less than 130 mmol/L. The rise in
the P_{Na}, however, should not exceed 4 mmol/L/day, given the risks
of the development of osmotic demyelination (i.e., poor nutrition
and K^+ depletion).

Are there new dangers to anticipate with therapy on admission?

- The new dangers in this setting are caused by a rapid rise in the P_{Na}. This may lead to osmotic demyelination because the patient has chronic hyponatremia and risk factors for osmotic demyelination (i.e., malnutrition, K^+ depletion).

There could be a sudden rise in his P_{Na} if the rate of excretion of water were to increase rapidly. The major reason for this would be a large increase in the distal delivery of filtrate owing to reexpansion of the effective arterial blood volume (i.e., there was a large input of NaCl). Examples include a large input of Na^+-rich food (e.g., pizza) or an infusion of saline to treat "dehydration" in the hospital. The P_{Na} rises as a result of both a positive balance of Na^+ and a negative balance for water, especially if water intake stops. To avoid this potential danger of osmotic demyelination, preventive measures are needed. Nevertheless, the specific plan for therapy in this group of patients is very challenging (see discussion to follow). The options for therapy of patients with chronic hyponatremia due to a low distal delivery of filtrate are described on page 341, in Table 10-9, and in Chapter 12, page 410.

What are the options for therapy after during admission?

- The emphasis is on measures to avoid an excessive rise in P_{Na}. The *safe* rate must be defined for each patient. If there is a larger risk of developing osmotic demyelination (i.e., malnutrition, K^+ deficit), the goal of therapy is to avoid a daily rise in the P_{Na} of more than 4 mmol/L. In the absence of these risk factors, the maximum allowable rise in the P_{Na} is 8 mmol/L/day.
- The possible dangers associated with each mode of therapy must be recognized and prevented.
- The first step is to define the balances for water, Na^+, and K^+ in quantitative terms in each body compartment.

TABLE 10-9 **OPTIONS FOR THERAPY FOR CHRONIC HYPONATREMIA AND A LOW DISTAL DELIVERY OF FILTRATE**

The goal of therapy is to raise the P_{Na} at a safe rate. The description here pertains to patients with chronic hyponatremia due to a low distal delivery of filtrate who drink a large volume of water and have a relatively large urine volume.

THERAPY	BENEFITS	DANGERS
1. Water restriction	• Creating a negative balance for water will raise the P_{Na}	• Rapid rise in the P_{Na} if urine output is much larger than water intake
2. Administer NaCl to reach the upper limit for rise in P_{Na}	• Replaces the deficit of Na^+ and improves hemodynamics	• Large water diuresis; if present and the rise in the P_{Na} is close to the daily upper limit, give dDAVP. Water intake must be restricted to prevent an acute and large ↓ in the P_{Na}

Composition of the body prior to the development of hyponatremia. The patient in this example weighed 50 kg and had 20 L of ICF and 10 L of ECF when his P_{Na} was normal (140 mmol/L). Hence, the content of Na^+ in his ECF compartment was 1400 mmol (140 mmol/L × 10 L). Although there was 200 mmol of Na^+ in his ICF compartment (10 mmol/L × 20 L), this does not change appreciably unless there is a significant deficit of K^+.

Since it is not possible to obtain a quantitative estimate of the ECF volume by physical examination, we are left with qualitative estimates unless the hematocrit or the concentrations of hemoglobin and/or total proteins in plasma were measured (i.e., assuming that these values were likely to be normal before hyponatremia developed). This is a major limitation for a quantitative analysis, but one can still obtain useful estimates for the balances of water and of Na^+ for clinical purposes.

Design of therapy for the first admission. Of note, the P_{Na} was 126 mmol/L, the urine output was 5 L/day, the U_{Osm} was 80 mOsm/kg H_2O, and the GFR was reasonably well preserved ($P_{Creatinine}$ was 0.7 mg/dL [60 μmol/L]). Nevertheless, the osmole excretion rate was low and the concentrations of Na^+ and of Cl^- in the urine were 10 mmol/L.

Define the balances in the extracellular fluid compartment

Water. The ECF volume was likely to be somewhat contracted even though the physical examination does not provide conclusive evidence when the degree of contraction of this volume is modest. Although the concentrations of Na^+ and Cl^- in the urine were only 10 mmol/L (as one cannot reabsorb all the Na^+ from each liter of urine during a water diuresis), recall that the urine flow rate was very high (i.e., 5 L/day vs. the expected 0.5 L/day in a patient with a contracted effective arterial blood volume). Hence, the rate of excretion of Na^+ and Cl^- is appreciable. Although the P_{Urea} and P_{Urate} could be helpful to suggest that the effective arterial blood volume is contracted, we think that the relatively low urine output (i.e., 5 L/day vs. the expected 15 L/day in a patient who lacks actions of vasopressin) suggests that there is an appreciably low distal delivery of filtrate, and this is the strongest evidence for a contracted effective arterial blood volume.

Because the deficit of water in the ECF compartment is almost impossible to quantitate at the bedside, we must make an educated guess of the degree of contraction of the ECF volume—that is, there could be a 15% contraction of this volume. *Hence, we shall assume that there is a 1.5-L deficit of water in the ECF compartment in this patient.*

Na^+. This deficit is equal to the difference between the normal content of Na^+ in the ECF compartment (1400 mmol) and the present content of Na^+. The latter is equal to the product of the current P_{Na} (126 mol/L) and the current ECF volume (8.5 L), which is 1071 mmol. *Hence, the deficit of Na^+ in the ECF compartment was somewhat greater than 300 mmol.*

Define the balances in the intracellular fluid compartment

Water

> • The percent expansion of the ICF volume is close to the percent fall in the P_{Na}.

Because the P_{Na} was 126 mmol/L (a reduction in the P_{Na} that is 14 mmol/L is a 10% fall) the ICF volume was expanded by close to 10%. Hence, the new ICF volume was 22 L (the original 20 L plus 10% of this volume).

Overall. This patient has a small positive balance of water of 0.5 L (i.e., a 2-L expansion of the ICF compartment and a 1.5-L deficit in the ECF compartment) and a deficit of 300 mmol of Na^+.

Specific therapy

> • Because the patient is malnourished, he has a greater risk for osmotic demyelination. In this setting, the goal is to avoid a rise in the P_{Na} that exceeds 4 mmol/L/day.

The initial dilemma is that one cannot be sure that the measured P_{Na} represents a steady-state value (*see margin note*). For example, if there was no water intake and an ongoing excretion of water in the past 12 hours, there could have been an appreciable and unknown rise in the P_{Na}. If this were the case, the goal of therapy should be to prevent a further rise in the P_{Na} for the next 12 hours or more (i.e., dDAVP should be given). If dDAVP is given, be certain that the patient will not drink water, as there would be a risk of developing acute hyponatremia.

On the other hand, the initial P_{Na} may reflect his usual steady-state value. In this case, the goal of therapy would be to avoid a rise in the P_{Na} that is higher than an upper limit (not a target to be achieved) of 4 mmol/L over the next 24 hours.

Create a negative balance for water. In total body water terms, his positive balance of water is small. Therefore, the major strategy to raise his P_{Na} is a positive balance of Na^+. Nevertheless, one must prevent a positive water balance, which requires careful monitoring of input and output of water. The danger of osmotic demyelination may be appreciable if this patient decreased his intake of water by more than 1 L/day compared to his urine output that day (see the following equation).

One may have to decrease his urine output by giving dDAVP if there is a large water diuresis. There would be a large risk of acute hyponatremia, however, if the patient, were to drink more water or if he were to sign himself out of the hospital while dDAVP is acting.

STEADY STATE VALUE FOR THE P_{Na}
- In a strict definition, the input and output of Na^+ and water must be equal over the time period of interest to define a steady state.
- Obviously, there is not a steady state using this strict definition because there are times when intakes exceed output and vice versa.
- Clinically, we use the term *steady state* to indicate that the P_{Na} will remain in a relatively narrow but low range.
- Of importance, be cautious when assuming that the first measured P_{Na} represents a steady-state value when defining the upper limit for the rise in the P_{Na} for the first day of therapy.

$$(1 \div \text{total body water}\,[31\,\text{L}]) \times P_{Na}\,[126\,\text{mmol/L}] = 4\,\text{mmol/L}$$

Create a positive balance for Na$^+$

> • This offers the best leverage to raise his P_{Na}, because the main reason for the low P_{Na} is the deficit of Na$^+$.
> • Administer enough NaCl to raise his P_{Na} by the desired amount and prevent a water diuresis by giving dDAVP.

To raise the patient's P_{Na} by 4 mmol/L, he would need a positive balance of 124 mmol of Na$^+$ (31 L × 4 mmol/L). Because this expands the ECF volume by close to 1 L, it could induce a rise in distal delivery that may be several liters and thereby a rapid water diuresis with the danger of an excessive increase in his P_{Na}. Thus, this therapy has a major risk of inducing osmotic demyelination if one does not prevent the water diuresis with the administration of dDAVP.

It is important to be sure that the patient does not drink more water than what is needed to maintain a nil balance for water. Accordingly, the P_{Na} must be followed closely (*see margin note*).

Other forms of therapy. The administration of urea or aquaretics is not beneficial when the major basis for the hyponatremia is a deficit of Na$^+$.

Na$^+$ RETENTION
The patient also needs to be advised that excessive quantities of NaCl will be retained for a period of time after consuming this load of NaCl and edema may develop.

Design of therapy for the second admission

His current P_{Na} was 112 mmol/L, the urine output was 1 to 1.5 L/day, the U_{Osm} was 350 mOsm/kg H$_2$O, and the $P_{Creatinine}$ was 1.8 mg/dL (150 µmol/L), which indicated that the GFR was considerably reduced (~50 L/day). The osmole excretion rate was somewhat low and the concentrations of Na$^+$ and Cl$^-$ in the urine were 5 mmol/L. Hence, there is an appreciable degree of contraction of his effective arterial blood volume.

Define the balances for water, Na$^+$, and K$^+$ in the extracellular and intracellular fluid compartments

Extracellular fluid compartment

Water. At this stage of the illness, the ECF volume would be close to 7 L (a best guess). Hence, there is a 3-L deficit of water in this compartment.

Na$^+$. Because the P_{Na} was 112 mmol/L and the ECF volume was close to 7 L, the content of Na$^+$ in the ECF compartment was 784 mmol. *Hence, the deficit of Na$^+$ in the ECF compartment was close to 600 mmol (1400 − 784 mmol).*

Intracellular fluid compartment

Water. Because the P_{Na} was 112 mmol/L, a 28-mmol/L fall in the P_{Na} (i.e., 20%), the ICF volume was expanded by close to 20%. Hence, the new ICF volume was 24 L (the original ICF volume of 20 L plus 20% of this volume), which is *a positive balance of 4 L.*

K$^+$. While hypokalemia was not present, the patient may have a deficit of K$^+$ and hypokalemia that is masked by a shift of K$^+$ out of cells. This shift of K$^+$ could be due to a degree of contraction of the effective arterial blood volume that is large enough to cause an important adrenergic surge, in which the α-adrenergic component will lead to inhibition of the release of insulin. This will become clear after enough NaCl is given to reexpand the effective arterial blood volume sufficiently to remove the hemodynamic stress.

Overall. This patient has a small positive balance of about 1 L of water (a deficit of 3 L of ECF volume and a gain of 4 L of ICF volume), a deficit of 600 mmol of Na^+, and an unknown deficit of K^+.

Specific therapy

> • Because the main danger is osmotic demyelination and the patient is even more likely to be malnourished, our goal is to avoid a rise in the P_{Na} that exceeds 4 mmol/L.

As discussed above, there is a concern about whether the initial P_{Na} represents a steady-state value (this is discussed on page 341).

Create a negative balance for water. The positive water balance is not a major component of the hyponatremia in this patient. Nevertheless, water restriction is important to prevent a positive balance for water. It is important to recognize, however, that it is not prudent to rely on this patient to restrict his intake of water by a specific volume.

Create a positive balance for Na^+

> • This offers the best leverage to raise his P_{Na}, because the main reason for the low P_{Na} is the large deficit of Na^+.

To raise the patient's P_{Na} by 4 mmol/L, he must have a daily positive balance of 124 mmol of Na^+ (31 L of total body water × 4 mmol/L). Again, this will expand his ECF volume by close to 1 L/day. Accordingly, it should take close to 5 days in theory before his ECF volume is reexpanded (but this includes a degree of expansion of his ECF volume, which is needed to induce a stimulus for a natriuresis). Hence, expect that his distal delivery of filtrate will rise and a water diuresis may occur before there is full reexpansion of his ECF volume. Thus, this therapy has a major risk of inducing osmotic demyelination if one does not curtail the water diuresis as the upper limit for the rise in the P_{Na} for that day is approached. If dDAVP is given, it is important to be sure that the patient does not drink more than 1 L/day to avoid the development of acute hyponatremia. Accordingly, the P_{Na} must be followed closely.

At this stage, therapy to raise the P_{Na} is a deficit of water if the patient still has a significant degree of hyponatremia. Therefore, on the next day, create a sufficient negative balance of water to raise the P_{Na} by the desired amount (i.e., 4 mmol/L; *see margin note*). Discontinue dDAVP temporarily to permit a negative balance of the desired volume of water to occur.

Other forms of therapy. The administration of urea or aquaretics is not beneficial when the basis for hyponatremia is a deficit of Na^+.

MINI-CASE 10-2: HYPONATREMIA WITH BROWN SPOTS

A 22-year-old woman has myasthenia gravis. In the past 6 months, she has noted a marked decline in her energy and in her weight (from 50 kg to 47 kg). She often felt faint when she stood up quickly. She denied having a large recent intake of water. On physical examination, her blood pressure was 80/50 mm Hg, pulse rate was

RAISE THE P_{Na} BY CREATING A NEGATIVE BALANCE OF WATER
- Assume that the patient weighs 50 kg and has 30 L of body water while the P_{Na} is 120 mmol/L. The goal is to raise the P_{Na} by 4 mmol/L in a specific time period.
- A negative balance of water of 1 L in this period will cause the P_{Na} to rise by 4 mmol ([1 L/30 L total body water] × 120 mmol/L = 4 mmol/L).

SIAD
- This case is presented to illustrate that a low distal delivery of filtrate can cause an impaired excretion of water that is large enough to induce chronic hyponatremia.
- The hyponatremia should be analyzed in terms of Na^+ and water balances.

126 beats per minute, jugular venous pressure was below the level of the sternal angle, and there was no peripheral edema. Brown pigmented spots were evident in her buccal mucosa. The EKG was unremarkable. The biochemistry data presented in the following table are consistent with a diagnosis of adrenal insufficiency.

		PLASMA	URINE
Na+	mmol/L	112	130
K+	mmol/L	5.5	24
BUN (Urea)	mg/dL (mmol/L)	28 (10)	130 mmol/L
Creatinine	mg/dL (μmol/L)	1.7 (150)	6.0 mmol/L
Osmolality	mOsm/kg H$_2$O	242	450

Questions

Are there emergencies present on admission?

What dangers should be anticipated during therapy, and how can they be avoided?

What is the most likely basis for the very low effective arterial blood volume?

What are the options for therapy?

Discussion of Mini-Case 10-2

- The loss of excessive quantities of Na+ in the urine is a major reason for the presence of hyponatremia; this results from the lack of aldosterone.
- Water may also be retained because of low distal delivery of filtrate (secondary to a low effective arterial blood volume, which in addition to Na+ loss is due in part to a lower degree of contraction of venous capacitance vessels because of the low glucocorticoid levels).
- Vasopressin may be released as a result of a very low effective arterial blood volume and/or the high corticotropin-releasing factor production in response to low glucocorticoid levels (*see margin note*).
- dDAVP should be given before reexpanding the effective arterial blood volume and administering glucocorticoids to prevent a large and potentially dangerous water diuresis.

CORTISOL AND VASOPRESSIN
- Because of lack of cortisol, the release of corticotropin-releasing factor from the hypothalamus is enhanced. This leads to the production of the precursor compound containing both ACTH and vasopressin.
- This nonosmotic release of vasopressin is reversed by the administration of glucocorticoids, which inhibit the release of corticotropin-releasing factor and hence this nonosmotic production of vasopressin may cease. An unwanted large water diuresis should be prevented with the administration of dDAVP.

Are there emergencies present on admission?

There are two potential emergencies that dominate the initial management: a very contracted effective arterial blood volume and the lack of cortisol. To deal with the former, the patient needs an infusion of a solution that is isotonic to the patient to reexpand the effective arterial blood volume without changing the P$_{Na}$. We would infuse this saline solution quickly at the outset (1 L/hr) and then at a slower rate once the hemodynamic state is improved. The second potential emergency is not life threatening at this moment, and it can be dealt with by administering a glucocorticoid.

There is one other possible emergency on admission—the presence of an acute element to her hyponatremia. This did not seem to be the case because the patient denied a recent large water intake and she did not have significant symptoms that could be related to an acute component of hyponatremia.

What dangers should be anticipated during therapy, and how can they be avoided?

Reexpansion of the patient's effective arterial blood volume can lead to an increased excretion of water due to an increased distal delivery of filtrate and suppression of the release of vasopressin. In addition, the administration of glucocorticoids will improve her hemodynamic state and also inhibit the release of corticotropin-releasing factor and hence of vasopression. The net result of this therapy is to cause a large excretion of water and thereby a dangerous rise in the P_{Na} (see later discussion). Because the patient has a small muscle mass (and hence a small total body water volume), a relatively small excretion of water can lead to a rapid rise in her P_{Na}. In addition, because of her poor nutritional state, which becomes even more evident if one interprets her weight loss in conjunction with water balance (i.e., a large gain of water in her cells but a contracted ECF volume), one should set a much lower daily upper limit for the maximum allowable rise in her P_{Na}. Accordingly, we would administer dDAVP to prevent a water diuresis early during therapy.

What is the most likely basis for the very low effective arterial blood volume?

In this case, the very contracted effective arterial blood volume (manifested by the low blood pressure and tachycardia), the low P_{Na}, the high P_K of 5.5 mmol/L, and the renal Na^+ wasting strongly suggest that the most likely diagnosis is adrenal insufficiency. This is likely due to autoimmune adrenalitis, as the patient has myasthenia gravis. The basis for the renal wasting of Na^+ is a lack of aldosterone. The low effective arterial blood volume is also caused in part by a lower degree of contraction of venous capacitance vessels because of the low glucocorticoid levels.

What are the options for therapy?

The design of therapy will depend on a quantitative analysis of the composition of the ECF and ICF compartments (see Table 10-9). This analysis is identical to the one used in Mini-Case 10-1 during the later admission of the patient to the hospital (see page 361).

Water. There is a 3-L water deficit in the ECF compartment and a 4-L positive balance of water in the ICF compartment. Hence, overall, there is a 1-L positive balance of water. The major difference in this patient is that vasopressin is almost certainly acting to lower rate of excretion of water.

Na^+. There is a 600-mmol negative balance of Na^+ in the ECF compartment and an unknown charge in the ionic charge in the ICF compartment.

1. *Water restriction*: Because there is only a small positive balance of water, this mode of therapy does not have a large impact. Nevertheless, because we would administer dDAVP at the outset to prevent a water diuresis, water intake must be limited to avoid an acute large fall in the patient's P_{Na} as long as dDAVP acts.

2. *Administer saline*: On the first day, our goal is to restore hemodynamic stability by infusing saline that is isotonic to the patient and administering glucocorticoids. Because this therapy should increase the distal delivery of filtrate and remove the actions of corticotropin-releasing factor to stimulate the release of vasopressin, it could lead to a large water diuresis and thereby an excessive rise in the P_{Na}, which may lead to osmotic demyelination. Therefore, dDAVP should be administered to prevent this water diuresis.

On the second day, the maximum limit for the rise in the P_{Na} is 4 mmol/L because of the high risk of osmotic demyelination owing to the catabolic state. We would create a positive balance of Na^+ and Cl^- of 4 mmol NaCl per liter of total body water (e.g., 120 mmol NaCl, if total body water is 30 L). Once a water diuresis begins, we would administer dDAVP to prevent a further rise in the P_{Na} on this day (see page 343 for details).

On day 3, if a water diuresis did not occur on day 2, repeat the therapy with NaCl as on day 2. On the other hand, if a water diuresis occured on day 2, we would create a further rise in the P_{Na} by inducing a negative balance of water. Once the P_{Na} reaches 135 mmol/L, one can simply stop the dDVAP.

There are two additional points to be made. First, do not try to increase the ECF volume to that of an individual who eats a higher amount of salt, because that person has an expanded ECF volume to cause the excretion of the daily salt load. Second, if a water diuresis does not occur, look for additional causes for the release of vasopressin.

MINI-CASE 10-3: TEA AND TOAST HYPONATREMIA

A 72-year-old astute, alert woman has been in excellent health until her physician prescribed a thiazide diuretic to treat hypertension (blood pressure ~160/85 mm Hg). After one month of therapy, her blood pressure was 130/80 mm Hg, but there were some disquieting symptoms: She had become lethargic and had difficulty concentrating, which was not usual for her. In addition, she did not look forward to the usual meetings with her friends where they would have their lively discussions over their traditional large cups of hot tea and biscuits. Moreover, because her appetite had declined, she ate only toast with jam. She was concerned that she had cancer and went to the hospital. On physical examination, the effective arterial blood volume appeared to be low. The EKG did not reveal changes related to hypokalemia. Her laboratory data were as follows (*see margin note*):

TOOLS TO ASSESS THE EFFECTIVE ARTERIAL BLOOD VOLUME

- When there has been a prior long period with a contracted effective arterial blood volume, the kidney will continue to retain Na^+ and Cl^-, which results in an expanded ECF volume. Therefore, use of the urine Na^+ and Cl^- concentrations should not guide therapy in this setting.
- We use the occurrence of water diuresis when dDVAP wears off to indicate that effective arterial blood volume is restored enough to increase distal delivery of filtrate.

CONCENTRATION OF Na^+ AND Cl^- IN THE URINE

- The rate of excretion of Na^+ and of Cl^- may be low if the urine flow rate is very low.
- Higher than expected rates of excretion of Na^+ and Cl^- may reflect continued actions of a natriuretic agent (e.g., thiazides) and/or an intrinsic problem with maximal conservation of Na^+.

		PLASMA	URINE
Na^+	mmol/L	112	50
K^+	mmol/L	2.6	20
Cl^-	mmol/L	72	50
HCO_3^-	mmol/L	30	—
Creatinine	mg/dL (µmol/L)	1.0 (87)	—
BUN (Urea)	mg/dL (mmol/L)	14 (5.0)	—
Osmolality	mOsm/kg H_2O	240	340

Questions

Are there any emergencies present on admission?

What dangers do you anticipate during therapy, and how can they be avoided?

How large is the positive balance for water and the deficit of Na^+?

What are the options for therapy to raise the P_{Na}?

Discussion of Mini-Case 10-3

> • The most likely diagnosis is diuretic-induced hyponatremia and hypokalemia.

Are there any emergencies present on admission?

There is no evidence of a hemodynamic emergency. There are also no symptoms that could be related to acute hyponatremia, a history of a large recent intake of water, or a prior recent P_{Na} to suspect a significant element of acute hyponatremia. The degree of hypokalemia is of concern, although it is not an acute emergency as suggested by the paucity of findings in the EKG.

What dangers do you anticipate during therapy, and how can they be avoided?

Although this patient has a large deficit of Na^+ and Cl^-, she is hemodynamically stable. The major potential danger is a cardiac arrhythmia related to the hypokalemia. Therefore, the initial aim of therapy should be to raise the P_K to a safer range (~3 mmol/L). Of note, most of the K^+ deficit is from the ICF compartment, and there was primarily a gain of Na^+ in the ICF compartment with this deficit of K^+. Accordingly, the administration of KCl will cause K^+ entry and Na^+ exit from cells. This will reexpand the ECF volume (gain of Na^+ and Cl^-) and may increase the distal delivery of filtrate and cause a large water diuresis. In addition, if the patient does not have bowel sounds, KCl will have to be given via the intravenous route in a saline solution (e.g., as 40 mmol KCl in 1 L of half isotonic saline). Nevertheless, this will reexpand the ECF volume and the effective arterial blood volume and thereby increase the distal delivery of filtrate, creating a water diuresis.

If a large water diuresis were to occur, the P_{Na} will rise too quickly and osmotic demyelination could be the result, as this patient with K^+ depletion and poor nutrition is at increased risk for this complication. Therefore, dDAVP must be given if the urine flow rate rises to avoid a daily rise in the P_{Na} that exceeds 4 mmol/L. To be safe, we would give the dDAVP before giving the KCl but ensure that water intake is restricted to avoid a large fall in the P_{Na}.

With the correction of hypokalemia, there may be increased intestinal motility, and another danger should be anticipated, depending on the volume and electrolyte content of the fluid that may have been retained in the intestinal lumen. If this fluid was rich in Na^+ and K^+ salts, expansion of the effective arterial blood volume may cause a large water diuresis and an overly rapid rise in the P_{Na}. On the other hand, if the fluid in the intestine contained sugar and little Na^+, when this fluid is reabsorbed, acute hyponatremia could develop after the sugar is metabolized. If the fall in the P_{Na} was excessive, hypertonic saline would have to be given to maintain the P_{Na} in the desired range.

How large is the positive balance for water and the deficit of Na$^+$?

Extracellular fluid compartment

Water. There is no accurate way to assign a value for the patient's ECF volume, other than to say that it is contracted. A reasonable estimate is that it has declined from 10 L to 8 L, a deficit of 2 L.

Na$^+$. If the patient's ECF volume was 8 L and her P_{Na} was 112 mmol/L, the content of Na$^+$ in her ECF compartment was close to 900 mmol and the deficit of Na$^+$ was 500 mmol. Notwithstanding, it is likely that some Na$^+$ has shifted from the ECF into her cells in response to the large deficit of intracellular K$^+$. Accordingly, her total body deficit of Na$^+$ was actually less than 500 mmol. This Na$^+$ will shift back into the ECF compartment when KCl is administered and much of the deficit of K$^+$ is replaced in the ICF compartment.

Intracellular fluid compartment

Water. With a P_{Na} of 112 mmol/L (a 20% decline), the ICF volume should be increased by 20% or 4 L (20% of 20 L). Nevertheless, if her muscle mass is much smaller than expected for her weight, the surplus of water would be less than 4 L, because 50% of body water is normally located in muscle cells.

K$^+$. We simply do not know how large the negative balance of K$^+$ was at the outset. The total dose of K$^+$ needed to correct the hypokalemia is likely to be smaller than expected for the degree of hypokalemia because of her low muscle mass.

Overall balances

Water. There was a positive balance of 1 to 2 L of water; this consists of a deficit of about 2 L of ECF volume and a surplus of about 4 L of ICF volume.

Na$^+$. There was a deficit of close to 500 mmol of Na$^+$ in the ECF compartment, but some of these Na$^+$ are now located in the ICF compartment, and this may accompany much of the deficit of K$^+$ in cells. Hence, an appreciable, but unknown, part of the deficit of Na$^+$ in the ECF compartment will be replaced when KCl is given and K$^+$ are retained in cells.

What are the options for therapy to raise the P_{Na}?

There are two options for therapy to raise the P_{Na}.

Create a negative balance for water. This is not the main component of therapy, as the major cause of hyponatremia is a deficit of NaCl. Nevertheless, water restriction is needed to prevent an acute large fall in the P_{Na}, especially if dDAVP will be given to prevent a water diuresis.

Administer NaCl and KCl

- The goal is to raise the P_{Na} with an upper limit of 4 mmol/L per 24 hours initially, because the patient has many risk factors for osmotic demyelination.
- dDAVP should be considered to prevent a water diuresis.

We would try to create a positive balance for Na$^+$ + K$^+$ of 4 mmol/L of total body water. This would mean giving the patient a positive balance of close to 125 mmol of Na$^+$ + K$^+$ (largely as KCl) in the next 24 hours (*see margin note*). Her inputs and outputs must be monitored, and the P_{Na} and P_K should be measured at frequent intervals to be sure that the desired rate of rise in her P_{Na} is not exceeded.

PRINCIPLES OF K$^+$ THERAPY
- *Route of K$^+$ administration:* It is much safer to give K$^+$ by the oral route if feasible and if bowel sounds are present, because this avoids local endothelial injury from high concentration of K$^+$ in intravenous fluid (should not exceed 40 mmol/L). The oral route also enables the administration of KCl without a large volume of intravenous fluid.
- *Monitoring is essential:* The EKG should be monitored until the P_K rises to a safe level (e.g., 3.5 mmol/L).
- Do not attempt to replace the entire deficit of K$^+$, as some of this K$^+$ loss represents catabolism of RNA and the excretion of K$^+$ and $H_2PO_4^-$ in the urine. This can only be replaced when there is an anabolic response.

If a water diuresis were to occur, dDAVP must be given to stop the loss of water in the urine and prevent a rise in the P_{Na} that exceeds the daily upper limit of 4 mmol/L. A water diuresis, however, indicates that the effective arterial blood volume has been restored sufficiently to increase the distal delivery of filtrate. If the patient is still hyponatremic, the plan for therapy is to allow a daily negative balance of water to achieve the desired rise in the P_{Na} that day. We would give dDAVP to limit the urine output to ensure that the rise in P_{Na} does not exceed our daily maximum limit for the rise in the P_{Na}.

There are two additional points. First, do not try to increase her ECF volume to one that is equal to individuals who eat a higher amount of salt, because they need an expanded ECF volume to excrete their salt load. Second, if a water diuresis does not occur after the effective arterial blood volume has been expanded and dDAVP has been discontinued, look for other causes for the release of vasopressin.

To avoid recurrence of hyponatremia, the patient should restrict her water intake, be given a smaller dose of thiazide, and increase her intake of NaCl somewhat. Alternatively, her hypertension could be treated without using diuretics.

Syndrome of inappropriate antidiuretic hormone

SIADH is the second subgroup of patients with chronic hyponatremia; the primary pathophysiology is persistently high levels of vasopressin (*see margin note*).

BASIC DEFECT IN PATIENTS WITH SIADH
- These patients have a fixed value for their effective U_{Osm} (nonurea osmolality) owing to constant actions of vasopressin.
- To achieve balance, they must consume the same quantity of Na^+ plus K^+ salts and water as they excrete (i.e., the opposite of normal subjects, who adjust the composition of urine to match their intake).
- Owing to changes in their daily intake of salt and water, the P_{Na} will have fluctuations in its concentration.
- Another variable that affects their P_{Na} is the quantity of nonrenal losses.

- SIADH is a diagnosis of exclusion. Hence, it cannot be made in the presence of a low distal delivery of filtrate.
- In some patients, the stimulus for the release of vasopressin may not be permanent (e.g., secondary to a drug, pain, anxiety; see Table 10-5). If vasopressin disappears, dDAVP must be given once a water diuresis begins to prevent a rapid rise in the P_{Na} and osmotic demyelination.
- In patients with persistently high vasopressin levels, the major danger is acute hyponatremia when there is a large intake of water.
- The presence of vasopressin may indicate that a serious underlying disease is present (e.g., a neoplasm).

Diagnostic criteria

The first step is to rule out patients who may have a low distal delivery of filtrate because of a low effective arterial blood volume (e.g., patients with congestive heart failure, hypoalbuminemia, edema, renal wasting of Na^+ [diuretics, adrenal insufficiency], cortisol deficiency, hypothyroidism), or a very low GFR. In patients with SIADH, the U_{Osm} should exceed the P_{Osm}, and the concentration of Na^+ in the urine should be appreciable (e.g., usually >50 mmol/L). In addition, these patients generally have low P_{Urea} and P_{Urate} with high fractional excretion of urea and of urate. The next step is to establish why vasopressin is being released (see Table 10-2).

Subtypes of syndrome of inappropriate antidiuretic hormone

Autonomous release of vasopressin

- In these patients, there is no physiologic basis for the release of vasopressin (e.g., release of vasopressin from cancer cells).

Vasopressin levels in these patients are consistently high. This subtype is said to represent approximately one third of the patients with SIADH, but clearly this depends on the population of patients to which one is exposed.

"Reset osmostat"

- The key finding in this subgroup of patients is that they have a water diuresis when a water load is administered. In addition, the excretion of hypotonic urine stops before the P_{Na} rises to the normal range.
- The importance of making the diagnosis of this type of SIADH is that the patient is not in danger of developing a significant further fall in the P_{Na} when ingesting a larger water load.

These patients have normal regulation of vasopressin release but around a hypotonic threshold. This pathophysiology may account for approximately one third of the patients with SIADH. This diagnosis hinges on documenting that the patient can excrete dilute urine when the P_{Na} is lowered appreciably. Because of the danger, a reset osmostat should not be tested for if the degree of hyponatremia is severe.

One possible cause is a sick-cell syndrome. This assumes that cells of the osmostat have fewer effective osmoles because of a catabolic illness. Therefore, the volume of these cells is decreased, even at a lower than normal P_{Na}, and vasopressin is released. With a more severe degree of hyponatremia, these cells swell back to exceed their original size, and thus the release of vasopressin is suppressed. Hence, they now defend this lower P_{Na}.

Nonosmotic stimuli (afferent) overload

- In this putative model, nonosmotic afferent signals are perceived by cells of the osmostat or of the vasopression release center, which leads to release of vasopressin despite the low P_{Na}.

Findings that may be in keeping with this model are that it may occur in patients who have lesions involving the lungs (e.g., pneumonia) and/or the brain (e.g., following trauma or an intracerebral hemorrhage that involves an area in the brain that is remote from the osmostat and the vasopressin release center; Fig. 10-7). Although this is rather indirect evidence, it provides a way to imagine how this lesion may develop. These afferent impulses may act on the osmostat or the vasopressin release center. In the former, thirst would be stimulated when P_{Na} rises somewhat but is still in the hyponatremic range.

Other possible causes

- This represents a heterogeneous group of patients who lack vasopressin in their plasma; we are not certain that their disorder is truly SIADH (*see margin note*).

OTHER POSSIBLE CAUSES
- A low distal delivery of filtrate (which is not SIADH by definition) must be ruled out before the patient can be included in the SIADH diagnostic category.
- We have observed that normal subjects who eat little NaCl may have undetectable levels of vasopressin in plasma, yet they can lower their urine flow rate to very low values (~0.4 mL/min).
- This implies that the assay for vasopressin may not be sufficiently sensitive in the very low range. Furthermore, when there is a persistently low level of circulating vasopressin, there is up-regulation of its V_2 receptor in the late distal nephron and thus lower circulating levels of vasopressin may cause the excretion of concentrated urine.

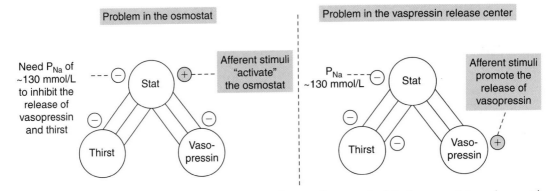

FIGURE 10-7 Reset osmostat due to nonosmotic stimulus. As shown to the *left*, the osmostat can be reset by afferent impulses such that it now defends a lower effective P_{Osm} (e.g., P_{Na} 130 mmol/L). If the problem is in the osmostat, thirst is stimulated when the P_{Na} is in the hyponatremic range. As shown to the *right*, the vasopressin release center can be reset by afferent impulses such that it now requires a lower effective P_{Osm} (e.g., P_{Na} 130 mmol/L) to fully inhibit the release of vasopressin; thirst is inhibited as long as hyponatremia persists.

The contention is that there is a normal release of vasopressin at high tonicity, but hyponatremia is present while vasopressin is not detectable in plasma. Some patients are said to have a vasopressin-like hormone present, whereas others may have an up-regulation of the V_2 receptors in the distal nephron.

MINI-CASE 10-4: DID MY P_{Na} RISE BY ACCIDENT?

(Discussion on page 355)

A young male had traumatic brain injury following an auto accident 3 years ago (*see margin note*). He does not have any obvious residual effects other than chronic hyponatremia. Since he has no evidence of a deficit of Na^+ and thereby a low distal delivery of filtrate, his chronic hyponatremia probably represents SIADH. His P_{Na} varied from 125 to 133 mmol/L. Typical values for his 24-hour urine were a volume close to 1.5 L, U_{Osm} 950 mOsm/kg H_2O, U_{Na} 200 mmol/L, and U_K 50 mmol/L.

When his P_{Na} was 126 mmol/L, he reduced his water intake to less than 1 L/day, but he did not change his dietary intake. There was no water diuresis, as his U_{Osm} in every urine collection was close to 950 mOsm/kg H_2O. Nevertheless, his P_{Na} rose progressively to 138 mmol/L over several days. The ability of water restriction alone to raise his P_{Na} was observed on a number of occasions.

COMMENTS
- This case is presented to illustrate that water restriction can raise the P_{Na} in certain patients with SIADH.
- A tonicity balance will help reveal why water restriction could raise the P_{Na} in certain patients with SIADH.

Questions

What are the hallmarks of SIADH?

Why did his P_{Na} rise with water restriction?

Why is water restriction not effective in most patients with SIADH?

Based on the above, is the major potential danger for this patient acute hyponatremia and/or osmotic demyelination?

Background to understand why water restriction may raise the P_{Na}

**TONICITY AFFECTING
CELL VOLUME**

- Tonicity is the osmolality due to the major electrolytes (i.e., $2 [(Na^+) + (K^+)]$).
- The osmolality due to urea and NH_4^+ salts in the urine is not included in this definition, as NH_4^+ were derived ultimately from glutamine in proteins (i.e., from a macromolecule). The osmolality due to urea is not included because urea is not an effective osmole in the body.

- The P_{Na} can be raised by water restriction if the tonicity of the input is greater than the tonicity of the outputs (via urine, sweat, and the GI tract; *see margin note*).

There are three points that merit emphasis with respect to the ability of water restriction to induce a rise in the P_{Na} (with apologies to the three bears).

1. *The effect may be too large.* In a subject who has a low distal delivery of filtrate and lacks actions of vasopressin (i.e., the U_{Osm} is considerably less than the P_{Osm}), it is very easy to have an intake with a higher tonicity than in the urine. Moreover, if the intake of water is considerably less than the output, there could be a large, rapid, and dangerous rise in the P_{Na}. Parenthetically, the output of sweat is hypotonic and the GI losses are very often isotonic or hypotonic solutions.

**URINE FLOW RATE IN A
PATIENT WITH SIADH**

- In this patient, the rate of excretion of electrolytes is high enough to ensure that urea is *not* an effective urinary osmole (i.e., urea diffuses rapidly from the lumen to the interstitial compartment in the terminal nephron).
- The urine flow rate is determined by the rate of excretion of effective or nonurea osmoles (which is the same as the osmolality due to electrolytes); their concentrations are always similar in the urine and in the interstitial compartment because vasopressin acts continuously.

2. *The effect may be too small.* It is very difficult to have an intake with a higher tonicity than in the output if the subject consumes little NaCl and K^+ unless that person has an extremely low concentration of $Na^+ + K^+$ in his or her urine and/or has a large nonrenal loss (e.g., sweat, which is a hypotonic solution).

3. *The effect may be just right.* In subjects with SIADH who consume a large quantity of NaCl and who restrict their intake of water, it is possible to make their intake have a higher tonicity than in their urine, as the latter has a maximum value of close to 600 mmol/L on a typical Western diet (*see margin note*; see the discussion of Mini-Case 10-4, page 355).

Design of therapy for the patient with syndrome of inappropriate antidiuretic hormone

- The first step is to calculate the balances for water and Na^+.

Case example: A 50-kg patient has SIADH due to the autonomous release of vasopressin from a cancer in her lung. Her total body water is 30 L, her ECF volume is 10 L, her ICF volume is 20 L, and her P_{Na} now is 126 mmol/L.

Extracellular fluid compartment

Water. It is likely that there is a small degree of expansion of her ECF volume from 10 L to 10.5 L. Hence, there is a gain of 0.5 L.

Na^+. The product of the P_{Na} and the new ECF volume is 1323 mmol (126 mmol/L × 10.5 L). Hence, there is a small deficit of Na^+ (77 mmol), which we shall ignore in the design of therapy.

Intracellular fluid compartment

Water. Since there is a 10% fall in the P_{Na}, there is close to a 10% positive balance of water in the ICF compartment, which is a gain of 2 L of water (10% of the 20 L of water in cells).

Na⁺ and K⁺. There is no important change in the content of electrolytes in all organs other than in the brain, where there is adaptive loss of osmoles to return the brain cell size toward normal.

Overall. There is a positive balance of 2.5 L of water.

Restrict water intake

> - The goal of therapy is to cause a negative balance of 2.5 L of water at a rate that does not cause the P_{Na} to rise by more than 8 mmol/L/day.
> - The major value of restricting the intake of water in most patients with SIADH is to prevent a further fall in the P_{Na}.

To raise the P_{Na} by just 1 mmol/L, the deficit of water should be 0.26 L (*see margin note*). Hence, the patient needs a negative balance of somewhat greater than 2 L of water in the next 24 hours to raise the P_{Na} by 8 mmol/L (i.e., 0.26 L × 8 mmol/L). It is obvious that simple restriction of water cannot be successful to raise the P_{Na} by the desired amount in 24 hours because this *exceeds* the usual daily intake of water.

Increase the excretion of water without electrolytes

> - There are several techniques that are used to create a negative balance of water while not changing the balance for Na⁺.

A loop diuretic is given to create a deficit of Na⁺ and water; the amount of water and Na⁺ lost in the urine after the diuretic acts must be measured. The patient is then given back all the Na⁺ and the K⁺ that was lost in the urine to have a net loss of "pure" water (Fig. 10-8). To create the desired negative balance of water, the patient would have to drink less water than he or she excretes during this therapy (calculate the volume of water intake based on the required negative

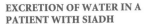

EXCRETION OF WATER IN A PATIENT WITH SIADH
- To calculate the negative balance of water that is needed to raise the P_{Na} by 1 mmol/L in this patient, multiply 1/126 mmol/L by her current total body water (32.5 L); the result is 0.26 L.
- A patient with SIADH is usually not able to excrete more electrolyte-free water because vasopressin acts throughout the 24-hour period.
- If the usual intake of Na⁺ and K⁺ salts is 450 mosmol/day, and if the effective medullary interstitial osmolality is 450 mOsm/kg H_2O, the urine volume will be 1.0 L/day.

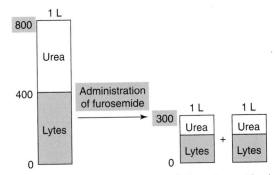

FIGURE 10-8 Excretion of water with a low concentration of electrolytes. The height of the rectangle indicates the osmolality of the urine. The *large rectangle* represents 1 L of urine excreted in a time period when vasopressin acts and the medullary interstitial osmolality is 800 mOsm/kg H_2O. When furosemide is acting, the U_{Osm} is close to 300 mOsm/kg H_2O. Since some of the urine osmoles are area, the concentration of Na⁺ + K⁺ in the urine will be less than its plasma. If all of these electrolyte osmoles are replaced, there will be a net loss of 2 L of water over this time period.

water balance to achieve a desired rate of rise in the P_{Na}). The P_{Na} must be followed closely to ensure that the upper limit set for the daily rise in the P_{Na} is not exceeded.

Use of aquaretics

- These drugs prevent vasopressin from binding to its V_2 receptor, and as a result, they prevent the insertion of AQP2 into the late distal nephron segments.
- To minimize the risk of a large water diuresis and thereby an excessive rise in the P_{Na}, their use should be restricted to patients with chronic hyponatremia and a low distal delivery of filtrate (i.e., they should not be used in patients with SIADH).
- This class of drugs inhibits the cytochrome P_{450} system (CYP3A4), and hence they may affect the metabolism of other drugs.

VOLUME OF WATER EXCRETED WHEN AQUARETICS BLOCK THE ACTIONS OF VASOPRESSIN
- Patients with chronic hyponatremia due to SIADH have a normal distal delivery of filtrate, which can be 1 L/hr. Hence, the excretion of water may be large enough to cause the rise in the P_{Na} to exceed its daily upper limit. The upper limit for the rise in the P_{Na} may be exceeded when aquaretics act for several hours in these patients. Thus, there could be a risk of developing osmotic demyelination.
- The only group of patients in whom aquaretics have a small risk are those who have disorders associated with a low effective arterial blood volume and edema (e.g., patients with congestive heart failure or hypoalbuminemia). These patients have a low distal delivery of filtrate and thus a much lower urine flow rate. Hence, the risk of inducing a large water diuresis and an excessive rise in P_{Na} should be less in this group of patients.

Aquaretics or "vaptans" is the generic name given to a family of drugs that cause a water diuresis despite the fact that vasopressin is present. *Said another way, they induce "true" nephrogenic diabetes insipidus!* Hence, the urine volume in this setting depends on the volume of water delivered to the distal nephron minus the volume of water reabsorbed by residual water permeability. The former depends on the avidity for the reabsorption of Na^+ in the proximal convoluted tubule and the GFR (*see margin note*).

Risks. Because many of the aquaretics are competitive inhibitors of vasopressin in terms of binding to its V_2 receptor, their effective dose in a given patient depends on the level of vasopressin at a particular moment, which is an unknown and not a constant value. Therefore, it is easy to have too large a water diuresis at some times and an inadequate water diuresis at other times with the same dose of the drug. Because the danger stems from too rapid a rise in the P_{Na} and the development of osmotic demyelination, it could be unsafe to use these drugs outside of a hospital. Moreover, whenever these agents are used, one must have the antidote at the bedside to stop an excessive water diuresis (vasopressin or dDAVP; be prepared to administer enough of this hormone to lower the urine flow rate to pretreatment levels to have a $U_{Osm} > P_{Osm}$).

Other possible side effects. All drugs have side effects as well as interactions with other medications or dietary constituents that may impair the clearance of that drug. In addition, the underlying disease itself might lead to reduced function of the organ that metabolizes and/or excretes the drug. With the aquaretics, there is a specific problem—they inhibit the cytochrome P450 system (CYP3A4). Hence, they can decrease the clearance of a number of medications (e.g., hepatic HMG-CoA reductase inhibitors, calcium channel blockers). The risk may be more evident in patients with liver disease.

QUESTIONS

(Discussions on pages 365 and 366)

10-5 *What role might K^+ depletion play in determining the severity of hyponatremia?*

10-6 *In what way might hyponatremia lead to a larger plasma volume?*

10-7 *Hyponatremic patients treated with oral capsules containing urea have a larger excretion of water without Na$^+$, which results in a rise in their P_{Na}, whereas similar patients eating a high-protein diet do not have a similar increase in their urine flow rate. Why might these responses be different?*

10-8 *What precautions are required to ensure that the use of aquaretics to raise the P_{Na} is safe?*

Discussion of Mini-Case 10-4

(Case presented on page 351)

What are the hallmarks of SIADH?

A diagnosis of SIADH cannot be made if there is a low distal delivery of filtrate. In patients with SIADH, there are continuous actions of vasopressin without a physiologic stimulus for its release (i.e., hypernatremia or a contracted effective arterial blood volume). Since vasopressin causes the insertion of AQP2 into the luminal membrane of principal cells in the late cortical and the medullary nephron segments and of urea transporters in the inner medullary collecting ducts, hyponatremia will develop if the intake has a lower tonicity than the urine.

One should extend the hallmarks of SIADH to the composition of the urine. Because AQP2 and urea transporters are present in the luminal membranes of late distal nephron segments owing to actions of vasopressin, water and urea will be in diffusion equilibrium between the lumen of the inner medullary collecting duct and the medullary interstitial compartment. This means that the osmolalities and the concentrations of urea will be equal in the final urine and in the inner medullary interstitial compartment.

Although there were daily variations in his P_{Na} over the past 3 years, this patient was in a virtual steady state over this period. Accordingly, his intake of water must be equal to the urine volume plus losses via nonrenal routes and the concentrations of Na$^+$ + K$^+$ must be similar in his dietary intake and in his urine (Na$^+$ 200 mmol/L, K$^+$ 50 mmol/L), as nonrenal losses are small. Thus, the total daily intake and excretions were 300 mmol NaCl and 75 mmol K$^+$ salts in 1.5 L of water. Since the sum of the *concentrations* of electrolytes in his urine was 250 mmol/L (or 500 mOsm/L, as these cations are excreted with monovalent anions), they are likely to be very similar in his medullary interstitial compartment. Thus he has little, if any, ability to change the nonurea osmolality in his urine in this setting (*see margin note*). Therefore, to raise his P_{Na}, his intake must be hypertonic to his urine.

Why did his P_{Na} rise with water restriction?

The key to answer this question is to examine a tonicity balance (*see margin note*). Since the patient has not changed his intake of NaCl and food (i.e., K$^+$ salts), the net effect of water restriction is to raise the tonicity of his input. If, for example, he halved his intake of water, the concentration of effective osmoles in his dietary intake (input) will be twice that in his urine (output). In balance terms, he will excrete all ingested osmoles while consuming less water than in his urine plus that by nonrenal routes. If his total body water were 30 L, his P_{Na} would rise by 3.2 mmol/L/day ([0.75 L/30 L] × 128 mmol/L). Hence, over 3 days, his P_{Na} would rise by close to 10 mmol/L.

EXCRETION OF NH$_4^+$
Since the quantity of NH$_4^+$ in his urine is small relative to the excretion of Na$^+$ + K$^+$, we have not included NH$_4^+$ salts in the urine in this analysis.

TONICITY BALANCE
In the table below, B = period before water restriction and A = period after water restriction.

	IN		OUT	
	B	A	B	A
Water (L/day)	1.5	0.75	1.5	1.5
Na$^+$ + K$^+$ (mmol/day)	375	375	375	375
[Na$^+$ = K$^+$] (mmol/L)	250	500	250	250

There are two possible mechanisms to explain why the P_{Na} rose: a positive balance of Na^+ or a negative balance for water (the urine volume is dictated by the rate of excretion of effective osmoles, and this did not change). In fact, both mechanisms are important, but their timing may be different—three possible events are considered below.

1. *Initial balance was achieved for Na^+*: Since the subject did not change his intake of NaCl, we shall assume for simplicity that the entire dietary input of NaCl was excreted.

2. *Initial consequences for water*: Since the urine composition is fixed in terms of nonurea osmolality, the urine volume will remain unchanged (1.5 L/day). Since the intake of water was lower than water loss, the patient has a negative balance of water and the volumes of the ECF and ICF compartments will fall—this will raise the P_{Na} and decrease body weight owing to a deficit of water.

3. *Later effects*: In response to less expanded ECF volume (and effective arterial blood volume), there will be a temporary decline in the rate of excretion of Na^+ and Cl^-, which leads to a positive balance of Na^+ and Cl^- and a rise in the P_{Na}. As a result of the rise in his P_{Na}, some water will shift from the ICF compartment to the ECF compartment.

Conclusions. These iterations will continue until the P_{Na} reaches 140 mmol/L. At this point, a new physiologic stimulus develops; thirst will be present. When this occurs, water restriction will fail, as thirst is such a powerful urge.

Why is water restriction not effective in most patients with SIADH?

To raise the P_{Na}, the tonicity of the input must be higher than the output. To raise the tonicity of the input to a value higher than the tonicity in the urine by reducing water intake, the intake of NaCl and K^+ salts must be relatively high because patients are unlikely to follow the instructions to drink a very small volume of water. When examined in quantitative terms, this limitation becomes clearer. For example, if the patient consumed 100 mmol of NaCl per day, the intake of water would have to be less than 0.33 L/day to have a tonicity of the intake that is greater than in the urine (using the maximum tonicity of 300 mmol/L or 600 mosmol/L of NaCl in the urine; *see margin note*).

Based on the above, is the major potential danger for this patient acute hyponatremia and/or osmotic demyelination?

1. *Osmotic demyelination*: A rapid rise in the P_{Na} is needed to cause osmotic demyelination; it may be due to a large positive balance of hypertonic saline or a large negative balance of water. Nevertheless, they are both unlikely for the following reasons.

   A. *Hypertonic saline administration*: Although, in theory, a hypertonic saline load could cause a large rise in the P_{Na}, this is unlikely unless these patients are treated incorrectly in the hospital.

   B. *Large negative balance of water*: There are three settings for patients with chronic hyponatremia in which a large negative balance of water may develop. Of note, only the latter two examples represent SIADH. In the first group, SIADH is not the correct diagnosis because the defect in water excretion is due to a low distal delivery of filtrate. Hence, a large water diuresis can develop when these patients are given a salt load, as they lack actions of vasopressin. The second group consists of patients with SIADH

URINE TONICITY

- It is possible for the urine tonicity to be somewhat lower or higher than 600 mOsm/L in normal subjects when vasopressin acts, as this upper limit applies to subjects eating a typical Western diet and a P_{Na} of 140 mmol/L.
- When the P_{Na} is considerably lower than 140 mmol/L, the maximum value for the urine tonicity is lower than when the P_{Na} was 140 mmol/L in animals and in humans.
- We have observed urine tonicities greater than 800 mOsm/kg H_2O in subjects who received very large infusions of saline following neurosurgery.
  - Alain Bombard survived at sea for 2 weeks while drinking seawater. Although he may have ingested some rainwater, it is possible that the nonurea osmolality in his medullary interstitial compartment was higher than 600 mOsm/kg H_2O in this setting.

who have a very large intake of NaCl. Nevertheless, as illustrated in Mini-Case 10-4, it would take several days to achieve a large rise in their P_{Na}. In the third group, patients with SIADH have renal actions of vasopressin that may disappear. This group includes patients with causes for the release of vasopressin that are reversible (i.e., discontinuing the administration of dDAVP or drugs that led to the secretion of vasopressin) or the administration of aquaretics to block the actions of vasopressin.

    Conclusion. Patients with SIADH of the variety in which there is continuous release of vasopressin will rarely develop osmotic demyelination unless treated incorrectly in the hospital (i.e., given hypertonic saline or an aquaretic).

2. *Acute hyponatremia*: In patients who have AQP2 inserted permanently in the luminal membranes of the late distal nephron, acute hyponatremia will result if they drink a sufficiently large quantity of water. Hence, this is the main danger and the patients should be warned about this risk. They should follow their weight closely and seek medical advice if there is a weight gain that exceeds 1 kg (that will reflect a fall of P_{Na} of above 4 mmol/L in a 50-kg subject if due to a water gain).

PART D
INTEGRATIVE PHYSIOLOGY

FACTORS THAT DECREASE THE MAXIMUM WATER DIURESIS

There are two factors that influence the maximum volume of urine in settings where there are no actions of vasopressin: the distal delivery of filtrate and the residual water permeability in the inner medullary collecting duct.

Distal delivery of filtrate

The distal delivery of filtrate is affected by the GFR and the quantity of Na^+ plus water reabsorbed in the proximal convoluted tubule (see the following equation). The major setting for a low distal delivery of filtrate is one where a low effective arterial blood volume augments the reabsorption of Na^+ and Cl^- in the proximal convoluted tubule. The usual cause for a low effective arterial blood volume is a true deficit of Na^+ and Cl^-, but in some patients, it is due to a cardiac problem (e.g., congestive heart failure) or states with a low $P_{Albumin}$ (e.g., cirrhosis of the liver, nephrotic syndrome).

    Distal delivery = GFR − Proximal reabsorbtion of filtrate

Low GFR

This is a later stage of the conditions that lead to a low distal delivery of filtrate. Nevertheless, the importance of the low GFR is shown in Table 10-10, where we illustrate the effects of reducing the GFR by 50% from 180 L/day to 90 L/day (called two kidneys and one kidney for simplicity).

TABLE 10-10 **MAXIMUM EXCRETION OF A WATER LOAD**

	TWO KIDNEYS (L/day)	ONE KIDNEY (L/day)
Glomerular filtration rate (GFR)	180	90
Delivery of filtrate to the DCT	27	13.5
Residual water reabsorption	5	5
Maximum water diuresis	22	8.5

A fall in GFR leads to a lower distal delivery of filtrate. Nevertheless, the fall must be significantly greater than 50% to be the sole factor to cause hyponatremia, as the intake of water must be considerably larger than most individuals are accustomed to ingesting.

Enhanced reabsorption of Na^+ and Cl^- in the proximal convoluted tubule

> • By extrapolation from micropuncture data in the fed rat, humans reabsorb five sixths of the GFR or 150 L/day of the filtered 180 L/day in the entire proximal convoluted tubule.

VENOUS TONE IN CAPACITANCE VESSELS
• When venous tone decreases, blood pools in venous capacitance vessels and this decreases the effective arterial blood volume.
• Cortisol acts to increase this venous tone.
• In patients with adrenal insufficiency, the lower venous tone leads to a lower effective arterial blood volume, but not the ECF volume. Conversely, administering a glucocorticoid may increase the effective arterial blood volume in this setting.

This enhanced reabsorption of Na^+ and Cl^- in the proximal convoluted tubule is due to a decreased effective arterial blood volume (*see margin note*). In this setting, the avidity for Na^+ reabsorption is increased. For example, if the reabsorption of Na^+ and water is increased from five sixths to seven eighths (83% to 87.5%) in a subject with a normal GFR, the delivery of filtrate to the loop of Henle and hence to the distal nephron would fall from 27 to about 22.5 L/day, a decrease of 4.5 L/day. Hence, distal delivery of filtrate is very sensitive to relatively small changes in Na^+ and water reabsorption in the proximal convoluted tubule.

Residual water permeability

> • The most important function of residual water permeability is to create a signal to desalinate the "future" urine during a maximal water diuresis.
> • The volume of filtrate delivered to the loop of Henle is about 27 L/day (see Chapter 9, page 263).
> • The maximum water diuresis in a 70-kg male with a high NaCl intake is close to 15 mL/min (extrapolates to close to 22 L/day).
> • Accordingly, about 5 L/day are reabsorbed via residual water permeability during a water diuresis.

The following features must be appreciated to understand the physiology of residual water permeability.
1. *The inner medullary collecting duct has a constitutive permeability to water.* The driving force for water reabsorption in the inner medullary collecting duct is the difference in osmolality between interstitial compartment and in the lumen of the inner medullary collecting duct (discussed in more detail in Chapter 9, page 278).
2. *When vasopressin is present, AQP2 water channels are abundant in the luminal membranes of late distal nephron segments.* In this setting, residual water permeability *cannot* mediate the reabsorption of water (i.e., there is no driving force for water reabsorption because the osmolalities are virtually identical in the lumen and in the interstitial compartment).

TABLE 10-11 **EFFECT OF A LOW INTAKE OF NaCl ON THE VOLUME OF URINE DURING A WATER DIURESIS**

All values are expressed per hour after consuming a large water load. In the subject who consumes a large amount of NaCl, there is a decreased reabsorption of NaCl and water in the proximal convoluted tubule and therefore a larger distal delivery of filtrate, whereas the subject with a low intake of NaCl has enhanced reabsorption of filtrate in the proximal convoluted tubule and thereby a lower distal delivery of filtrate. Note that the proportion of the volume of water reabsorbed by residual water permeability is larger in the subject with the low intake of NaCl.

NaCl INTAKE	HIGH	LOW
Distal delivery	1 L/hr	0.7 L/hr
Medullary interstitial osmolality	350 mOsm/L	350 mOsm/L
Water reabsorbed	0.3 L/hr	0.3 L/hr
Urine flow rate	0.7 L/hr (17 L/day)	0.4 L/hr (9.6 L/day)

3. *When vasopressin is absent, there are no AQP2 in luminal membranes.* In this setting, there is an enormous driving force for water reabsorption, because the luminal osmolality is close to 300 mOsm/L lower than in the interstitial compartment (Table 10-11).

4. *Water fails to reach osmotic equilibrium in the inner medullary collecting duct for a number of reasons.* First, the permeability to water via residual water permeability is not high. Second, the time of exposure is not long. Third, there is little stirring action to aid diffusion. The latter two limitations can be partially overcome by repeated renal pelvic contraction and reflux of urine from the renal pelvis into the medullary collecting duct. This reflux can occur more than once, in theory, before urine enters the ureter. There is one other issue of importance in this regard: The larger the volume in the renal pelvis, the more likely it is that a large proportion of the volume will enter the ureter when pressure rises due to renal pelvic contraction because only a limited volume can enter the medullary collecting duct. *Therefore, residual water permeability makes the urine flow rate much more sensitive to the distal delivery of filtrate* (see the following equation):

Urine flow rate = Distal delivery − Residual water permeability

"ESCAPE" FROM THE RENAL ACTIONS OF VASOPRESSIN

- "Escape" from the renal actions of vasopressin implies that the number of AQP2 in the late distal nephron does not permit the osmolality in the final urine to be as high as the osmolality in the medullary interstitial compartment in patients with chronic hyponatremia.

The reader should decide which of the following criteria is absolutely essential to support the concept that there is "escape" from the renal actions of vasopressin. Because one must make measurements directly in the kidney, the true test of this hypothesis is derived from experiments in animals.

1. *Rats treated with vasopressin have chronic hyponatremia and a lower U_{Osm} (~2000 mOsm/kg H_2O) than observed in normal rats (~3000 mOsm/kg H_2O). In these rats, there was a significant reduction in the number of AQP2 in the luminal membrane of the final functional nephron unit.*
2. *Under the same conditions as the experiments in which AQP2 channels were measured in rats, the maximum U_{Osm} was close to 2000 mOsm/kg H_2O (see margin note). When the osmolality was measured in the excised tip of the renal papilla in these rats, there was no significant difference between this osmolality and that in simultaneously excreted urine.*

The following issues will help the reader decide the merits of the two opposing views of escape from vasopressin actions.

Factors affecting the diffusion of water in the inner medullary collecting duct

• Diffusion depends on the driving force, the permeability to water, and the contact time.

Driving force

This driving force is *enormous* in this location. In quantitative terms, normal rats have a papillary interstitial osmolality of close to 3000 mOsm/kg H_2O. In contrast, rats with chronic hyponatremia have a urine osmolality of about 2000 mOsm/kg H_2O. If the medullary interstitial osmolality remained at 3000 mOsm/kg H_2O, there would be a difference in osmolality of 1000 mOsm/kg H_2O, which would exert an osmotic pressure of 19,300 mm Hg (19.3 mm Hg/mOsm/L); this is equivalent to the mean arterial pressure generated by pumping of blood by close to 200 beating hearts.

Permeability to water

Considering the enormous driving force, one would need the near total absence of AQP2 water channels to limit for the reabsorption of water.

Contact time

Every time the renal pelvis contracts, luminal fluid moves retrograde up the inner medullary collecting duct. Hence, these extra exposures make contact time and stirring, variables that are not accounted for when correlating the volume of water absorbed with the number of AQP2 water channels.

Conclusions

There is strong evidence against the hypothesis of "escape" from the renal actions of vasopressin in vivo in experimental animals. The lower U_{Osm} observed in these animals seems to result from the fact that the medullary interstitial osmolality has also fallen (not really an escape from the renal actions of vasopressin). Although there is a decrease in number of AQP2, this does not represent a true escape from the renal actions of vasopressin because water moved to osmotic equilibrium.

VALUE FOR THE MEDULLARY INTERSTITIAL OSMOLALITY

• The maximum urine osmolality in a human subject consuming a typical Western diet is ~1200 mOsm/kg H_2O. This osmolality is made up of equal proportions of urea and electrolytes.

• While the nonurea osmolality undergoes little change, the component due to urea can change appreciably with the urine flow rate because the latter affects the concentration of urea in the urine.

• The presence of urea transporters in the luminal membrane of the inner medullary collecting ducts permits the concentrations of urea in the urine and in the medullary interstitial compartments to be equal. Hence, the concentration of urea in the urine sets the upper limit on the concentration of urea in the medullary interstitial compartment.

• When hyponatremia is present, less water is abstracted in the cortical portion of the final nephron unit because of the lower P_{Osm}. As a result, there will be a lower concentration of urea in the luminal fluid throughout the medullary collecting ducts.

DISCUSSION OF CASES

CASE 10-1: THIS CATASTROPHE SHOULD NOT HAVE OCCURRED!

(Case presented on page 315)

What dangers are present on admission?

Because her P_{Na} yesterday was 125 mmol/L and today is 112 mmol/L, there is an acute component to the hyponatremia. Of great importance, the new symptom (headache) indicates that urgent therapy with hypertonic saline is needed. She should receive enough hypertonic saline to shrink the size of her brain cells to where they were before this acute element of hyponatremia developed (i.e., raise the P_{Na} to close to 125 mmol/L). The aim is to draw water out of the skull quickly by giving a bolus of hypertonic saline to raise her P_{Na} by 5 mmol/L rapidly. Follow this with a continuous infusion of hypertonic NaCl to raise the P_{Na} to 120 to 125 mmol/L over few hours.

What dangers should be anticipated during therapy, and how can they be avoided?

The first danger is the absorption of a large volume of water from her GI tract, which will acutely lower her arterial P_{Na}. Follow her P_{Na} to see if this danger is present. Also, be alert for even mild symptoms, because they may herald danger. Measuring the P_{Na} in arterial blood or blood drawn from a vein on the dorsum of the hand and comparing this value to the P_{Na} in brachial venous blood will help reveal whether water is currently being absorbed in the intestinal tract (see Chapter 9, page 280).

The second risk is the development of osmotic demyelination with a rapid rise in P_{Na} above 125 mmol/L because she has an element of chronic hyponatremia. This is most likely if she has a large water diuresis; therefore, extreme caution is needed to detect when the actions of dDAVP disappear. When a water diuresis occurs, dDAVP should be administered. If dDAVP is given, one must ensure that water restriction is imposed. If the patient cannot be followed closely, it is perhaps safer to give her dDAVP to prevent a water diuresis, water intake must also be restricted.

After the first 24 hours, we would limit the rate of rise in her P_{Na} to no more than 8 mmol/L/day. Therefore, she should be permitted to have a total negative balance of close to 2 L of water per day ([8 mmol/L ÷ 125 mmol/L] × total body water of somewhat greater than 30 L = 1.9 L). Control of the urine output by giving dDAVP after she voids the desired urine volume should prevent a rise in her P_{Na} above the upper limit set beforehand. The P_{Na} should be closely monitored to ensure that this upper limit is not exceeded.

CASE 10-2: THIS IS FAR FROM "ECSTASY"!

(Case presented on page 320)

Is this acute hyponatremia?

It is reasonable to presume that this is acute hyponatremia for two reasons. First, she has the recent ingestion of a large volume of water and second, she had the intake of a drug, Ecstasy, that leads to the secretion of vasopressin.

Importantly, in acute hyponatremia, the situation can become very serious in a very short period, even if symptoms are mild (e.g., headache, drowsiness, mild confusion). Therefore, this patient needs urgent therapy to shrink the size of her brain cells; this is discussed in more detail subsequently.

Why did she have a seizure if the P_{Na} was 130 mmol/L?

There are two possible explanations. First, she has an underlying central nervous system lesion that makes her more susceptible to develop a seizure with a smaller degree of brain cell swelling. Second, her P_{Na} was initially significantly lower than the value obtained after seizure. In more detail, because of the seizure, many new osmoles were generated in her skeletal muscle cells, which caused a shift of water from her ECF to her ICF and hence her P_{Na} measured now is significantly higher than what it was (see Fig. 9-30, page 309). There are at least four reasons why the number of osmoles in muscle cells may increase during a seizure. First, during muscle contraction, phosphocreatine is converted to creatine and phosphate, which increases the number of osmoles in these muscle cells. Second, the vigorous muscle contraction generates ADP that causes a rapid increase in anaerobic glycolysis with the production of L-lactic acid (*see margin note*). Third, the intracellular P_{CO_2} rises in this setting; therefore, the new H^+ produced are forced to bind to proteins rather than HCO_3^- and hence there is a gain of L-lactate anions without a loss of HCO_3^- osmoles. Fourth, these new osmoles accumulate in muscle cells because the rate of exit of L-lactate anions from these muscles cells is not as fast as their rate of formation.

There is another issue to consider. Blood drawn from the brachial vein shortly after the seizure reflects the changes in muscle. Hence, the measured P_{Na} in brachial venous blood would be higher than the arterial P_{Na}, and it is the latter that determines the brain cell volume (see the discussion of Case 9-1, page 308 for more details).

What role might anorexia nervosa have played in this clinical picture?

Approximately 50% of water in the body is located in skeletal muscle cells. This patient has a very small muscle mass, so a smaller positive water balance could cause a greater fall in her P_{Na} compared with another subject with a larger muscle mass.

What is your therapy for this patient?

The aim is to draw water out of the skull by raising the P_{Na} by 5 mmol/L to decrease the intracranial pressure. Give hypertonic saline rapidly, because the goal is to have water cross the blood-brain barrier faster than Na^+ (see the discussion of Question 10-2 for more details). This therapy should be enough to control the seizure. If seizures persist, another cause should be sought.

Watch for the reabsorption of water from a reservoir in the intestinal tract or water retained in muscle cells during the seizure. Follow the P_{Na} closely and continue to infuse hypertonic NaCl to keep this water out of the brain cells. The P_{Na} can be brought close to the normal range, but if there is a possibility of a degree of chronic

NEW ICF OSMOLES DURING A SEIZURE
If the $P_{L-lactate}$ is elevated, suspect that the higher P_{Na} is due to a gain in intracellular osmoles.

hyponatremia, do not exceed the maximum value set for the daily rise in her P_{Na} (*see margin note*).

- In this patient, these concerns may be of lesser importance because the initial P_{Na} was only 130 mmol/L.
- One has to be cautious if there is an element of chronic hyponatremia because a patient with anorexia nervosa is likely to be at higher risk of osmotic demyelination with a rapid rise in P_{Na}.

DISCUSSION OF QUESTIONS

10-1 *Some authorities determine the basis for the change in the P_{Na} using an analysis based on electrolyte-free water balance. Does this provide different information compared with an analysis based on tonicity balance?*

Electrolyte-free water in a solution is defined by performing an imaginary calculation, in which the solution is divided into a volume of isotonic saline, and if there is water left over, this is called *electrolyte-free water*. For example, if one has 3 L of a solution that has 50 mmol Na^+/L, the total 150 mmol of Na^+ accounts for 1 L of isotonic saline; the remaining 2 L is called *electrolyte-free water*. Thus, an infusion of hypotonic fluid adds electrolyte-free water to the body.

Electrolyte-free water can be generated even if the infusate is isotonic saline. In more detail, if 1 L of fluid that contains 150 mmol of Na^+ is infused, and all of its Na^+ is excreted in 0.5 L of urine at a concentration of 300 mmol/L, one is left with 0.5 L of electrolyte-free water; we call this process *desalination*. For this desalination to occur, the concentration of Na^+ plus K^+ in the urine must be higher than that in the infusate (or in the patient if there are no infusions).

An analysis based on electrolyte-free water balance correctly predicts the change in the P_{Na}, but it does not determine its basis or its appropriate therapy. For example, if a patient has a positive balance of 300 mmol of Na^+, from the electrolyte-free water analysis perspective, this is called a *negative balance* of 2 L of electrolyte-free water. This is identical to another patient who has a net loss of ingested and retained 2 L of water. The problem with making these analyses based on electrolyte-free water becomes obvious when making a decision for therapy.

In both cases, a positive balance of 2 L of electrolyte-free water is needed to return body fluid composition to normal, but the therapy differs in each patient. In the first patient, with a positive balance of 300 mmol of Na^+, one should create a negative balance of 300 mmol of NaCl. In contrast, in the second patient, who has a negative balance of 2 L of water, the specific therapy is to give a positive balance of 2 L of water. Therefore, the analyses performed in electrolyte-free water terms do not reveal which of the two options is the correct way to treat an individual patient. This is why separate balances for Na^+ and water are needed to plan ideal therapy for these two patients; we call this a *tonicity balance* (see Fig. 10-5).

10-2 *Does hypertonic saline reduce the intracranial pressure simply because it draws water out of brain cells?*

Because water cannot be compressed, a gain of water in a closed box (the skull) causes a rise in pressure. Simply shifting water between the ICF and ECF compartments of the brain within the skull does not lower the intracranial pressure. To lower this pressure, one must force water to leave the skull. This is achieved when hypertonic saline is infused rapidly because water crosses the capillary membrane faster than Na^+ (Fig. 10-9). To prevent water from returning into the skull, more hypertonic saline should be given or a deficit of water should be created.

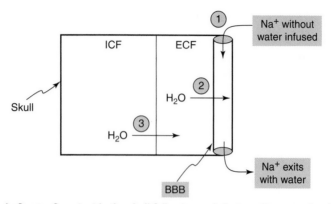

FIGURE 10-9 Removal of water from inside the skull following an infusion of hypertonic saline. When hypertonic saline reaches the blood-brain barrier (BBB; *site 1*), water is drawn from the extracellular fluid (ECF) compartment (*site 2*) across the BBB into the capillary, because movement of Na$^+$ out of this location is relatively slow. As a result, the concentration of Na$^+$ rises in the interstitial fluid compartment of the brain. This rise causes water to be drawn out of brain cells (*site 3*). The net effect is that the water that crossed the BBB is removed from the cranium. ICF, intracellular fluid.

10-3 *A young woman with low muscle mass is asked to drink a standard water load (20 mL/kg) in an experimental study designed to examine the ability to excrete water; her P_{Na} prior to ingesting this water load was 140 mmol/L. Thirty minutes later, she complained of a headache, which is very unusual for her. Is therapy required at this time?*

After she drinks 20 mL of water per kg body weight, the osmolality in all body fluid compartments falls. Hence, the volume of water in cells increases because there is no change in the number of osmoles in the ICF compartment in the acute setting. The cells we are concerned about are the brain cells. When the volume of brain cells increases, the intracranial pressure rises, unless there is other water that can be "squeezed" out of the ventricles of the brain.

The fact that she has a headache, which is very unusual for her, is a major concern. Therefore, we would give her hypertonic NaCl. Notwithstanding, her arterial P_{Na} is likely to be considerably lower than that calculated based on the positive water balance and her estimated total body water; this has serious implications for the degree of brain cell swelling. Her small muscle mass and the "gulping" of water add credence to the possibility that the headache represented a danger of brain cell swelling due to a low arterial P_{Na}.

The dose of hypertonic saline should be enough to raise her P_{Na} acutely by 5 mmol/L (i.e., 125 mmol NaCl [~250 mL of 3% saline] if she weighs 50 kg and has 25 L of body water).

10-4 *What may limit the ability of water to achieve diffusion equilibrium in the inner medullary collecting duct in a patient with chronic hyponatremia (P_{Na} 130 mmol/L, daily urine volume 5 L/day, U_{Osm} of 80 mOsm/kg H$_2$O) during a large water diuresis (see margin note)?*

- The volume of water reabsorbed by residual water permeability seems to be large, yet there are circumstances in which this system fails to achieve diffusion equilibrium for water.

> • In the answer to this conundrum, the authors have provided a speculation that may explain these observations (see page 359). Unfortunately, its tenets cannot be tested in vivo in human subjects.

The U_{Osm} is distinctly lower than the P_{Osm}, which suggests that vasopressin has not led to the insertion of AQP2 in the luminal membrane of principal cells in the distal nephron. This is not surprising, because the patient is hyponatremic and does not have an obvious reason for the release of vasopressin. Nevertheless, the relatively low 24-hour urine volume in this setting (5 L/day instead of 15 L/day) suggests that the basis for the inability to excrete the extra water is a low distal delivery of filtrate and reabsorption of some of the water in the inner medullary collecting duct via residual permeability. Despite this large reabsorption of water, the U_{Osm} is very low but diffusion equilibrium for water was not achieved. In fact, there may be additional factors at play, as described on page 359.

10-5 *What role might K^+ depletion play in determining the severity of hyponatremia?*

One needs to examine how electroneutrality is achieved when K^+ are lost from the body. Ninety-eight percent of K^+ in the body is in cells, so this is the compartment from which the vast majority of K^+ are lost.

First, if K^+ left cells accompanied by an intracellular anion, water would leave these cells and the P_{Na} will fall.

Second, if K^+ are lost from cells and cells gain an equivalent amount of Na^+, there is no change in the number of osmoles in cells. Now, if these K^+ are excreted along with Cl^-, the ECF has lost Na^+ and Cl^- and its volume becomes contracted because water is shifted into cells (this represents events when diuretics, like thiazides, are administered). This decrease in the effective arterial blood volume diminishes the distal delivery of filtrate and thereby the excretion of water. The net result is the development of hyponatremia due to a deficit of K^+ and Cl^- plus a shift of Na^+ into cells.

Third, patients who have a severe degree of hypokalemia may have muscle weakness and low motility of their small intestine. As a result, ingested fluid may be retained in the lumen of the GI tract (see Fig. 10-6, page 328). Because the intestinal wall is permeable to Na^+ (between the cells), Na^+ are lost into this fluid, and this causes the P_{Na} to fall. At a later time, when K^+ are given in therapy, intestinal motility increases and there is a sudden absorption of a hypotonic saline solution (i.e., because luminal fluid has other osmoles, which would reexpand the ECF volume). This in turn may both diminish the release of vasopressin and increase the distal delivery of filtrate, thus potentially causing a large water diuresis. This can be very dangerous because patients who are K^+ depleted are more susceptible to osmotic demyelination when the P_{Na} rises too quickly. Hence, the upper limit for the daily allowable rise in the P_{Na} should be much smaller in these patients (~4 mmol/L). A water diuresis must be avoided in these patients; consider giving dDAVP to avoid an excessive rise in the P_{Na} once the P_{Na} has risen by close to 4 mmol/L.

10-6 *In what way might hyponatremia lead to a larger plasma volume?*

If the hyponatremia was due to water retention (e.g., SIADH), the ECF and ICF volumes will be increased. If the patient has chronic hyponatremia, the resulting increase in Na^+ excretion would return the ECF volume toward normal.

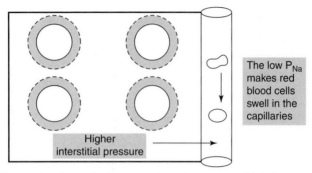

FIGURE 10-10 Effect of hyponatremia on the intravascular volume. The *solid circles* represent the normal cell volume, and the *dashed circles* represent the expanded intracellular fluid volume during hyponatremia. The *rectangle* represents the capsule surrounding some organs of the body. As the tissue pressure rises, interstitial fluid enters the vascular compartment, as illustrated by the *horizontal arrow*. Hyponatremia also causes red blood cells to swell, which also increases the intravascular volume by a small amount.

There are two other factors that lead to an expanded blood volume in a patient with hyponatremia. First, because of the low P_{Na}, red blood cells swell. Because these cells account for 40% of blood volume, their gain in water expands the circulating volume. Second, in an organ that has a capsule, such as the kidney or the liver, the swelling of their cells increases the pressure in the interstitial compartment. Owing to Starling forces, there is a net entry of fluid from the interstitial fluid compartment of these organs into the vascular space (Fig. 10-10).

10-7 *Hyponatremic patients treated with oral urea have a larger excretion of water without Na^+, which results in a rise in their P_{Na}, whereas similar patients eating a high-protein diet do not have a large increase in their urine volume. Why might these responses be different?*

When vasopressin acts, both AQP2 and a urea transporter are inserted into the luminal membrane of the inner medullary collecting duct. As a result, urea and water can be reabsorbed in this nephron segment. Notwithstanding, urea can become an effective osmole in the lumen of the inner medullary collecting duct and cause the excretion of extra water if the distal delivery of urea is high enough to *exceed the capacity* for its reabsorption in the inner medulla, as may occur when urea is ingested as a large bolus. This setting differs from the high rate of urea production following ingestion of a large protein load because there is now a continuous, slow, steady production of urea. Accordingly, the amount of this nitrogenous waste that is excreted at any instant is not enough to exceed the reabsorptive capacity of the urea transporter in the inner medullary collecting duct and thereby cause an extra excretion of water. Rather, there is simply a higher concentration of urea in each liter of urine.

10-8 *What precautions are required to ensure that the use of aquaretics to raise the P_{Na} is safe?*

The following three principles must be followed to use this class of drugs safely.
1. The P_{Na} must not rise above the limit set for the maximum value on a given day to minimize the risk of osmotic demyelination.

2. The rise in the P_{Na} must not be due to a positive balance for Na^+ in patients in whom an expansion of their effective arterial blood volume may be dangerous (i.e., those with a high blood pressure or those in congestive heart failure).
3. A water diuresis must be terminated with dDAVP if it is larger than the volume that is required to achieve the desired rise in the P_{Na}.

Some of the dangers when using this class of drugs have been derived from published data, which emphasized their safety.

- Some patients have had a rise in their P_{Na} that was greater than 12 mmol/L/day, which is the upper limit for the rise in P_{Na} that most investigators consider acceptable. This rise would definitely be excessive in some patients (e.g., those with a degree of malnutrition, K^+ depletion due to the use of diuretics for underlying hypertension or congestive heart failure).
- A rise in the P_{Na} that occurs in a matter of just a few hours because of a brisk water diuresis may be more dangerous than a steady slower rise over a 24-hour period. Recall that one is measuring the P_{Na} in venous blood and not the arterial P_{Na}, which may have a much higher value in this setting.
- Balance studies must demonstrate unequivocally that these drugs induce a negative balance for water and *not* a positive balance for Na^+. In fact, some of the published data are disquieting in this regard because they suggest that this class of drugs does lead to retention of Na^+ in the longer term. This is likely because the initial weight loss (a rise in the P_{Na} due to a negative balance of water) did not persist while the rise in the P_{Na} was sustained (i.e., the subsequent rise in body weight suggests that water was again retained with Na^+, as there was no fall in the P_{Na}). Hence, we cannot be certain from data available that continued use of these drugs does not lead to retention of Na^+. This may be dangerous in patients who have hypertension or congestive heart failure.

chapter

11

Hypernatremia

Introduction

Hypernatremia is defined as a P_{Na} that is greater than 145 mmol/L. Hypernatremia is not a final diagnosis; rather it is a laboratory finding that occurs in other disorders. Hence, one must discover its underlying cause.

Although the concentration of Na^+ is a ratio of Na^+ to water in the extracellular fluid (ECF) compartment, in the majority of patients, hypernatremia is due primarily to a deficit of water.

The first step in the clinical approach to the patient with hypernatremia is to deal with emergencies and to anticipate and prevent dangers induced by therapy. Because the P_{Na} is inversely related to the intracellular fluid (ICF) volume, *acute* hypernatremia is associated with a decrease in the size of cells in the body. The organ that is most adversely affected is the brain because, as its volume declines, vessels coming from the inner surface of the skull become stretched and thus are at risk for rupture. In patients with *chronic* hypernatremia, cells in the brain gain effective osmoles, and this returns their volume back toward normal. After this occurs, the danger for the patient is a rapid decrease in the P_{Na}, because this causes these cells to swell, as they cannot lose these extra newly gained osmoles quickly. This may result in a rise in intracranial volume, and thereby pressure, which can lead to herniation of the brain.

The next step in the clinical approach is to examine for the presence of the expected responses in this setting, which are thirst and the excretion of the smallest volume of urine with the highest concentration of effective osmoles due to renal actions of vasopressin.

Hypernatremia that develops outside the hospital is usually caused by a large deficit of water. Although patients who develop hypernatremia in the hospital may also have a deficit of water, in many, hypernatremia is due in large part to a positive balance of Na^+ owing to the administration of intravenous solutions with a higher concentration of $Na^+ + K^+$ than that patient is excreting in the urine. Therefore, it is essential to assess balances for water and for $Na^+ + K^+$ to determine the basis of hypernatremia—we call this a *tonicity balance.*

The issues for therapy are similar in principle to those that were discussed in patients with hyponatremia in Chapter 10. If there is reliable evidence that the rise in the P_{Na} has occurred in less than 24 hours, the P_{Na} should fall rapidly in the initial period of therapy (*see margin note*). In contrast, if the duration of hypernatremia is definitely greater than 48 hours, one should not permit the P_{Na} to fall by more than 8 mmol/L in 24 hours to prevent a sudden rise in brain cell volume and therefore in intracranial pressure, with possible disastrous consequences. This is particularly important if there are other disorders that may lead to an increase in the intracranial volume (e.g., meningitis, encephalitis, or a space-occupying lesion such as a malignancy or a hemorrhage).

It is important to stress that there are times when the development of hypernatremia can be beneficial (e.g., to maintain a constant high effective plasma osmolality ($P_{Effective\,osm}$) during therapy of patients with diabetic ketoacidosis, especially in children, because this may help prevent the development of cerebral edema; see Chapter 5, page 129 for more discussion).

RELIANCE ON 48-HOUR PERIOD TO DISTINGUISH BETWEEN ACUTE AND CHRONIC HYPERNATREMIA

- Some patients may have virtually completed this adaptive response in much less than 48 hours.
- During therapy of a patient in whom the P_{Na} rose from 140 mmol/L to 168 mmol/L over 48 hours, we observed that lowering the P_{Na} quickly led to symptoms of acute brain cell volume.
- Hence, do not try to lower the P_{Na} by a large amount if the P_{Na} was close to 160 mmol/L or if the duration of hypernatremia was clearly greater than 24 hours.

OBJECTIVES

- ■ **Pathogenesis:** To emphasize that hypernatremia represents an increase in the amount of Na^+ relative to the volume of water in the ECF compartment. This almost always means that the ICF volume is contracted. If hypernatremia is chronic (>48 hours), brain cells gain enough effective osmoles that their volume is close to normal. To determine why the P_{Na} has risen, examine balances for Na^+ and water if data are available rather than relying simply on inputs or outputs of water or an analysis based on electrolyte-free water balance.

■ **Expected responses:** To emphasize that if the thirst center is intact and the patient has access to water, a severe degree of hypernatremia should not develop. The expected renal response to hypernatremia is to excrete the smallest volume of water with the highest effective urine osmolality. One must evaluate the concentrations of $Na^+ + K^+$ in the urine and *not* the U_{Osm} to deduce the impact of this excretion on cell volume.

■ **Diagnosis:** To provide a diagnostic approach to the patient with hypernatremia based on an evaluation of thirst, assessment of the ECF volume, changes in body weight and of the urine composition to determine whether the major basis of hypernatremia is a deficit of water or a gain of Na^+.

■ **Therapy:** To provide the basis for rational decision making in the treatment of patients with hypernatremia emphasizing whether the disorder has an acute element. If data are available, we prefer to calculate tonicity balance rather than an electrolyte-free water balance to provide the information needed to design therapy to restore both the volume and composition of the ECF and ICF compartments.

CASE 11-1: CONCENTRATE ON THE DANGER

(Case discussed on page 396)

A 16-year-old man (weight: 50 kg; total body water: 30 L) had a craniopharyngioma resected. During surgery, his urine flow rate rose to 10 mL/min over 5 hours (i.e., 3 L in 300 minutes) and his P_{Na} rose from 140 mmol/L to 150 mmol/L. During this time period, he received 3 L of isotonic saline. His U_{Osm} was 120 mOsm/kg H_2O, and his $U_{Na} + U_K$ was 50 mmol/L. Following the administration of dDAVP, his U_{Osm} rose quickly to 375 mOsm/kg H_2O, and his U_{Na} was 175 mmol/L.

Questions

For a discussion of the basis for polyuria in this case, see the discussion of Case 12-2, page 420.

Why did hypernatremia develop (*see margin note*)?
What are the changes in his ECF and ICF compartment volumes?
What are the goals for therapy of his hypernatremia?

CASE 11-2: WHAT IS "PARTIAL" ABOUT PARTIAL CENTRAL DIABETES INSIPIDUS?

(Case discussed on page 397)

A 32-year-old healthy man fell while snowboarding and suffered a basal skull fracture. His urine output has been close to 4 L/day. He complained of thirst. His P_{Na} has varied between 137 mmol/L and 143 mmol/L, and his 24-hour U_{Osm} was usually close to 200 mOsm/kg H_2O while he was in the hospital. When his P_{Na} was 141 mmol/L, vasopressin was undetectable in plasma. Of note, his urine flow rate was distinctly lower overnight, and his sleep was not interrupted by a need to urinate; in fact, his U_{Osm} was close to 425 mOsm/kg H_2O on multiple occasions in overnight urine samples. When he was given dDAVP, his urine flow rate decreased to 0.5 mL/min and the U_{Osm} rose to 900 mOsm/kg H_2O. An infusion of hypertonic saline led to the release of vasopressin and the excretion of very concentrated urine.

Questions

What is the basis for the high urine flow rate in this patient?
What are the options for therapy?

CASE 11-3: WHERE DID THE WATER GO?

(Case discussed on page 399)
A 55-year-old man who weighed 80 kg has had type 2 diabetes mellitus for 15 years. In the past several months, a new, but intermittent, problem developed: the acute onset of thirst after meals; this usually lasted for several hours and then subsided. This time, however, 12 hours after a large meal in which he added more NaCl than usual to his food, the thirst was more intense and lasted longer. On this occasion, he drank a larger volume of fluid, but he did not pass a large volume of urine. He was alert and responded appropriately to questions. His blood pressure was 150/90 mm Hg, his pulse rate was 96 beats per minute (usual values for this patient), and his weight was 1 kg (2.2 lb) higher than usual; his ECF volume appeared to be normal. His fundi had changes consistent with diabetic retinopathy; he also had signs of peripheral neuropathy. Laboratory findings are listed for blood drawn at presentation; these results were unchanged in blood drawn 2 hours later. The hematocrit was similar to values noted on previous laboratory results.

P_{Na}	mmol/L	169	P_{Cl}	mmol/L	133
P_K	mmol/L	5.2	P_{HCO_3}	mmol/L	25
$P_{Glucose}$	mg/dL (µmol/L)	180 (10)	pH [H^+]	(nmol/L)	7.40 (40)
$P_{Creatinine}$	mg/dL (µmol/L)	1.8 (157)	P_{Urea}	mg/dL (mmol/L)	22 (8)
$P_{Albumin}$	g/dL (g/L)	3.8 (38)	Hemoglobin	g/dL (g/L)	12.5 (125)
Hematocrit		0.36			

Questions

What is the basis for the hypernatremia (in quantitative terms)— a positive balance for Na^+ and/or a negative balance of water?
Why does he have such a severe degree of hypernatremia?
What is the therapy of hypernatremia in this patient?

PART A
BACKGROUND

SYNOPSIS OF THE PERTINENT PHYSIOLOGY

The plasma Na^+ concentration

- The P_{Na} is the ratio of the amount of Na^+ to the volume of water in the ECF compartment.

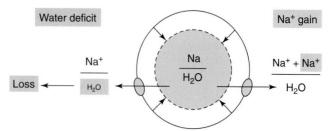
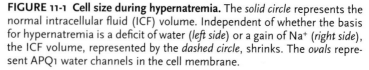

FIGURE 11-1 Cell size during hypernatremia. The *solid circle* represents the normal intracellular fluid (ICF) volume. Independent of whether the basis for hypernatremia is a deficit of water (*left side*) or a gain of Na^+ (*right side*), the ICF volume, represented by the *dashed circle*, shrinks. The *ovals* represent APQ1 water channels in the cell membrane.

The actual Na^+-to-water ratio in plasma is 152 mmol/kg H_2O. If measured per liter of plasma, however, the P_{Na} is 140 mmol/L, because each liter of plasma is 6% to 7% nonaqueous by volume (lipids and proteins), and Na^+ is distributed only in its aqueous phase. The normal range for the P_{Na} is 136 to 145 mmol/L; thus hypernatremia is defined as a P_{Na} that is greater than 145 mmol/L. Hypernatremia can be due to a positive balance for Na^+ and/or a negative balance for water, although both are often present in the same patient to varying degrees (Fig. 11-1; Table 11-1).

Hypernatremia is associated with a low ICF volume unless its basis is a shift of water into cells secondary to a gain of effective osmoles in the ICF compartment (e.g., owing to seizures or rhabdomyolysis; see Fig. 10-3, page 323). The ECF volume, on the other hand, may be increased (due to positive Na^+ balance) or decreased (due to negative water balance), depending on the basis for the rise in the P_{Na}.

TABLE 11-1 **CAUSES FOR HYPERNATREMIA**

Hypernatremia is usually due to a deficit of water. In some circumstances, however, its basis may be primarily a gain of Na^+. In both instances, look for the reason for a low intake of water.

Primary water deficit

Reduced water intake for many days
- Lack of water
- Inability to gain access to, or to drink, water
- Defective thirst due to altered mental state, psychological disorder, or diseases involving the osmoreceptor and/or the thirst center

Increased water loss
- Renal loss: central DI, tissue necrosis and the release of vasopressinase, nephrogenic DI, osmotic diuresis
- Gastrointestinal loss: vomiting, osmotic diarrhea
- Cutaneous loss: excessive sweating (*see margin note*)
- Respiratory loss: hyperventilation (this is a *net* water loss only if it came from the upper respiratory tract; see page 384 for more details)

Shift of water into cells
- Gain of "effective" osmoles in the intracellular fluid compartment (e.g., due to seizures, rhabdomyolysis)

Primary gain of Na^+

- Administration of intravenous saline with a higher concentration of $Na^+ + K^+$ than their concentration in the urine during an osmotic or a water diuresis
- Infusion of hypertonic NaCl or $NaHCO_3$ in oliguric patients
- Ingestion of sea water or replacing sugar by NaCl in feeding formula in infants

COMPOSITION OF SWEAT
- Sweat is always hypotonic; its volume can be as high as 2 L/hr during vigorous exercise in a hot environment.
- The concentration of Na^+ in sweat is usually ~25 mmol/L, but in patients with cystic fibrosis, the concentration of Na^+ is higher (~60 mmol/L).

DI, diabetes insipidus.

Responses to hypernatremia

- When the P_{Na} rises, the water control system elicits two responses that are designed to lower the P_{Na} to prevent a further decrease in brain cell size. There is an input response (stimulation of thirst) and an output response (minimizing the loss of water in the urine).

The rise in the P_{Na} is sensed in a group of cells in the hypothalamus (called the *osmostat*, or better, the *tonicity receptor*). In response to a high P_{Na}, this tonicity receptor sends messages to the thirst center and to a second site for the production and release of vasopressin (Fig. 11-2). Vasopressin causes the insertion of aquaporin 2 (AQP2) water channels in the luminal membranes of principal cells of the late cortical distal nephron and the medullary collecting duct. Each of these responses is discussed in the paragraphs to follow.

Thirst

- It is virtually impossible to have the P_{Na} increase above the normal range if the thirst response is intact and water is available.

In patients with a significant degree of hypernatremia, look for a reason why they cannot appreciate thirst or gain access to water. Examples include an unconscious patient, those with disorders involving the osmostat or the thirst center, those with primary hypodipsia (e.g., following a subarachnoid hemorrhage), patients who are unable to communicate their desire for water (e.g., infants, patients with a stroke), or patients who may not have access to water (e.g., inability to move). At times, the basis for the reduced intake of water is recurrent vomiting or mechanical obstruction of the upper gastrointestinal (GI) tract (e.g., an esophageal tumor).

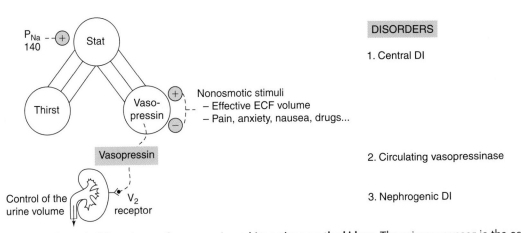

FIGURE 11-2 Control of the release of vasopressin and its actions on the kidney. The primary sensor is the osmostat, which consists of a group of cells that detect a change in their volume in response to a change in the P_{Na}; thus "tonicity receptor" is a better description than "osmostat." These cells are linked to a group of cells that control the intake of water (thirst center) and to others that are responsible for the release of vasopressin, which then acts on the kidney to cause the excretion of the smallest volume of urine with the highest concentration of effective osmoles. Other factors, such as a decrease in the effective arterial blood volume and a number of afferent stimuli (e.g., pain, nausea, anxiety, and a number of drugs), also cause the release of vasopressin. DI, diabetes insipidus; ECF, extracellular fluid.

Renal response

> • The expected central response in a patient with hypernatremia is to release vasopressin, which makes the late distal nephron permeable to water. Hence, the urine flow rate should be as low as possible and the effective U_{Osm} should be as high as possible (equal to the effective osmolality in the renal medullary interstitial compartment). The low urine flow rate is the more important of these two effects.

If vasopressin is not present or if it fails to act, late distal nephron segments lack AQP2 water channels and hence are largely impermeable to water; therefore, a water diuresis ensues. In this setting, the urine flow rate is determined principally by the volume of filtrate delivered to the distal nephron minus the volume of water reabsorbed via residual water permeability in the inner medullary collecting duct (Fig. 11-3). The volume of filtrate delivered distally is a function of the glomerular filtration rate and the volume of fluid reabsorbed in the proximal convoluted tubule. The rate of excretion of osmoles during a water diuresis influences the U_{Osm}, but *not* the urine flow rate.

When vasopressin acts, the urine flow rate is determined by the rate of excretion of effective osmoles ($2 [Na^+ + K^+ + NH_4^+]$) and the effective ("nonurea") osmolality in the inner medullary interstitial compartment (~600 mOsm/kg H_2O). On a typical Western diet, the rate of excretion of effective osmoles is close to 450 mosmol/day. Hence, the minimum urine flow rate is close to 0.75 L/day or 0.5 mL/min when the effective U_{Osm} is close to 600 mOsm/kg H_2O (*see margin note*). When vasopressin acts, the urine flow rate is higher when the rate of excretion of effective osmoles rises.

The value for the effective U_{Osm} is virtually identical to the effective inner medullary interstitial osmolality when vasopressin acts. Notwithstanding, this later osmolality can be lower because of drugs that compromise the function of the loop of Henle (e.g., loop diuretics or ligands that bind to the calcium-sensing receptor such

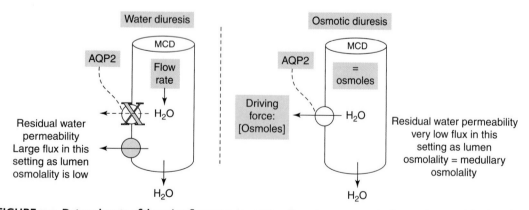

FIGURE 11-3 Determinants of the urine flow rate. In a water diuresis, vasopressin does not act and the late distal nephron segments lack AQP2 water channels. In this setting, the urine flow rate is determined primarily by the volume of filtrate delivered to the distal nephron (*left portion*). When vasopressin acts and causes the insertion of AQP2 into the luminal membrane of collecting duct cells, the urine flow rate is determined by the rate of excretion of effective osmoles and the effective osmolality ("nonurea" osmolality) in the inner medullary interstitial compartment (*right portion*). MCD, medullary collecting duct.

as calcium in patients with hypercalcemia or cationic drugs (e.g., gentamicin or cationic proteins in patients with dysproteinemias), diseases that cause medullary interstitial damage, and/or when the renal medulla is "washed out" by a prior waters diuresis (see the discussion of Question 11-1, page 401).

Regulation of brain cell volume

- Acute hypernatremia is associated with shrinkage of brain cells.
- When hypernatremia is present for more than 48 hours (*see margin note*), adaptive changes have proceeded sufficiently to reexpand the volume of brain cells back toward their normal size.

CAUTION
The time frame that separates acute from chronic hypernatremia is not known with certainty and may differ from patient to patient.

In response to chronic hypernatremia, cells in the brain (mostly non-neuronal cells) gain effective osmoles (Na^+ and K^+ and their accompanying anions as well as organic osmoles; see Chapter 9, page 250 for more discussion). As a result, water shifts from the ECF compartment (and from other cells in the body) into brain cells, which returns their volume toward normal (Fig. 11-4). It is important to appreciate this adaptive change because if the P_{Na} were to fall quickly, brain cells would swell and this could cause a dangerous rise in intracranial pressure, akin to what occurs in acute hyponatremia (see Chapter 10, page 321 for more discussion).

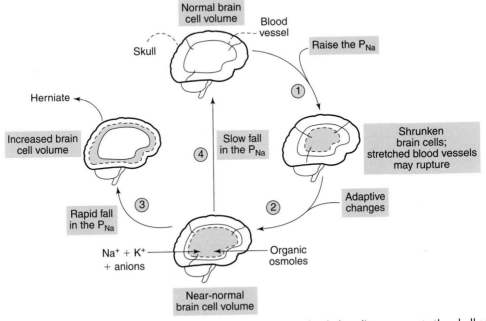

FIGURE 11-4 Regulation of brain cell volume during hypernatremia. The *dark outline* represents the skull and the *lighter line* represents brain cell volume. The *convoluted lines* from the skull to the brain represent blood vessels. When the P_{Na} rises acutely (*site 1*), the brain cell volume decreases, which causes blood vessels to stretch and possibly rupture. Over a 48-hour period, adaptive changes are almost complete, and they return brain cell size toward normal—this involves a gain of osmoles in brain cells (*site 2*). If the P_{Na} were to fall acutely at that time, brain cell volume will increase and brain herniation may result (*site 3*). This danger is avoided if the P_{Na} falls slowly (*site 4*).

PATHOPHYSIOLOGY OF HYPERNATREMIA

• Hypernatremia can be caused by a deficit of water and/or a gain of Na+.

Hypernatremia due to a deficit of water

Reduced water intake

Hypernatremia may develop if the patient has a generalized or localized lesion in the central nervous system involving the thirst mechanism or if the patient is unable to obtain enough water (i.e., water loss is not matched by water intake). Infants may also be at risk for hypernatremia from nonrenal water loss because they cannot specifically complain of thirst; they also \have a reduced capacity to decrease their urine volume in the first month of life (see page 394 for more discussion).

Water loss

Although water loss is the most frequent cause of hypernatremia, an inadequate intake of water contributes to the clinical picture. The sites of water loss are discussed below.

Nonrenal water loss

Sweat

• The evaporation of 1 L of water causes a loss of 500 to 600 kcal (heat of evaporation); any sweat that drops on the ground is *not* useful for heat dissipation.

The concentration of Na+ in sweat is close to 20 to 30 mmol/L. Since the water that is lost is derived from total body water rather than solely from the ECF compartment this minimizes the danger of a significant degree of effective arterial blood volume contraction. The usual volume of sweat is close to 0.5 L/day in an adult. Losses in sweat, however, can increase dramatically in a hot environment during exercise and in febrile patients.

QUESTION

(Discussion on page 401)
11-1 *Why must sweat always contain some Na+ and Cl-?*

Respiratory tract. Alveolar air is humidified with body water because inspired air is not fully saturated with water at body temperature. Nevertheless, the source of this water is ultimately from the oxidation of fuels. In more detail, oxidation of food yields water and CO_2 in a 1:1 proportion. Because the partial pressures of water and CO_2 in alveolar air are similar (47 and 40 mm Hg), H_2O and CO_2 are also lost in almost a 1:1 proportion. Hence, there is no decrease in total body water as a result of loss of water in the alveolar air (Fig. 11-5).

Evaporation of water in the upper respiratory tract causes local cooling. The source of this evaporated water is humidified alveolar

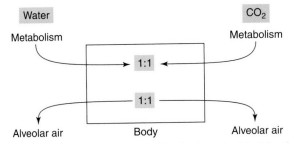

FIGURE 11-5 Fate of metabolic water. The body is depicted by the large rectangle. Events describing water are shown to the *left*, whereas events describing CO_2 are shown to the *right*. Both the production of water and CO_2 from the oxidation of fuels (*top arrows*) and their loss in alveolar air (*bottom arrows*) are close to a 1:1 proportion. Hence, there is no net change in water balance as a result of metabolism and alveolar ventilation.

air. The volume of water loss is greater when the rate of ventilation is high *and* the volume of inspired air is low because the percentage of dead space ventilation rises (*see margin note*).

Gastrointestinal tract. The loss of gastric secretions containing HCl is a loss of hypotonic solution because at a pH of 1, the concentration of Cl^- is 100 mmol/L *and* for every Cl^- lost, one new HCO_3^- is added to the body (see Fig. 7-2, page 198). Conversely, if 1 L of iso-osmotic HCl in gastric fluid reacts with 1 L of iso-osmotic $NaHCO_3$ from the fluid secreted in the small intestine, there is now 150 mmol of Na^+ and 150 mmol of Cl^- in a total volume of 2 L. Therefore, the loss of this fluid results in the loss of 2 L of half-isotonic NaCl. Hypotonic fluid can be lost in diarrhea fluid if this fluid contains organic osmoles (e.g., lactulose) because the resultant fluid, although iso-osmotic to plasma, has a low concentration of Na^+.

Renal water loss

- Patients with hypernatremia who excrete large volumes of dilute urine suffer from diabetes insipidus (see Fig. 11-2).

If the urine volume can be decreased and the urine osmolality can be raised appreciably following the administration of a physiologic dose of vasopressin, the defect is in the release of vasopressin from the posterior pituitary gland (central diabetes insipidus; Table 11-2). Diabetes insipidus may also be due to deficiency of vasopressin because of its destruction in the circulation by an enzyme (vasopressinase). This diagnosis is established by finding a renal response to a synthetic derivative of vasopressin that is not hydrolyzed by this enzyme (called *dDAVP; see margin note*), but not to the usual dose of vasopressin. If the urine, however, remains hypo-osmolar after dDAVP is given, the patient has nephrogenic diabetes insipidus (see Part C, page 385 for more discussion).

Hypernatremia due to Na^+ gain

Hypernatremia due to a gain of Na^+ rarely occurs in an outpatient setting (e.g., ingestion of sea water, replacing sugar with salt in preparation of a pediatric feeding formula, inducing abortion with hypertonic saline, suicide/murder attempts). In contrast, hypernatremia due to a gain of Na^+ commonly occurs in a hospital setting as a result

SELECTIVE BRAIN COOLING
- When humidified alveolar air loses some of its water by evaporation on the roof of the palate, this will cool the region of the brain that is immediately above it (i.e., the midbrain).
- This cooling is especially important during vigorous exercise, as a considerable amount of heat is generated in the muscles that are involved in the work. There is also a major degree of hyperventilation in this setting, which helps to increase evaporative loss from the upper respiratory tract and thereby cooling of the brain.

dDAVP
This vasopressin analogue lacks a terminal amino group and has D-arginine instead of L-arginine. Hence, it cannot be hydrolyzed by vasopressinase.

TABLE 11-2 **ETIOLOGY OF DIABETES INSIPIDUS**

Central diabetes insipidus

- Trauma (especially basal skull fractures)
- Neurosurgery (e.g., hypophesectomy)
- CNS space-occupying lesions (e.g., craniopharyngioma, granulomas [e.g., sarcoidosis])
- CNS infections (e.g., meningitis, encephalitis)
- CNS vascular disease (e.g., aneurysm)
- Post-brain hypoxia
- Idiopathic (may be familial)

Vasopressin is destroyed by vasopressinase(s) released from necrotic tissues

- Most often with retained placenta, but may be due to other tissue injury

Nephrogenic diabetes insipidus

- **AQP2-deficient type of nephrogenic diabetes insipidus**
  - Drugs (usually lithium, rarely dimethylchlortetracycline)
  - Congenital nephrogenic diabetes insipidus
- **Normal AQP2 type of nephrogenic diabetes insipidus (i.e., low medullary interstitial tonicity)**
  - Interstitial disorders, obstructive uropathy
  - Loop diuretics
  - Occupancy of Ca-SR in the loop of Henle (e.g., by calcium in a patient with hypercalcemia, by cationic drugs such as aminoglycosides, by cationic proteins in patients with dysproteinemias)

Ca-SR, calcium-sensing receptor; CNS, central nervous system.

of the administration of hypertonic Na^+ salt intravenously (e.g., $NaHCO_3$ to treat a cardiac arrest) or when hypotonic Na^+ losses are replaced with isotonic saline infusion (e.g., during the treatment of diabetic ketoacidosis, diabetes insipidus, or osmotic diuresis due to organic solutes).

PART B
CLINICAL APPROACH

The steps to take in the clinical approach to patients with hypernatremia are similar to those with all other fluid, electrolyte, and acid-base disorders. First, recognize if there are emergencies prior to therapy; second, anticipate and prevent dangers due to each option for therapy; and third, proceed with the diagnostic approach. The tools to use in the clinical diagnosis in each setting are provided in the more detailed descriptions of the specific disorders.

IDENTIFY EMERGENCIES PRIOR TO THERAPY

- In the presence of an emergency, therapy takes precedence over diagnostic issues.

To be succinct, we consider only those emergencies that are directly related to the presence of hypernatremia, independent of its cause. An emergency prior to therapy may be present in a patient who has an element of acute hypernatremia

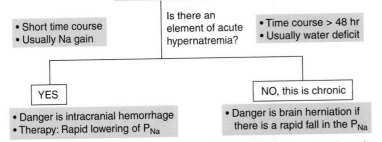

HYPERNATREMIA

Is there an element of acute hypernatremia?

• Short time course
• Usually Na gain

• Time course > 48 hr
• Usually water deficit

YES

NO, this is chronic

• Danger is intracranial hemorrhage
• Therapy: Rapid lowering of P_{Na}

• Danger is brain herniation if there is a rapid fall in the P_{Na}

FLOW CHART 11-1 Emergencies associated with hypernatremia. The emergencies in patients with acute hypernatremia are caused by brain cell shrinkage and a resultant intracranial hemorrhage, whereas the danger in the patient with chronic hypernatremia is a rapid and large fall in the P_{Na}, which results in brain swelling and possibly herniation of the brain.

(occurred in the past 48 hours; Flow Chart 11-1). In the patient with chronic hypernatremia who has a deficit of water and a deficit of Na^+, there can be a hemodynamic emergency due to a markedly reduced effective arterial blood volume. Therefore, our focus will be on acute hypernatermia in this section on emergencies on admission.

The typical setting for the development of a severe degree of acute hypernatremia in the hospital is in the patient who is undergoing surgery and is receiving isotonic saline to avoid a fall in the blood pressure (*see margin note*), while the concentration of electrolytes in the urine is low because of diabetes insipidus. In addition, this patient does not sense thirst or have the ability to drink.

The emergency in patients with acute hypernatremia arises because the brain is in a confined rigid space and it receives some of its blood supply from vessels attached to the skull. When the size of brain cells decreases, the brain shrinks, and this stretches blood vessels that are attached to the inner surface of the skull. This may cause the vessels to rupture and lead to an intracranial hemorrhage, with possible devastating results (see Fig. 11-4, page 375).

If hypernatremia is severe and/or if there are significant symptoms that could be due to acute hyponatremia (e.g., confusion, convulsion), the goal of treatment is to lower the P_{Na} by an appropriate degree. The measures include giving dDAVP if there is an ongoing water diuresis and inducing a rapid loss of Na^+ and/or a gain of water.

Induce a negative balance of Na^+

It is almost impossible to induce a rapid and large loss of Na^+ in hypertonic form by using diuretics alone. In more detail, the administration of a loop diuretic causes a high rate of excretion of Na^+ *with* water, and this urinary loss is *not* hypertonic to the patient. To create a negative balance of Na^+ in hypertonic form, one would need to replace all the water lost when the loop diuretic acts (Fig. 11-6). Conversely, the urine may have a concentration of Na^+ that is hypertonic to plasma, but this loss is not large enough to cause a rapid fall in the P_{Na}.

Induce a positive balance for water

- The safest way to administer water quickly is to use the oral route (unless the splanchnic blood flow rate is very slow).

BLOOD PRESSURE DURING ANESTHESIA
Anesthetic agents cause a reduced vasoconstrictor tone in capacitance blood vessels. As a result, there is a fall in blood pressure, and this is minimized by overexpansion of the vascular (and interstitial) fluid compartments.

LIMITED RATE OF GLUCOSE METABOLISM
The maximum rate of glucose oxidation in an ill patient is close to 0.25 g/kg/hr, which is equivalent to close to 0.3 L of D_5W in a 70-kg person. Therefore, administration of a large volume of D_5W could result in hyperglycemia. The resulting osmotic diuresis could aggravate the degree of hypernatremia.

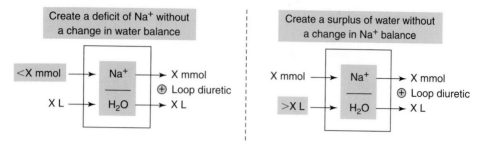

FIGURE 11-6 Create a fall in the P_{Na} using a loop diuretic. The *rectangles* represent the body, with its Na^+ and H_2O content in the extracellular fluid compartment. To lower the P_{Na} by inducing a deficit of Na^+ (*left portion*), create a loss of $Na^+ + H_2O$ with a loop diuretic and replace all the water, but administer less Na^+ than was excreted. To create a positive balance of water after giving a loop diuretic (*right portion*), replace all the Na^+ and give more water than was lost (e.g., give 2 L of 75 mmol/L saline when 1 L of 150 mmol/L NaCl was lost).

RAPID ADMINISTRATION OF WATER

- To administer water rapidly, a central vein must be used to minimize the risk of hemolysis.
- If the goal were to lower the P_{Na} by 10% in a 50-kg patient with acute hypernatremia, one would have to infuse 10% of total body water (30 L) or 3 L of water. If one wanted half of this fall in the P_{Na} to occur in 5 hours (300 minutes), the infusion rate would have to be 10 mL/min.
- Parenthetically, when the P_{Na} is very high, there is usually a major element of Na^+ gain and/or a large shift of water into the lumen of the GI tract and/or into skeletal muscle because the urine flow rate declines when the effective arterial blood volume is low.

It is difficult to administer a large volume of water rapidly by the intravenous route because there is a limited amount of glucose in D_5W that can be administered intravenously without causing hyperglycemia and thereby inducing an osmotic diuresis (*see margin note*). Moreover, if the oral route is used, GI absorption may be too slow to have a major decline in the P_{Na} in a short period. The only way to lower P_{Na} rapidly by inducing a gain of water is to infuse distilled water through a central vein because this solution should not be given via a peripheral vein, as it will enter a small volume of plasma, which will be diluted sufficiently to cause hemolysis. Nevertheless, even with this *drastic* therapy, there is a great difficulty in causing a large and rapid fall in the P_{Na} (*see margin note*; see the discussion of Case 11-3). In some cases, hemodialysis may be the only option to cause a large and rapid fall in P_{Na} (see the discussion of Case 11-3 for an example).

If hypernatremia is acute but not symptomatic, one should lower the P_{Na} more slowly. The choice of therapy (induce a loss of Na^+ or a gain of water) depends on the basis of hypernatremia, which follows from a tonicity balance (Fig. 11-7; Table 11-3). In fact, the input and output volumes and the quantity of Na^+ and K^+ infused are usually available if hypernatremia has developed in the hospital, especially in the critical care setting. The concentrations of Na^+ and K^+ in the urine should be measured; if not, they can be calculated if the P_{Na} was measured before hypernatremia developed and if the volume and composition of fluids administered and the volume of urine are known (see the discussion of Question 11-2). To illustrate this point, examine the balance data provided in Case 11-1 and decide why acute hypernatremia has developed in this patient.

Example: In Case 11-1, the basis for the acute rise in the P_{Na} to 150 mmol/L is a positive balance of 300 mmol of Na^+ (see Fig. 11-7). The current rate of Na^+ excretion after dDAVP in this patient is close to 1 mmol/min (urine flow rate is 6 mL/min × U_{Na} of 175 mmol/L). Accordingly, in 1 hour, he excretes only 60 mmol of Na^+, so it would take 5 hours (300 minutes) to excrete the 300 mmol of Na^+, providing that no additional Na^+ are administered. One method to induce a negative balance for Na^+ is provided in Figure 11-6; you must administer all the water excreted to maintain the normal body water content. Nevertheless, because of the edema in the brain associated with surgery, it may be advantageous

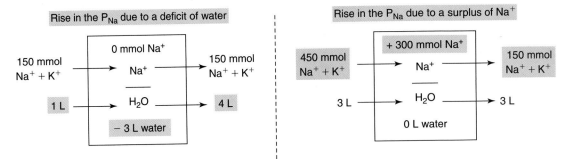

FIGURE 11-7 Use of a tonicity balance to determine the basis for a rise in the P_{Na}. The patient weighs 50 kg and has 30 L of body water. To perform a tonicity balance, the input and output volumes and the quantity of Na^+ and K^+ infused and excreted in the urine are required. Two examples of an acute rise in the P_{Na} from 140 mmol/L to 150 mmol/L are illustrated; a negative balance of 3 L of water is shown to the *left of the vertical dashed line* while a positive balance of 300 mmol of Na^+ is shown to the *right*.

TABLE 11-3 COMPARISON OF AN ELECTROLYTE-FREE WATER AND A TONICITY BALANCE IN PATIENTS WITH HYPERNATREMIA

Three situations are illustrated in which the P_{Na} rises from 140 to 150 mmol/L. The only difference is the volume of isotonic saline infused in each setting. In all three examples, there is a negative balance of 2 L of electrolyte-free water (EFW; *see margin note.*) Notwithstanding, the balances for Na^+ and for water are very different in these three examples. Accordingly, the goals for therapy to correct the hypernatremia and the composition of the extracellular fluid and intracellular fluid compartments are clear only after a tonicity balance is calculated.

	$Na^+ + K^+$ (mmol)	WATER (L)	EFW (L)
Infusion of 3 L of isotonic saline			
Input	450	3	0
Output	150	3	2
Balance	**+ 300**	**0**	**−2**
Infusion of 4 L of isotonic saline			
Input	600	4	0
Output	150	3	2
Balance	**+450**	**+1**	**−2**
No intravenous fluid infusion			
Input	0	0	0
Output	150	3	2
Balance	**−150**	**−3**	**−2**

ELECTROLYTE-FREE WATER (EFW)
This requires an imaginary separation of all the $Na^+ + K^+$ and water into a solution of isotonic (150 mmol/L) saline. Hence, for every 150 mmol of $Na^+ + K^+$, we remove 1 L of water to make it a solution of isotonic saline. Remaining water is called *EFW*, whereas remaining $Na^+ + K^+$ is called *negative EFW* (a very awkward term).

to maintain a higher P_{Na} even though this is acute hypernatremia in this patient.

Select the desired rate of fall in the P_{Na}

- It is important to recognize that the data for selecting a dividing line of 48 hours to define acute versus chronic hypernatremia in humans are not robust.

Although it is stated that the volume regulatory increase in brain cell volume in response to acute hypernatremia requires 48 hours (see Fig. 9-3, page 250), the time course is not known with certainty (discussed later). Therefore, even if hypernatremia is known to be acute, it may be advisable not to bring the P_{Na} back to the normal range if the patient is not symptomatic.

Recognize settings where the development of acute hypernatremia may be advantageous

Maintaining a degree of acute hypernatremia may be beneficial in patients with other reasons for increased water in the skull (e.g., edema fluid following recent neurosurgery or with brain trauma, hemorrhage, encephalitis, or meningitis). The intracranial pressure should be monitored. The goal of therapy is to maintain a degree of hypernatremia that is sufficient to minimize the rise in intracranial pressure. The long-term goal of therapy is to have a slow fall in the P_{Na} once this pressure is close to the normal range.

In a young patient with DKA, it is essential to maintain a constant high $P_{Effective\ osm}$ during therapy to help prevent the development of cerebral edema. Therefore, when the $P_{Glucose}$ falls, the P_{Na} must rise by half of the fall in $P_{Glucose}$ to keep the $P_{Effective\ osm}$ from decreasing. To achieve this aim, it is often necessary to create a degree of hypernatremia (see Chapter 5, page 130 for more discussion).

ABBREVIATIONS
DKA, diabetic ketoacidosis
$P_{Effective\ osm}$, effective osmolality in plasma
$P_{Glucose}$, concentration of glucose in plasma

DANGER FOLLOWING SEIZURE
- It is possible that an acute seizure may cause a gain of effective osmoles in brain cells. If a large enough number of these cells have gained particles, there could be a gain of water in these cells and thereby an increase intracranial pressure.
- Conversely, the intense contraction of skeletal muscle cells may cause a large transient rise in intracellular solutes (see Chapter 10, page 323) and thereby a rise in the P_{Na}, which would shrink the size of normal brain cells. Since the P_{Na} falls very quickly once phosphocreatine is regenerated after the seizure, there could be a delay in the rise in intracranial pressure.

DANGERS TO ANTICIPATE DURING THERAPY

The danger to anticipate during therapy of acute hypernatremia is a sudden rise in intracranial pressure owing to a large shift of water into brain cells (*see margin note*). This could occur if hypotonic fluid was infused too rapidly, as the infusate is diluted in a relatively small volume of plasma before reaching the arterial compartment (see Chapter 9, page 280 for a more detailed discussion of this topic). This danger could be even greater in the portal capillary blood following a large oral water load once the stomach contracts and propels its hypotonic contents into the intestinal tract. If reabsorption is rapid, hemolysis could occur and this could, in theory, lead to acute renal failure.

There is no major emergency related to initial therapy for hypernatremia in the patient with chronic hypernatremia, because when hypernatremia has been present for longer than 48 hours, brain cells have gained effective osmoles and their size has returned toward normal values (see Fig. 11-4). Thus, the danger in this setting is provoked by an error in therapy that leads to a rapid and large fall in the P_{Na}, which may result in brain swelling and possibly herniation. Hence, one should not permit the P_{Na} to fall by more than 8 mmol/L per 24-hour period. Specific issues related to the treatment of chronic hypernatremia are discussed later in this chapter (page 391).

DIAGNOSTIC ISSUES

Patients with chronic hypernatremia, like those with chronic hyponatremia, often have a variety of nonspecific symptoms such as lassitude, difficulty concentrating, and generalized malaise. These symptoms often markedly improve when the P_{Na} returns close to the normal range.

TABLE 11-4 **FACTORS TO ASSESS IN THE PATIENT WITH HYPERNATREMIA**

- Thirst
- Urine flow rate and effective osmolality, comparing findings to the "expected" responses to hypernatremia
- Extracellular fluid volume
- Body weight

The factors to assess to determine the basis of hypernatremia are summarized in Table 11-4 . The most common cause of chronic hypernatremia is a negative balance of water. There are three sources for this water loss: sweat; the GI tract; and, most commonly, the kidneys when a large volume of urine with a low concentration of $Na^+ + K^+$ is excreted (i.e., a large water diuresis or an osmotic diuresis caused by glucose or urea). If the cause is a negative balance of water, the ECF volume is likely to be contracted and there should be an appropriate loss of weight. Conversely, if the cause of hypernatremia is a water shift (e.g., because of mild rhabdomyolysis or a shift of water into the lumen of the intestinal tract), the ECF volume may be contracted, but weight loss is not present. To shift water into the lumen of the small intestine, there must be a large accumulation of products of digested food from a slow GI transit time or obstruction of the intestinal tract. An example of this pathophysiology is illustrated in Case 11-3, page 399. Although chronic hypernatremia is rarely due to a positive balance of Na^+, it should be suspected if there is an expanded ECF volume. In addition, if this is the sole cause for hypernatremia, there should not be a loss of weight. One should also look for the source of the added Na^+.

There are two expected responses to hypernatremia. First, thirst is the most important response to hypernatremia. Second, the expected renal response is to excrete the smallest volume of urine with the highest effective osmolality. If this is not present, the basis for this abnormal renal response must be sought.

Assess the hypothalamic responses

- For hypernatremia to develop, there must be a problem with water intake.

Thirst may be absent if the patient has a generalized problem with cognition or a localized lesion in the hypothalamus affecting the osmostat, the thirst center, and/or the neural links between them (see Fig. 11-2). Alternatively, thirst may be present but cannot be acted on or the patient cannot communicate the need for water.

Assess the renal response to hypernatremia

In response to hypernatremia, vasopressin should be released and the urine output should be close to 0.5 mL/min (30 mL/hr) in an adult who consumes a typical Western diet (Flow Chart 11-2). If the urine flow rate is much higher than this value, proceed to Flow Chart 11-3 to determine the reason for the inappropriate renal response.

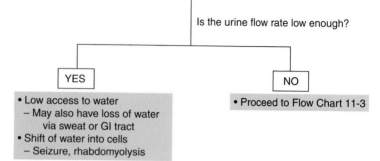

HYPERNATREMIA

Is the urine flow rate low enough?

YES

• Low access to water
  – May also have loss of water
    via sweat or GI tract
• Shift of water into cells
  – Seizure, rhabdomyolysis

NO

• Proceed to Flow Chart 11-3

FLOW CHART 11-2 Hypernatremia: Assessing the renal response. The objective is to assess whether vasopressin is present and acting on the kidney.

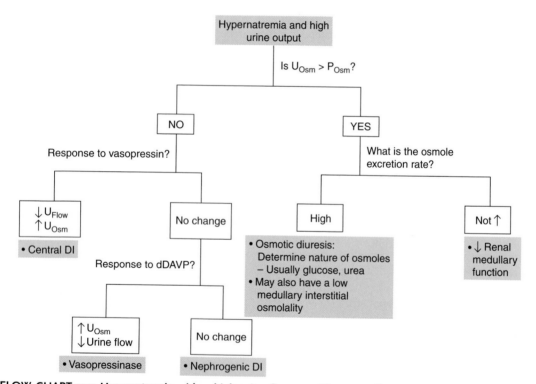

Hypernatremia and high
urine output

Is $U_{Osm} > P_{Osm}$?

NO

Response to vasopressin?

$\downarrow U_{Flow}$
$\uparrow U_{Osm}$

• Central DI

No change

Response to dDAVP?

$\uparrow U_{Osm}$
$\downarrow$ Urine flow

• Vasopressinase

No change

• Nephrogenic DI

YES

What is the osmole
excretion rate?

High

• Osmotic diuresis:
  Determine nature of osmoles
  – Usually glucose, urea
• May also have a low
  medullary interstitial
  osmolality

Not $\uparrow$

• $\downarrow$ Renal
  medullary
  function

FLOW CHART 11-3 Hypernatremia with a high urine flow rate. The steps illustrated permit the clinician to separate a water diuresis from an osmotic diuresis. The principal tools are assessment of both the urine flow rate and the U_{Osm} and then calculation of the osmole excretion rate (high if >0.6 mOsm/min). From a clinical perspective, we would administer dDAVP first unless there was a strong suspicion of the presence of retained necrotic tissue. DI, diabetes insipidus.

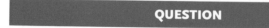

QUESTION

(Discussion on page 401)

11-2 *A 50-kg man received 3 L of isotonic saline (150 mmol/L) and excreted 3 L of urine with an unknown concentration of Na+ and K+. In this period, his P_{Na} rose from 140 mmol/L to 150 mmol/L. If there are no other inputs or outputs during this period, what is the concentration of Na+ and K+ in mmol/L in this urine?*

PART C
SPECIFIC CAUSES OF
HYPERNATREMIA

DIABETES INSIPIDUS

> • An appreciable degree of hypernatremia develops only if there
> is a problem with water intake in this setting.

This is a disorder in which there is a lack of actions of vasopressin. Therefore, the kidney cannot conserve water because there is an absence of AQP2 in the luminal membrane of principal cells in the late cortical distal nephron and in the medullary collecting duct. Hence, all the water delivered to the late distal nephron (minus the amount of water reabsorbed in the inner medullary collecting duct via its residual water permeability) is excreted in the urine. There are three major categories to consider.

Central diabetes insipidus

In this disorder, there is a failure to synthesize vasopressin because of an inborn error or because of a lesion that compromises the osmostat, the site where vasopressin is synthesized (paraventricular and supraopric nuclei in the hypothalamus), the neural pathway connecting the osmostat to these nuclei (see the discussion of Case 11-3), and the tracts connecting these nuclei to the posterior pituitary, where vasopressin is stored and/or to a lesion that involves the posterior pituitary.

Circulating vasopressinase

> • Vasopressin released from the posterior pituitary must travel in
> the blood to exert its effect on the kidney.
> • Necrotic tissues may release an enzyme (vasopressinase) that
> destroys vasopressin (*see margin note*).

This has been reported for the most part in patients with retained necrotic placenta, but it may be also seen with other diseases where there is extensive tissue damage (e.g., a large abscess). This group of peptidases targets the N-terminal amino group of vasopressin and/or its L-arginine. The hallmark of this diagnosis is that the kidney does not respond to a physiologic dose of vasopressin, but it does respond to a small dose of the vasopressin analogue dDAVP, as vasopressinase does not hydrolyze this compound.

RELEASE OF VASOPRESSINASE EARLY IN PREGNANCY
- This enzyme is released by the liver in relatively low amounts.
- Its probable function is to destroy oxytocin, a pituitary hormone that causes contraction of the uterus, which may abort the pregnancy.

Nephrogenic diabetes insipidus

It is common to group the following two types of disorders that lead to polyuria into a single category called nephrogenic diabetes insipidus. The authors do not favor this approach; instead we use the classification used in the following box.

- *AQP2-deficiency type of nephrogenic diabetes insipidus*: Although vasopressin levels are high, AQP2 cannot be inserted into the luminal membrane of the late distal nephron.
- *Normal-AQP2 type of nephrogenic diabetes insipidus*: AQP2 are present in the luminal membrane of the late distal nephron. The major reason for the higher urine flow rate is a major decrease in the renal medullary interstitial osmolality (e.g., in patients with renal insufficiency).

AQP2-deficiency type of nephrogenic diabetes insipidus

We use the term *nephrogenic diabetes insipidus* to describe only the group of disorders in which the late distal nephron is unable to synthesize and/or insert functional AQP2 water channels into the luminal membranes of principal cells. The hallmark for this diagnosis is a failure of either vasopressin or dDAVP to cause an appreciable fall in the urine flow rate and a rise in the U_{Osm} to values greater than the P_{Osm}.

The central clinical feature of this type of nephrogenic diabetes insipidus is the enormous daily urine volume—typically as much as 15 L/day in a 70-kg adult (200 mL/kg body weight). Nevertheless, this daily volume of urine can be smaller in three settings. First, there can be factors that lead to a low distal delivery of filtrate, such as a low effective arterial blood volume due to a negative balance for Na^+ (e.g., the combination of a low-salt diet plus the use of thiazide diuretics as therapy). Second, there can be more water reabsorbed by residual water permeability if a person has a low osmole excretion rate (see Chapter 9, page 278 for more discussion of this topic) or develops an acquired disorder later in life (*see margin note*). Third, in one variant of congenital nephrogenic diabetes insipidus there are mutations in the region of the gene that encodes for the carboxy terminal region of AQP2. Nevertheless, it appears that a residual small number of functioning AQP2 channels are inserted into the lumen of the medullary collecting duct and thereby there is reabsorption of some of the water that is delivered to the distal nephron. Of note, this is the only variant of congenital nephrogenic diabetes insipidus in which patients may have lower urine volume (close to half that in patients with the other types of congenital nephrogenic diabetes insipidus). These patients may have a renal response to large doses of dDAVP (i.e., a fall in the urine flow rate and a rise in the U_{Osm}).

Congenital nephrogenic diabetes insipidus

- To make this diagnosis in a newborn, one must wait until after the first month of life, as there is a physiologic developmental delay in the insertion of AQP2 into the late distal nephron (see page 394 for more discussion).

In newborn animals and humans, there is a period of time before they synthesize and insert AQP2 into the luminal membranes of the late cortical and all the medullary collecting duct nephron segments. This is a physiologic form of nephrogenic diabetes insipidus.

There are two broad classes of defects in water permeability that cause congenital nephrogenic diabetes insipidus: mutations affecting

URINE VOLUME IN ACQUIRED NEPHROGENIC DI

- In patients with congenital renal nephrogenic DI, the renal pelvis may have lost much of its muscular tone. Hence, a much smaller volume of urine travels in a retrograde direction into the inner MCD. Thus the urine volume is larger than in patients with acquired nephrogenic DI.
- In patients with acquired nephrogenic DI, the musculature in the renal pelvis may be stronger. Hence, a larger proportion of the volume in the pelvis can travel in a retrograde fashion up the inner MCD and be absorbed via residual water permeability. Thus, the urine volume may be lower.

the gene encoding for the V_2 receptors for vasopressin and those affecting the gene that encodes for AQP2.

Mutations in the V_2 receptor gene. These mutations are responsible for the majority of patients with inherited nephrogenic diabetes insipidus. The mode of inheritance is X-linked. These patients have a very large urine flow rate.

Mutations in the AQP2 gene. This is an autosomal recessive condition. In patients with mutations that involve the carboxy terminus of the AQP2 molecule, the pattern of inheritance is autosomal dominant. In more detail, the mutation of a single base results in a frame shift that results in elongation of the C-terminal tail of AQP2. Three properties characterize this latter group of patients:

1. The mutated AQP2 has little capability of causing water permeability.
2. There is a dominant negative effect due to association of the mutated AQP2 with wild-type AQP2. Therefore, the vast majority of the normally produced AQP2 cannot reach the membrane site where they can permit the reabsorption of water in the distal nephron (a trafficking disorder in which AQP2 cannot move into the cell membrane). Nevertheless, it seems that a few functioning units of AQP2 may reside in these luminal membranes, because the patients typically have a lower daily urine output; hence, it is called *"partial" nephrogenic diabetes insipidus* (this name adds to the confusion rather than being helpful).
3. Polyuria develops somewhat later in the first years of life rather than in the first months after birth (*see margin note*).

Lithium-induced nephrogenic diabetes insipidus. One possible mechanism for this type of nephrogenic diabetes insipidus is that lithium leads to a diminished transduction of signals elicited by vasopressin. A second possibility stems from experiments performed in vitro, where lithium causes a decrease in mRNA levels for AQP2 in cortical collecting duct cells, which suggests that lithium reduces AQP2 gene transcription or mRNA stability. Regardless of the actual mechanism, it is interesting that these effects of lithium may last for a very long time and may persist for years after the drug is discontinued, especially in patients who haven been on the drug for more than 2 years; the basis for this is not clear (*see margin note*).

Unique to patients with lithium-induced nephrogenic diabetes insipidus is the fact that their urine flow rate is lower and their U_{Osm} is higher (although always less than their P_{Osm} in the presence of hypernatremia) than in patients with central diabetes insipidus or in patients with congenital nephrogenic diabetes insipidus.

It is difficult to imagine that a limited number of AQP2 channels are retained in the luminal membrane of the late distal nephron that never vary in amount. Moreover, there is a very large driving force for the reabsorption of water (an osmotic difference of more than 300 mOsm/kg H_2O, which is equivalent to close to 6000 mm Hg). Hence, it is unlikely that the number of AQP2 channels is actually rate limiting for water reabsorption. We provide the following speculations to account for this conundrum.

1. *Lithium causes a low distal delivery of filtrate to the distal nephron.* Although there is no consistent evidence for a low glomerular filtration rate, there could be an enhanced reabsorption of filtrate in the proximal convoluted tubule; nevertheless there is

USE OF PHOSPHODIESTERASE INHIBITORS
- Inhibitors of the enzyme that destroys cAMP and cyclic GMP (phosphodiesterases of the type 4 class) appear to lead to a greater insertion of AQP2 into luminal membranes in vitro.
- Although greeted with great enthusiasm, disappointingly, treatment of humans with this autosomal dominant mutation with the same phosphodiesterase inhibitor did not result in an appreciable decrease in their urine flow rate and increase in their U_{Osm}.

LITHIUM AND PERSISTENT NEPHROGENIC DIABETES INSIPIDUS
- It is possible, but highly unlikely, that cells affected by lithium in the late distal nephron never die. More likely, they are replaced by newly synthesized cells.
- Obviously, lithium does not change the genetic code for the synthesis of AQP2 or the proteins involved in their insertion in the luminal membrane of principal cells.
- Perhaps lithium has an indirect effect that modifies the gene encoding for AQP2 (e.g., methylation of cytosine bases or by another epigenetic mechanism) that causes a secondary long-lasting form of inactivation of this gene.

no evidence for a lower effective arterial blood volume in every patient who has this disorder. Hence, we do not favor this speculation.

2. *The defect induced by lithium is present mainly in the late cortical distal nephron and* not *in the medullary collecting duct.* This is a distinct possibility because the modest lumen-negative voltage and open epithelial Na^+ channel would permit some lithium to enter principal cells in the late cortical distal nephron. Although there is no lumen voltage in the medullary collecting duct there are far fewer epithelial Na^+ channels in this location. Hence, there may be little lithium reabsorption in this location. Thus, the reabsorption of water in the medullary collecting duct could occur, but it may be small because the flow rate would be very high.

3. *There is an increased reabsorption of water in the inner medullary collecting duct.* Water can be reabsorbed in the inner medullary collecting duct in the absence of AQP2 by residual water permeability. For this to occur, there must be a driving force (already present because of the higher interstitial osmolality compared with the luminal osmolality). In addition, urine will reflux into the inner medullary collecting duct each time the renal pelvis contracts because of preservation of muscular function of the renal pelvis. This would increase the contact and enhance water reabsorption via residual water permeability.

Normal AQP2 type of nephrogenic diabetes insipidus

- The primary defect is a low medullary interstitial osmolality.
- Typically, these patients have a U_{Osm} close to 300 mOsm/kg H_2O and the volume of urine is close to 3 L/day if they ingest a diet that results in the excretion of 900 mosmol/day (*see margin note*).

Although the late distal nephron becomes permeable to water when vasopressin acts, the U_{Osm} in these patients is not appreciably higher than the P_{Osm} because the medullary interstitial osmolality is much lower than that in normal subjects. As a result, the daily osmole load must be excreted in a larger volume of urine. The urine volume in these patients is determined by the rate of excretion of effective osmoles and the medullary interstitial osmolality. Because urea typically represents half of the urinary osmoles, patients with this disorder must have a concentration of Na^+ ($+ K^+$) in the urine that is close to 75 mmol/L when the U_{Osm} is 300 mOsm/kg H_2O. Hence, if their intake of water does not match this obligatory water loss, their P_{Na} will rise initially (*see margin note*). Because the thirst mechanism is intact, and they have a desire to prevent the development of thirst, patients in this setting increase their intake of water and their P_{Na} may be somewhat less than 140 mmol/L.

The causes for destruction of the renal medullary interstitial compartment include infections, infiltrations or hypoxia (e.g., sickle cell disease), and/or disorders that lead to chronic renal diseases. At times, the defect is attributed to hypokalemia or hypercalcemia; these disorders are discussed in more detail subsequently.

EFFECTIVE URINE OSMOLES WHEN VASOPRESSIN ACTS IN THE MEDULLARY COLLECTING DUCT DURING A POLYURIC STATE

- *Electrolytes:* These are always effective osmoles in the urine, as they are not permeable in the medullary collecting duct.
- *Urea:* Urea is sparingly permeable in the medullary collecting duct when the ionic strength of the urine is low. In addition, when polyuria is not due to a urea-induced osmotic diuresis, the concentration of urea is very low in the urine and thereby in the papillary interstitial compartment. Moreover, the fast flow rate per medullary collecting duct and the low retrograde reflux with pelvic contraction all lead to making urea act as an effective osmole in this setting.
- In patients with chronic renal insufficiency, although the total flow rate is similar to normal individuals eating the same diet, the flow per nephron is much faster, as there are far fewer nephrons. Hence urea will diffuse move slowly from the lumen to the papillary interstitial compartment.

BALANCE
The concentration of $Na^+ + K^+$ in the input and outputs must be equal, as must these volumes to have a steady-state value for the P_{Na}.

Hypokalemia

- Hypokalemia is often listed as a cause of nephrogenic diabetes insipidus. This is based largely on data from studies in animals.

Hypokalemia diminishes cAMP formation in response to vasopressin in medullary collecting duct segments from rats in vitro. In addition, rats with hypokalemia have a decreased density of AQP2 water channels in the luminal membrane of the distal nephron. Nevertheless, in vivo data to demonstrate that the osmolality of luminal fluid in the terminal medullary collecting duct of the rat is distinctly lower than the osmolality in the interstitial compartment have not been published; this is required to conclude that the observed lower levels of AQP2 are actually rate limiting for the reabsorption of water in this location. On the other hand, since many patients with hypokalemia do not develop hypernatremia when water intake is diminished, they do not seem to have AQP2-deficient type of nephrogenic diabetes insipidus. Moreover, there are possible reasons why these patients may have a larger urine output. For example, they may have a lower medullary interstitial osmolality resulting from the effect of chronic hypokalemia to cause medullary interstitial damage. In addition, they may have a larger water intake.

Hypercalcemia

- Hypercalcemia is associated with higher urine flow rates and U_{Osm} values close to the P_{Osm} when vasopressin acts; accordingly, it is thought to cause nephrogenic diabetes insipidus.
- Human subjects with the highest concentrations of calcium in the urine have very high U_{Osm} values and a very low urine flow rate.

The impression that hypercalcemia causes nephrogenic diabetes insipidus was supported by in vitro findings that the calcium-sensing receptor colocalizes with AQP2 in vesicles derived from the inner medullary collecting duct. Furthermore, perfusion of inner medullary collecting duct segments of the rat with a solution that has a high concentration of calcium resulted in a small decrease in their water permeability and a somewhat lower luminal osmolality. Many investigators and clinicians believe that if hypercalcemia and/or hypercalciuria causes nephrogenic diabetes insipidus, this would be beneficial because it would minimize the risk of precipitation of calcium-containing stones. Nevertheless, as shown in Table 9-10 (page 292), one needs only a small increment in urine flow rate to virtually eliminate the risk due to growth of precipitates of calcium-containing stones in the terminal nephron. Notwithstanding, it is extremely difficult to achieve small increments in the urine flow rate by decreasing the number of AQP2 water channels given the enormous osmotic driving force to reabsorb water in this location (*see margin note*).

A large body of clinical data suggests that the observed higher urine flow rates and lower U_{Osm} in subjects with hypercalcemia are not the result of true nephrogenic diabetes insipidus. First, the U_{Osm} in patients with hypercalcemia is not lower than the P_{Osm} when vasopressin acts. Second, in human subjects, the *highest* concentrations of calcium are present in urines with the *lowest* flow rate.

A PALEOLITHIC PERSPECTIVE
Inducing a large water diuresis when the rate of excretion of ionized calcium is high would be very dangerous in a setting where there is limited availability of water.

The most likely mechanism for why polyuria occurs with hypercalcemia begins with a high ionized calcium concentration in the renal medullary interstitial compartment; this in turn causes more Ca^{2+} to bind to its receptor on the basolateral membrane of cells of the medullary thick ascending limb of the loop of Henle. Accordingly, this causes an effect akin to actions of a loop diuretic, with a higher rate of excretion of Na^+ and Cl^- as well as a lower renal medullary interstitial osmolality.

QUESTIONS

(Discussion on page 402)

11-3 *Why may the degree of polyuria be so much greater when the interstitial renal disease results from sickle cell anemia compared with other causes of renal medullary damage?*

11-4 *A patient with AQP2-deficient type of nephrogenic diabetes insipidus is treated with a loop diuretic to create a deficit of Na^+. His U_{Osm} rose from 100 mOsm/kg H_2O to 200 mOsm/kg H_2O. Did his nephrogenic diabetes insipidus improve with this therapy?*

HYPERNATREMIA DUE TO A SHIFT OF WATER

In some circumstances, hypernatremia may be due to a shift of water from the ECF compartment into cells. The basis for this water shift is a gain of effective osmoles in cells. The cells involved are almost always skeletal muscle cells because this is where most of the water in the body exists. The usual causes are seizures or mild rhabdomyolysis. A second example of this phenomenon is a shift of water into the lumen of the intestinal tract following the digestion of food in a patient with slow intestinal motility (see discussion of Case 11-3, page 399).

This type of acute hypernatremia may occur inside or outside the hospital. The diagnosis is suspected from the clinical history, the absence of a change in body weight, and the presence of contraction of the ECF volume if the rise in P_{Na} is sustained and severe in degree. Notwithstanding, the threat for brain cell shrinkage is just as important as when hypernatremia is due to a Na^+ gain or a total body water deficit.

HYPERNATREMIA AND POLYURIA IN GERIATRIC PATIENTS

- There are three settings where chronic hypernatremia may be seen in geriatric patients: First, when there is a low intake of water; second, when there is a high protein intake and a urea-induced osmotic develops; and third, when loop diuretics are given to patients who have congestive heart failure.

Low water intake

It is not uncommon to find elderly patients in a nursing home or in a hospital setting who have the combination of a cause of water loss (e.g., fever) and an inability to complain of thirst and/or gain access to water (e.g., because of a previous stroke). If this goes on for a period of time, hypernatremia will develop. The degree of hypernatremia will be even more severe if there is also a reason to have a large urine output (discussed in the following paragraph).

Urea-induced osmotic diuresis

> - There are usually three components to the development of a urea-induced osmotic diuresis in these patients.
>   - First, they are given supplements of protein.
>   - Second, urea may become an effective osmole in the lumen of the lumen of the inner medullary collecting duct.
>   - Third, there is a lower medullary interstitial osmolality.

When protein supplements are given to these patients, there is an increased production and excretion of urea. Nevertheless, the amount of urea excreted is less than that in subjects who consume a typical Western diet. Hence, there must be other reasons for the urea-induced osmotic diuresis to be large enough to lead to the development of hypernatremia. First, these patients often have a degree of medullary interstitial disease, which diminishes the ability to maximally concentrate the urine. Second, these patients consume little salt and K^+; thus, their urine contains little Na^+ and K^+. As a result, urea is reabsorbed much more slowly in the inner medullary collecting duct, even though vasopressin is released in response to the high P_{Na}. Hence, urea is now an effective urine osmole, and it obligates the excretion of water (see Chapter 9, page 289 for more discussion of why urea may become an effective urine osmole). For the patient to develop hypernatremia, there is also a reason for an inability to appreciate or communicate thirst and/or gain access to water.

Use of a loop diuretic in a patient who has congestive heart failure

The basis for hypernatremia has two major components. First, there may be the excretion of a large volume of urine with a relatively low concentration of $Na^+ + K^+$. This results from the actions of the loop diuretic, which cause the excretion of a large volume of urine (especially with mobilization of edema fluid) with a maximum U_{Osm} that is similar to the P_{Osm} (Fig. 11-8). In fact, the effective U_{Osm} must be low in this setting because the U_{Osm} is close to 350 mOsm/kg H_2O owing to the actions of the loop diuretic and the fact that a significant proportion of these osmoles are urea. The second component contributing to the hypernatremia in these patients is the failure to appreciate or communicate thirst and/or an inability to obtain water.

TREATMENT OF PATIENTS WITH HYPERNATREMIA

> - The dangers are different in acute versus chronic hypernatremia.
> - There is no treatment for hypernatremia that is effective in all patients because the basis for this electrolyte disorder may be a deficit of water and/or a positive balance for Na^+.

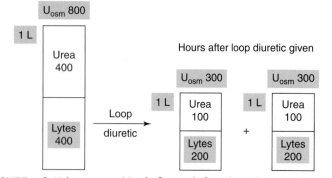

FIGURE 11-8 Urine composition before and after a loop diuretic. The height of the rectangles represents the urine osmolality (U_{Osm}). The *rectangle to the left* represents the 24-hour urine volume on the day prior to administering the loop diuretic; its U_{Osm} is 800 mOsm/kg H_2O. The *two rectangles to the right* represent 2 L of urine that are produced after the loop diuretic acted. As expected, their U_{Osm} is much lower (close to 300 mOsm/L). Since the concentration of urea is 100 mmol/L in this urine, the osmolality due to electrolytes is 200 mOsm/L. Thus the concentrations of Na^+ plus K^+ are 100 mmol/L. Therefore, there was a loss of one third of a liter of electrolyte-free water in each liter of urine.

Acute hypernatremia

This topic was discussed earlier in this chapter, on page 379.

Chronic hypernatremia

• The danger to the patient is brain swelling due to a rapid fall in the P_{Na}; hence, the fall in the P_{Na} should not exceed 8 mmol/L/day.

Chronic hypernatremia is most commonly caused by a deficit of water. The initial step in therapy in these patients is to stop ongoing water loss (e.g., give dDAVP to the patient with central diabetes insipidus or circulating vasopressinase). The design of therapy should be to restore the volume and composition of both the ICF and ECF compartments; this can be achieved by performing a separate analysis for the ICF and ECF compartments. Although there is a water deficit in the ICF that should be replaced, therapy for the ECF compartment depends on the status of the ECF volume. To illustrate these points, consider two 50-kg women (each has a total body water of 30 L; one patient has a normal ECF volume of 10 L while the other has contracted ECF volume of 7 L). They both have a P_{Na} of 154 mmol/L.

Intracellular fluid analysis

A high P_{Na} indicates that there is a water deficit in the ICF compartment with rare exceptions (e.g., a patient with a seizure or rhabdomyolysis). The amount of water needed to restore the ICF tonicity and volume can be estimated using the following calculation. For this calculation, we have made two assumptions: First, the normal ICF volume is two thirds of the total body water; second, the number of particles in the ICF does not change appreciably.

ICF H_2O deficit = normal ICF volume

$$\times (\text{current } P_{Na} - 140 \text{ mmol/L} \div 140 \text{ mmol/L})$$

This is similar for both patients in this example. Because the P_{Na} is now 10% higher, each has close to a 10% decrease in ICF volume. Hence, they each need a positive balance of water that is close to 10% of normal ICF volume of 20 L (2 L of water). Use the oral route if possible. Intravenous solutions must have a lower concentration of Na^+ than ongoing losses in the urine during a polyuric state. The two options are 5% glucose in water (limited by the rate of glucose metabolism; do not exceed 0.3 L/hr) or hypotonic saline (50 to 75 mmol/L, the limit being the Na^+ load that the patient can tolerate).

Extracellular fluid analysis

One patient has a normal ECF volume (10 L). With a P_{Na} of 154 mmol/L and a normal ECF volume of 10 L, there is a positive balance of 140 mmol of Na^+ (154 − 140 mmol/L × 10 L). Hence, a deficit of 140 mmol of Na^+ corrects her ECF composition and volume. The methods used to cause a loss of this quantity of Na^+ have been described previously in the treatment of acute hypernatremia, page 380.

The other patient has an estimated ECF volume of 7 L instead of 10 L. Because the content of Na^+ in the ECF compartment is 1078 mmol (154 mmol/L × 7 L), a positive balance of 322 mmol of Na^+ (1400 − 1078 mmol) plus a positive balance of 3 L of water is required to restore the tonicity and the volume of the ECF compartment to normal.

Therapy for patient 1

Recall that there is a negative balance of 2 L of water and a positive balance of 140 mmol of Na^+. If the goal on day one is to lower the P_{Na} by about 7 mmol/L (half of the rise in P_{Na} of 14 mmol/L) and there is not a special need to change the ECF volume, we would replace half of the deficit of water (create a positive balance of 1 L of water) and cause a negative balance of 70 mmol of Na^+ to lower the P_{Na} by the desired amount. This therapy will be repeated on the second day to bring the compositions of the ECF and ICF back to their usual values. Parenthetically, the positive balance of 1 L of water should account for about 5 of the 7 mmol/L fall in P_{Na} in this patient (*see margin note*).

FALL IN THE P_{Na} FROM 154 DUE TO A POSITIVE BALANCE OF 1 L OF WATER IN A 50-kg PERSON
- Total body water ~30 L
- An extra 1 L of water will lower the P_{Na} by 1/30 x current P_{Na}.
- 1/30 x 154 mmol/L = ~5 mmol/L (this calculation is not intended to be precise).

Therapy for patient 2

Recall that there is a negative balance of 5 L of water (2 L from the ICF compartment and 3 L from the ECF compartment) and a negative balance of about 320 mmol Na^+ in this patient; there are also a significantly contracted ECF and effective arterial blood volumes. We would first reexpand the ECF compartment initially by infusing 2 L of isotonic saline over 5 to 10 hours, which would replace close to the entire deficit of Na^+ with little change in the P_{Na}. The net result is that the balances will change to a negative balance of 3 L of water and a nil balance for Na^+. Therefore, we would give this patient a positive balance of 1.5 L of water per day for 2 days to lower the P_{Na} by about 8 mmol/L/day.

PART D
INTEGRATIVE PHYSIOLOGY

AQP2-DEFICIENCY TYPE OF NEPHROGENIC DIABETES INSIPIDUS IN THE NEWBORN

- Newborn infants fail to insert AQP2 water channels into their inner medullary collecting duct even when vasopressin is present (or after it is administered).
- The analysis of an important process often begins with a very fundamental issue: its essential requirement for survival. In this example, survival depends on having enough ATP to perform essential biologic work.
- Important control systems developed in Paleolithic times—it is unlikely that evolutionary pressures in modern times would have resulted in major modifications in these control systems.

ATP must be regenerated as quickly as possible because it is used in vital organs (e.g., the brain). The main (almost only) fuel that the brain can oxidize to regenerate ATP in the brain of the newborn is glucose. In fact, hypoglycemia poses a unique threat in the first month of life because the metabolic requirements of the brain are large, the availability of circulating ketoacids is low (*see margin note*), and the size of storage pools of glucose is quite small. Therefore, the newborn needs a constant supply of sugar from its only exogenous caloric intake, mother's milk, to avoid neuroglucopenia. This source of brain fuel provides a large water load that the newborn must eliminate promptly. Although some of this water is used for evaporative heat dissipation, a large volume of water must be excreted in the urine and this could lead to both thirst and a wet diaper, which could produce signals for early arousal and a call for a source of sugar.

LOW KETOACID CONCENTRATIONS IN THE NEWBORN
This is an advantage because if ketoacid levels rise between meals, the newborn might be less able to remove glucose derived from milk after it is ingested, resulting in a severe degree of hyperglycemia.

Control of water excretion in the newborn

- A well-developed and safe system to have a water diuresis is essential for survival. A physiologic form of the AQP2-deficiency type of nephrogenic diabetes insipidus is present in the first month of life, and it may provide a survival advantage as it permits a large and rapid excretion of water from milk, as well as providing a warning sign of an impending low supply of glucose for the brain.

There are two important additional physiologic processes that operate to make the water diuresis a safer response.

Low distal delivery of filtrate

> • A low glomerular filtration rate and avid reabsorption of Na^+ in the proximal convoluted tubule are part of the renal physiology in the newborn to decrease the distal delivery of filtrate.

A reduction in the effective arterial blood volume enhances the reabsorption of Na^+ in the proximal convoluted tubule. The sensitivity of this control is likely to be much greater when there is little intake of NaCl. Parenthetically, the caloric input of the newborn contains little NaCl (*see margin note*). Accordingly, a small deficit of water may lead to a sufficient degree of contraction of the effective arterial blood volume in the newborn to stimulate proximal reabsorption of Na^+ and water, which limits the distal delivery of filtrate.

Residual water permeability

The presence of residual water permeability in the newborn could limit the magnitude of a water diuresis by permitting a fall in the urine volume when a modest degree of contraction of the effective arterial blood volume is superimposed on the already low glomerular filtration rate. Thus, it could account for a somewhat higher U_{Osm} once a small deficit of water is lost in the urine, making this a safer signal system.

Moreover, having a neonatal renal concentrating system that does not respond to vasopressin may provide two advantages.

1. If an infant had a nonosmotic stimulus for the release of vasopressin (e.g., nausea, pain, distress), a severe degree of acute hyponatremia would not develop. Although a small degree of brain cell swelling can easily be accommodated by the large open fontanelle in the skull, there could be problems for two reasons. The daily intake of water is very large, and there could be rapid absorption of water in the intestine, which lowers the arterial P_{Na} (i.e, akin to gulping of water; see Chapter 9, page 280 for more discussion).

2. Residual water permeability could also limit the magnitude of the loss of Na^+ in the urine by desalination of luminal fluid in the medullary thick ascending limb of the loop of Henle. In more detail, this added water lowers the concentration of ionized calcium in the outer medullary interstitial compartment by dilution. Therefore, inhibition of the reabsorption of Na^+ in the medullary thick ascending limb of the loop of Henle does not occur in the newborn (see Chapter 9, page 266 for more discussion).

Maternal/fetal integrative physiology

> • During pregnancy, the P_{Na} falls from 140 mmol/L to close to 136 mmol/L.

A pregnant woman has a mild degree of hyponatremia compared with the nonpregnant state. This is, in effect, a reset type of osmostat condition in that a water load can be excreted promptly but stops when the P_{Na} rises to close to 136 mmol/L. In addition, concentrated urine can be excreted if she is water deprived.

COMPOSITION OF MILK
• To have the highest concentration of sugar, milk must have very low electrolyte concentrations (its concentration of Na^+ is ~10 mmol/L) because the osmolality of milk is similar to that in plasma.
• The sugar in milk is a disaccharide (lactose) to provide a larger energy supply without having a higher osmolality or volume.
• A newborn drinks close to 150 mL of milk per kg of body weight, which is 15% of body weight (i.e., equivalent to 7.5 L/day in a 50-kg adult). Hence, this water must be excreted promptly to avoid a serious degree of acute hyponatremia (i.e., retention of this daily intake of water would cause the P_{Na} to fall from 140 to 120 mmol/L).

THE P_{Na} IN THE NEWBORN
The P_{Na} in the mother at term and in the newborn will be equal because water moves across the placenta, and it should reach osmotic equilibration.

How maternal hyponatremia is beneficial becomes obvious when examined in conjunction with the hyponatremia in the newborn infant (*see margin note*). Because of the low P_{Na}, cells of the newborn are swollen. Accordingly, the newborn has a reserve of water after losing circulatory continuity with the mother. Given that there is an AQP2-deficiency type of nephrogenic diabetes insipidus in the newborn, this can be advantageous to provide the source of water loss until the time when the lactation occurs to provide enough water for the newborn.

DISCUSSION OF CASES

CASE 11-1: CONCENTRATE ON THE DANGER

(Case presented on page 370)

Why did hypernatremia develop?

Several facts are obvious. The man has diabetes insipidus because he is excreting dilute urine (U_{Osm} 120 mOsm/kg H_2O) despite the presence of hypernatremia (P_{Na} 150 mmol/L). This indicates that vasopressin has not been released, has been destroyed by vasopressinase released from damaged tissues, and/or has failed to act. The most likely diagnosis is central diabetes insipidus because he had neurosurgery; nephrogenic diabetes insipidus does not have such an abrupt onset and he had a prompt response to dDAVP. Although it is tempting to conclude that the basis for hypernatremia is a deficit of water due to the excretion of a large volume of dilute urine, data are available to evaluate balances for Na^+ and water (tonicity balance) to determine the basis of hypernatremia. As shown in Figure 11-9, the volumes of input and output of water were equal. Therefore, the basis for hypernatremia is a positive balance for Na^+. This is confirmed because the concentration of Na^+ in the infusate was 150 mmol/L, whereas the concentration of Na^+ was only 50 mmol/L in the urine, yielding a positive balance of 300 mmol of Na^+. With a body weight of 50 kg, he had 30 L of total body water; the rise in his P_{Na} should be 10 mmol/L (300 mmol/30 L), and in fact, his P_{Na} rose from 140 mmol/L to 150 mmol/L.

What are the changes in his ECF and ICF compartment volumes?

Because his P_{Na} rose to 150 mmol/L, his ICF volume was contracted. With a total body water of 30 L, the original ICF volume was 20 L. Therefore, his ICF volume has decreased to 18.7 L ([(150 − 140 mmol/L) ÷ 150 mmol/L] × 20 L = 1.3 L).

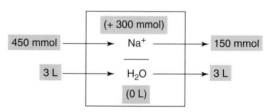

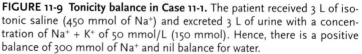

FIGURE 11-9 Tonicity balance in Case 11-1. The patient received 3 L of isotonic saline (450 mmol of Na^+) and excreted 3 L of urine with a concentration of Na^+ + K^+ of 50 mmol/L (150 mmol). Hence, there is a positive balance of 300 mmol of Na^+ and nil balance for water.

With respect to his ECF compartment, there was a gain of 300 mmol of Na^+, and all of this Na^+ should have remained in this compartment (see Fig. 11-9). Because there was no change in his total body water, his ECF volume was expanded by 1.3 L.

What are the goals for therapy of his hypernatremia?

Because hypernatremia was due to a positive balance of 300 mmol of Na^+, efforts should be made to cause the patient to lose 300 mmol of Na^+ while maintaining a nil balance for water. Since this is acute hypernatremia, the goal is to lower the P_{Na} quickly at first. Nevertheless, it is possible that there has been edema of the brain after surgery. Therefore, it might be advisable to aim for a P_{Na} that is close to 145 mmol/L for the next 24 hours. If intracranial pressure is being monitored, this may provide a useful guide to therapy.

To lower P_{Na} by creating a negative balance of 300 mmol of Na^+, the concentration of Na^+ in the infusate should be lower than that in the urine while maintaining water balance. After dDAVP was given, the patient's U_{Na} was 175 mmol/L. Hence, half-isotonic saline (75 mmol/L) was infused for the time needed for the patient to excrete 3 L of urine. This therapy should return his P_{Na} to 140 mmol/L.

CASE 11-2: WHAT IS "PARTIAL" ABOUT PARTIAL CENTRAL DIABETES INSIPIDUS?

(Case presented on page 370)

What is the basis for the high urine flow rate in this patient?

- One cannot have a water diuresis and an osmotic diuresis at the same time, because the former requires an absence of AQP2 and the latter demands that AQP2 be present in the luminal membrane of the late distal nephron.

Because the U_{Osm} is 200 mOsm/kg H_2O and the daily urine volume is 4 L, this patient has a water diuresis. The P_{Na} is high enough to stimulate the release of vasopressin; therefore, this rules out primary polydipsia as the current diagnosis.

To rule out nephrogenic diabetes insipidus or a circulating vasopressinase due to tissue injury as the cause of water diuresis, the patient was given a physiologic dose of vasopressin. In fact, in response to this hormone, his U_{Osm} rose to 900 mOsm/kg H_2O—this rules out both of these diagnoses. Therefore, the final diagnosis was central diabetes insipidus. Because his urine volume was only 4 L/day (a much *lower than expected* urine flow rate in a patient with central diabetes insipidus), the diagnosis was partial central diabetes insipidus, but we ask, "What is the meaning of the word 'partial' in physiologic terms?"

Although the diagnosis of central diabetes insipidus is straightforward, there are three findings that provide insights into the site of the lesion and the possible pathophysiology that has caused partial central diabetes insipidus. Understanding this pathophysiology has important implications in designing the appropriate therapy for this patient.

1. *He was thirsty.* This suggests that his osmostat and thirst center as well as the fibers connecting these two areas were functionally intact (Fig. 11-10).

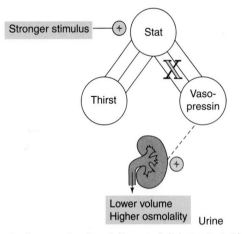

FIGURE 11-10 Lesion causing "partial" central diabetes insipidus. The *upper circle* labeled "osmostat" is the sensor, the *lower left circle* is the thirst center, and the *lower right circle* is the vasopressin release center. The *X* represents a hypothetical lesion that causes severing of some but not all of the fibers connecting the "osmostat" to the vasopressin release center.

2. *He was able to sleep for 8 hours without having to void.* This is a surprise because 8 hours is one third of a day, and one third of the 4-L urine volume is 1.33 L; this exceeds normal urinary bladder capacity and suggests that his urine flow rate is likely much lower during the night. This could be caused by either a higher U_{Osm} or a lower osmole excretion rate during the nocturnal period (see equation). When measured, his overnight U_{Osm} was 425 mOsm/kg H_2O (*see margin note*), suggesting that vasopressin is present during most of the overnight period. This challenges the diagnosis of central diabetes insipidus, or at least our concept of what that diagnosis really means, because it suggests that the vasopressin release center is also functioning but needs a "stronger" stimulus for the release of vasopressin. Perhaps this was achieved during the night; his P_{Na} rose because he continued initially to have a water diuresis, but he stopped drinking water. This impression was supported by the findings that his urine volume was very low and his U_{Osm} was 900 mOsm/L after he received an infusion of hypertonic saline. Therefore, his lesion may involve destruction of some but not all of the fibers linking his osmostat to his vasopressin release center.

> **U_{Osm} OF 425 mOsm/kg H_2O**
> This is the average value for all the urine that may be in his bladder while sleeping; hence it does not represent his maximum U_{Osm}.

$$\text{Urine volume} = \text{number of mosmol excreted} / U_{Osm}$$

3. *He had polyuria during the daytime.* His P_{Na} was 136 mmol/L during the day and his U_{Osm} was 90 mOsm/kg H_2O. This suggests that primary polydipsia was present while he is awake. Its basis probably reflects a learned behavior to avoid the very uncomfortable feeling of thirst.

What are the options for therapy?

A higher P_{Na} in this patient could stimulate the release of vasopressin. There are two ways to raise the P_{Na}, an input of Na^+ or a deficit of water (Table 11-5). The patient selected the intake of oral NaCl tablets to raise his P_{Na} during working hours because the onset of action

TABLE 11-5 **OPTIONS FOR THERAPY IN CASE 11-2**

Option 1 is designed to have actions of vasopressin. Options 2 and 3 are designed to raise the P_{Na} and thereby cause the release of endogenous vasopressin.

OPTION	ADVANTAGES	DISADVANTAGES
dDAVP	• Avoids thirst • Rapid onset • Long duration	• Acute hyponatremia after a water load • May down-regulate V_2 receptors
Water restriction	• Duration: until water intake • May conserve V_2 receptor level	• Thirst develops • Slow onset
Hypertonic NaCl	• Rapid onset • Duration: until water intake • May conserve V_2 receptor level	• Thirst develops

would be quick and it avoids the need for polyuria, which could interrupt business meetings. In contrast, he selected water deprivation to raise his P_{Na} overnight to permit him to have undisturbed sleep. In both settings, he needed to be able to tolerate the thirst that developed. He preferred not to use dDAVP because of the danger of acute hyponatremia if he were to drink an excessive quantity of water while dDAVP acts and because it also may cause down-regulation of his V_2 receptors and thereby lead to a dependence on hormone replacement.

CASE 11-3: WHERE DID THE WATER GO?

(Case presented on page 371)

What is the basis for the hypernatremia (in quantitative terms)— a positive balance for Na^+ and/or a negative balance of water?

Na⁺ gain: In quantitative terms, if Na^+ gain is the basis of hypernatremia, there should be a positive balance of more than 1100 mmol of NaCl (*see margin note*), but it is highly unlikely that the patient has consumed this much NaCl. Both the physical examination and the unchanged value for his hematocrit (0.36), hemoglobin (125 g/L), and $P_{Albumin}$ (38 g/L) indicate that his ECF volume was not grossly expanded as would be expected from this large gain of Na^+. Therefore, it is highly unlikely that a large positive balance of Na^+ is the major cause of his hypernatremia.

Water deficit: Because there was no obvious source of water loss and the ECF volume was not contracted, a water deficit is not a sole cause of his hypernatremia (*see margin note*). In addition, he had a weight gain of 1 kg instead of a loss of 20% of total body water (~8 L or 8 kg) if the cause of hypernatremia was a water deficit.

Why does he have such a severe degree of hypernatremia?

Because the sudden rise in the P_{Na} cannot be explained simply by a gain of Na^+, a deficit of water (or even half owing to a gain of Na^+ and half owing to a deficit of water), there must be an internal shift of Na^+ or water to explain the acute and large rise in the P_{Na}.

Shift of water: There are two considerations to explain a large shift of water to a hidden compartment.

1. This compartment must be large to accommodate about 8 L of water. Based on this consideration, the only organ in the body that is large enough is skeletal muscle. As discussed previously in this

Na GAIN AS A CAUSE OF A P_{Na} OF 169 mmol/L

- The calculation is based on total body water of 40 L (50% of 80 kg owing to a degree of obesity).
- With an acute rise in P_{Na} of 29 mmol/L, his positive balance for Na^+ would have to be greater than 1000 mmol (40 L × 29 mmol/L = 1160 mmol). This is greater than 50% increase in the content of Na^+ in his ECF compartment (~14 L × 140 mmol/L = ~2000 mmol).
- His ECF volume should be expanded by almost 7 L (2000 + 1160) mmol ÷ 169 mmol/L). This is unlikely in view of the absence of overt signs of ECF volume expansion.

WATER DEFICIT AS A CAUSE OF P_{Na} OF 169 mmol/L

The rise in his P_{Na} is 29 mmol/L, which is a 20% rise (29 ÷ 140 mmol/L). Hence, the water deficit should be 20% of his total body water of 40 L, or 8 L.

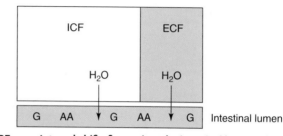

FIGURE 11-11 Internal shift of water into the intestinal lumen. The key to this analysis is that the compartment where the water is redistributed has to be large, with the capacity to expand considerably. The lumen of the intestinal tract is depicted as a *narrow rectangle below the intracellular fluid* (ICF; *white rectangle*) and the extracellular fluid (ECF; *green rectangle*) compartments, and it contains amino acids (AA) and glucose (G) from the digestion of food, but prior to the absorption of the large amount of these solutes.

chapter (see page 390), the driving force for a shift of water is a gain of solutes in muscle cells during a seizure or rhabdomyolysis. Against this possibility, the patient did not have a seizure and there was no accumulation of H^+ or L-lactate anions; his P_{HCO3} was 25 mmol/L and his $P_{L\text{-lactate}}$ was 1 mmol/L. In addition, it is unlikely that he had rhabdomyolysis because his creatine kinase (CK) level was not elevated in plasma.

2. Not only must the compartment into which water enters must be large, it must also be able to "stretch" to accommodate this huge volume (*see margin note*). Accordingly, another possible site for a large water shift is the lumen of the intestinal tract. The force to move water is an osmotic one—a large rise in the number of effective osmoles in the intestinal lumen (Fig. 11-11).

The fact that water can shift into the intestinal lumen in normal subjects after a meal has been demonstrated by measuring the P_{Na} before and during digestion of a meal containing little Na^+—a typical rise in the P_{Na} is 3 mmol/L, even though there is secretion of Na^+ into the lumen of the intestine. To have a much larger rise in the P_{Na}, one would need a longer time period (e.g., owing to low intestinal motility, perhaps the result of autonomic neuropathy secondary to long-standing type 2 diabetes mellitus) and a larger number of osmoles produced by digestion of dietary constituents (e.g., glucose and amino acids) that remain in the intestinal lumen. In this regard, the usual dietary intake of 270 g of carbohydrate (1500 mmol of glucose) and 1.5 g protein per kg body weight (~1000 mmol of amino acids in an adult) are within the range of number of osmoles needed to cause a sufficiently large acute shift of water to be responsible for the very high P_{Na}.

Because there was no obvious contraction of the ECF and effective arterial blood volumes when water shifted into the lumen of the small intestine, it appears that some effective osmoles were absorbed from his dietary intake (i.e., Na^+ and Cl^-). Therefore, we suspect that the rise in P_{Na} reflects the combination of absorbed Na^+ and Cl^- along with the movement of water from the body into the lumen of the intestinal tract.

What is the therapy of hypernatremia in this patient?

- The major threat on admission is the shrinkage of brain cell volume because this stretches the blood vessels that come from the inner lining of the skull and hence they may rupture.

Before addressing the specific therapy, it is important to recognize that we do not know with certainty whether his P_{Na} will rise further as the result of a continuing osmotic-driven shift of water into the lumen of his intestinal tract, or whether just the opposite may happen. In more detail, there may be an increase in GI motility that leads to the absorption of glucose, amino acids, and water, and therefore there would be a danger of inducing an acute and large fall in his P_{Na}. Hence, the most important initial therapy is to remove the contents of his stomach and upper intestinal tract and place an emphasis on the major threat at this moment, the danger of an intracranial hemorrhage. Although this is just an opinion, we would prefer to lower his P_{Na} by close to 10 mmol/L and then reevaluate the situation.

Add water

Once the contents of the stomach and small intestine have been removed, it is advisable to give water. If the patient is not symptomatic, we would give water through the GI tract. The volume of water needed to cause a fall in the P_{Na} by 10 mmol/L is about 2.5 L. We would follow the P_{Na} closely and create a positive water balance to lower his P_{Na} toward 140 mmol/L over 24 hours.

Remove a large quantity of Na⁺

It is very likely that there is a positive balance of Na^+. In fact, this positive balance of Na^+ was valuable because it helped prevent an enormous degree of contraction of his ECF volume owing to the very large internal shift of water. Accordingly, we would not remove much of this Na^+ load by the administration of a natriuretic agent until a large volume of water has been added to his body, unless the patient suffered from an expanded arterial blood volume.

DISCUSSION OF QUESTIONS

11-1 Why must sweat always contain some Na⁺ and Cl⁻?

The driving force to reabsorb Cl^- in the sweat gland is a lumen-negative voltage, which is created by reabsorbing Na^+ faster than Cl^-. This lumen-negative voltage pushes Cl^- across both the luminal and basolateral membranes because they each have Cl^- ion channels. The magnitude of the transepithelial negative voltage must be large to push Cl^- against a large Cl^- concentration difference (i.e., Cl^- must be "pushed" by this negative voltage to enter the ECF, where the concentration of Cl^- is 103 mmol/L).

Now consider the effect of a large lumen-negative voltage on cations. Na^+ enters cells via the epithelial Na^+ channel because the concentration of Na^+ in cells is low and the voltage is negative in cells, as a result of the actions of the Na-K-ATPase on the basolateral membrane. Notwithstanding, the luminal negative voltage places a constraint on the reabsorption of Na^+. Hence, not all the Na^+ and Cl^- in the sweat duct can be reabsorbed.

11-2 A 50-kg man receives 3 L of isotonic saline (150 mmol/L) and excretes 3 L of urine with an unknown concentration of Na⁺ and K⁺. In this period, his P_{Na} rises from 140 mmol/L to 150 mmol/L. If there are no other inputs or outputs during this period, what is the concentration of Na⁺ and K⁺ in mmol/L in this urine?

To answer this question, examine the balances for water and for Na^+ and K^+. Because water balance is nil, and the P_{Na} rises by 10 mmol/L, this patient retains 300 mmol of Na^+ ($[150 - 140\ mmol/L = 10\ mmol/L$, multiplied by total body water of 30 L = 300 mmol]). Because 450 mmol of Na^+ were infused of ($3\ L \times 150\ mmol/L$) and 300 mmol are retained, the urine must contain 150 mmol of Na^+. With a urine volume of 3 L, the concentration of $Na^+ + K^+$ is 50 mmol/L (150 mmol ÷ 3 L).

11-3 *Why may the degree of polyuria be much greater when the interstitial renal disease results from sickle cell anemia compared with other causes of renal medullary damage?*

The volume of an osmotic diuresis is inversely proportional to the osmolality of the medullary interstitial compartment and directly proportional to the number of effective osmoles being excreted. With respect to the medullary interstitial osmolality, it makes no difference whether this osmolality is reduced because of sickle cell anemia or a different etiology. Conversely, in patients with sickle cell anemia, the number of effective urine osmoles may be increased without an increase in the excretion of total osmoles. This occurs because red blood cells sickle in a hypoxic, hyperosmolar environment (e.g., in the inner medulla). As a result, this area may become damaged. Because this is the major site of luminal urea transporters in the medullary collecting duct, less urea is reabsorbed; hence, urea is now an effective urine osmole. This can cause the rate of excretion of effective osmoles to double as urea is typically half of the urine osmoles (*see margin note*).

11-4 *A patient with AQP2-deficient type nephrogenic diabetes insipidus is treated with a loop diuretic to create a deficit of Na^+. His U_{Osm} rose from 100 mOsm/kg H_2O to 200 mOsm/kg H_2O. Did his nephrogenic diabetes insipidus improve with this therapy?*

When a loop diuretic acts, there is a large increase in the quantity of Na^+ delivered to the distal nephron because the reabsorption of Na^+ and Cl^- in the medullary and the cortical thick ascending limbs of the loop of Henle is inhibited by the loop diuretic (*see margin note*). As a result of having more osmoles to excrete, the U_{Osm} rises, but this rise in U_{Osm} does not indicate that more water was reabsorbed in the late distal nephron.

QUANTITY OF Na^+ AND Cl^- REABSORBED IN THE MEDULLARY AND CORTICAL THICK ASCENDING LIMBS OF THE LOOP OF HENLE

- In the mTAL, there are two types of Na^+ reabsorption: ~1600 mmol/day during Na^+ recycling in the loop of Henle and ~1000 mmol/day to restore the composition of the medullary interstitial compartment after water was reabsorbed from the MCD and from the DtL of juxtamedullary nephrons (see Table 9-11, page 305 for more details).
- There is a larger amount of Na^+ and Cl^- reabsorbed daily for "desalination" of luminal fluid in the cortical thick ascending limb of the loop of Henle and the early distal convoluted tubule because the luminal Na^+ concentration declines by ~80 mmol/L (i.e., from 120 mmol/L to ~40 mmol/L) and 27 L/day flow through these water-impermeable nephron segments (27 L/day × 80 mmol/L = 2160 mmol/day).

chapter 12

Polyuria

Introduction

Polyuria is due to either a water or an osmotic diuresis. Many patients who present with polyuria also have hypernatremia because they excrete a large volume of urine with a low concentration of Na^+ plus K^+ (e.g., patients with diabetes insipidus or a urea-induced osmotic diuresis). Hence, there are areas of overlap between this chapter and the previous one on hypernatremia. Nevertheless, there are a number of issues that are pertinent to polyuria, and they are the focus of this chapter.

■ To illustrate that polyuria should be defined based on principles of physiology that determine the urine volume in a certain setting rather than be defined by a larger than usual urine volume.

■ To illustrate that a large water diuresis can occur only if the distal nephron is virtually impermeable to water (lacks actions of vasopressin). In this setting, the magnitude of the water diuresis depends on the volume of hypotonic fluid delivered to the distal nephron and how much water is reabsorbed via residual water permeability in the inner medullary collecting duct.

■ To emphasize that because actions of vasopressin must be present during an osmotic diuresis, the urine flow rate depends directly on the number of effective osmoles excreted and inversely on the medullary interstitial effective osmolality.

CASE 12-1: OLIGURIA WITH A URINE VOLUME OF 4 LITERS PER DAY

(Case discussed on page 410)

A 22-year-old woman lives in a hot climate and runs each day to keep fit. She is very careful not to eat "unhealthy" foods, and she restricts her salt intake. She typically drinks a large volume of water. Her daily urine volume is 4 L. On repeated measurements done on visits to the office of her physician, her P_{Na} was close to 130 mmol/L and her U_{Osm} was close to 80 mOsm/kg H_2O.

Questions

Does this patient have polyuria?

What dangers related to Na^+ and water may develop in this patient?

PART A
BACKGROUND

SYNOPSIS OF THE PHYSIOLOGY

Following a large intake of water that lowers the P_{Na} sufficiently to inhibit the release of vasopressin, virtually all of the AQP2 water channels are removed from the luminal membrane of the late distal nephron. Because these nephron segments are now impermeable to water (except for residual water permeability in the inner medullary collecting duct; see Chapter 9, page 278 for more discussion of this topic), the expected response is that the majority of the volume of filtrate delivered to the late distal nephron will be excreted in the urine (Fig. 12-1). Typical values for peak urine flow rates in a normal adult are 10 to 15 mL/min, and they occur 60 to 90 minutes after the rapid ingestion of a large water load. If this volume is extrapolated to 24 hours, the urine volume is usually 10 to 20 L (*see margin note*).

Conversely, for a high rate of excretion of osmoles to be the *cause* of polyuria, vasopressin must be acting (Fig. 12-2). The urine flow rate during an osmotic diuresis is determined by the rate of excretion of effective osmoles and the medullary interstitial effective osmolality.

EXPECTED U_{Osm} DURING A WATER DIURESIS OF 10 LITERS PER DAY

The rate of excretion of osmoles influences the U_{Osm} but not the urine flow rate when actions of vasopressin are absent as shown below.

FLOW RATE (L/day)	mOsmol/ day	U_{Osm} (mOsm/L)
10	800	80
10	400	40

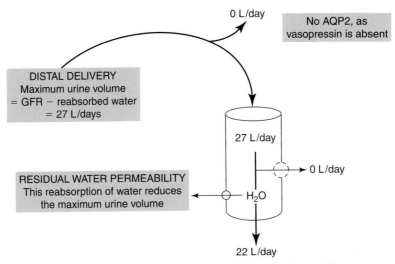

FIGURE 12-1 Determinants of the urine volume during a water diuresis. The *cylinder* represents the medullary collecting duct. The actions of vasopressin on the final functional unit of the nephron must be absent. Thus the urine flow rate is determined by the volume of filtrate delivered to the distal nephron minus the volume of water reabsorbed via residual water permeability in the inner medullary collecting duct (*see margin note*). The latter is relatively large because of the large difference in osmolality between the luminal fluid in the inner medullary collecting duct and the medullary effective interstitial compartment. AQP2, aquaporin 2.

FLUX THROUGH AQP2 WATER CHANNELS

- To have a water diuresis, virtually all of the AQP2 water channels must be removed from the luminal membrane in the late distal nephron.
- Given the enormous osmotic force, even if there are some AQP2 in the luminal membranes of the late distal nephron, a large volume of water should be reabsorbed.

DISTAL DELIVERY OF FILTRATE
- Most of the descending thin limbs of the loop of Henle lack AQP1 and hence are likely to be impermeable to water.
- A minor exception is the descending thin limbs of loop of Henle that descend into the inner medulla (~15% of all nephrons).
- Based on a GFR of 180 L/day and that five sixths of this volume is reabsorbed in the proximal convoluted tubule, we estimate that 30 L exit the pars recta of the convoluted tubule, and about 27 L are delivered to the distal convoluted tubule.

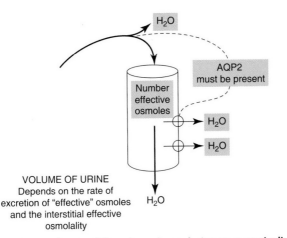

FIGURE 12-2 Determinants of the urine volume during an osmotic diuresis. The structures are the same as in Figure 12-1. The requirement for an osmotic diuresis is a large distal delivery of osmoles (>900 mosmol/day) in the presence of actions of vasopressin. The urine flow rate is higher during an osmotic diuresis if there is a lower medullary interstitial effective osmolality (*see margin note*).

MAXIMUM MEDULLARY INTERSTITIAL OSMOLALITY
The maximum U_{Osm} is lower during an osmotic diuresis or when there has been a prior water diuresis due to a lower osmolality in the medullary interstitial compartment.

Because each milliosmole exerts an osmotic pressure of 19.3 mm Hg, a difference in osmolality between the lumen of the medullary collecting duct and the medullary interstitial compartment of 400 mOsm/kg H_2O results in a driving force of almost 8000 mm Hg. Therefore, AQP2 must be virtually absent in the luminal membranes in the final functional unit of the nephron during a water diuresis.

DEFINITION OF POLYURIA

• Polyuria is present if the urine volume is greater than expected for the clinical setting.

There are two different ways to define polyuria. The commonly used definition compares the urine output in the patient to the usual urine volume in normal subjects who consume a typical Western diet. Therefore, polyuria is commonly defined as a 24-hour urine output that is greater than 2.5 L or 3 L.

We prefer, however, to define polyuria based on physiologic principles that determine the urine flow rate. In this case, polyuria is present if the urine volume is *greater than what is expected* for the clinical setting. If the P_{Na} is lower than 136 mmol/L, the release of vasopressin should be inhibited and the urine flow rate should be as high as possible (i.e., ~10 to 15 mL/min in an adult). A lower urine flow rate in this case indicates that oliguria (rather than polyuria) is present even if the urine volume is relatively large. In contrast, polyuria is present if the urine volume is higher than what is expected for the rate of excretion of effective osmoles when vasopressin acts even if it does not exceed 2.5 L or 3 L/day (e.g., in a patient with a very low distal delivery of filtrate). The advantages of this physiology-based definition of polyuria will become clearer after reading the discussion of Case 12-1, page 410, and the discussion of Questions 12-1 and 12-2, page 421. The differential diagnosis of polyuria is outlined in Table 12-1.

TABLE 12-1 **DIFFERENTIAL DIAGNOSIS OF POLYURIA**

BASIS	KEY FEATURE	DIAGNOSTIC TOOLS
Water diuresis		
• Primary polydipsia	• P_{Na} < 136 mmol/L	• ↑ U_{Osm} and ↓ $U_{Flow\ rate}$ if stop water intake
• Central DI	• Central nervous system pathology	• ↑ U_{Osm} and ↓ $U_{Flow\ rate}$ after ADH is given
• Vasopressinase	• Necrotic tissue	• Responds to dDAVP and not to ADH
• Nephrogenic DI	• Often due to lithium	• No response to dDAVP
Osmotic diuresis		
• Organic compounds (e.g., urea, glucose) or electrolytes (Na + Cl)	• U_{Osm} > 300 mOsm/L and osmole excretion > 900 mosmol/day	• Calculate osmole excretion rate • Establish nature of the urine osmoles
Renal concentrating defect		
• Low osmolality in the renal medulla	• Maximum U_{Osm} is < 600 mOsm/kg H_2O	• Diseases or drugs that affect the renal medulla

ADH, antidiuretic hormone or vasopressin; DI, diabetes insipidus.

CLINICAL TOOLS

Urine flow rate

> • Polyuria is present if the urine flow rate is *higher than expected* for the clinical setting.

During a water diuresis, the urine flow rate is determined by the volume of hypotonic fluid delivered to the distal nephron minus the volume reabsorbed through residual water permeability in the inner medullary collecting duct (see Fig. 12-1). In subjects who consume more than 100 mmol (6 g) of NaCl, the distal flow rate is about 20 mL/min, and the peak urine flow rate in the absence of vasopressin actions is close to 15 mL/min. If the urine volume is considerably less than 15 L/day, determine why there is a low distal delivery of filtrate (e.g., low glomerular filtration rate [GFR] and/or enhanced reabsorption of filtrate in the proximal convoluted tubule) and/or increased reabsorption of water via residual water permeability in the inner medullary collecting duct. For example, subjects who eat a very small quantity of NaCl should have a lower distal delivery of filtrate than subjects who have a larger intake of NaCl because they should have an enhanced reabsorption of Na^+, Cl^-, and water in the proximal convoluted tubule.

During an osmotic diuresis, the major factor that influences the urine flow rate is the number of effective osmoles to be excreted and the medullary interstitial effective osmolality.

Urine osmolality

When polyuria is caused by a water diuresis, the U_{Osm} is considerably less than the P_{Osm}. Nevertheless, the absolute value for the U_{Osm} is determined by the rate of excretion of osmoles (*see margin note*). Hence, subjects consuming little protein and little salt should have a much lower U_{Osm} than those consuming a typical Western diet or those who have a high rate of excretion of osmoles (e.g., high rate of excretion of NaCl due to infusion of large volumes of saline or renal salt wasting, high excretion of urea due to a catabolic state). In an osmotic diuresis, the U_{Osm} is greater than 300 mOsm/kg H_2O. In this setting, U_{Osm} is determined by the tonicity of the medullary interstitium, which may vary in different clinical states (e.g., in a prior water diuresis, the U_{Osm} is low because of medullary washout). The effect of ethanol on the U_{Osm} is described in a margin note.

Osmole excretion rate

> • This is the product of the U_{Osm} and the urine flow rate.

In subjects eating a typical Western diet, the osmole excretion rate is 600 to 900 mosmol/day. Electrolytes and urea each account for half of these osmoles. Although the rate of excretion of osmoles does not directly influence the urine flow rate in the absence of vasopressin actions, it should be calculated in every patient with polyuria because this excretion rate will influence the urine flow rate if desmopressin (dDAVP) acts in a patient with central DI. The nature of the excess osmoles (e.g., urea, glucose, electrolytes) should also be established by measuring the composition of the urine.

USE OF THE U_{Osm} DURING A WATER DIURESIS
• The expected U_{Osm} during a water diuresis on a typical Western diet is close to 60 mOsm/kg H_2O because there are 15 L/day and 900 mosmol are excreted per day.
• The U_{Osm} may be higher if there is a high rate of excretion of osmoles and/or a low distal delivery of filtrate.
• Beware! At times, the U_{Osm} may not represent a steady-state value because of mixing of urines with a higher and lower U_{Osm}.

ETHANOL AND THE OSMOLALITY OF THE URINE
• Ethanol is not an effective osmole in plasma or in the urine. Hence, it does not influence the urine flow rate when vasopressin acts. The higher U_{Osm} in this setting should not be misinterpreted to reflect vasopressin action.
• Ethanol does not inhibit the release of vasopressin sufficiently to cause a water diuresis unless its concentration in plasma is greater than 100 mmol/L.

PRODUCTION OF GLUCOSE AND UREA FROM PROTEIN CATABOLISM
Breakdown of 100 g of protein leads to the net production of 60 g (333 mmol) of glucose and 572 mmol of urea (see Chapter 16, page 550 for more discussion).

CEREBRAL SALT WASTING
In the vast majority of these patients, there is an adrenergic surge and a higher than expected blood pressure. Because it is really the effective arterial volume that must be low to diagnose salt wasting, this diagnosis is not correct in many patients.

EXPECTED RESPONSE TO dDAVP
- Normal subjects have a medullary interstitial effective osmolality of 600 mOsm/kg H_2O and excrete 450 effective mosmol/day. Hence, their average urine flow rate is close to 0.6 to 0.8 mL/min.
- Because the renal medullary osmolality falls to close to 400 mOsm/kg H_2O during a water diuresis, the expected urine flow rate is greater than 2 mL/min when dDAVP acts. If the effective osmole excretion rate is significantly elevated, the urine flow rate will be even higher (see the discussion of Case 11-1, page 396).
- On the other hand, despite the absence of luminal AQP2, a fall in the blood pressure after the administration of dDAVP may lead to a fall in the GFR and an enhanced proximal reabsorption of Na^+ and Cl^- water. Therefore the distal delivery of filtrate will fall and the urine flow rate will be much lower despite an absence of a renal response to dDAVP.

To deduce which solute may be responsible for the osmotic diuresis, the concentration of likely compounds in plasma (e.g., glucose and urea) should be measured. In a patient with a urea-induced osmotic diuresis, it is important to determine if these osmoles are derived from catabolism of endogenous proteins (*see margin note*). Patients are rarely given a sufficiently large amount of mannitol for it to be the sole cause of a sustained osmotic diuresis.

A saline-induced osmotic diuresis may occur if there is a large infusion of saline or if the patient has cerebral or renal salt wasting (*see margin note*). Another common setting of polyuria due to a saline-induced osmotic diuresis is the patient with an edema state who is treated with a loop diuretic. To confirm that salt wasting is present (e.g., renal or cerebral salt wasting, adrenal insufficiency), there must be an appreciable excretion of Na^+ at a time when the effective arterial blood volume is *definitely* low.

Renal response to vasopressin or dDAVP

> - In the diagnostic approach to the patient with polyuria, for safety, dDAVP should be given only if the P_{Na} is elevated and water intake must be restricted if dDAVP is given.

If the urine volume declines and the U_{Osm} rises to be equal to or greater than the P_{Osm} when vasopressin is given, the reason for the water diuresis is central diabetes insipidus. In patients with a water diuresis due to the presence of a circulating vasopressinase (released from necrotic tissue), there is a response to dDAVP, but not to the dose of vasopressin that is usually administered. On the other hand, a lack of response to dDAVP indicates that AQP-deficient type of nephrogenic diabetes insipidus is present. Two cautionary points should be kept in mind in assessing the renal response to dDAVP. First, patients who have a lower medullary osmolality (e.g., due to washout of the renal medulla after a water diuresis; *see margin note*) will have a much higher urine flow rate even though dDAVP has acted (see the discussion of Case 12-2, page 420). Second, when the effective osmole excretion rate is high, there is a much higher minimum urine flow rate when dDAVP acts.

Effective osmoles in the urine

> - Only osmoles that have a restricted permeability across the luminal membrane of the late distal nephron influence the volume of water in the lumen of that nephron segment when vasopressin acts.

Upstream in the distal nephron, both urea and electrolytes are *not* permeable, and they are effective osmoles in this location. In the inner medullary collecting duct, electrolytes are effective urine osmoles, but urea may or may not be an *effective* urine osmole. Cells in the inner medullary collecting duct have urea transporters in their luminal membrane when vasopressin acts. Hence, urea is *not* an effective osmole (i.e., the concentration of urea on both sides of that membrane is equal; see Chapter 9, page 289). The net result of excreting a small *extra* amount of urea is a higher U_{Osm}, but not a higher effective U_{Osm} or a higher urine flow rate. Urea becomes an effective osmole under two major conditions. First, when the rate of excretion of urea rises sufficiently so that it cannot be absorbed fast enough to achieve equal concentrations on both sides of the inner medullary collecting duct membrane. Second, even though the rate of excretion of urea may not be high, urea can become a partially effective urine osmole when vasopressin acts if the rate of excretion of electrolytes is low (see Chapter 9, page 290 for more discussion). This permits the excretion of a minimum safe urine volume to avoid the risk of forming precipitates in the urine.

Effective urine osmoles with respect to cell volume

Because Na^+ and K^+ and their attendant anions have a restricted permeability across cell membranes, the $U_{Na} + U_K$ influences the P_{Na} and hence the volume of water in cells. Urea moves across cell membranes and achieves concentration equilibrium; therefore, it does not influence movement of water. One can ignore U_{NH4} plus its attendant anions in this analysis because the U_{NH4} was derived from a macromolecule (glutamine in proteins).

PRECAUTIONS TO AVOID MISINTERPRETATIONS

There are a few ways that one can be misled when examining the composition and volume of the urine to determine the basis for a large urine output.

1. If values from a single urine collection are used to deduce excretion rates over a long period of time, this can lead to a problem if the composition of the urine is not constant throughout the entire time period. Therefore, one should examine multiple short urine collections (see the discussion of Question 12-4, page 422).

2. When interpreting the urine flow rate after administering dDAVP, one should not be misled by thinking that there is an incomplete response to dDAVP if the urine flow rate does not decrease to what is expected in normal subjects. Two examples of this are if the patient has a prior water diuresis causing medullary washout, or if the rate of excretion of osmoles is high (see the discussion of Question 12-5, page 423). On the other hand, a lower than expected urine flow rate may be caused by a large fall in the blood pressure due to the administration of dDAVP, which leads to a fall in the GFR and a decrease in the distal delivery of filtrate.

3. One cannot have a water diuresis and an osmotic diuresis at the same time because the rate of excretion of effective osmoles does not directly influence the urine flow rate in the absence of vasopressin actions. In a patient with central diabetes insipidus, a high rate of excretion of effective osmoles causes a much higher than expected urine flow rate *after* dDAVP acts.

QUESTIONS

(Discussions on page 421)

12-1 *An obese patient has been fasting for 2 weeks in a weight reduction program. His P_{Na} is 145 mmol/L, his urine flow rate is 0.6 L/day, his U_{Osm} is 700 mOsm/kg H_2O, and the concentration of urea in his urine is 100 mmol/L. Does this patient have a renal concentrating defect?*

12-2 *A patient with cirrhosis of the liver was placed on a diet with little protein and salt. While in the hospital, his urine flow rate was 0.4 L/day, his U_{Osm} was 375 mOsm/kg H_2O, and his osmole excretion rate was 150 mosmol/day. Does this patient have oliguria, polyuria, and/or a renal concentrating defect?*

DISCUSSION OF CASE 12-1

CASE 12-1: OLIGURIA WITH A URINE VOLUME OF 4 LITERS PER DAY

(Case presented on page 404)

Does the patient have polyuria?

Conventional interpretation

Polyuria is present because the urine volume is greater than 3 L/day. This is a water diuresis because the U_{Osm} is considerably less than the P_{Osm}. The presence of a low P_{Na} indicates that the patient has primary polydipsia.

Physiology-based interpretation

The *observed* urine flow rate (~3 mL/min, 4500 ÷ 1440 minutes) is *much lower than expected* when vasopressin is absent. In more detail, because of the low P_{Na} of 130 mmol/L, the expected urine flow rate is 10 to 15 mL/min. Hence, this patient does *not* have polyuria in physiologic terms.

The lower than expected urine flow rate could result from the fact that vasopressin was present intermittently due to a nonosmotic stimulus for its release. Alternatively, there may be a low delivery of filtrate to the distal nephron because of an enhanced proximal tubular reabsorption due to a degree of contraction of the effective arterial blood volume with a somewhat lower GFR (see Fig. 12-1, page 405). There may also be enhanced residual water permeability due to the low luminal osmolality in the inner medullary collecting duct (see Chapter 9, page 278). The low osmole excretion rate becomes obvious after this parameter is calculated (80 mOsm/kg H_2O × 4 L/day or 320 mosmol/day instead of the usual 600 to 900 mosmol/day).

What dangers related to Na⁺ and water may develop in this patient?

Acute hyponatremia

Understanding that this patient does not have polyuria, but rather diminished ability to excrete water, makes one realize that this patient is at risk for a substantial gain of water if she were to ingest more water and/or if her loss of water were to decrease. The latter may occur if she has a nonosmotic stimulus for the release of vasopressin (e.g., pain, nausea, and/or the intake of a drug such as Ecstasy; see Table 10-2, page 320). Alternatively, her nonrenal loss of water in sweat would decrease if she fails to run one day (sweat volume may be as large as 1 to 2 L/hr). The resulting acute fall in her P_{Na} places her at risk of developing acute brain cell swelling with possible herniation.

Osmotic demyelination because of a rapid rise in the P_{Na}

If she were to have a large intake of NaCl, there could be a large increase in the distal delivery of filtrate and thereby a large and acute excretion of urine with a low Na⁺ concentration because vasopressin is absent (hyponatremia is still present). In addition, the higher rate of excretion of osmoles could decrease the volume of water reabsorbed owing to residual water permeability. This very rapid rise in the P_{Na} in this patient, who has chronic hyponatremia, could place her at risk for osmotic demyelination, especially if her dietary intake is poor and/or if K^+ depletion is present (*see margin note*). Alternatively, if she had a chronic nonosmotic stimulus for the release of vasopressin and it disappeared, there could also be a large water diuresis with the risk of osmotic demyelination.

PART B
WATER DIURESIS

DIAGNOSTIC ISSUES

The following issues must be kept in mind in a patient with a water diuresis. One must seek the cause for absence of vasopressin actions on the distal nephron. At times, the magnitude of the water diuresis may be much smaller than expected because of a low distal delivery of filtrate. It is also important to estimate the rate of excretion of osmoles because this will influence the urine flow rate if there is a renal response to the administration of dDAVP.

If hypernatremia is present, assess thirst to help evaluate the function of the hypothalamus. On the other hand, hypernatremia may not be present if the patient drinks excessively to avoid thirst. If the patient develops acute polyuria in the hospital, calculate a tonicity balance to determine the basis for a change in the P_{Na} (and thereby the intracellular fluid [ICF] volume) to design appropriate therapy to restore ICF and extracellular fluid (ECF) volumes and composition.

CLINICAL APPROACH

The differential diagnosis is provided in Table 12-1, and the steps to take to determine the diagnosis are outlined in Flow Chart 12-1

RISK OF OSMOTIC DEMYELINATION IN A PATIENT WITH A P_{Na} OF 130 mmol/L
Although her P_{Na} is 130 mmol/L, one might conclude that there is little risk of osmotic demyelination from a rapid rise in P_{Na} in this setting. On the other hand, because only severe cases of osmotic demyelination with evident neurologic defects are reported, we may be missing less severe and hence less obvious defects, and perhaps a rapid rise in the correction with P_{Na} from 130 mmol/L is not without risk, especially if minor deficits from repeated insults are cumulative.

FLOW CHART 12-1 **Approach to the patient with a water diuresis.** The final diagnostic categories are shown in the *green shaded boxes*. If a diagnosis of primary polydipsia is made, the patient might still have one of the forms of diabetes insipidus if the water diuresis persists when the P_{Na} exceeds 140 mmol/L (see Case 11-2, page 397).

DIAGNOSTIC APPROACH
- On the left side of the flow chart, we test with dDAVP first, as this will stop the water diuresis and be effective treatment for both central DI and DI due to the presence of vasopressinase.
- The vasopressin test need not be performed if the diagnosis of central DI is obvious and there is no evidence of necrotic tissue to suggest that vasopressinase is the cause of the DI.

(*see margin note*). The list of causes for central and nephrogenic diabetes insipidus can be found in Chapter 11, page 385.

Step 1

> - A large water diuresis is the expected physiologic response to a water intake that is large enough to cause the arterial P_{Na} to fall below 136 mmol/L.

In this case, the diagnosis is primary polydipsia. Once the P_{Na} has returned to the normal range, the urine flow rate should decrease and the U_{Osm} should rise appropriately, keeping in mind that the prior water diuresis may have caused a lower medullary interstitial osmolality due to medullary washout. In contrast, diabetes insipidus is present when there is a water diuresis that is accompanied by a P_{Na} that is greater than 140 mmol/L. This disorder could be due to a lesion in the hypothalamic-posterior pituitary axis that controls the production and/or release of vasopressin (central diabetes insipidus), a circulating vasopressinase, or a renal lesion that prevents vasopressin from causing the insertion of luminal AQP2 in the final functional unit (nephrogenic diabetes insipidus; see Fig. 11-2, page 373).

> - At this point, calculate the osmole excretion rate (U_{Osm} × urine flow rate)—the usual value is close to 0.5 mosmol/min in subjects consuming a typical Western diet.

If the osmole excretion rate is more than double this rate, be careful, because an osmotic diuresis will ensue if the patient has a renal response to the administration of a vasopressin analogue. This may lead to significant changes in P_{Na} and hence brain cell volume depending on the concentrations of Na^+ and K^+ in the urine and the tonicity of administered fluids.

Step 2

CLASSIFICATION OF NEPHROGENIC DIABETES INSIPIDUS
- We use the term *"true" nephrogenic DI* to indicate a disorder in which there is a failure to insert AQP2 in the luminal membrane of principal cells in the distal nephron in response to vasopressin.
- The other form of nephrogenic DI is the result of a lesion that lowers the medullary interstitial osmolality. Our view is that this should not be called *nephrogenic DI*, as, from a pathophysiologic perspective, it is a different disorder.

> - If the water diuresis is curtailed by dDAVP, but not vasopressin, look for a cause for the release of an enzyme that hydrolyzes vasopressin in plasma (vasopressinase).

If there is no response to dDAVP, this is "true" nephrogenic diabetes insipidus.

Step 3

> - If dDVAP fails to cause the appropriate decrease in urine flow rate (depending on the rate of excretion of osmoles) and the appropriate rise in U_{Osm} (depending on the value of medullary interstitial osmolality, which is usually lower from prior water diuresis), the diagnosis is "true" nephrogenic diabetes insipidus (*see margin note*).
> - The most common cause in an adult is the use of lithium to treat a bipolar affective disorder.

At this point, examine the central water control system (see Fig. 11-2, page 373) for a lesion that has caused the defect in vasopressin biosynthesis or release. An important part of this workup is to determine whether thirst is present; its absence suggests that the defect involves the hypothalamic osmostat (discussed in more detail in Chapter 11, page 373).

ISSUES IN THERAPY

- There is no specific therapy for polyuria per se.
- One requires individualized therapy for each patient depending on the cause of the water diuresis.

Hypernatremia is not common because of the thirst response. If a patient does not have a normal thirst response, he or she will need to drink a given volume of water at frequent time intervals and monitor body weight to provide an index of a significant change in total body water, and thereby the P_{Na}. This is a very difficult problem to manage if the patient does not sense thirst or does have a disorder that makes him or her unable to be actively involved in this therapy. If the cause of the water diuresis is central diabetes insipidus, the cornerstone of therapy is to administer the lowest possible dose of a long-acting preparation of vasopressin—dDAVP. The indicator of its effect is a decline in the urine flow rate to close to 1 mL/min (if the patient is consuming a typical Western diet). Early on, patients may be more sensitive to low doses of dDAVP because of up-regulation of V_2 receptors for vasopressin in late distal nephron segments. The risk of this therapy is water retention, which would lead to the development of acute hyponatremia if the patient were to drink more water than can be excreted. To minimize this risk, daily water intake should be limited to close to 1 L/day, but compliance may be an issue.

If water intake is considerably greater than the recommended amount, there should be a time period in the day during which patients are free of dDAVP actions to permit the excretion of extra water; development of thirst will indicate that this extra water was probably excreted. To prevent the occurrence of hyponatremia, patients should check their weight each morning before drinking. If there is a gain in weight of more than 1 kg, the P_{Na} should be measured.

An example of how to treat a patient who has "partial" central diabetes insipidus is provided in the discussion of Case 11-2, page 397. In a patient with AQP2-deficiency type of nephrogenic diabetes insipidus, lowering the volume of distal delivery of filtrate decreases the urine flow rate. This requires a negative balance of Na^+, which can be created by the combination of a low intake of NaCl and the intake of a diuretic that does not lower the osmolality in the medullary interstitial compartment (e.g., a thiazide diuretic; *see margin note*). Nonsteroidal anti-inflammatory drugs may also decrease the distal delivery of filtrate via a hemodynamic effect that reduces the GFR. The concern about their chronic use is the potential for the development of chronic renal insufficiency. The use of other drugs such as chlorpropamide seems to be of little benefit in patients with nephrogenic diabetes insipidus.

USE OF A THIAZIDE DIURETIC IN A PATIENT WITH NEPHROGENIC DI
This class of natriuretic agents may offer an advantage of having a higher medullary interstitial osmolality to drive the reabsorption of water by residual water permeability and by AQP1 in the descending thin limbs of the nephron that enter the inner medulla (this may conserve ~3 L/day).

The use of amiloride in patients with lithium-induced nephrogenic diabetes insipidus is a suggested therapy, but it does not seem to cause a clinically significant decrease in the daily urine volume. Notwithstanding, to obtain a sufficiently high luminal concentration of amiloride for it to be an effective blocker of epithelial Na^+ channels, very high doses are needed because of the high flow rate in the distal nephron. In patients who have taken lithium for more than 2 years, the polyuria persists even after years of discontinuing lithium (see Chapter 11, page 387).

QUESTIONS

(Discussions on page 422)

12-3 *A patient with central diabetes insipidus has polyuria, a low U_{Osm} (50 mOsm/kg H_2O), and a P_{Na} of 137 mmol/L. What does this imply for diagnosis and therapy?*

12-4 *A patient excreted 6 L of urine in the past 24 hours, and he did not receive any infusions or complain of thirst. The last urine aliquot in this 24-hour period was sent for analysis; the U_{Osm} was 500 mOsm/kg H_2O, U_{Urea} was 250 mmol/L, and the $U_{Na + K}$ was 125 mmol/L. In addition, the values for $P_{Glucose}$ and P_{Urea} were normal. Does the patient have a water diuresis and/or an osmotic diuresis?*

PART C
OSMOTIC DIURESIS

CASE 12-2: MORE THAN JUST SALT AND WATER LOSS

(Case discussed on page 420)

A 70-kg man had a recent bone marrow transplant, and his treatment included high doses of glucocorticoids. He became septic over the past 24 hours. His 24-hour urine volume today is 6 L and the U_{Osm} is 500 mOsm/kg H_2O. He has not received mannitol. His $P_{Glucose}$ is 180 mg/dL (10 mmol/L) and his P_{Urea} is 75 mmol/L (BUN 210 mg/dL).

Questions

Does he have an osmotic diuresis?
What is the major aim of therapy with respect to urea excretion?

DIAGNOSTIC ISSUES

The rate of excretion of osmoles must be calculated in every patient with polyuria. An osmotic diuresis is present when the osmole excretion rate significantly exceeds 900 mosmol/day and the U_{Osm} is greater than the P_{Osm} (see Flow Chart 12-2). In a patient with central diabetes insipidus, however, the rate of excretion of osmoles will influence the urine flow rate only after vasopressin is given.

Before the composition of the urine is known, one should establish whether a sufficient number of organic osmoles (glucose or urea) have been filtered to cause the osmotic diuresis and if

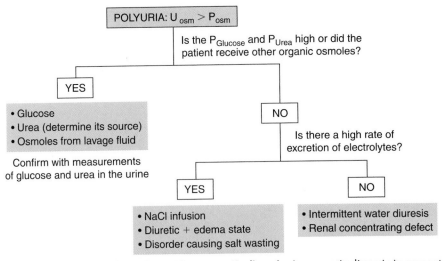

FLOW CHART 12-2 Approach to the patient with an osmotic diuresis. An osmotic diuresis is present when the osmole excretion rate is considerably greater than 900 mOsm/day (0.7 mOsm/min). The final diagnostic categories are shown below the *boxes*.

solutes such as mannitol or lavage fluid have been administered. The presumptive diagnosis should be confirmed by measuring the individual urine osmoles. In the case of a urea-induced osmotic diuresis, identifying the source of urea may provide clues to reveal a very large endogenous protein catabolism.

In a patient who develops acute polyuria in the hospital, it is necessary to calculate a tonicity balance to determine the basis for a change in the P_{Na} (and thereby the ICF volume) and to design therapy to restore ICF and ECF volumes and composition to normal (see the discussion of Case 11-1, page 396 for an illustration of the value of this calculation).

CLINICAL APPROACH

During an osmotic diuresis, the U_{Osm} should be greater than the P_{Osm}. Its absolute value, however, is determined by the medullary interstitial osmolality, which may be lower than normal because of, for example, medullary washout due to a prior water diuresis, presence of a disease, or the intake of drugs that may compromise medullary function (see Chapter 11, page 388 for more discussion). The causes for an osmotic diuresis are the excessive excretion of organic solutes (glucose, urea, or mannitol [if a sufficiently large amount of mannitol has been administered]) or a very high rate of excretion of electrolytes.

Step 1. Calculate the osmole excretion rate

If the U_{Osm} is greater than the P_{Osm} and the osmole excretion rate exceeds 1000 mosmol/day (or 0.7 mosmol/min), an osmotic diuresis is present.

Step 2. Assess which solute is likely to be the cause of the polyuria

One can make a reasonable assessment of a solute's likelihood to cause polyuria if its concentration in plasma is measured, the GFR is estimated, and the renal handling of that solute is known (*see margin note*).

QUANTITATIVE EXAMPLE
- Consider a patient who has a P_{Urea} of 50 mmol/L and a GFR of 100 L/day.
- The filtered load of urea is the product of the P_{Urea}, and the GFR equals 5000 mmol/day.
- Because close to 50% of the filtered load of urea is reabsorbed (2500 mmol), the excretion of 250 mmol of urea will cause the urine volume to be 5 L if the concentration of urea remains at 500 mmol/L. For this to occur, there must be a very high rate of production of urea.

One should also determine if enough mannitol or lavage fluid was administered to cause the observed degree of polyuria. If Na^+ and Cl^- are excreted at very high rates and if they represent the vast majority of the urine osmoles, this could be the basis for the osmotic diuresis.

Step 3. Identify the source of excess osmoles in the urine

Urea

In a patient with a urea-induced osmotic diuresis, determine whether the source of urea is from exogenous protein and/or from tissue catabolism.

Glucose

When there is a glucose-induced osmotic diuresis, one must assess the $P_{Glucose}$ and the GFR to assess the magnitude of the possible osmotic diuresis. Be aware of "hidden" glucose in lumen of the gastrointestinal tract, because this may soon be absorbed and contribute to the osmotic diuresis (see Chapter 16, page 562 for more discussion). In most cases, the quantity of glucose produced from the catabolism of protein is not large.

Electrolytes

In a patient with a saline-induced osmotic diuresis, one must determine why so much NaCl is being excreted. Some potential causes are prior excessive saline administration (a common situation in a hospital setting), administration of a loop diuretic in a patient with significant degree of edema, cerebral salt wasting (discussed in Chapter 9, page 271), and renal salt wasting.

A special example in which polyuria can be due to multiple factors is postobstructive diuresis, which is discussed below.

Postobstructive diuresis

> • In postobstructive diuresis, polyuria is due to a constellation of abnormalities that occur as a result of an increase in intraluminal pressure in renal tubules for a sustained period of time.

One of the defects is a loss of AQP2 water channels in the luminal membrane of the final fuctional nephron unit. This causes a water diuresis due to "true" AQP2-deficiency type of nephrogenic diabetes insipidus. In this setting, the urine volume is determined primarily by factors affecting the volume of distal delivery of filtrate.

Other lesions that may contribute to postobstructive diuresis in the absence of "true" AQP2-deficiency type of nephrogenic diabetes insipidus include expansion of the effective arterial blood volume by prior infusion of saline and possibly a distal defect in the reabsorption of Na^+ and Cl^-. Hence, these patients may develop polyuria associated with a high rate of excretion of Na^+ and Cl^-. The urine volume may also be higher than expected because of a low osmolality in the renal medullary interstitial compartment. Because patients with a prolonged obstruction may have a low rate of excretion of urea, their P_{Urea} could rise. Once the urinary tract obstruction is relieved and if the GFR rises, they could undergo a urea-induced osmotic diuresis if urea becomes an effective urine osmole—that is, if its excretion is very high or if there is failure to insert urea transporters into the luminal membrane of the inner medullary collecting duct. In addition, if the concentration of electrolytes in the urine is low, urea will be an effective urine osmole, which increases the volume of the urine (see page 290 for more discussion).

ISSUES IN THERAPY

There are two important issues in patients with an osmotic diuresis that should be considered in therapy (*see margin note*).

First, one must determine the impact of the loss of solutes plus water on the ECF volume and body tonicity (and hence brain cell volume). Second, one must ask, "What is the cost to the body for excreting these solutes (i.e., determine their source)?"

Impact of the urine composition on body tonicity and ICF volume

One needs to examine the concentrations of Na^+ and K^+ in the urine. The concentrations of Na^+ and K^+ in the urine are low during an osmotic diuresis caused by high rates of excretion of glucose, urea, or mannitol. Thus, one must also examine the volume and the tonicity of the input and perform a tonicity balance to deduce which direction the P_{Na} and ICF volume will change (see Fig. 11-7, page 381). If the concentration of $Na^+ + K^+$ in urine is hypotonic to the infusate, the urinary excretion tends to raise the P_{Na} and shrink the ICF volume. In addition, balance data for $Na^+ + K^+$ indicate the changes in the ECF volume and K^+ balance; the latter may not be revealed by the P_K because of other factors that may cause a shift of K^+ into cells.

Source of excreted osmoles

This is important during a urea-induced osmotic diuresis because the precursor can be endogenous proteins. The impact of this catabolic state is illustrated in the discussion of Case 12-2, page 420.

OSMOTIC DIURESIS
- A detailed discussion of an osmotic diuresis due to excreting glucose is provided in Chapter 16, page 552.
- A urea-induced osmotic diuresis is examined further in the discussion of Case 12-2, page 420.
- The impact of a saline-induced osmotic diuresis on the ECF volume and tonicity is illustrated in the discussion of Case 11-1, page 396.

PART D
INTEGRATIVE PHYSIOLOGY

CREATININE AS A MARKER OF CATABOLISM OF BODY PROTEIN

It is important to determine the source of urea in a patient with urea-induced osmotic diuresis because it may be due to catabolism of body proteins. Clearly, early identification of tissue catabolism is of major clinical importance not only to determine the adequacy of nutritional therapy, but also as a marker for an acute superimposed stress situation (e.g., sepsis) and possibly dysfunction in many organs. Moreover, products of catabolism of proteins in the body can have serious consequences.

The breakdown of tissue proteins causes the release of amino acids, which, if oxidized, yield urea as the major nitrogen end product. In addition, other intracellular constituents such as potassium, phosphate, and magnesium are released with a predictable stoichiometry.

There are data to suggest that the rate of appearance of creatinine may be an early indicator of endogenous protein catabolism, because there is an appreciable increase in the excretion of creatinine that is coincident with the rise in the rate of appearance of urea. An understanding of metabolism of the creatinine is required to comprehend how the excretion of creatinine may be an early marker for catabolism of body proteins.

Metabolism of creatinine

The source of urinary creatinine is the nonenzymatic conversion of phosphocreatine to creatinine. Each day, close to 2% of phosphocreatine in skeletal muscle is converted to creatinine, and this occurs at a relatively constant rate. Accordingly, approximately 20 mg or 200 µmol of creatinine per kg body weight is excreted each day. To achieve balance, this same quantity of phosphocreatine must be synthesized per day. How this is controlled is discussed in the following paragraphs, where the focus is on the metabolism of arginine.

Metabolism of dietary arginine

- The initial step to synthesize the creatine backbone of phosphocreatine is the conversion of arginine to the precursor of creatine, guanidinoacetic acid, in the cortex of the kidney.
- The most important objective in control of arginine metabolism is to prevent an oversupply of arginine to the *systemic* circulation after meals and hence the excessive production of nitric oxide that may cause hemodynamic instability. It is also necessary to have a sufficient supply of arginine to the kidney between meals to synthesize the creatine needed to replenish phosphocreatine in skeletal muscle on a continuing basis.
- A higher rate of excretion of creatinine may occur when the concentration of arginine rises in the *systemic* circulation owing to an excessive endogenous protein catabolism.

ARGININE-RICH PROTEIN
- It has been known that the liver synthesizes arginine-rich protein (ARP), a very large protein that is enriched in arginine. Despite being abundant, it is mainly destroyed without being released. Later, ARP was identified as an important lipoprotein.
- The net effect may be to control the concentration of arginine in systemic plasma and to have a reserve of this amino acid that can be made available for protein synthesis throughout the day.

Events in the liver

Arginine is delivered to the liver after digestion of dietary protein followed by absorption of amino acids in the small intestine. While passing through the enterocytes, 40% of dietary arginine is catabolized. Hence, the liver is supplied with an arginine-poor amino acid mixture plus a precursor of arginine (ornithine) if the liver needs to synthesize more arginine. The major fates of arginine in hepatocytes are protein synthesis and its hydrolysis by hepatic arginase to produce urea. *The net effect of this is to ensure that there is very little entry of free arginine into the systemic circulation* (see margin note).

Events in the cortex of the kidney

The cortex of the kidney is the second site of the enzyme arginase in the body. The major function of this enzyme is the synthesis of the precursor of creatine, guanidinoacetic acid. When endogenous (nonhepatic) proteins are hydrolyzed, there is a steady release of their constituent amino acids, including arginine, into the systemic circulation throughout the 24-hour period. To achieve daily balance for

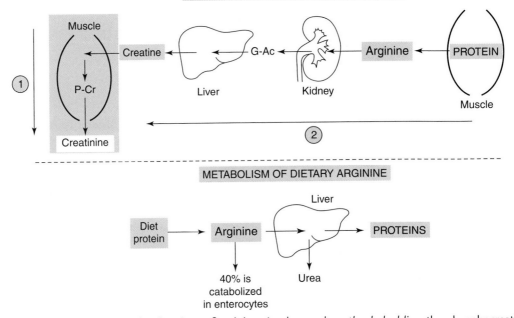

METABOLISM OF ENDOGENOUS ARGININE

METABOLISM OF DIETARY ARGININE

FIGURE 12-3 Overview of the biochemistry of arginine. As shown *above the dashed line*, the phosphocreatine (P-Cr)/arginine cycle begins with the degradation of P-Cr in skeletal muscle to produce creatinine (*site 1*), which is excreted (shown in the *green shaded portion on the left*). To replenish muscle P-Cr (*site 2*), arginine must be added to the systemic circulation during hydrolysis of endogenous proteins (*far right*). This arginine is converted to guanidinoacetate (G-Ac) by renal arginase; this G-Ac is then converted to creatine in the liver, and the uptake of creatine by muscle completes the cycle. As shown *below the dashed line*, the overriding principle is that dietary arginine does not directly become free arginine in the *systemic* circulation. Rather, a significant proportion of dietary arginine is catabolized by enterocytes, yielding ornithine for disposal in the liver. The liver produces a variety of proteins that contain arginine, some of which are released into the systemic circulation and virtually all of the remaining free arginine is converted to urea by hepatic arginase.

arginine without marked changes in its concentration in systemic blood, this amino acid must be degraded at a rate that closely matches its rate of appearance.

Once guanidinoacetic acid is synthesized in the kidney cortex, it is delivered to the liver, where methyl groups (CH_3) are added to it to form creatine. The stoichiometry of this synthesis is the catabolism of one molecule of arginine per molecule of creatine synthesized (Fig. 12-3), which uses approximately one third of the usual daily intake of arginine. Therefore, it is critical that there is a continuing and controlled supply of arginine to the kidney cortex.

> • Of clinical importance, measuring the rate of appearance of creatinine can reflect the renal rate of metabolism of arginine, which is related to the concentration of arginine in systemic plasma and thereby the protein catabolic rate (*see margin note*).

Integrative physiology

Because the liver and the kidneys each receive 25% of the cardiac output at rest, close to half of the circulating pool of arginine can be removed each minute. Therefore, there are three possible causes of high systemic arginine levels: a very rapid rate of endogenous protein catabolism, a slower rate of protein synthesis in skeletal muscles, and reduced renal and/or hepatic function. Hence, it is not surprising

EXCRETION OF CREATINE
- There is very little excretion of creatine in the urine unless its plasma level rises markedly from its very low concentration in blood (~10 µmol/L).
- In studies in patients with traumatic injury, there was a delay of several days before the rate of excretion of creatine rose unless there was extensive injury to skeletal muscle. This probably reflects the fact that the kidney has a large capacity to reabsorb filtered creatine.

that excessive protein catabolism due to the failure to provide adequate nutritional support in patients with sepsis, especially if there is reduced renal function, may lead to hyperargininemia with increased production of nitric oxide and thereby hemodynamic instability.

Therapeutic implications

There are several potential strategies that may help decrease the concentration of arginine in the systemic circulation. This understanding of arginine metabolism may provide theoretical reasons to use the enteral route rather than the parenteral route to administer amino acids because this should result in a lower concentration of arginine in the systemic circulation. It has been shown that the supply of both exogenous protein by the enteral route and a source of calories are usually sufficient to induce a positive balance of protein in the days after a surgical stress. A marker for reversal of a high rate of protein catabolism may be a decrease in the rate of excretion of creatinine to control values. Of great importance, despite adequate nutritional support, a high rate of appearance of creatinine may be a marker for a catabolic state (e.g., sepsis that may not yet be clinically evident). Further, the return of creatinine excretion to its basal rate may be a useful marker that excessive catabolism is no longer present and that therapy for sepsis is effective.

DISCUSSION OF CASE 12-2

CASE 12-2: MORE THAN JUST SALT AND WATER LOSS

(Case presented on page 414)

Does he have an osmotic diuresis?

This high urine flow rate is the result of an osmotic diuresis because his U_{Osm} is greater than 300 mOsm/kg H_2O and his calculated osmole excretion rate is 3000 mosmol/day. The next step in Flow Chart 12-2 is to define the nature of the urine osmoles. Before the urine data are available, one can deduce whether glucose, urea, and/or mannitol is the cause of the polyuria. In this patient, there would not have been enough glucose or mannitol filtered to cause this osmotic diuresis. In contrast, because his P_{Urea} was very high, he could have a urea-induced osmotic diuresis; this was confirmed by the laboratory results: The concentration of urea in the urine was 400 mmol/L.

What is the source of urea?

In quantitative terms, he excreted approximately 2400 mmol of urea that day (6 L/day × 400 mmol urea/L). For every 100 g of protein oxidized, 16 g of nitrogen are converted to 572 mmol of urea. Therefore, the amount of urea excreted represents the breakdown of close to 400 g of protein (Fig. 12-4). On that day, the patient was given only 60 g of protein by the enteral route. Therefore, he catabolized approximately 340 g of endogenous protein.

What is the major aim of therapy with respect to urea excretion?

Each kg of lean body mass has 800 g of water and close to 180 g of protein. Therefore, the amount of urea excreted on that day represents the catabolism of close to 4 lb or 2 kg of lean body mass.

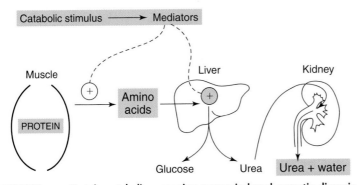

FIGURE 12-4 Protein catabolism causing a urea-induced osmotic diuresis. This patient was given a large dose of glucocorticoids and had sepsis, both of which lead to catabolic signals favoring the net breakdown of proteins in muscle. When amino acids are released and delivered to the liver, they are converted to glucose plus urea and the P_{Urea} rises. The higher filtered load of urea leads to an increased excretion of water (a urea-induced osmotic diuresis). The loss of lean body mass is particularly dangerous for this patient.

Should this continue, he would undergo marked muscle wasting. This could compromise respiratory muscle function and lead to bronchopneumonia. Furthermore, this catabolic state could affect his immunologic defense mechanisms. Therefore, look for the cause of this catabolic state (e.g., sepsis). Therapy should include a strong emphasis on nutrition. More exogenous calories *and* protein should be given to decrease catabolism of his lean body mass. Anabolic hormones (e.g., high-dose insulin with glucose to prevent hypoglycemia) or anabolic steroids and/or the provision of nutritional supplements such as glutamine may minimize endogenous protein catabolism (*see margin note*). In addition, one should reevaluate the need for continuing the use of drugs that can augment catabolism (e.g., high-dose glucocorticoids; see Fig. 12-4).

MINIMIZE PROTEIN CATABOLISM
- On one hand, one might say that there is no evidence that some of these measures clearly decrease the rate of protein catabolism, so do not use them.
- On the other hand, we are desperate! We would use any measure that does not have a major risk, as time is too short to do a study.
- The degree of protein catabolism is unusually large and the data in a heterogeneous group of patients may have obscured a benefit in a subgroup. Said another way, large clinical studies apply only to an "average" patient in that study.

DISCUSSION OF QUESTIONS

12-1 *An obese patient has been fasting for 2 weeks in a weight reduction program. His P_{Na} is 145 mmol/L, his urine flow rate is 0.6 L/day, his U_{Osm} is 700 mOsm/kg H_2O, and the concentration of urea in his urine is 100 mmol/L. Does this patient have a renal concentrating defect?*

If one considers only the U_{Osm} of 700 mOsm/kg H_2O, one might think that this patient has a concentrating defect, but the control of the urine flow rate should be examined in effective osmolality terms. Since the nonurea or effective U_{Osm} is 600 mOsm/kg H_2O, the patient does not have a concentrating defect. Rather, this is the expected U_{Osm} because of a low rate of production and excretion of urea (0.6 L/day × 100 mmol/L = 60 mmol/day). The low urine flow rate (0.6 L/day) indicates that his medullary interstitial osmolality is appropriately high.

12-2 *A patient with cirrhosis of the liver was placed on a diet with little protein and salt. While in the hospital, his urine flow rate was 0.4 L/day, his U_{Osm} was 375 mOsm/kg H_2O, and his osmole excretion rate was 150 mosmol/day. Does this patient have oliguria, polyuria, and/or a renal concentrating defect?*

Although the patient's urine flow rate appears to be low, a major factor that contributes to the low urine flow rate is his low osmole excretion rate, which reflects his dietary intake (low protein, low salt). Notwithstanding, his low U_{Osm} while vasopressin acts (375 mOsm/kg H_2O) raises the suspicion that he has an underlying lesion that compromises his ability to have a maximum effective medullary interstitial osmolality (~600 mOsm/kg H_2O). Therefore, this patient may have a concentrating defect and hence polyuria (rather than oliguria) in physiologic terms.

12-3 *A patient with central diabetes insipidus has polyuria, a low U_{Osm} (50 mOsm/kg H_2O), and a P_{Na} of 137 mmol/L. What does this imply for diagnosis and therapy?*

The polyuria is a water diuresis because the U_{Osm} is so low. Because the P_{Na} is 137 mmol/L, this indicates that the patient also has a high water intake that is not driven by thirst. The usual basis for the excessive water intake is to avoid the uncomfortable sensation of thirst. This illustrates why the P_{Na} cannot be relied on to determine whether diabetes insipidus is present in this patient.

To reach a final diagnosis, water intake should be curtailed and the P_{Na} and U_{Osm} should be monitored. If the U_{Osm} remains low, and the P_{Na} rises above normal, the diagnosis of diabetes insipidus is established. This is important to consider because if this patient is treated with vasopressin and continues the high water intake, acute hyponatremia may be a serious risk.

12-4 *A patient excreted 6 L of urine in the past 24 hours, and he did not receive any infusions or complain of thirst. The last urine aliquot in this 24-hour period was sent for analysis; the U_{Osm} was 500 mOsm/kg H_2O, U_{Urea} was 250 mmol/L, and the $U_{Na + K}$ was 125 mmol/L. In addition, the values for $P_{Glucose}$ and P_{Urea} were normal. Does the patient have a water diuresis and/or an osmotic diuresis?*

To decide whether this is really an osmotic diuresis, determine whether the patient could have filtered enough nonelectrolyte osmoles (at least 3000 mOsm in 24 hours) to cause this marked polyuria. Because he does not have a high $P_{Glucose}$ or P_{Urea} and did not have an infusion of mannitol, the only type of osmotic diuresis that could be present is a saline-induced one. Nevertheless, the sum of the U_{Na} and U_K is not high enough for this diagnosis; moreover, he did not receive a large saline infusion and does not appear to have a significant degree of effective arterial blood volume contraction (there was no rise in his hematocrit). Hence, all causes for an osmotic diuresis are unlikely.

As it turned out, he had a water diuresis for most of that day because of central diabetes insipidus but also intermittent release of vasopressin resulting from nonosmotic stimuli (e.g., nausea, pain, intake of a drug that stimulated the release of vasopressin). Thus, he has a defect involving his osmostat and possibly his thirst center, leaving enough capacity to secrete vasopressin if there are nonosmotic stimuli for its release. This illustrates that one can be misled if the urine is collected for a long period of time and a spot urine is analyzed and the findings extrapolated to the entire urine volume because the composition of the urine may have changed over time. Therefore, one needs to examine multiple short urine collections to determine the basis of polyuria.

section three
Potassium

Potassium Physiology

Introduction

Regulation of total body potassium (K$^+$) homeostasis is vital. Changes in the concentration of K$^+$ in plasma (P$_K$) are inversely related to changes in the negative voltage across cell membranes, and this in turn influences many essential functions in the body. On the one hand, a change in the negative voltage across cell membranes may have direct and dangerous consequences (e.g., altered cardiac impulse conduction causing cardiac arrhythmias). On the other hand, subtle changes in this negative voltage across cell membranes have important physiologic functions in an indirect way by altering the concentration of ionized calcium in cells (e.g., the release of insulin from β-cells of the pancreas, contractility in vascular smooth muscle cells).

The vast majority of K^+ in the body is located in cells where this cation balances the negative charge on intracellular anions—primarily organic phosphates. Specific ion channels for K^+ in cell membranes permit K^+ to enter or exit cells.

The body deals with an intake of K^+ in two phases. First, the K^+ load is stored temporarily in cells, which is essential for short-term K^+ homeostasis. Second, with the usual intake of K^+, this extra K^+ must ultimately be excreted in the urine, but there may be a long lag time before this renal process can be carried out.

The major site where the renal excretion of K^+ is regulated is in the late cortical distal nephron. Secretion of K^+ in these nephron segments requires the generation of a lumen-negative voltage via the electrogenic reabsorption of Na^+ and the presence of open K^+ channels in the luminal membranes of their principal cells.

To gain insights into the regulation of K^+ homeostasis, it is very helpful to examine this process from a Paleolithic perspective. The Paleolithic diet had a large but episodic intake of K^+, and this K^+ was provided with sugar in berries. In addition, there was little NaCl in the Paleolithic diet, and this created a potential difficulty to be overcome—the need for a large enough distal delivery of Na^+ to secrete K^+. This has implications for the extrarenal K^+ homeostasis and the regulation of the excretion of K^+ by the kidney.

It is important to realize that hyperkalemia and hypokalemia are not specific diseases; rather, they result from many disorders with different underlying pathophysiology. Therefore, an understanding of the physiology of K^+ is critical for the diagnosis and design of specific therapy for patients with these "electrolyte symptoms."

ABBREVIATIONS

P_K and U_K, concentrations of K^+ in plasma and in urine

P_{Na} and U_{Na}, concentrations of Na^+ in plasma and in urine

P_{Cl} and U_{Cl}, concentrations of Cl^- in plasma and in urine

$P_{Creatinine}$ and $U_{Creatinine}$, concentrations of creatinine in plasma and in urine

P_{Osm} and U_{Osm}, osmolality in plasma and in urine

OBJECTIVES

- To illustrate the common strategy used to ensure that K^+ will enter or leave a given compartment. This requires a driving force to cause K^+ movement (a negative voltage in the area K^+ must be retained) and channels with a high conductance for K^+.
- To consider how the voltage across cell membranes is regulated and its implications for the control of a shift of K^+ into cells.
- To illustrate how the kidneys adjust the rate of excretion of K^+ to maintain balance for K^+ and keep the P_K in the normal range.
- To illustrate that examining this process from a Paleolithic perspective provides insights into the control of K^+ homeostasis.

INTRODUCTORY CASE 13-1: WHY DID I BECOME SO WEAK?

(Case discussed on page 454)

A very fit, active, 27-year-old Caucasian woman was in excellent health until 1 year ago. Her past medical history revealed mild asthma, for which she took a bronchodilator on an intermittent basis.

In the past year, she had three episodes of extreme weakness; each lasted up to 12 hours; she felt perfectly well between attacks. On more detailed questioning, she said that she had ingested a large amount of sugar before the first attack. Each subsequent attack, however, was not preceded by the use of a bronchodilator, performance of exercise, or the ingestion of a large amount of sugar or caffeinated beverages. She denied the use/abuse of diuretics or laxatives, bulimic symptoms, glue sniffing, substance abuse (no needle marks), or the ingestion of licorice or over-the-counter drugs. She was not overly concerned about her body weight. There was no family history of hypokalemia, hypertension, or paralytic episodes. In the emergency room on each occasion, she was clearly very concerned, but other than the paralysis, the only findings of note were tachycardia (130/min) and mild systolic hypertension with a wide pulse pressure (150/70 mm Hg). There were no signs of hyperthyroidism. Because of the very low P_K (~2.1 mmol/L), an intravenous infusion of KCl was started, and, as on the other occasions, she recovered promptly with the administration of relatively little K^+. The laboratory data are provided below. While not shown, all tests of thyroid function were in the normal range and the tests for a pheochromocytoma were negative. On the last admission, her $P_{Insulin}$ was in the normal range and the C-peptide level in blood was not elevated. In addition, the levels of cortisol, renin, and aldosterone and the ratio of renin to aldosterone were all in the normal range.

Na^+	mmol/L	141	Glucose	mg/dL (mmol/L)	133 (7.4)
K^+	mmol/L	2.1	Creatinine	mg/dL (µmol/L	0.9 (77)
HCO_3^-	mmol/L	22	BUN (Urea)	mg/dL (mmol/L)	10 (3.4)
Arterial pH		7.38	P_{CO_2}	mm Hg	38
Urine K^+	mmol/L	8	Urine creatinine	(g/L) (mmol/L)	0.8 (7)

Questions

What is the most likely basis for the repeated episodes of acute hypokalemia?

Was an adrenergic effect associated with the acute hypokalemia?

After the laboratory results were examined, were there any clues to suggest what the cause of acute hypokalemia might be?

Would your treatment be different for her next attack?

What tests should be performed in the emergency room if she has another episode of acute hypokalemia to reveal the correct diagnosis?

PART A
PRINCIPLES OF PHYSIOLOGY

- Close to 98% of total body K^+ is inside cells, where it balances the anionic valance inside cells.
- Although only 2% of total body K^+ is in the extracellular fluid (ECF) compartment, changes in the concentration of K^+ in this compartment are critical, because they reflect the changes in resting membrane potential (i.e., the voltage difference across cell membranes).

DIURNAL VARIATION IN THE EXCRETION OF K⁺
The bulk of K⁺ is excreted close to noontime. This does not seem to be related to a rise in the $P_{Aldosterone}$ or the delivery of Na⁺ to the late cortical distal nephron. While the mechanism is still open to debate, it is possible that it is due to increased delivery of HCO_3^- to the distal nephron during an increase in the alkaline tide.

The concentration of K⁺ in cells is very high relative to its concentration in the ECF compartment, and it does not vary appreciably in most circumstances. K⁺ in cells balances the charge on intracellular anions; intracellular anions cannot exit from cells because they are macromolecules. Moreover, these anions are essential for cell functions (DNA, RNA, phospholipids, compounds for energy provision such as ATP and phosphocreatine). Hence, the vast majority of K⁺ is retained in cells. Only 2% of body K⁺ is in the ECF compartment. Changes in this concentration of K⁺ in the ECF compartment are, however, extremely important because the *ratio* of concentrations of K⁺ across cell membranes largely reflects changes in the magnitude of the negative voltage difference across cell membranes. The P_K is determined on a minute-to-minute basis by the distribution of K⁺ between the intracellular fluid (ICF) and ECF compartments (acute internal K⁺ balance) and on a day-to-day basis by the renal excretion of K⁺ (long-term external K⁺ balance). With the usual intake of K⁺, the kidney excretes the majority of the K⁺ load close to noontime (*see margin note*); therefore, there must be sensitive regulatory mechanisms to minimize transient changes in the P_K before renal K⁺ excretion occurs.

GENERAL CONCEPTS FOR THE MOVEMENT OF K⁺ ACROSS CELL MEMBRANES

There are two requirements for movement of K⁺ across cell membranes. First, there must be sufficient electrochemical driving force across that membrane; and second, there must be open K⁺ channels in that membrane.

Driving force to shift K⁺ across cell membranes

- This driving force is a more negative voltage in the compartment where K⁺ will be located.
- The active pumping of cations by the Na-K-ATPase initiates the process to create this voltage because it is an electrogenic pump, as it causes 3 Na⁺ to exit and 2 K⁺ to enter cells.

There are two ways to generate a negative voltage across a cell membrane: import anions or export cations. The usual mechanism is to export Na⁺, in part because of its abundance (Fig. 13-1). The Na-K-ATPase is responsible for electrogenic exit of Na⁺, because it extrudes 3 Na⁺ and imports only 2 K⁺ into cells. Export of intracellular, macromolecular phosphate does not occur; therefore, the net result is the generation of a more negative intracellular voltage, which limits the exit of K⁺ from cells.

The same principle for the movement of K⁺ applies to principal cells in the late cortical distal nephron, but the details are different. A transepithelial lumen-negative electrical voltage drives the secretion of K⁺. This is generated when Na⁺ is reabsorbed in an electrogenic fashion (i.e., more Na⁺ than its accompanying anions, usually Cl⁻). Reabsorption of Na⁺ occurs via the epithelial Na⁺ channel (ENaC); it is driven by the low concentration of Na⁺ and the negative voltage in principal cells (created by the Na-K-ATPase in their basolateral membrane; see Part C for more discussion).

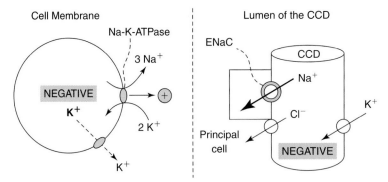

FIGURE 13-1 Concept for the movement of K⁺ across cell membranes. The *circle on the left* represents a cell membrane and the *cylinder on the right* represents the CCD (*see margin note*). There is a much higher concentration of K⁺ in cells than in the ECF compartment owing to the negative voltage inside cells, which is generated in part because more Na⁺ are extruded than K⁺ are imported by the Na-K-ATPase. For the passive movement of K⁺, there must be open K⁺ channels in the cell membrane. To cause a redistribution of K⁺ across cell membranes, there must be either a change in the magnitude of the negative voltage inside cells or in the number, open probability, and conductance of K⁺ channels (because the concentration of K⁺ in cells is higher than the predicted value from the electrochemical equilibrium). Similarly, K⁺ will enter the lumen of the CCD when it has a negative voltage and if there are open K⁺ channels in the luminal membrane of principal cells in the CCD.

Pathways for the movement of K⁺ across cell membranes

- There are several different types of K⁺ channels that permit K⁺ to cross cell membranes.
- Some of these channels are regulated by voltage, others by ligands such as calcium ions, and yet others by metabolites such as ADP—these are called K_{ATP} *channels.*
- Movement of K⁺ through the specific K⁺ channels depends on the driving force, the number of K⁺ channels, whether they are in an open configuration, and how quickly K⁺ can move through them (called their *conductance*).

K⁺ channels are composed of a diverse family of membrane-spanning proteins that selectively conduct K⁺ across cell membranes. K⁺ channels have a pore that permits K⁺ to cross the cell membrane, a selectivity filter that specifies K⁺ as the ion species to move through the channel (*see margin note*), and a gating mechanism that serves to switch between open and closed channel conformations.

When K⁺ move out of cells (Fig. 13-2), there is an increase in the net negative voltage in cells. Because the concentration of K⁺ in cells is higher than the predicted value from its electrochemical equilibrium, control of the open probability of K⁺ channels in cell membranes is critical to regulate the magnitude of cell voltage, which in turn influences many essential cell functions. As illustrated in Figure 13-2, regulation of K^+_{ATP} channels influences the gating of calcium ion channels as a result of a change in the voltage in cells (more negative if K^+_{ATP} channels are open—the converse is

ABBREVIATION
CCD, late cortical distal nephron including the late distal convoluted tubule, the connecting segment, and the cortical collecting duct
ENaC, epithelial Na⁺ channels

BASIS FOR THE SELECTIVITY OF THE K⁺ CHANNEL FOR K⁺
- Na⁺ are much smaller than K⁺, yet the K⁺ channels are specific for K⁺.
- Ions in solution have layers of water surrounding them; hence, we must think in terms of their hydrated size.
- The chemical structure of the K⁺ channel at its mouth strips off the water shells surrounding K⁺. Thus, K⁺ becomes smaller than Na⁺ and can pass through the channel, whereas Na⁺ cannot do so.

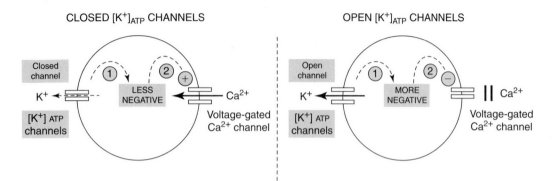

CLOSED [K⁺]$_{ATP}$ CHANNELS   OPEN [K⁺]$_{ATP}$ CHANNELS

FIGURE 13-2 Regulatory roles for [K⁺]$_{ATP}$ channels in cell function. The goal of this process is to adjust the concentration of ionized calcium in cells, because this regulates many important cellular events. Begin the analysis with the [K⁺]$_{ATP}$ channels in each setting. As shown on the *left*, when the [K⁺]$_{ATP}$ channels are closed, positive voltage (K⁺) cannot exit from cells and the interior of the cell becomes less negative. As a result, the voltage-gated ionized calcium channels open, and the concentration of ionized calcium rises in that cell. In contrast, as shown on the *right*, when the [K⁺]$_{ATP}$ channels are opened, positive voltage (K⁺) can exit from cells and the interior of the cell becomes more negative. As a result, the concentration of ionized calcium falls in that cell.

ABBREVIATION
ROMK, rat outer medullary K⁺
channels

also true). Clinical examples where control of K⁺$_{ATP}$ channels has important effects on physiologic functions are discussed in the answers to Question 13-1.

From a renal perspective, secretion of K⁺ in principal cells of the late cortical distal nephron requires that open K⁺ channels (primarily ROMK) must be present in the luminal membrane of these cells to permit K⁺ to enter the luminal fluid.

(Discussion on page 456)

QUESTION

13-1 *Is the [K⁺]$_{ATP}$ channel regulated in fact by ATP?*

PART B
SHIFT OF POTASSIUM ACROSS CELL MEMBRANES

ALTERING THE NEGATIVE VOLTAGE IN CELLS

- K⁺ shift into cells when there is an increase in the negative voltage in cells.
- The components of the system that regulates intracellular voltage include the Na-K-ATPase, the Na⁺/H⁺ exchanger (NHE), the Cl⁻/HCO₃⁻ anion exchanger (AE), and the open probability of K⁺$_{ATP}$ channels in cell membranes.

There are three mechanisms to increase the negative voltage in cells via augmenting flux through the Na-K-ATPase.

Raise the intracellular concentration of Na⁺

> • More Na⁺ is pumped out of cells by the Na-K-ATPase when the concentration of Na⁺ rises in cells. This leads to an increase in cell negative voltage only if the source of Na⁺ is Na⁺ that existed in the cell or Na⁺ that entered the cell in an electroneutral fashion.

The first and quickest mechanism to increase the flux of Na⁺ through the Na-K-ATPase is to raise the intracellular concentration of Na⁺, because the extracellular concentration of K⁺ is always high enough for maximal activity of the Na-K-ATPase. The impact of this increase in Na⁺ pumping on the net cell voltage, however, depends on whether the Na⁺ entry step into cells is electrogenic or electroneutral.

Electrogenic entry of Na⁺ into cells

The Na⁺ channel in cell membranes is normally closed by the usual magnitude of the negative intracellular voltage. If the Na⁺ channel in skeletal muscle cell membranes were to open (e.g., by nerve impulses that lead to the release of acetylcholine), the resting membrane potential quickly becomes less negative. In more detail, one cationic charge enters the cell per Na⁺ transported. Because only one third of a charge exits per Na⁺ pumped via the Na-K-ATPase (Fig. 13-3), this diminishes the degree of intracellular negative voltage. This promotes the entry of ionized calcium and thereby muscle contraction. There is also a net *exit* of K⁺ from cells through open K⁺ channels in the cell membrane and thus a rise in the [K⁺] in the ECF compartment.

Clinical implications

An abnormally large increase in the entry of Na⁺ via Na⁺ channels in cell membranes of skeletal muscle and its subsequent exit via the Na-K-ATPase diminishes the magnitude of the intracellular negative

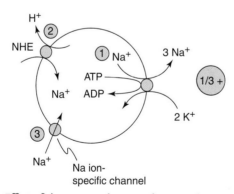

FIGURE 13-3 Effect of electroneutral versus electrogenic entry of Na⁺ on the negative voltage in cells. A more negative voltage in cells is generated by the Na-K-ATPase, providing that the source of Na⁺ pumped out is either Na⁺ that exist in cells (*site 1*) or Na⁺ that enter cells in an electroneutral fashion via the Na⁺/H⁺ exchanger (NHE; *site 2*). In contrast, if the source of Na⁺ pumped out of cells is Na⁺ that enters cells via the Na⁺-specific ion channel (*site 3*), the voltage in cells becomes less negative (count the charges). Although flux of K⁺ through K⁺ channels may be limited to some degree by their open probability, a higher concentration of K⁺ in the ICF compartment due to ion pumping by the Na-K-ATPase drives the electrogenic exit of K⁺.

voltage. This is the underlying pathophysiology of hyperkalemia in some patients with hyperkalemic periodic paralysis.

Electroneutral entry of Na⁺ into cells

> • If Na⁺ enters the cell in an electroneutral fashion, its subsequent electrogenic exit via the Na-K-ATPase results in a more negative cell interior voltage and hence less net exit of K⁺ from cells.

This occurs when Na⁺ enter cells in exchange for H⁺ via the NHE (see Fig. 13-3). The NHE in cell membranes is normally *inactive*. This can be deduced from the fact that it is an electroneutral exchange and that the concentrations of its substrates (Na⁺ in the ECF compartment and H⁺ in the ICF compartment) are considerably higher than that of its products (Na⁺ in the ICF compartment and H⁺ in the ECF compartment) in steady state. There are two major activators of NHE: a sudden spike in the release of insulin and a higher concentration of H⁺ in the ICF compartment.

Role of insulin

> • Insulin plays an important role to cause K⁺ uptake by the liver before it enters the systemic circulation.

MAJOR SETTINGS WHERE A RAPID SHIFT OF K⁺ INTO CELLS IS NEEDED
• *After the ingestion of a large K⁺ load:* The major hormone involved is insulin.
• *After a vigorous sprint:* The major hormones involved are β_2-adrenergics, which are released in the "fight-or-flight" response.

ABBREVIATION
$P_{Glucose}$, concentration of glucose in plasma

One major physiologic setting where there is a need to shift K⁺ into cells and do so quickly is when there is a large dietary K⁺ intake (*see margin note*). Fruit and berries were the major sources of calories in the Paleolithic diet. Accordingly, this diet provided a large quantity of sugar (fructose and glucose), K⁺, and a family of organic anions (e.g., citrate) that are metabolized promptly to produce HCO_3^- in the liver. To remove this K⁺ before it can enter the systemic circulation where it can be dangerous, the first line of defense is to shift K⁺ into liver cells. The trigger for this control mechanism is by the sugar content of the diet. When the concentration of glucose in plasma ($P_{Glucose}$) rises, there is a sudden spike in the release of insulin from β-cells of the pancreas. This high concentration of insulin activates NHE in cell membranes of hepatocytes after a meal rich in K⁺. As a result, Na⁺ enters these cells in an electroneutral fashion. When this Na⁺ is pumped out of cells by the Na-K-ATPase (see Fig. 13-3), there is an export of positive voltage and the interior of the cells becomes more negative; this negative voltage keeps some extra K⁺ in cells (for more discussion of this topic, see Part D, page 453).

Clinical implications

Because insulin activates NHE, this hormone has been used clinically in the emergency treatment of patients with hyperkalemia. On the other hand, a lack of actions of insulin results in a shift of K⁺ out of cells and the development of hyperkalemia in patients with diabetic ketoacidosis despite having a total body K⁺ deficit.

Activate preexisting Na-K-ATPase by hormones

> • The second mechanism for increasing flux through Na-K-ATPase is also a rapid one; it involves activation of existing Na-K-ATPase units in the cell membrane by β_2-adrenergic actions.

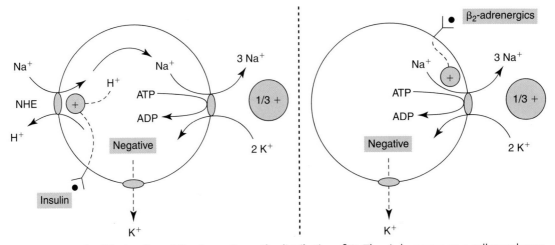

FIGURE 13-4 Role of the insulin and β₂-adrenergics on the distribution of K⁺. The *circle* represents a cell membrane. The Na-K-ATPase generates the electrical driving force for net K⁺ entry into cells, providing that the source of the Na⁺ pumped out is either Na⁺ that exist in cells or Na⁺ that enter cells in an electroneutral fashion via the Na⁺/H⁺ exchanger (NHE). Two hormones that cause more Na⁺ pumping by the Na-K-ATPase are shown; one is insulin, which activates NHE, and the other is β₂-adrenergics, which activate Na-K-ATPase by phosphorylation. The increase in negative voltage in cells diminishes the exit of K⁺ from cells via K⁺ channels.

β₂-Adrenergic agonists activate the Na-K-ATPase via a cyclic AMP–dependent mechanism, which phosphorylates this ion pump and leads to the export of preexisting intracellular Na⁺ (Fig. 13-4). This mechanism is particularly important during vigorous exercise in the second major physiologic setting where there is a need to shift K⁺ into cells quickly. In the fight-or-flight response, the stimulus for muscle contraction is the entry of Na⁺ through its voltage-gated Na⁺ channel. This entry of positive voltage diminishes the cell interior negative voltage (called *depolarization*). As a result, K⁺ are released from exercising muscles, and there is a danger of acute hyperkalemia (*see margin note*). To minimize this risk, the β₂-adrenergic effect of adrenaline released in this setting is exerted on hepatocytes and possibly on resting muscle cells, which obligates them to take up much of this K⁺ and thereby prevent a dangerous rise in the P_K (see the discussion of Question 13-2 for a discussion of the mechanisms involved).

If the release of adrenaline is especially large, its α-adrenergic effect would inhibit the release of insulin, even if the $P_{Glucose}$ is high. This has the advantage of preventing working muscle cells from consuming the most valuable brain fuel, glucose, from the circulation. On the other hand, this α-adrenergic effect may override the β₂-adrenergic effect, permitting a more severe degree of hyperkalemia to develop (*see margin note*).

Clinical implications

It should not be surprising that an acute shift of K⁺ into cells causing hypokalemia is seen in conditions associated with a surge of catecholamines (e.g., patients with a subarachnoid hemorrhage, myocardial infarction, and/or an extreme degree of anxiety). On the other hand, β₂-agonists may be used to shift K⁺ into cells in patients with an emergency associated with hyperkalemia. In states with a very low effective arterial blood volume, the large α-adrenergic response leads to hyperkalemia because of a shift of K⁺ out of cells despite large losses of K⁺ (e.g., patients with cholera). The shift of K⁺ out of cells is valuable to prevent a severe degree of hypokalemia because there is a large loss of K⁺ in diarrhea fluid.

BENEFIT OF ACUTE HYPERKALEMIA
An acute rise in the P_K helps increase local blood flow in working skeletal muscles.

MECHANISMS FOR THE RELEASE OF K⁺ FROM MUSCLE CELLS DURING A SPRINT
• A diminished magnitude of the negative voltage in cells occurs when Na⁺ enter muscle cells via open Na⁺ channels.
• Intracellular alkalinization when phosphocreatine is hydrolyzed activates the extrusion of HCO_3^- and, secondarily, the exit of K⁺ (see Chapter 1, page 32, and Fig. 13-5, page 435).

EFFECT OF AN ADRENERGIC SURGE ON K⁺ DISTRIBUTION ACROSS CELL MEMBRANES
• β₂-Adrenergics activate the Na-K-ATPase and thereby make voltage in cells more negative, which causes K⁺ to be retained in cells.
• α-Adrenergic actions inhibit the release of insulin, and thereby lead to the exit of K⁺ from cells. A very large adrenergic surge is needed to have the α-effect dominate.

(Discussion on page 458)

13-2 *What mechanisms permit nonexercising cells to take up K^+ during a sprint?*

Increase in the number of Na-K-ATPase units in cell membranes

- Thyroid hormone and insulin lead to the synthesis of more Na-K-ATPase units.

The third mechanism to augment flux of K^+ via the Na-K-ATPase takes time to develop because it involves the synthesis of more Na-K-ATPase units and their insertion into cell membranes. Having more Na-K-ATPase units in the cell membrane of skeletal muscle cells is not important at rest, but it is very important during vigorous exercise. In this latter setting, there is a strong positive correlation between the activity of this ion pump, which is essential for recovery from cell depolarization, and the maximum ability for skeletal muscle to contract during vigorous exercise. Hyperthyroidism is also associated with a higher content of Na-K-ATPase units in the membrane.

Clinical implications

A severe degree of hypokalemia due to a shift of K^+ into cells is seen in Asian patients with the thyrotoxic subtype of hypokalemic periodic paralysis. These patients can be managed effectively during their attacks with the use of nonselective β-blockers and the administration of a small dose of KCl (see Chapter 14, page 478 for more details). It is also interesting to note that many of these patients have attacks of acute hypokalemia and paralysis after eating a large amount of carbohydrates. Perhaps the effect of high levels of insulin to activate NHE in addition to the effect of thyroid hormone to cause the synthesis of more Na-K-ATPase units may lead to the severe degree of hypokalemia (see Part D for a more detailed discussion of this topic).

METABOLIC ACIDOSIS AND A SHIFT OF POTASSIUM ACROSS CELL MEMBRANES

The effect of an acid load on the P_K depends on whether the anions accompanying the H^+ can cross cell membranes in an electroneutral fashion (i.e., on the monocarboxylic acid transporter).

Acids that can be transported by the monocarboxylic acid transporter

- Monocarboxylic acids (e.g., L-lactic acid or ketoacids) enter cells in an electroneutral fashion. Therefore, they do not cause a change in cell voltage.
- L-lactic acid produced in enterocytes can contribute to an important shift of K^+ into liver cells after meals because of the large influx of H^+ into these cells, which can activate their NHE.

For example, when L-lactic acid is formed in exercising skeletal muscles during a sprint, many of these H^+ along with L-lactate anions are removed by entering cells that are not involved in the exercise via their monocarboxylic acid transporter; this minimizes the fall in the intracellular pH and the rise in the P_K. Because this entry of H^+ is electroneutral, it does *not* change the magnitude of the negative voltage in these cells and hence does not result directly in a shift of K^+. Nevertheless, both the high concentration of H^+ inside these cells (by activating the NHE) and the β_2-adrenergic response to exercise (by activating the Na-K-ATPase) may cause a shift of K^+ into these resting muscle cells, thus diminishing the degree of hyperkalemia caused by release of K^+ from exercising muscles. The close proximity of NHE and the monocarboxylic acid transporter could lead to a much stronger activation of NHE by the rise in the local ICF concentration of H^+ (see Part D, page 453 for more discussion).

Acids that cannot be transported by the monocarboxylic acid transporter

- These acids cause K^+ to shift out of cells when much of their H^+ load is titrated by HCO_3^- in the ECF compartment; thus the Cl^-/HCO_3^- anion exchanger likely participates in this mechanism.

Inorganic acids (e.g., HCl) or nonmonocarboxyl organic acids (e.g., citric acid) cannot be transported by the monocarboxylic acid transporter. Moreover, their H^+ cannot enter cells via NHE, because this exchanger can cause only the *export* of H^+ from, and *not* the entry of H^+ into, cells (Fig. 13-5). Hence, a different mechanism is needed to permit some of these H^+ to be titrated by HCO_3^- in the ICF compartment. The mechanism has two steps. First, with a low P_{HCO3}, there is activation of the anion exchanger (the exact mechanism is not known) and an electroneutral shift of HCO_3^- out of cells and Cl^- into cells. Because this exchange of anions in a 1:1 stoichiometry

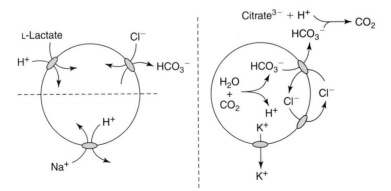

FIGURE 13-5 Shift of K^+ out of cells in patients with metabolic acidosis. The *circles* represent cell membranes. Shown on the *left* are the transport mechanisms for the entry of H^+ into and the exit of HCO_3^- from cells. The two transport mechanisms for net gain of H^+ in cells, the monocarboxylic acid transporter and the Cl^-/HCO_3^- anion exchanger, are shown *above the horizontal dashed line*. The Na^+/H^+ exchanger, which is activated by intracellular acidosis and *catalyzes* only the exit of H^+ from cells, is shown *below the horizontal dashed line*. As shown on the *right*, when there is an H^+ load with anions that cannot enter cells (e.g., citric acid), the fall in the P_{HCO3} is associated with more flux through the HCO_3^-/Cl^- anion exchanger, which accelerates the electroneutral exit of HCO_3^- from, and the entry of Cl^- into, cells. The subsequent exit of Cl^- via Cl^- channels decreases the net negative intracellular voltage, leading to the exit of K^+ from cells via K^+ channels.

is electroneutral, it does not change the magnitude of the negative voltage in these cells. Second, as a result of the combination of the higher concentration of Cl^- in cells, the negative intracellular voltage, and the presence of open Cl^- ion channels in cell membranes, Cl^- is forced out of cells in an electrogenic fashion, and therefore the voltage in these cells becomes less negative and K^+ exit.

Clinical implications

If hyperkalemia is present in a patient with metabolic acidosis owing to an increased production of a monocarboxylic organic acid, causes of hyperkalemia other than the acidemia should be sought (e.g., lack of insulin in patients with diabetic ketoacidosis, tissue injury, or a decreased availability of ATP to drive the Na-K-ATPase in patients with L-lactic acidosis due to hypoxia).

Although inorganic acidosis (addition of HCl) causes a shift of K^+ out of cells, patients with chronic hyperchloremic metabolic acidosis may have a low P_K because of excessive loss of K^+ in the diarrhea fluid in patients with chronic diarrhea or in the urine (e.g., patients with renal tubular acidosis; see Chapter 4, page 96 for more discussion).

There are only small changes in the P_K in patients with respiratory acid-base disorders because there is little movement of Na^+ or Cl^- across cell membranes and hence no change in the ICF voltage.

PHYSIOLOGY OF A SHIFT OF K^+ INTO CELLS: A PALEOLITHIC PERSPECTIVE

The Paleolithic diet consisted primarily of fruit and berries; hence, it provided sugar, K^+, and organic anions (potential HCO_3^-). Therefore, it is not surprising that one of the stimuli to shift K^+ into cells is insulin, which is released after carbohydrate intake.

There are three phases in the process of handling a load of K^+ and HCO_3^-, and this depends on its magnitude.

- *Low intake of K^+ and HCO_3^-*: In this setting, the entire load of K^+ and HCO_3^- can be shifted into cells. The key in this process is activation of NHE in cell membranes by insulin.
- *Somewhat larger intake of K^+ and HCO_3^-*: In this setting, as more HCO_3^- has accumulated in cells, intracellular alkalinization will inhibit NHE. As a result, some of the Na^+ that exist in cells are exported via Na-K-ATPase, which is also activated by insulin. Accordingly, there is a net gain of some Na^+ and HCO_3^- in the ECF compartment.
- *Even larger intake of K^+ and HCO_3^-*: In this setting, there is a problem causing a further deficit of intracellular Na^+. As a result, some K^+ cannot enter cells despite the continuing actions of insulin. The net result is a gain of K^+ and HCO_3^- in the ECF compartment.

Low intake of K^+ and HCO_3^-

Let us examine the net removal of an arbitrary three units of $KHCO_3$. The process begins when 3 Na^+ enter and 3 H^+ exit from cells on NHE, which is activated by insulin. H^+ that exit from cells neutralize all the new HCO_3^- in the ECF compartment. The source of H^+ for NHE in cells is the conversion of $CO_2 + H_2O$ to $H^+ + HCO_3^-$, catalyzed by the enzyme carbonic anhydrase; hence, there is a gain of HCO_3^- in cells. When 3 Na^+ are pumped out of cells by the Na-K-ATPase, 2 K^+ enter, and there is a more negative voltage in cells, which draws the remaining 1 K^+ into the ICF compartment. The net result is that all the added K^+ and HCO_3^- are now inside these cells.

A somewhat larger intake of K^+ and HCO_3^-

When more HCO_3^- enter cells, the concentration of H^+ falls, which inactivates NHE. To shift more K^+ into cells, some of the Na^+ that existed in cells is exported via the Na-K-ATPase, which is also activated by insulin. As a result, there is a net gain of some Na^+ and HCO_3^- in the ECF compartment. There is one other component to the picture: This newly gained Na^+ and HCO_3^- must be retained temporarily in the body—that is, hidden from the kidney (Fig. 13-6). Once a lower limit for intracellular Na^+ concentration is reached, the ability to cause K^+ to enter cells is compromised. Hence, to avoid a significant degree of hyperkalemia, the excess K^+ load must be excreted.

A much larger input of K^+ and HCO_3^-

- This represents the diet of vegetarians and of our Paleolithic ancestors.
- Not all of the K^+ and HCO_3^- can be shifted into cells; accordingly, this excess K^+ and HCO_3^- must be excreted in the urine.

The ion pumping by the Na-K-ATPase declines when the intracellular Na^+ concentration falls. This, together with the low NHE activity resulting from the intracellular alkaline pH, leads to a decreased capacity to transfer K^+ and HCO_3^- into cells. Accordingly, there is a rise in the P_K and in the P_{HCO3}. Both of these effects help the kidney excrete the K^+ and the HCO_3 loads.

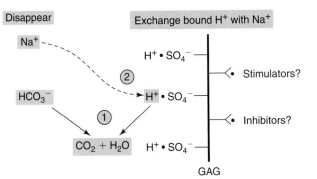

The process described in this figure is a speculation, but it could help explain why our Paleolithic ancestors did not waste Na^+ in their urine. The absence of a natriuresis has been observed in the Yanomamo Indians whose diet is also virtually devoid of NaCl but rich in K^+ and organic anions (potential HCO_3^-).

FIGURE 13-6 "Hiding" Na^+ and HCO_3^- in the extracellular fluid (ECF) compartment. After the consumption of a large load of K^+ and potential HCO_3^-, there is a net gain of Na^+ and HCO_3^- in the ECF compartment. To prevent the loss of Na^+ (and HCO_3^-) in the urine in subjects consuming little NaCl, the higher P_{HCO3} may draw H^+ from a bound form (glycosaminoglycans [GAG]) in connective tissue (*the structure on the right*), leaving a net anionic charge, which attracts Na^+ (keeps them in bound form), completing the process to "hide" $NaHCO_3$ in the ECF compartment. There is uncertainty about what may stimulate and what may lead to reversal of this process.

Exit of K^+ and HCO_3^- from cells after excretion begins

- The process of exit of K^+ and HCO_3^- from cells should begin once the kidneys begin to excrete the K^+ and potential HCO_3^- in the urine.
- The mechanisms responsible for this shift of K^+ and HCO_3^- out of cells are not clear.

There is probably a process that results in the exit of K^+ and HCO_3^- from cells after the excretion of K^+ is underway. Its first step is likely to be activation of the Cl^-/HCO_3^- anion exchanger in cell membranes where K^+ and HCO_3^- were stored. This anion exchanger is both electroneutral and normally held in an inactive form in cell membranes (see Fig. 13-5, page 435). When activated, there is an electroneutral exit of HCO_3^- and entry of Cl^- into these cells, which raises the concentration of Cl^- in the ICF compartment (*see margin note*). Because of the presence of open channels for Cl^- in the cell membrane and a higher concentration of Cl^- in cells, there is an electrogenic exit of Cl^-, which diminishes the magnitude of the intracellular negative voltage. Hence, this electrical driving force that retains K^+ in cells is diminished, and K^+ exit from these cells down their concentration difference via open K^+ channels in the cell membrane. The net effect of all of these steps is to cause the export of K^+ and HCO_3^- from cells.

FUNCTION/CONTROL ANALYSIS
It appears that the intracellular alkalinization facilitates, but does not initiate, this exit of K^+ and HCO_3^-, because it is present before the excretion of K^+ and HCO_3^- begins. It is possible that a signal related to a transient fall in the arterial P_K initiates this process.

PART C
RENAL EXCRETION OF POTASSIUM

Most of the secretion of K^+ occurs in the late distal convoluted tubule and the connecting segment; the cortical collecting duct (CCD) also participates in this process when the K^+ load is large.

COMPONENTS OF THE EXCRETION OF K^+ IN THE CORTICAL COLLECTING DUCT

- Although the usual intake of K^+ in adults eating a typical Western diet is close to 1 mmol/kg body weight, the rate of excretion of K^+ can rise or fall by close to a factor of five to match the intake of K^+ with only a minor change in the P_K. While most of this K^+ intake occurs during the evening meal, its excretion typically occurs around noon the next day.
- The kidneys must be able to excrete a K^+ load with any anion that may accompany it; the strategy used, however, may differ with individual anions.

Arguably the most important immediate function of the kidney is to excrete a large K^+ load to avoid the development of hyperkalemia and the risk of a cardiac arrhythmia. Control of K^+ secretion occurs primarily in the cortical distal nephon, which includes the late distal convoluted tubule, the connecting segment and the cortical collecting duct (*see margin note*).

ABBREVIATION
For simplicity, we use the abbreviation CCD for all of these nephron segments.

Although there are two components that affect the rate of excretion of K^+, the flow rate in the CCD and the net secretion of K^+ by principal cells, which raises the luminal concentration of K^+ ($[K^+]_{CCD}$; see equation), it is the latter that controls the rate of excretion of K^+. Therefore, we focus on factors that contribute to the regulation of the $[K^+]_{CCD}$.

$$K^+ \text{ excretion} = \text{flow rate}_{CCD} \times [K^+]_{CCD}$$

K⁺ SECRETION IN THE LATE CORTICAL DISTAL NEPHRON

- The net secretion of K^+ destined for excretion occurs in the late cortical distal nephron.

Overview

Although a large quantity of K^+ are filtered daily (720 mmol in an adult; 4 mmol/L × 180 L GFR/day), very little will be excreted, as five sixths is reabsorbed in the proximal convoluted tubule when a similar proportion of filtered Na^+ and water are reabsorbed (i.e., the concentration of K^+ remains equal to the P_K). Therefore, 120 mmol of filtered K^+ are delivered to the loop of Henle (4 mmol/L × 30 L/day). Although there is a large passive entry of K^+ into the lumen of the loop of Henle via its ROMK, the concentration of K^+ in the fluid entering the early distal convoluted tubule, as measured during micropuncture studies in the fed rat, is about 1.5 mmol/L. Hence, there is net reabsorption of K^+ in the loop of Henle and about 40 mmol of K^+ are delivered to the CCD, the nephron sites where K^+ secretion occurs (*see margin note*).

Two elements are required for the process whereby K^+ is secreted in the CCD: the presence of K^+ channels in an open configuration in the luminal membranes for cells that perform this secretion (principal cells) and a lumen-negative voltage in these nephron segments. This voltage is generated by reabsorbing more Na^+ than Cl^-. For this to occur, separate pathways for the reabsorption of Na^+ and Cl^- must be present in the CCD, and the reabsorption of Na^+ must be by an electrogenic pathway (i.e., an epithelial Na^+ channel [ENaC]). The driving force for Na^+ reabsorption is a higher concentration of Na^+ in the lumen of the CCD than in principal cells (~10 to 15 mmol/L), and a negative cell interior voltage owing to the actions of the Na-K-ATPase at the basolateral membrane in these cells.

There are two other features of this process of generating lumen-negative voltage. First, since aldosterone is the major hormone that causes an increase in the number of open ENaC units in the luminal membrane of principal cells, these cells must have a receptor for aldosterone in their cytosol. Second, these cells also must have a way to prevent cortisol from reaching this aldosterone receptor, as the level of cortisol in plasma is more than an order of magnitude higher than the $P_{Aldosterone}$ and both of these adrenal steroids bind avidly to this receptor (*see margin note*).

There are two steps in the secretory process that leads to the net secretion of K^+. We shall describe them beginning with a setting where there is a large intake of K^+ following a prolonged period of little intake of K^+, which caused a deficit of K^+ and thereby

REABSORPTION OF K⁺ IN THE LOOP OF HENLE
- This occurs via the Na^+, K^+, 2 Cl^- cotransporter in the medullary and cortical thick ascending limbs.
- In micropuncture experiments in the rat, the $[K^+]$ in the luminal fluid at the earliest part of distal convoluted tubule is ~1.5 mmol/L. A reasonable estimate of the volume of filtrate delivered to the distal nephron in humans is ~27 L/day. Hence ~40 mmol of K^+ are delivered to the late cortical distal nephron (1.5 mmol/L × 27 L/day).
- Therefore, there is net reabsorption of ~80 mmol of K^+ per day in the loop of Henle.

SPECIFICTY OF THE MINERALOCORTICOID RECEPTOR FOR ALDOSTERONE
- The way to make these receptors have specificity for aldosterone is to prevent cortisol from being present in their cytosol.
- Cortisol is "destroyed" by a pair of enzymes called 11β-hydroxysteroid dehydrogenase (11β-HSDH), which converts it to cortisone, which does not bind this receptor.

the removal of K^+ channels from the luminal membrane of the CCD.

K^+ channels

> • The main channel for K^+ secretion in the CCD is ROMK.
> • In terms of regulation of K^+ secretion, one should think of these channels as being absent or present because control of K^+ secretion by modulation of the number of channels does not provide control with enough sensitivity.

ROMK channels

A family of ROMK channels permits the secretion of K^+ in the CCD when there is a negative voltage in the lumen of these nephron segments. These channels recycle; by this we mean that they can be removed from the luminal membrane and stored in vesicles inside the cytoplasm of principal cells when the P_K declines to the lower end of its normal range. This process involves the dephosphorylation of ROMK. On the other hand, when the P_K rises, this leads to a set of signals to phosphorylate ROMK channels, and this results in the insertion of open ROMK channels in the luminal membrane. *One should consider ROMK channels as preventing K^+ secretion when a deficit of K^+ is imminent and giving "permission" for K^+ secretion when the P_K rises above 4.0 mmol/L (i.e., after eating a K^+ load).*

The phosphorylation/dephosphorylation system involves a complicated mixture of kinases and phosphatases including the WNK kinases (*see margin note;* see Part D), tyrosine kinases, and serum and glucocorticoid kinase. The details concerning their importance for the secretion of K^+ is discussed on page 447.

Maxi-K^+ channels

> • The physiologic importance of maxi-K^+ channels is not clear. On the one hand, they could be important when there are insufficient ROMK channels to permit high rates of excretion of K^+ (e.g. while consuming a Paleolithic diet). On the other hand, if these channels are always present in the CCD, they obscure the importance of the control mechanisms related to the abundance of ROMK.
> • If these channels are present in the medullary collecting duct, they cannot play an important role in K^+ secretion, because this nephron segment lacks a lumen-negative voltage.

The medullary collecting ducts and the CCD in rats and mice have another K^+ channel called *maxi-K^+ channels.* Maxi-K^+ channels are open when the flow rate in the collecting ducts is high; this is mediated by an increase in the intracellular concentration of ionized calcium concentration. Their possible function depends on their location.

Maxi-K^+ channels in the cortical distal nephron. When present in the CCD, maxi-K^+ channels have the same function as ROMK channels—they permit high rates of K^+ secretion to occur. They may have been important in Paleolithic times when there was a very high

WNK KINASES
• K is the single-letter symbol for the amino acid lysine, which is important for catalytic actions of kinases (in these kinases, lysine is near but not in the active site).
• WNK stands for With No Lysine (i.e., K).

intake of K⁺ providing that there were insufficient ROMK channels in this setting. Nevertheless, there is a problem with this putative role of maxi-K⁺ channels because one would lose the advantages described above for limiting the excretion of K⁺ by removing ROMK when there is a deficit of K⁺ if the same control does not apply to these channels. In addition, since maxi-K⁺ channels in the CCD are activated by a high flow rate, this could increase renal K⁺ wasting unless they too are removed from the luminal membrane or inactivated in states with a high flow rate in the CCD. One other comment merits emphasis: Maxi-K⁺ channels are located in intercalated cells rather than in principal cells. Hence, this may pose a problem for coordinated regulation.

Maxi-K⁺ channels in the medullary collecting duct. In this location, maxi-K⁺ channels could not be involved in K⁺ secretion because this nephron segment lacks the appropriate lumen-negative electrical driving force.

There is one disease state where maxi-K⁺ channels may permit an excessive quantity of K⁺ to be excreted and cause hypokalemia (i.e., in patients with Bartter's syndrome caused by a truncating mutation in the gene encoding ROMK that results in failure to have active ROMK units). Affected infants present initially with a severe degree of hyperkalemia during the first month of life, because maxi-K⁺ channels have a developmental delay (similar to AQP2). After this time, these channels are present in the CCD. Hence, the clinical picture changes to one of hypokalemia.

Generation of a lumen-negative voltage

A lumen-negative voltage in the late cortical distal nephron is generated by reabsorbing more Na⁺ than Cl⁻ in this nephron segment (Fig. 13-7). The maximum concentration of K⁺ that can be achieved in the lumen of the CCD is influenced by several factors (*see margin note*).

MAXIMUM VALUE OF THE [K⁺]$_{CCD}$
- Because the osmolality of luminal fluid is close to 300 mOsm/L and if all the luminal osmoles are K⁺ and an anion such as Cl⁻, the maximum value for the [K⁺]$_{CCD}$ would be 150 mmol/L.
- When half the osmoles are urea plus Na⁺ and Cl⁻, the maximum value for the [K⁺]$_{CCD}$ would be 75 mmol/L.
- Since it is more likely that 75% of the osmoles in the fluid traversing the terminal CCD are urea (due to urea recycling), the maximum concentration of Na⁺ plus K⁺ is 37.5 mmol/L (¼ × 300 mOsm/L, and half of these osmoles are cations). Therefore the maximum value for [K⁺]$_{CCD}$ is ~40 mmol/L.
- With a volume of 6 L/day delivered to the terminal CCD, K⁺ excretion can rise to 240 mmol/day without a rise in the flow rate in the CCD (6 L × ~40 mmol/L).

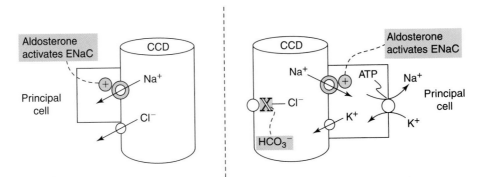

FIGURE 13-7 Electrogenic reabsorption of Na⁺ in the late cortical distal nephron (CCD). The *barrel-shaped structures* represent the CCD, and the *rectangles* represent its principal cells. Na⁺ is reabsorbed via the epithelial Na⁺ channel (ENaC); this reabsorption is increased when aldosterone binds to its receptor in principal cells, leading to more open ENaC units in the luminal membrane of these cells (*shaded enlarged circle*). Net secretion of K⁺ occurs through ROMK channels. An example of electrogenic reabsorption of Na⁺ (presence of HCO₃⁻ or an alkaline luminal pH causing a decrease in the apparent permeability for Cl⁻ in the CCD) is shown on the *right*.

Reabsorption of Na⁺ in the late cortical distal nephron

- Na⁺ is reabsorbed separately from Cl⁻ in the late cortical distal nephron segments.
- One Na⁺ must be delivered and reabsorbed without its accompanying anion (usually Cl⁻) for every K⁺ secreted in the late cortical distal nephron.
- Under most circumstances, the usual variations in the luminal Na⁺ concentration in the CCD do not regulate the net secretion of K⁺.
- There are more open ENaCs in the luminal membranes of principal cells when aldosterone acts.

The principal pathway for the reabsorption of Na⁺ in the CCD is via ENaC (Fig. 13-8). Aldosterone increases the number of open ENaC units in the luminal membrane of principal cells in the CCD. It also has other actions to increase flux through ENaC (*see margin note*).

Mechanism of action of aldosterone

The first step is the binding of aldosterone to its receptor in the cytoplasm of principal cells. The second step is entry of this hormone-receptor complex into the nucleus, where it acts as a transcription factor and induces the synthesis of new proteins, including SGK (Fig. 13-9). SGK increases the number of open ENaC units in the luminal membrane of principal cells (*see margin note next to Fig. 13-9*).

The concentration of cortisol in plasma is more than an order of magnitude higher than that of aldosterone and these two hormones bind to the aldosterone receptor with equal avidity. Nevertheless, cortisol does not exert mineralocorticoid actions because it is converted into an inactive form (cortisone) by the 11β-hydroxysteroid dehydrogenase 1 and 2 enzyme system (11β-HSDH) before it can reach this receptor (see Fig. 14-8, page 497 for more details).

ALDOSTERONE AND PROTEOLYTIC CLEAVAGE OF ENaC
Aldosterone induces the production of "channel-activating serine proteases," which activate ENaC units by proteolytic cleavage. This increases the open probability of the channels but not their expression at the cell surface.

ABBREVIATION
SGK, serum and glucocorticoid-regulated kinase

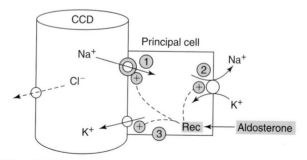

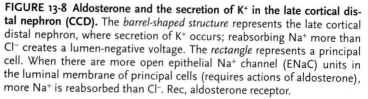

FIGURE 13-8 Aldosterone and the secretion of K⁺ in the late cortical distal nephron (CCD). The *barrel-shaped structure* represents the late cortical distal nephron, where secretion of K⁺ occurs; reabsorbing Na⁺ more than Cl⁻ creates a lumen-negative voltage. The *rectangle* represents a principal cell. When there are more open epithelial Na⁺ channel (ENaC) units in the luminal membrane of principal cells (requires actions of aldosterone), more Na⁺ is reabsorbed than Cl⁻. Rec, aldosterone receptor.

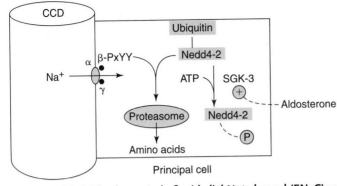

FIGURE 13-9 Model for the control of epithelial Na⁺ channel (ENaC) units in the cortical collecting duct (CCD). The *barrel-shaped structure* represents the CCD, and the *rectangle* represents a principal cell. The *oval* in the principal cell's luminal membrane is ENaC, with its α-subunit (the channel pore); the β- and γ-subunits with their PxYY motif face the interior of the cell. When Nedd4-2 binds to these latter subunits, ENaC are removed from the luminal membrane by endocytosis *(see margin note)*. SGK-3 phosphorylates Nedd4-2, causing its inactivation and thereby increasing the number of open ENaC units in the luminal membrane of principal cells.

ALDOSTERONE, Nedd4-2, AND SGK
- Nedd4-2 binds to subunits of ENaC, and this causes the removal of ENaC from the luminal membrane by endocytosis.
- Nedd4-2 ligates ubiquitin to ENaC, which results in its targeting to the proteasome, where it is destroyed.
- Phosphorylation of Nedd4-2 by SGK causes its inactivation, leading to an increased number of open ENaC units in the luminal membrane, and thereby, an increased Na⁺ transport.

Reabsorption of Cl⁻ in the late cortical distal nephron

- The components responsible for the reabsorption of Cl⁻ in the cortical distal nephron are less clearly defined than those for Na⁺.

The major pathway for reabsorption of Cl⁻ in the late cortical distal nephron is paracellular (Cl⁻ moves between cells), and this pathway appears to be regulated. The concentration of HCO_3^- and/or an alkaline luminal fluid pH seem to increase the quantity of K⁺ secreted in the CCD (see Fig. 13-7). Although the mechanism has not been fully validated, this may result from a decrease in the apparent permeability of Cl⁻.

The maximum capacity for the reabsorption of Cl⁻ in these nephron segments is *less* than that for Na⁺, providing that aldosterone acts and causes the insertion of more open ENaC units in the luminal membranes of principal cells. Hence, there is more electrogenic reabsorption of Na⁺ when there is a stimulus for the release of aldosterone (e.g., a low effective arterial blood volume where the stimulus is a high level of angiotensin II), providing that the delivery of Na⁺ and Cl⁻ to the CCD is high. This may explain the renal K⁺ wasting and hypokalemia with pharmacologic and osmotic diuretics, as well as that caused by ligand binding to the calcium-sensing receptor in the loop of Henle. A similar pathophysiology occurs with inborn errors that affect the transporters for the reabsorption of Na⁺ in upstream nephron segments to the CCD (e.g., Bartter's or Gitelman's syndrome).

When a subject has a much larger intake of NaCl with the same 70 mmol of K⁺ plus organic anions, balance for Na⁺, Cl⁻, and K⁺ must be achieved in steady state. Focusing on the excretion of K⁺, this requires that 70 mmol more Na⁺ than Cl⁻ must be reabsorbed each day. Nevertheless, the volume of fluid in the lumen of the CCD will be larger owing to the extra Na⁺ and Cl⁻ in this fluid (Fig. 13-10). Hence, the voltage need in the lumen of the CCD is less negative as the concentration of K⁺ is 28 mmol/L with a total volume of 2.5 L on the high-salt diet whereas it was 47 mmol/L in a volume of 1.5 L before the NaCl was ingested in the example in Figure 13-10. The lower $P_{Aldosterone}$ while consuming more NaCl could mediate this response (less open ENaC).

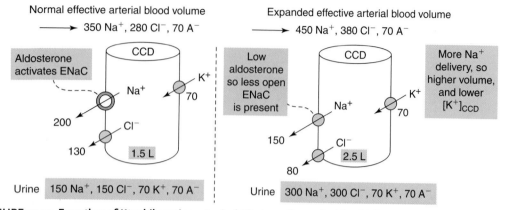

FIGURE 13-10 Excretion of K⁺ while eating a typical Western diet and with a higher intake of NaCl. The *barrel-shaped structure* represents the nephron segments responsible for the secretion of K⁺. In both settings, there is an intake of 70 mmol of K⁺, and since each subject is in balance for K⁺, 70 mmol of K⁺ will be excreted. The *values on the left* represent the typical Western diet, which contains 150 mmol NaCl and 70 mmol K⁺ with 70 mEq of anions other than Cl⁻ (organic anions, inorganic phosphate [$H_2PO_4^-$] and SO_4^{2-} (summarized as A⁻). There are 70 mmol more Na⁺ reabsorbed than Cl⁻. The *values on the right* represent events when the diet contains 300 mmol NaCl, but no other changes. Because of the expanded effective arterial blood volume, there are fewer Na⁺ and Cl⁻ reabsorbed upstream and thus more Na⁺ and Cl⁻ are delivered to the CCD. Since the luminal osmolality is equal to the P_{Osm} because vasopressin acts, there is a larger volume traversing the CCD. Hence, while the same quantity of K⁺ is secreted into a larger volume, the [K⁺]$_{CCD}$ is lower in each liter (lower $P_{Aldosterone}$ overall due to lower P_{Renin}, but the $P_{Aldosterone}$ is increased when dietary K⁺ is absorbed). The imaginary numbers for delivery of Na⁺ Cl⁻, A⁻ are shown at the top of the CCD.

There are disease states that result in low [K⁺]$_{CCD}$, a low rate of excretion of K⁺, and hyperkalemia because there are near-equal rates of Na⁺ and Cl⁻ transport in the CCD. For example, the delivery of Na⁺ and Cl⁻ to the CCD can be very low because their reabsorption is augmented in the distal convoluted tubule as a result of increased activity of the Na⁺, Cl⁻ cotransporter (Gordon's syndrome). Alternatively, Na⁺ and Cl⁻ can be reabsorbed at comparable rates when the delivery of Na⁺ and Cl⁻ is normal, but the reabsorption of Cl⁻ in the CCD is increased (Cl⁻ shunt disorder). A steady state is eventually achieved, but the price is the presence of a degree of hyperkalemia needed to stimulate the release of aldosterone and lead to more electrogenic reabsorption of Na⁺ in CCD by increasing the number of open ENaC in luminal membranes of principal cells.

Aldosterone paradox

- There are more open ENaC units in the luminal membranes of principal cells, which permits both NaCl conservation and K⁺ secretion. Thus, when aldosterone acts, there must be another signal to select either of these possible effects.
- We suggest that the secretagogue for the release of aldosterone (angiotensin II or a high P_K) via modulating the delivery of HCO_3^- to the CCD, and hence the apparent permeability for Cl⁻ in these nephron segments could provide the signal to select the appropriate renal response once there are more open ENaC units in the luminal membrane of principal cells.

Aldosterone can be a NaCl-retaining or a kaliuretic hormone. The paradox derives from the fact that aldosterone is under the control of two separate stimuli, angiotensin II when there is a low effective arterial blood volume and a higher P_K following a large intake of K^+. Each of these stimuli for the release of aldosterone has an identical effect on ENaC in the CCD—they lead to a larger number of open ENaC units in the luminal membrane of principal cells. Therefore, the kidney must "know" whether the appropriate response is to reabsorb more NaCl or to secrete more K^+ when the $P_{Aldosterone}$ is high.

An increased distal delivery of HCO_3^- and/or the rise in the pH of luminal fluid in the CCD may provide the signal to augment the secretion of K^+ in the late cortical distal nephron. The net effect may be to decrease the reabsorption of Cl^-, which would increase the magnitude of the luminal negative voltage and thereby promote the secretion of K^+. Alternatively and/or in addition, the luminal alkalinization may increase the number of open luminal ROMK channels in these cortical distal nephron sites.

When the P_K is high, the reabsorption of HCO_3^- in the proximal convoluted tubule is inhibited. Accordingly, the kaliuretic actions of aldosterone are selected. In contrast, when there is a low effective arterial blood volume, angiotensin II, the other secretagogue for aldosterone, is released. Angiotensin II is a potent activator of the reabsorption of HCO_3^- in the proximal convoluted tubule (see Chapter 7, page 202 for more discussion). The net result is an electroneutral reabsorption of Na^+ and Cl^-, with little kaliuresis (Fig. 13-11). Another reason for the low excretion of K^+ in this setting is that Na^+ cannot be reabsorbed faster than Cl^- because the reabsorption of Na^+ and Cl^- is stimulated in upstream nephron segments by the low effective arterial blood volume, which lowers their distal delivery and therefore the capacity to generate a lumen-negative voltage in the CCD.

Implications for hypertension

- This concept of the regulatory role of HCO_3^- in K^+ excretion provides insights into the pathophysiology of certain forms of "low renin" hypertension.

There is experimental and epidemiologic evidence to support the notion of a role of K^+ depletion in the pathogenesis of hypertension. A possible explanation is that a deficiency of K^+ leads to an acidified proximal cell pH, which increases the reabsorption of HCO_3^- in the proximal tubule and diminishes its distal delivery. This has the advantage of diminishing an unwanted kaliuresis by promoting the electroneutral reabsorption of NaCl when ENaC is activated. As a result, the effective arterial blood volume may become expanded, and low-renin hypertension could ensue in patients whose blood pressure is more sensitive to their effective arterial blood volume than to angiotensin II levels. In experimental studies in which these patients were given KCl supplementation, a negative balance for NaCl and a drop in blood pressure was observed.

Clinical issues

- In a patient with hypokalemia, a higher than expected rate of K^+ excretion (assessed by the $U_K/U_{Creatinine}$ in a spot urine) implies a more negative luminal voltage and open luminal ROMK channels are present in the CCD.

A higher than expected rate of excretion of K^+ in a patient with hypokalemia is caused by reabsorbing more Na^+ than Cl^- in the

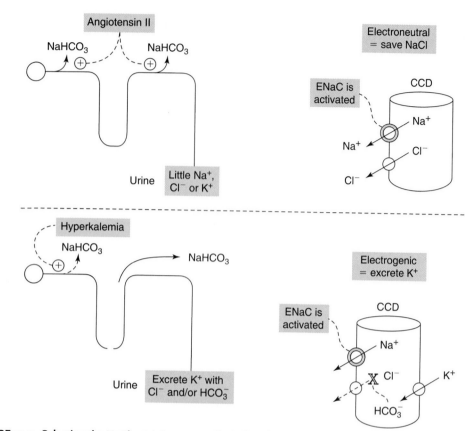

FIGURE 13-11 Selecting the NaCl-retaining versus the kaliuretic actions of aldosterone. The stylized drawings on the *left* represent a nephron, and the cylindrical structures on the *right* represent its late cortical distal nephron (CCD). When aldosterone acts, more open epithelial Na⁺ channel (ENaC) units are present in the luminal membrane of the CCD. The NaCl-retaining actions of aldosterone are shown above the *line,* and the kaliuretic actions of this hormone are shown below the *line.* High levels of angiotensin II and hyperkalemia influence the net effects of aldosterone by altering the reabsorption of HCO_3^- in the proximal convoluted tubule and thereby the distal delivery of HCO_3^- to select the desired renal response. Angiotensin II diminishes the distal delivery of HCO_3^-, which leads to retention of NaCl. Hyperkalemia leads to inhibition of $NaHCO_3$ reabsorption in the proximal convoluted tubules. Hence, there is increased delivery of $NaHCO_3$ to the CCD, which results in a kaliuresis.

CCD; the converse is true in a patient with hyperkalemia and a lower than expected rate of excretion of K⁺. The task for the clinician is to explain why this excretion rate is abnormally high or low.

The indices that help in the differential diagnosis of the pathophysiology of the abnormal rate of electrogenic reabsorption of Na⁺ in the CCD are an assessment of the effective arterial blood volume and blood pressure as well as the ability to conserve Na⁺ and Cl⁻ in response to a contracted effective arterial blood volume. Measuring the activity of renin (P_{Renin}) and the level of aldosterone in plasma ($P_{Aldosterone}$) is helpful in this setting (see Chapter 14, page 474, and Chapter 15, page 527). One should also assess the flow rate in the late cortical distal nephron (*see margin note*).

ABBREVIATIONS

P_{Renin}, the activity or mass of renin in plasma

$P_{Aldosterone}$, the concentration of aldosterone in plasma

FLOW RATE IN THE CCD

- When vasopressin acts, the flow rate in the CCD is determined by the number of osmoles in its lumen.
- The major osmole in the lumen of the CCD is urea. In fact, 75% of these osmoles are urea owing to urea recycling (see Chapter 9, page 291 for more details).

FLOW RATE IN THE LATE CORTICAL DISTAL NEPHRON

- The flow rate in the CCD does not regulate the rate of secretion of K⁺ (*see margin note*).

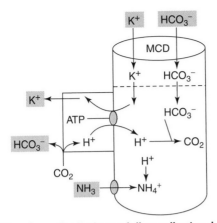

FIGURE 13-12 K⁺ reabsorption in the medullary collecting duct (MCD). The *barrel-shaped structure* represents the MCD. The reabsorption of K⁺ is mediated by an H⁺/K⁺-ATPase, which is electroneutral and requires H⁺ acceptors in the luminal fluid (i.e., HCO_3^- and/or NH_3). HCO_3^- is present in the lumen if its reabsorption was not complete in upstream nephron segments. NH_3 could act as an H⁺ acceptor to form NH_4^+ (*lower left*).

The only setting where the flow rate in the CCD may be important is when there is a very large quantity of K⁺ to excrete. Nevertheless, it is difficult to determine whether this increase in K⁺ excretion results from a high flow rate in CCD per se or an increase in delivery of Na⁺ to the CCD (see the section Control of the Excretion of K⁺: A Paleolithic Analysis, page 447). A low flow rate, however, may raise the concentration of drugs that block ENaC in the luminal fluid in the CCD and lead to a decrease in the rate of excretion of K⁺ (see the discussion of Case 15-3, page 539).

REABSORPTION OF K⁺ IN THE MEDULLARY COLLECTING DUCT

K⁺ reabsorption occurs primarily in the medullary collecting duct (Fig. 13-12). It is stimulated by K⁺ depletion and the transporter is an H⁺/K⁺-ATPase (see Chapter 1, page 21, Fig. 1-12). This exchange is electroneutral and requires H⁺ acceptors in the luminal fluid (i.e., HCO_3^- and/or NH_3; *see margin note*; see Fig. 1-17, page 27).

PART D
INTEGRATIVE PHYSIOLOGY
CONTROL OF THE EXCRETION OF K⁺: A PALEOLITHIC ANALYSIS

- Virtually all our major control mechanisms developed in Paleolithic times; the important ones provided an advantage for survival.
- There have been no pressures in modern times that had enough control strength to override these control mechanisms.

LUMINAL ACCEPTORS FOR THE H⁺/K⁺-ATPase

- HCO_3^- is present in the lumen if its reabsorption is not complete in upstream nephron segments (see Part D for more details) and/or if it is secreted into the lumen via an active Cl⁻/HCO_3^- anion exchanger. If NH_3 is to be the luminal H⁺ acceptor, it must be produced in the proximal convoluted tubule and transferred across the medullary interstitial compartment to form NH_4^+ in the luminal fluid of the medullary collecting duct.
- When there is a deficit of K⁺ and hypokalemia, there is an enhanced reabsorption of HCO_3^- and an increased production of NH_4^+ in the proximal convoluted tubule. As a result, NH_3 rather than HCO_3^- is the most likely H⁺ acceptor in the lumen of the collecting duct in this setting.

**COMPOSITION OF THE
DIET IN RATS CONSUMING
LABORATORY CHOW**
- Rats that consume their usual
  chow excrete 10 times more K+
  than a 70-kg human while consuming a typical Western diet on
  a per-kg per-day basis (700 vs. 70
  mmol). It follows that the mechanisms to excrete an additional
  K+ load in the rat can reveal only
  how to raise a very large rate of K+
  excretion to an even bigger one.
  They may *not*, however, indicate
  how to initiate a modest, episodic
  increment in K+ excretion while
  maintaining very low rates of
  excretion of K+ at other times.
- The need for a mechanism to
  increase the delivery of Na+ to the
  late cortical distal nephron may
  not be present in rats consuming
  their regular chow, because these
  rats consume almost four times
  more Na+ than humans eating
  a typical Western diet when
  expressed in per-kg weight.

The diet of our most ancient ancestors consisted mainly of fruit and berries, which is a diet that provides sugar, K+, and organic anions (potential HCO_3^-), but little NaCl. In addition, this intake was probably large and episodic. Hence, control mechanisms were required for disposal of a large dietary K+ load at times and for prevention of hypokalemia when dietary K+ was not available. In addition, the Paleolithic diet had very little NaCl, but 1 mmol of Na+ must be delivered to the cortical distal nephron to secrete 1 mmol of K+. Therefore, there must be a mechanism to increase the delivery of Na+ to the CCD when there is a large intake of K+. Notwithstanding, it was essential to minimize the excretion of Na+ and Cl− to remain in balance. The components of this control system will be described subsequently.

A word of caution is needed in this regard. Most of our understanding of how the excretion of K+ is regulated in vivo has come from experiments in rats because invasive procedures are required. Nevertheless, because of the large difference in intake of NaCl and K+ per kg body weight in rats and humans (*see margin note*), control mechanisms in rats may not resemble those in humans in Paleolithic times.

Control of K+ excretion in Paleolithic times

Prevent the excretion of K+ when little K+ is consumed

- When the P_K is at the nadir of the normal range, ROMK channels are removed from the luminal membrane of the CCD.

If the P_K is at the nadir of the normal range, the excretion of K+ must be very low. This is largely the result of removing ROMK from the luminal membrane of principal cells in the CCD. Therefore, none of the usual factors, including high levels of aldosterone, the presence of HCO_3^- in luminal fluid, a lumen-negative voltage, and a high distal delivery of Na+, can increase the net secretion of K+ when ROMK are absent in the luminal membranes of principal cells.

In addition, there is an active reabsorption of K+ (and HCO_3^-) in the medullary collecting duct via the H+/K+-ATPase in this setting.

Initiate the excretion of K+ when there is a large intake of K+

- When this Paleolithic diet is consumed, the large intake of K+ causes a rise in the P_K and thereby ROMK channels are inserted into the luminal membrane of principal cells.
- It is important to recall that the families of organic anions, which accompanied the K+ in the diet (e.g., citrate), are usually converted to HCO_3^- in the liver. Accordingly, there may be a role for HCO_3^- in the control of K+ excretion in this setting.

When open ROMK channels are present in the luminal membrane of principal cells, K+ are secreted if a lumen-negative voltage is generated in the CCD. This requires the presence of open ENaC units in the luminal membrane and thereby the ability to reabsorb more Na+ than Cl−. When rats consuming a diet containing little NaCl and K+ salts were given a supplement of KCl, the P_K rose somewhat and the calculated $[K^+]_{CCD}$ rose to near-maximal levels very quickly. There was a modest initial increase in the rate of excretion of K+ that was caused, almost exclusively, by the rise in the $[K^+]_{CCD}$ (Fig. 13-13).

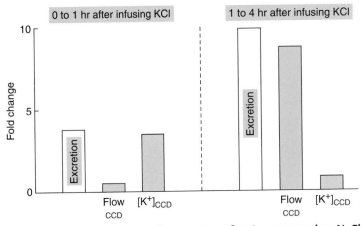

FIGURE 13-13 Time course for the excretion of K$^+$ in rats on a low NaCl intake and given KCl. On the *left*, the data represent a comparison of K$^+$ excretion, the flow rate in the terminal cortical collecting duct (CCD), and the [K$^+$]$_{CCD}$ up to 1 hour after KCl is given to rats consuming a diet with little NaCl and K$^+$ salts. On the *right*, the data represent a comparison of the same parameters at 1 to 4 hours after KCl is given. Notice how the rise in the rate of K$^+$ excretion mirrors the change in the [K$^+$]$_{CCD}$ at the earlier time, whereas it is influenced primarily by the rise in flow rate in the terminal CCD at the later time, which implies that there was increased delivery of Na$^+$ and Cl$^-$ to the CCD.

This reflected the generation of a lumen-negative voltage and the presence of open ROMK in the luminal membrane. The signal could have been the higher P_K (*see margin note*).

Achieving maximal rates of excretion of K$^+$ after a large intake of K$^+$

In the following 4 hours in the above experiment, the rate of excretion of K$^+$ rose by close to a factor of six (see Fig. 13-13). This rise in K$^+$ excretion was accompanied by a large increase in the rate of delivery of Na$^+$ to the CCD, as reflected by a rise in the calculated flow rate in the terminal CCD. *Hence, once K$^+$ channels are inserted into the luminal membrane and a luminal negative voltage is generated, increasing the delivery of Na$^+$ and Cl$^-$ to the CCD have an important degree of control strength on the rate of excretion of K$^+$.*

Mechanism to raise the distal delivery of Na$^+$

- The delivery of Na$^+$ and Cl$^-$ to the late cortical distal nephron and K$^+$ secretion rose within the 3 hours after the rats received a supplement of KCl.
- Since the Paleolithic diet contained little NaCl, it is of great importance that the increase in Na$^+$ delivery is sufficient to augment K$^+$ excretion but not large enough to cause a natriuresis.

To increase the distal delivery of Na$^+$, one must make an "investment." By this we mean that some of the K$^+$ and HCO$_3$$^-$ delivered to the medullary collecting duct is likely to be reabsorbed owing to the fact that the H$^+$/K$^+$-ATPase is still in the luminal membrane because of the prior state of K$^+$ depletion (see Fig. 13-12). Although it seems counterproductive to have an active process to lower the rate of K$^+$ excretion, this

CONTROL OF K$^+$ EXCRETION BY ROMK
- Removal of ROMK is the most effective way to prevent the excretion of K$^+$.
- Modulation of the rate of K$^+$ excretion by adjusting the number of open luminal ROMK channels is a very insensitive way to control K$^+$ excretion. Rather, controls by luminal voltage are more likely to achieve fine regulation once the luminal membrane contains ROMK. Hence the role of ROMK is "permissive" in this setting.

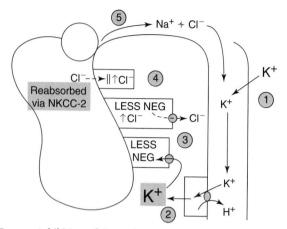

FIGURE 13-14 Inhibition of the reabsorption of NaCl in the loop of Henle by a K⁺ load. The *stylized structure* represents a nephron. Shortly after K⁺ is ingested, there is a somewhat higher secretion of K⁺ in the cortical collecting duct (*site 1*). As a result, more K⁺ is delivered to the medullary CCD, where some of the K⁺ is reabsorbed by the H⁺/K⁺-ATPase, which is still active because of the prior K⁺ depletion (*site 2*). Recall that diet provides a family of organic anions that can be converted to HCO_3^- and that a rise in P_K diminishes the reabsorption of HCO_3^- in the proximal convoluted tubule. As a result, an H⁺ acceptor is available when the H⁺/K⁺-ATPase is active. The higher concentration of K⁺ in the medullary interstitial compartment leads to a diminution in the negative voltage in cells of the medullary thick ascending limb (mTAL; *site 3*). This negative voltage in mTAL cells provides the driving force for the exit of Cl⁻ from these cells. As a result of this diminished driving force, the concentration of Cl⁻ rises in cells of the mTAL (*site 4*). This higher intracellular concentration of Cl⁻ diminishes reabsorption of NaCl via the Na⁺, K⁺, 2 Cl⁻ cotransporter (NKCC-2), which then increases the delivery of Na⁺ to the late cortical distal nephron (*site 5*). The net result is that K⁺ reabsorption in the medullary collecting duct provides the signal (a high medullary interstitial [K⁺]) to increase the delivery of Na⁺ to the cortical distal nephron segments, thus leading to a large kaliuresis. NEG, negative.

PHYSIOLOGY OF THE WNK KINASES

- While the WNK kinases participate in the switch between the NaCl conservation and the kaliuretic effects described in this section, it is not certain whether they are the primary controllers or whether there are components to this regulatory system.

- In a control system, there must be a signal, a process to recognize the signal, the delivery of the message (perhaps the WNK kinases are operating at this step), and response elements, which include the early distal convoluted tubule for the conservation of NaCl, and principal cells in the CCD for adjusting the secretion of K⁺.

- There is a potential parallel with cyclic AMP in the cascade for water conservation/excretion and the WNK kinase system in the shift between NaCl conservation and K⁺ excretion. For the former, the signal, messenger, and response elements are more clearly defined.

causes a higher rate of K⁺ excretion owing to the following effects: The concentration of K⁺ rises in the medullary interstitial compartment, which depolarizes the basolateral membrane of cells of medullary thick ascending limb of the loop of Henle. Thus, there is a smaller intracellular negative voltage, which diminishes the exit of Cl⁻, and as a result, Cl⁻ accumulates in these cells, and this decreases the net reabsorption of Na⁺ and Cl⁻ in the medullary thick ascending limb (Fig. 13-14).

With time, as the rise in the P_K is sustained, there are fewer luminal H⁺/K-ATPase units in the medullary collecting duct, so the rate of K⁺ reabsorption declines somewhat and the interstitial concentration of K⁺ is less elevated. Hence, the inhibition of reabsorption of NaCl in the medullary thick ascending limb is not as marked. As a result, there can be enough distal delivery of Na⁺ and Cl⁻ to maintain high rates of K⁺ secretion in the CCD but not to induce a large natriuresis.

WNK KINASE SIGNAL SYSTEM

One way to think about the WNK kinase system is from the perspective of what was required in Paleolithic times, when the diet contained very little NaCl. Moreover, there were relatively frequent periods when there was an obligatory and possibly large loss of

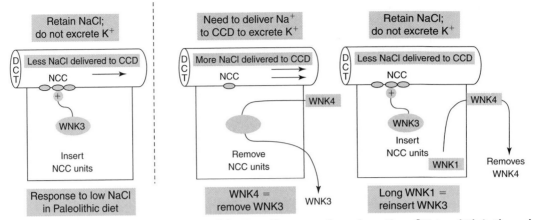

FIGURE 13-15 Influence of the components of the WNK kinases on the reabsorption of Na+ and Cl− in the early distal convoluted tubule. The *horizontal cylinders* represent the lumen of the early distal convoluted tubule (DCT) and the *rectangles* below these cylinders represents cells of this nephron segment. As shown at *far left*, WNK-3 is present in their cytoplasm when little NaCl is consumed (i.e., the Paleolithic diet). As a result, more Na+, Cl− cotransporters (NCC) reside in the luminal membrane of these cells. When there is a large intake of K+ salts while little NaCl is consumed, WNK-3 is removed by WNK-4. NCC thus is internalized, and there is a larger delivery of Na+ and Cl− to the CCD to facilitate the excretion of K+ (*middle panel*). As shown in the *right panel*, NaCl must be retained when there is no longer a need for K+ secretion. Thus NCC must be reinserted in the early DCT. This is achieved by having WNK-1 remove WNK-4 and thus reestablish the effects of WNK3.

NaCl (i.e., loss of NaCl sweat when exercise was performed in a hot environment). Hence, the kidneys must be programmed to retain virtually all filtered Na+ and Cl− in this setting.

Interspersed with this low intake of NaCl were periods when there was an intermittent large intake of fruit and berries (foods rich in K+ and a family of organic anions that will be converted promptly into HCO_3^- in the liver). At these times, there was a critical need to excrete K+ as quickly as possible. This will include mechanisms to decrease the reabsorption of Na+ and Cl− in upstream nephron segments to deliver the requisite quantity of Na+ for the secretion of K+ in the CCD, as well as the insertion of the needed elements of the K+ secretory system. Moreover, once there was no longer a threat of hyperkalemia, there was a need to reestablish the mechanisms to prevent the excretion of the increased delivery of Na+ and Cl− to the CCD. Hence, it is not surprising that a very complex regulatory system would be involved; it is in this context that we shall examine the WNK kinases (Fig. 13-15 and Table 13-1).

Period when retention of NaCl is required

- The WNK kinase that is most important for this effect is WNK kinase-3 (WNK-3).

WNK-3 is present in the cytoplasm of cells of the distal convoluted tubule. The expected effect of this kinase is to ensure that there will be an abundant quantity of the Na+, Cl− cotransporter in the luminal membrane of these cells (see Fig. 13-15). In addition, WNK-3 is also present in the medullary thick ascending limb of the loop of Henle, where it may contribute to stimulation of the reabsorption of Na+ and Cl− in this nephron segment.

TABLE 13-1 **SYNOPSIS OF THE WNK KINASE SYSTEM AND THE REGULATION OF NCC AND ROMK**

To facilitate understanding of this complex signaling system, we provide a function/control analysis based on the changing needs in a Paleolithic setting when the intake of Na^+ was low and the intake of K^+ was very large but episodic. Hence, a control system is needed to conserve Na^+, but also to allow for the excretion of K^+ when faced with a large K^+ load. Once the threat of a K^+ load is dealt with, the signal to secrete K^+ must be removed to reestablish the salt conservation mode. The basic premise of this signaling system is to enhance the electroneutral reabsorption of NaCl in the distal tubule to conserve salt, which also increases the delivery of NaCl to the CCD, where Na^+ is reabsorbed in an electrogenic fashion and to insert ROMK into the luminal membrane of the CCD when there is a need to excrete K^+.

FUNCTION	CONTROL IN DISTAL NEPHRON	SPECIFIC WNK KINASES
• Must minimize NaCl excretion when there is a low NaCl intake	• Increase the presence of NCC in the early distal convoluted tubule	• WNK-kinase-3 ensures that NCC is present in the DCT luminal membrane.
• Must excrete the large dietary intake of K^+	• Remove NCC from DCT: deliver Na^+ for electrogenic reabsorption of Na^+ in CCD	• WNK-4 counters WNK-3: NCC is removed in the DCT and ROMK is inserted in CCD
• Conserve NaCl after K^+ load is excreted	• Must reinsert NCC in the DCT and remove ROMK in the CCD	• Long form of WNK-1 removes WNK-4, which allows WNK-3 to reinsert NCC into the DCT and to remove ROMK from the CCD.

Period when there is a need to excrete K^+

- When there is a need to secrete a large quantity of K^+, a different member of the WNK kinase family (WNK-4) has the task of removing the Na^+, Cl^- cotransporter from the luminal membrane of cells in the distal convoluted tubule (via removing the actions of WNK-3), while inserting K^+ channels (ROMK) in the luminal membrane of principal cells in the CCD.

The actions of WNK kinase 4 (WNK-4) removes the effects of WNK-3 in the early distal convoluted tubule (see Fig. 13-15) and thereby promotes the delivery of Na^+ and Cl^- to the CCD. Since aldosterone is released in response to the higher P_K, there will be more open ENaC units in the luminal membrane of principal cells and thereby more electrogenic reabsorption of Na^+ in these nephron segments. WNK-4 leads to the insertion of ROMK into the luminal membrane of principal cells in the CCD. As a result, there will be an increased rate of secretion of K^+ in the CCD.

LONG WNK-1 AND KS-WNK-1
- This interaction is complex, but it is also important. Hence it is provided here.
- The *WNK-1* gene produces two major products: a full-length or long WNK-1 and a truncated form that is expressed only in the kidney. It is called *kidney-specific WNK-1 (KS-WNK-1)*.
- KS-WNK-1 inhibits the long form of WNK-1 and thus it reestablishes the effects of WNK-4 to inhibit WNK-3, which results in augmented secretion of K^+.
- Dietary K^+ loading increases the abundance of KS-WNK-1 relative to the long form of WNK-1, while K^+ depletion has the opposite effect.

Effects of stopping the intake of K^+

- The effects of WNK-4 must be removed to reestablish the NaCl-retaining effect of WNK-3; this is accomplished by the long form of WNK-1 kinases (*see margin notes*).

The long form of WNK-1 inhibits WNK-4, which leads to higher levels of WNK-3 and thereby to the insertion of the Na^+, Cl^- cotransporter into the luminal membrane of cells in the early distal convoluted tubule. As a result, there is stimulation of NaCl reabsorption in this nephron segment (*see margin note*). The short form of WNK-1 inhibits the effects of its long form. If the long and the short forms of WNK-1 are products of the same gene, this may provide a rapid way to modulate the system to enhance the excretion of K^+ should the need arise.

Clinical implications

Mutations in genes encoding for WNK-1 and WNK-4 are associated with the development of Gordon's syndrome; this is discussed in more detail in Chapter 15, page 526.

MEDULLARY RECYCLING OF K⁺: IMPLICATIONS FOR KIDNEY STONE FORMATION

- When there is a large flux rate through the H^+/K^+-ATPase, this can lead to medullary alkalinization, which may increase the risk of developing calcium oxalate kidney stones.

The H^+/K^+-ATPase in Paleolithic times provided a means to increase the medullary interstitial K^+ concentration and the distal delivery of Na^+—a survival advantage when faced with a large K^+ load. Nevertheless, modern diets provide much less K^+. Accordingly, this transporter now has a different major function because it is needed to prevent K^+ depletion rather than to generate the signal for the excretion of a large quantity of K^+. This adaptive change, however, comes with a "price." Increased reabsorption of K^+ via the H^+/K^+-ATPase also adds HCO_3^- to the interstitial compartment (Fig. 13-16). This alkalinization can lead to a rise in the concentration of carbonate and thereby the deposition of calcium carbonate, which may cause a local high pH and calcium concentration at its surface. Of interest, the initial solid phase in the formation of calcium oxalate stone may be a precipitate of calcium phosphate (apatite; Randall's plaques) on the basolateral aspect of the ascending thin limbs of the loops of Henle. This precipitate subsequently erodes into the collecting duct and provides a nidus for deposition of calcium oxalate in patients with idiopathic hypercalciuria and calcium oxalate stones. To prevent medullary interstitial alkalinization, other processes that add H^+ to this compartment are likely to be present (*see margin note*).

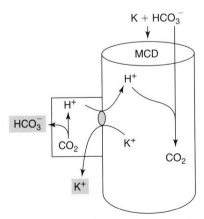

FIGURE 13-16 Possible influence of increased H^+/K^+-ATPase flux on acid-base balance in the renal medulla. The *cylindrical structure* represents the medullary collecting duct (MCD). When more K^+ are reabsorbed by the H^+/K^+-ATPase in the MCD, HCO_3^- are added to the interstitial compartment. This alkalinization raises the concentration of CO_3^{2-}, which may ultimately lead to local precipitation of $Ca_3(PO_4)_2$ on the basolateral aspect of the thin limbs of the LOH and thereby be the initial solid phase that leads to deposition of calcium oxalate precipitates.

MECHANISM TO SHIFT K⁺ INTO LIVER CELLS AFTER A MEAL

- K⁺ will shift into cells when there is an increased negative voltage in their ICF compartment. This voltage is generated by an increase in ion flux through the Na-K-ATPase because it is an electrogenic pump (i.e., it exports 3 Na⁺ while importing only 2 K⁺).
- The combined actions of insulin and flux of L-lactic acid through the monocarboxylic acid transporter lead to activation the NHE and thereby the electroneutral uptake of Na⁺ into hepatocytes which drives flux through the Na-K-ATPase.

Our Paleolithic ancestors consumed a diet of fruit and berries that led to a large input of sugar, K⁺, and organic anions (potential HCO_3^-; *see margin note*). If this K⁺ load were to enter the systemic circulation, it could lead to hyperkalemia and thereby a cardiac arrhythmia. Therefore, a mechanism is needed to shift this K⁺ into hepatocytes to minimize this risk.

The mechanism that is most likely to account for this shift of K⁺ is depicted in Figure 13-17, and it requires a stimulus for the release of insulin and a high local concentration of H⁺ in hepatocytes near the NHE. The flux through the Na-K-ATPase is increased owing to a higher concentration of Na⁺ in cells.

Stimuli for the release of insulin

This is easy to understand, as the absorption of sugar from the diet provides the stimulus to the β-cells of the pancreas to release insulin and deliver it at a high concentration to the liver (i.e., the insulin is

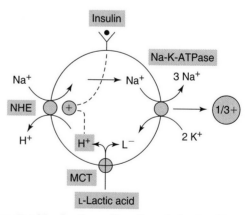

FIGURE 13-17 Combined actions of insulin and L-lactic acid on a shift of K⁺ into hepatocytes. The *circle* represents the cell membrane of hepatocytes. When L-lactic acid enters hepatocytes on the monocarboxylic acid transporter (MCT), this leads to the release of H⁺ immediately adjacent to the NHE. When these H⁺ bind to the H⁺ modifier site of the NHE, this cation exchanger is activated, providing that insulin is present and binds to its receptor on the cell membrane. As a result, Na⁺ enter cells in exchange for H⁺ (an electroneutral exchange), and this higher concentration of Na⁺ in these cells drives the exit of Na⁺ through the Na-K-ATPase (an electrogenic export), which increases the negative voltage in these cells. Thus there is a shift of K⁺ into these cells.

added to the portal circulation so it is diluted in only one fifth of the plasma volume).

Source of L-lactic acid

To have a large delivery of L-lactic acid to the liver, this mono-carboxylic acid must be generated in the cells of the small intestine (*see margin note*). In addition, glycolysis produces L-lactic acid in these cells because this pathway is much faster than the rate of oxidation of pyruvate in the citric acid cycle, possible because the entry of glucose is so high and because these cells do a large amount of work. In more detail, the reabsorption of glucose occurs by a Na^+-linked glucose transporter (SLGT1), which requires the export of Na^+ by the Na-K-ATPase. This intestinal SLGT1 uses 2 Na^+ per glucose, so there is an even larger generation of ADP, which stimulates intestinal glycolysis. In fact, there is a rise in the L-lactate concentration to the 3- to-4 mmol/L range in plasma in the portal vein in rats following a meal. The uptake of L-lactic acid into hepatocytes uniquely raises the local H^+ concentration near the NHE at the inner aspect of the cell membrane. This together with high insulin levels leads to the uptake of K^+ into liver cells (see Fig. 13-17).

DISCUSSION OF INTRODUCTORY CASE 13-1

INTRODUCTORY CASE 13-1: WHY DID I BECOME SO WEAK?

(Case presented on page 426)

What is the most likely basis for the repeated episodes of acute hypokalemia?

Since the time course was only a matter of hours, the excretion of K^+ was low ($U_K/U_{Creatinine}$ was ~1), there was no major acid-base disorder, and the recovery was so rapid and required only a small infusion of KCl, the diagnostic category is an acute shift of K^+ into cells.

Was an adrenergic effect associated with the acute hypokalemia?

It appears that the answer is yes, as the patient had tachycardia, systolic hypertension, and a wide pulse pressure on physical examination on each episode. Notwithstanding, there was no obvious source of the adrenergic surge. In more detail, she denied an exogenous source of a long-acting β_2-adrenergic (e.g., the intake of amphetamines), drugs with adrenergic actions (she had stopped using bronchodilators), caffeine, or drugs that could inhibit cytochrome P_{450}. There was no evidence of an endogenous disease that has a similar hormonal milieu (e.g., hyperthyroidism, pheochromocytoma). Therefore, the source of the surge of β_2-adrenergics was still a mystery.

After the laboratory results were examined, were there any clues to suggest what the cause of acute hypokalemia might be?

There were two signs that could be associated with a shift of K^+ into cells owing to the coordinated actions between the monocarboxylic acid transporter and NHE. First, there was a sign of an elevated $P_{L-lactate}$ (i.e., the P_{HCO3} was 22 mmol/L [later the $P_{L-lactate}$ was measured and it was 3 mmol/L]). Second, the $P_{Glucose}$ was a little higher

GLUCOSE CONVERSION TO L-LACTIC ACID
If all the ingested glucose were converted to L-lactic acid (which is extremely unlikely), the production of L-lactic acid from this glucose load would be 1500 mmol (750 mmol × 2).

than expected at 133 mg/dL (7.4 mmol/L), and this is associated with a stimulus for the release of insulin. Hence, with the synergistic actions of the monocarboxylic acid transporter and NHE, this could be the basis for a shift of K^+ into hepatocytes (see Fig. 13-17). Finally, the last clue is the presence of an adrenergic surge that must be explained. Perhaps the attacks were initiated by the release of insulin from an insulinoma, which caused a sustained period of hypoglycemia and thereby an adrenergic surge. The metabolic consequence could be hypoglycemia, which is followed by both an increased production of glucose and more rapid stomach emptying. If the stomach contained sugar, the net result would be a higher $P_{Glucose}$. One reason that the high $P_{Insulin}$ and the C-peptide in plasma were not observed is that the blood tests were drawn the next day after this association was considered.

Would your treatment be different for her next attack?

Based on the signs of an adrenergic surge on physical examination, the therapy of the next attack would include a nonselective β-blocker if the patient does not have evidence of bronchospasm.

What tests should be performed in the emergency room if she has another episode of acute hypokalemia to reveal the correct diagnosis?

The likely duration of the disorder is that its initiating cause may have been present for many hours earlier; hence, the blood that was drawn on admission may not reveal the factors responsible for the fall in the P_K (Fig. 13-18). In addition, if an organ produces or removes a substance that influences a shift of K^+ across cell membranes, the results in venous blood draining that organ may not reveal the etiology of the hypokalemia. In more detail, if there was a large uptake of glucose in muscle owing to the effects of insulin, the $P_{Glucose}$ may be considerably less than its concentration in arterial blood that was delivered to the kidneys.

Based on the above, the clues for the basis of the shift of K^+ into cells may be present in the bladder urine—this urine should be saved and analyzed for glucose (i.e., to detect prior glucosuria), signs of a high prior $P_{Insulin}$ (i.e., a high excretion of C-peptide), signs of new glucose production during gluconeogenesis (a higher urea to creatinine ratio in the urine on admission as compared to subsequent values), and signs of the adrenergic response to the hypoglycemia (ketonuria, metabolic products that may indicate an adrenergic surge [e.g., urinary metanephrines or catecholamines]).

DISCUSSION OF QUESTIONS

13-1 *Is the $[K^+]_{ATP}$ channel regulated in fact by ATP?*

- ADP acts as an "opener" of $[K^+]_{ATP}$ channels in an indirect way.
- Ionized Ca^{2+} is a major signal for regulation of many intracellular processes.

The name of this channel is incorrect because K^+_{ATP} channels are not regulated by the intracellular concentration of ATP, as the

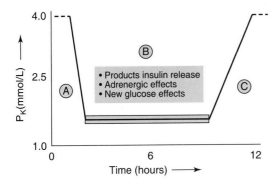

FIGURE 13-18 Possible sequence of events in a patient with acute hypokalemia due to an insulinoma. The P_K is shown on the y-axis, and the time course for the change in the P_K is shown on the x-axis. The *dashed lines* represent the times when the P_K is in the normal range. Very early on, there is a stimulus to cause a shift of K^+ into hepatocytes and perhaps other cells (e.g., prolonged release of insulin from an insulinoma, a β_2-adrenergic response to hypoglycemia, and possibly a high $P_{L-lactate}$; *site A*). Some time later (perhaps ~8 hr), the $P_{Insulin}$ falls, the $P_{Glucose}$ rises, and the β_2-adrenergic hormone levels begin to decline. In this interval, a clue to the etiology of the acute hypokalemia may be in the urine (*site B*) including the C-peptide reflecting proinsulin, the presence of ketonuria as part of the adrenergic response to hypoglycemia, and evidence of protein conversion to glucose (high urea/creatinine in the urine as compared to later urine samples). When she arrives at the hospital (~10-hr time), clues may not be detected in the blood sample (*site C*).

concentration of ATP in cells never rises or falls sufficiently in health to modulate these channels. In fact, the prevailing concentration of ATP ensures that this channel is closed. Nevertheless, if one includes the effects of ADP, which opens this channel, under the usual ATP concentration, the channel may have a certain degree of open probability. Thus, when the concentration of ADP rises, there is a higher degree of open probability of this channel; conversely, when the ADP concentration falls, this channel closes.

To understand what the change in voltage in cells is when the K^+_{ATP} channel opens, recall that a cationic charge leaves the cell; hence, the voltage in cells becomes more negative, which may affect the gating of voltage-gated ion channels. The best example is the voltage-gated Ca^{2+} channel, which is closed when there is a more negative voltage in cells. Conversely, when fewer K^+ leave the cell because the K^+_{ATP} channel is closed, the voltage in cells becomes less negative. This less negative intracellular voltage opens the voltage-gated Ca^{2+} channel and thereby causes a higher intracellular ionized calcium concentration. By modulating the concentration of ionized Ca^{2+} in cells, many other functions are controlled because ionized Ca^{2+} is a major signal for regulation of many intracellular processes.

K^+_{ATP} *channel and the release of insulin:* Closing the K^+_{ATP} channel by a fall in the concentration of ADP plays a critical role in the release of insulin from β-cells of the pancreas (Fig. 13-19). In more detail, when the $P_{Glucose}$ is high, more glucose enters β-cells because of their nonregulated glucose transporter (GLUT-2). Hence, some ADP is converted to ATP and the intracellular concentration of ADP falls, which causes the K^+_{ATP} channels to close. The voltage in the ICF compartment thus becomes less

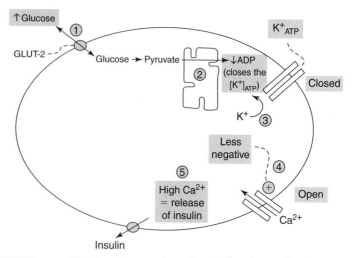

FIGURE 13-19 Signal system to release insulin from beta cells of the pancreas. The *large oval* represents a beta cell of the pancreas. When the $P_{Glucose}$ rises, the intracellular fluid $(ICF)_{Glucose}$ rises to the same extent because of the type of glucose transporter (GLUT-2; *site 1*) in these cells. The concentration of ADP falls when glucose is oxidized (*site 2*), and this permits K_{ATP} channels to be closed. The ICF compartment becomes less negative when K^+_{ATP} channels close (*site 3*). This opens voltage-gated Ca^{2+} channels and raises the ionized Ca^{2+} concentration in the cytosol (*site 4*). A higher ionized Ca^{2+} level in these cells causes the release of insulin (*site 5*).

negative, which increases the conductance of voltage-gated Ca^{2+} channels. The resultant rise in the intracellular ionized Ca^{2+} concentration provides the final signal for the release of insulin from β-cells.

K^+_{ATP} channel and vasodilatation: A similar logic can be used to deduce how the blood flow to exercising muscle may be controlled using intracellular Ca^{2+} as the signal (Fig. 13-20). During a sprint, L-lactic acid is released from exercising skeletal muscle cells. When L-lactic acid enters vascular smooth muscle cells, the concentrations of H^+ and L-lactate rise, which leads to opening of the K^+_{ATP} channels independent of the effect of ADP. As a result, K^+ exit and the voltage in these cells becomes more negative. This causes closure of voltage-gated Ca^{2+} channels and less entry of extracellular calcium ions into cells and hence vasodilatation.

Clinical implications: Using a drug that closes K^+_{ATP} channels (e.g., sulfonylureas) can be a useful adjunct for therapy of patients with shock due to vasodilatation (e.g., septic shock).

PHOSPHOCREATINE AND THE EXIT OF K⁺ FROM MUSCLE CELLS DURING SPRNT

- The hydrolysis of phosphocreatine yields an alkali load in cells (see Chapter 1, page 32 for more discussion).
- The exit of HCO_3^- causes a fall in the ICF negative voltage (see Fig. 13-5, page 435).
- This fall in negative voltage leads to a shift of K⁺ out of cells.

13-2 *What mechanisms permit nonexercising cells to take up K⁺ during a sprint?*

During depolarization of exercising skeletal muscle cells, K⁺ is released into the spaces in the exterior of these muscles (called the *t-tubules*; *see margin note*). Nevertheless, a small quantity of this K⁺ that is released enters the circulation, and this raises the P_K to close to 6.0 mmol/L. The cooperation of resting cells is needed to prevent much larger and dangerous rises in the P_K. The mechanisms involved include activation of the Na-K-ATPase by the β₂-adrenergic component of the fight-or-flight response, which pumps endogenous

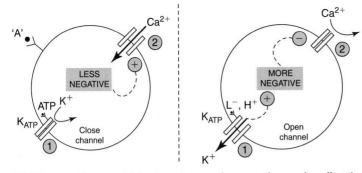

PROMOTE VASOCONSTRICTION   PROMOTE VASODILATION

FIGURE 13-20 Vasoconstrictor tone in vascular smooth muscle cells. The *circles* represent vascular smooth muscle cells. When the intracellular fluid (ICF) has a less negative voltage because its K^+_{ATP} channels are closed and actions of the hormones symbolized by the A (adrenaline, arginine vasopressin, and angiotensin II) cause the voltage-gated Ca^{2+} channel to be in a more open configuration, permitting a sustained rise in the intracellular ionized calcium concentration. Hence, vasoconstriction is the dominant response (shown on the *left*). In contrast, during a sprint, K^+_{ATP} channels are open because of a high concentration of L-lactate anions (L^-) and H^+ (shown on the *right*). This leads to a more negative ICF voltage and closure of the voltage-gated Ca^{2+} channels.

Na^+ out of cells and thereby creates a negative voltage inside cells. A second mechanism is the activation of the NHE by a high intracellular concentration of H^+, which is the result of L-lactic acid uptake by the monocarboxylic acid transporter in nonexercising cells.

chapter 14

Hypokalemia

Introduction

Hypokalemia, usually defined as a P_K of less than 3.5 mmol/L, is a common electrolyte disorder that is present in a number of disease states. When faced with a patient with hypokalemia, the first step is to determine whether an emergency is present. The most serious emergency due to hypokalemia is a cardiac arrhythmia; this threat and the absolute P_K, however, are not tightly correlated. The other major risk that is directly related to hypokalemia is muscle weakness, and this can be serious if respiratory muscles are affected, especially if there is a need for deep and frequent respirations (e.g., in a patient with metabolic acidosis). If an emergency is present, therapy to raise the P_K must begin without delay.

If the time course for the development of hypokalemia is short and/or if there is no obvious cause for K+ loss, suspect that the major basis of the hypokalemia is a shift of K+ into cells. Chronic hypokalemia in the absence of large loss of K+ in diarrhea fluid implies that there is a defect that causes renal K+ wasting. This is detected by finding that the rate of excretion of K+ is inappropriately high for the presence of hypokalemia, and one must identify why the net secretion of K+ may be increased in the late cortical distal nephron. Useful clues to determine the underlying pathophysiology are provided by the medical history, an assessment of the effective arterial blood volume, the blood pressure, and the acid-base status. It is important to recognize that hypokalemia is a sign of a number of diseases with diverse etiologies; hence, the diagnosis of the underlying disease may be made, as this may have implications for therapy.

ABBREVIATIONS

P_K and U_K, concentration of K+ in plasma and in the urine
P_{Na} and U_{Na}, concentration of Na+ in plasma and in the urine
P_{Cl} and U_{Cl}, concentration of Cl− in plasma and in the urine
P_{Osm} and U_{Osm}, osmolality in plasma and in the urine
P_{HCO3}, concentration of HCO_3 in plasma
$P_{Aldosterone}$, concentration of aldosterone in plasma
CCD, late cortical distal nephron; this includes the late distal convoluted tubule, the connecting segment, and the cortical collecting duct
$[K^+]_{CCD}$, concentration of K+ in the lumen of the CCD
NHE, Na+/H+ cation exchanger
AE, Cl−/$HCO_3^−$ anion exchanger

OBJECTIVES

- To emphasize that hypokalemia is a common electrolyte abnormality, which may pose a major threat to survival. Hypokalemia, however, is not a diagnosis; rather it is a laboratory finding that occurs in many different diseases.
- To provide a clinical approach to the patient with hypokalemia based on an understanding of the physiology of a shift of K+ into cells and regulation of the excretion of K+.
- To provide an approach to the therapy of the patient with hypokalemia.

Case 14-1: Why Did Hypokalemia Develop So Quickly?

(Case discussed on page 468)

A 52-year-old previously healthy man fell five stories at a construction site; this resulted in multiple fractures, soft tissue injuries, and acute traumatic brain injury. He was transported quickly to a hospital, and his P_K was 3.2 mmol/L. Within the first hour, his P_K fell to 1.3 mmol/L and ventricular tachycardia developed. The basis of the decline in P_K was a sudden and marked shift of K^+ into cells caused by the extreme adrenergic response due to the fall and the adrenergic agents that were administered to maintain hemodynamics.

Questions

What is the emergency therapy for the acute, severe hypokalemia in this patient?

How much K^+ do you anticipate the patient will need to bring his P_K to a safe range?

What therapy will be needed to deal with the K^+ load that was given after K^+ started to shift out of cells?

Case 14-2: Hypokalemia with Paralysis

(Case discussed on page 505)

A 45-year-old man developed profound weakness in both his lower and upper extremities over the past several hours. He had two similar episodes in the preceding two months; prior to each of these episodes, he had a very large intake of sweetened soft drinks. He was not taking any medications, including laxatives or diuretics. There was no family history of hypokalemia, periodic paralysis, or hyperthyroidism. On physical examination, he was alert and oriented. His blood pressure was 150/70 mm Hg, heart rate was 124 beats per minute, and respiratory rate was 18 breaths per minute. The only neurologic findings were symmetrical flaccid paralysis with areflexia in all four limbs; fasciculations, myoclonus, and muscular atrophy were not present. Laboratory data on admission are summarized in the following table; tests of thyroid function were normal.

		PLASMA	URINE
Na^+	mmol/L	138	103
K^+	mmol/L	1.9	10
Cl^-	mmol/L	102	112
HCO_3^-	mmol/L	26	—
Phosphate	mg/dL (mmol/L)	2.0 (0.7)	1.3 (0.4)
pH		7.41	—
Glucose	mg/dL (mmol/L)	90 (5.0)	—
Creatinine	mg/dL (μmol/L)	0.6 (52)	1 g/L (9.0 mmol/L)

Questions

Is there a medical emergency in this patient?

What is the basis of hypokalemia in this patient?

What effects cause a prolonged shift of K^+ into cells?

What is the best therapy for the acute hypokalemia in this patient?

CASE 14-3: HYPOKALEMIA WITH A SWEET TOUCH

(Case discussed on page 507)

A 76-year-old Asian man became very weak this morning and was unable to walk for the past 6 hours. He denied nausea, vomiting, and diarrhea. He did not take diuretics or laxatives. Hypokalemia (P_K 3.3 mmol/L) and hypertension were present 1 year ago but were not investigated further. There was no previous history or family history of similar episodes. His blood pressure was 160/96 mm Hg, and his heart rate was 70 beats per minute. The only positive finding was symmetric flaccid paralysis with areflexia. His electrocardiogram showed U waves and a prolonged Q-T interval. The laboratory data on admission are presented in the following table:

		PLASMA	URINE
Na^+	mmol/L	147	132
K^+	mmol/L	1.8	26
Cl^-	mmol/L	96	138
HCO_3^-	mmol/L	38	—
pH		7.50	—
Pco_2 (arterial)	mm Hg	45	—
Creatinine	mg/dL (µmol/L)	0.8 (70)	0.6 g/dL (5 mmol/L)

The patient was given a large quantity of KCl; his weakness improved when his P_K reached 2.5 mmol/L. Over the following 2 weeks, his P_K and blood pressure returned to normal levels and his body weight decreased from 78 to 74 kg. When the results became available, his renin activity in plasma was low, his $P_{Aldosterone}$ was low, and his $P_{Cortisol}$ was in the normal range.

Questions

Is there a medical emergency in this patient?
Is there a danger to anticipate during therapy?
What is the basis of hypokalemia in this patient?

CASE 14-4: HYPOKALEMIA IN A NEWBORN

(Case discussed on page 508)

A young boy, who is now 2 years of age, is the first child of consanguineous marriage (his parents are first cousins). His mother's pregnancy was complicated by severe polyhydramnios, for which amniocentesis was performed on two occasions early in the pregnancy. Delivery occurred in the 26th week; he weighed 2.2 lb (1 kg). His urine flow rate was very large, which resulted in a loss of more than 20% of his weight in the first 24 hours. The concentration of Na^+ in his urine was very high (98 mmol/L; expected, <10 mmol/L). His P_K was high at the 24-hour time (5.5 mmol/L), but after aggressive infusion of isotonic saline, persistent hypokalemia was consistently present (P_K ~3.3 mmol/L).

Over the first month of life, he required a large daily fluid volume to replace his urine output (250 mL/kg/day). There was also a huge excretion of NaCl (~12 mmol/kg/day), and he required supplements of NaCl to maintain hemodynamic stability. He was treated with a prostaglandin synthesis inhibitor (indomethacin), and his renal salt wasting largely disappeared. Notwithstanding, this uncovered a second abnormality, a large water diuresis (urine flow rate was ~10% of his glomerular filtration rate as judged by the urine-to-plasma creatinine concentration ratio) with a U_{Osm} less than 100 mOsm/kg H_2O. When he was given vasopressin, his urine flow rate did not fall and his U_{Osm} did not rise. The laboratory data during his first week of life are presented in the following table:

		PLASMA	URINE
Na^+	mmol/L	133	89
K^+	mmol/L	3.3	26
Cl^-	mmol/L	96	92
Osmolality	mOsm/kg H_2O	276	250
Creatinine	mg/dL (µmol/L)	1.1 (90)	10 mg/dL (850 µmol/L)

Questions

Is there a medical emergency in this patient?

Is there a danger to anticipate during therapy?

What is the basis of hypokalemia in this patient?

Why did the patient have nephrogenic diabetes insipidus?

Why did his U_{Osm} fall after indomethacin was given?

In what nephron segment might indomethacin have acted to curtail the natriuresis?

Why is antenatal Bartter's syndrome not a lethal abnormality?

PART A
SYNOPSIS OF K⁺ PHYSIOLOGY

A detailed discussion of the physiology of K^+ is presented in Chapter 13; we shall provide a brief synopsis of this physiology in this chapter.

MOVEMENT OF K⁺ ACROSS CELL MEMBRANES

- K^+ move across cell membranes in response to an electrochemical driving force providing that there are open K^+ channels.

Negative voltage inside cells

K^+ are shifted and retained in cells when there is an increase in the intracellular negative voltage. This increase in negative voltage is generated by an increase in ion flux through the Na-K-ATPase because it is an electrogenic pump (i.e., it exports 3 Na^+ while importing only 2 K^+). Flux through the Na-K-ATPase may be increased if the concentration of Na^+ in cells rises (i.e., when there is a spike of insulin to activate the Na^+/H^+ exchanger [NHE]), if existing Na-K-ATPase units are activated (occurs with high levels of β_2-adrenergic hormones), and/or if there is an increased number of Na-K-ATPase pump units (occurs with high levels of thyroid hormone and/or insulin). The impact of this increase in Na^+ pumping on the net cell voltage, however, requires that the source of Na^+ is Na^+ that existed in the cell or Na^+ that entered the cell in an electroneutral fashion. In more detail, when Na^+ enter cells in an electroneutral fashion, its subsequent electrogenic exit via the Na-K-ATPase results in a more negative cell interior voltage, and hence there is less net exit of K^+ from these cells. This occurs when Na^+ enter cells in exchange for H^+ on the NHE (*see margin note*).

ACTIVATION OF NHE
Although NHE is normally *inactive* in cell membranes, it can become active if there is a spike of insulin or a higher concentration of H^+ in cells.

Clinical implications

An acute shift of K^+ into cells occurs when insulin is given to a patient with diabetic ketoacidosis (DKA). An initial spike of insulin may also explain why a high carbohydrate load is a risk factor for development of an acute attack in patients with hypokalemic periodic paralysis. For the same reason, KCl should not be administered in a solution that contains glucose in a patient with a severe degree of hypokalemia, because even a small degree of an acute shift of K^+ into cells due to the release of insulin can be dangerous in this setting (*see margin note*). In patients with a severe degree of hypokalemia and acidemia due to metabolic acidosis, the P_K should be raised to at least 3 mmol/L *before* administering $NaHCO_3$, because even a small acute shift of K^+ into cells can be dangerous in this setting (*see margin note*).

An acute shift of K^+ into cells can be seen in conditions associated with an adrenergic surge (e.g., acute myocardial infarction, acute pancreatitis, subarachnoid hemorrhage, and traumatic brain injury; see discussion of Case 14-1). Acute hypokalemia may also occur in patients who are given a large dose of β_2-agonists to treat asthma or in patients who are given amphetamines for weight reduction. Because large doses of caffeine result in an adrenergic surge, acute hypokalemia may be also seen in this setting. Nonselective β_2-antagonists should be used in the emergency therapy of patients with acute hypokalemic precipitated by an adrenergic surge.

Patients with catabolic states such as DKA have a deficit of K^+ and phosphate anions because these ions were released from cells and excreted in the urine. There is also a shift of K^+ into cells when patients with DKA are treated with insulin and phosphate is provided from the diet; hypokalemia may develop if enough K^+ is not given. A similar caution is merited for patients early in the course of therapy for pernicious anemia with vitamin B_{12} and also in cachectic patients who are treated with parenteral nutrition.

EFFECT OF A SMALL SHIFT OF K^+ ON THE P_K IN PATIENTS WITH HYPOKALEMIA
- There are 20 mmol of K^+ in the extracellular fluid (ECF) compartment in a 50-kg person with the usual 10 L of ECF and a P_K of 2.0 mmol/L.
- A shift of only 4 mmol of K^+ into cells lowers the P_K by 20% to 1.6 mmol/L.

REGULATION OF RENAL EXCRETION OF K^+

Control of the renal excretion of K^+ maintains overall daily K^+ balance, and this occurs primarily in the late cortical distal nephron. Most of the secretion of K^+ occurs in the late distal convoluted tubule, and the connecting segment, but the cortical collecting duct also participates in this process when the K^+ load is large. We shall use the abbreviation CCD to represent all of these nephron segments. The major process that influences the rate of excretion of K^+ is net secretion of K^+ by principal cells, which raises the concentration of K^+ in the lumen of the CCD ($[K^+]_{CCD}$; *see margin note*).

FLOW RATE IN THE CCD
A high flow rate in the CCD is not likely to be a sole cause of hypokalemia.

Secretion of K^+ in the late cortical distal nephron

- The driving force for the secretion of K^+ in the CCD is a lumen-negative voltage, which is generated by reabsorbing more Na^+ via epithelial Na^+ channel (ENaC) than its accompanying anion (usually Cl^-).

ABBREVIATIONS
ROMK, rat outer medullary K$^+$ channels
11β-HSDH, 11β-hydroxysteroid dehydrogenase
ACTH, adrenocorticotrophic hormone

- The secretory process for K$^+$ in principal cells is also dependent on having a sufficient number of open ROMK channels in the luminal membrane of principal cells.

Actions of aldosterone increase the number of open ENaC units in the luminal membranes of principal cells and thus may increase renal excretion of K$^+$. Notwithstanding, when the secretagogue for aldosterone is angiotensin II and the effective arterial blood volume is contracted for nonrenal reasons, the net result is conservation of NaCl rather than the excretion of K$^+$ (see the Aldosterone Paradox in Chapter 13, page 444).

The concentration of cortisol in plasma is an order of magnitude higher than that of aldosterone. Moreover, cortisol binds to the intracellular aldosterone receptor with the same avidity as aldosterone. Nevertheless, cortisol does not normally act as a mineralocorticoid because cortisol is converted to an inactive form (cortisone) by the 11β-HSDH 1 and 2 enzyme system before it can reach the intracellular receptor for aldosterone. There are three circumstances, however, when cortisol acts as a mineralocorticoid: first, when 11β-HSDH is lacking (e.g., in patients with apparent mineralocorticoid excess syndrome); second, when 11β-HSDH is inhibited (e.g., by glycyrrhetinic acid in licorice); and third, when the activity of 11β-HSDH is overwhelmed by a large excess of cortisol (e.g., in a patient with an ACTH-producing tumor).

The major pathway for Cl$^-$ reabsorption in the CCD is paracellular, and it appears to be regulated. The concentration of HCO$_3^-$ and/or an alkaline luminal fluid pH increases the secretion of K$^+$ in the CCD. The mechanism has not been fully clarified, but it may be the result of a decrease in the apparent permeability of Cl$^-$ and/or an increase in the number of open ROMK channels residing in the luminal membrane of principal cells in this nephron segment.

In addition to control by the lumen-negative voltage, the secretory process for K$^+$ in principal cells is dependent on having a sufficient number of open ROMK channels in the luminal membrane of principal cells. A decreased number of open luminal ROMK channels limits the net secretion of K$^+$ in rats on a low-K$^+$ diet.

Basis of a high [K$^+$]$_{CCD}$

ABBREVIATIONS
WNK, with no lysine
P$_{Renin}$, mass or activity of renin in plasma
P$_{Aldosterone}$, level of aldosterone in plasma

- The most common explanation for a high [K$^+$]$_{CCD}$ is a more negative voltage in the lumen of the CCD due to a higher rate of "electrogenic" reabsorption of Na$^+$ (i.e., more Na$^+$ is reabsorbed than Cl$^-$).
- There are two major groups of disorders that lead to a high lumen-negative voltage in the CCD: those that cause more reabsorption of Na$^+$ and those that lead to diminished reabsorption of Cl$^-$.

In a patient with chronic hypokalemia, a higher than expected rate of excretion of K$^+$ implies that an abnormally high lumen-negative voltage is present in the CCD. This could be due to more reabsorption of Na$^+$ or relatively less reabsorption of Cl$^-$ in the CCD. The clinical tools that are most useful in this differential diagnosis include an assessment of the effective arterial blood volume, whether or not Na$^+$ and Cl$^-$ can be conserved adequately when the effective arterial blood volume is contracted, and whether the blood pressure is elevated.

TABLE 14-1 **PLASMA RENIN AND ALDOSTERONE TO ASSESS THE BASIS OF HYPOKALEMIA DUE TO A LESION WITH MORE REABSORPTION OF Na⁺ THAN Cl⁻**

	RENIN	ALDOSTERONE
Lesions in the adrenal gland		
Primary hyperaldosteronism	Low	High
Glucocorticoid remediable hyperaldosteronism	Low	High
Lesions in the kidney		
Renal artery stenosis	High	High
Malignant hypertension	High	High
Renin-secreting tumor	High	High
Liddle's syndrome	Low	Low
Disorders involving 11β-HSDH	Low	Low

Measurements of the P_{Renin} and the $P_{Aldosterone}$ are often helpful to determine the cause of a higher rate of reabsorption of Na⁺ than Cl⁻ in the CCD (Table 14-1).

PART B
CLINICAL APPROACH

DEALING WITH EMERGENCIES ON ADMISSION

- The first step is to deal with medical emergencies that may be present on admission and to anticipate and prevent risks that may arise during therapy.

The major emergencies related to hypokalemia are cardiac arrhythmias and respiratory muscle weakness leading to respiratory failure; these must be dealt with very quickly (Flow Chart 14-1). Because the administration of large doses and high concentrations of K⁺ are likely needed, K⁺ may have to be administered via a large central vein; cardiac monitoring is also essential in this setting (see the discussion of Case 14-1, page 468).

Anticipate and prevent dangers due to therapy

Overaggressive K⁺ replacement therapy can induce acute hyperkalemia; it is a grave error to replace the entire K⁺ deficit too quickly, because one does not know how much of the hypokalemia is due to a shift of K⁺ into cells. Therapy should not contain compounds that may cause K⁺ to shift into cells. Hence, the initial infusion should not contain glucose or $NaHCO_3$, and β_2-adrenergic agonists should be avoided because they may increase the severity of hypokalemia. In patients who also have hypomagnesemia, hypokalemia may be refractory to the administration of KCl until supplements of magnesium salts are given. This should be kept in mind, especially in patients with a cardiac arrhythmia.

There are a number of reasons why the administration of KCl may induce a water diuresis in a patient with chronic hyponatremia. Accordingly, be prepared to administer dDAVP to prevent a rapid

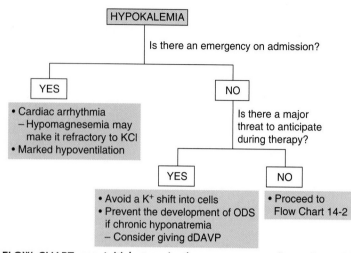

FLOW CHART 14-1 Initial steps in the management of a patient with hypokalemia. The steps are to deal with emergencies and to anticipate and prevent dangers during therapy.

ABBREVIATIONS
dDAVP, desamino, D-arginine, vasopressin
ODS, osmotic demyelination syndrome

rise in the P_{Na} in patients with hypokalemia or malnutrition, as they are at high risk for the development of osmotic demyelination syndrome (e.g., patients who are K^+ depleted or malnourished; see Chapter 10, page 341 for more discussion).

DISCUSSION OF CASE 14-1

CASE 14-1: WHY DID HYPOKALEMIA DEVELOP SO QUICKLY?

(Case presented on page 462)

What is the emergency therapy for acute, severe hypokalemia in this patient?

- Because the patient has a life-threatening cardiac arrhythmia, the goal is to raise his P_K quickly. We would infuse a solution with high concentration of KCl via a central line.

K+ CONCENTRATION IN THE INTERSTITIAL FLUID IN THE HEART
As discussed in Mini-Case 14-1, page 503, diffusion of ions between capillaries of the heart and myocardial cells is likely to be quite rapid due to "stirring" of the interstitial fluid by myocardial contraction once mycardial contractility improves.

Our immediate aim is to have a sustained rise in the P_K by 1 mmol/L. Therefore, we would infuse 3 mmol K^+ per minute for the first few minutes. The rationale for selecting this dose is that blood volume is 5 L, cardiac output is 5 L/min, and 60% of the blood volume is plasma (i.e., 3 L). A smaller infusion rate would be selected if the cardiac output is obviously less than 5 L/min. The increase in the concentration of K^+ in the interstitial fluid bathing cardiac myocytes (which is really what is needed to deal with the cardiac arrhythmia) would be much smaller (*see margin note*). Following this initial K^+ bolus, we would reduce the rate of infusion of K^+ and measure the P_K (stopping the infusion for at least 1 minute to avoid a spuriously high P_K). If the electrocardiographic changes do not improve and/or the P_K is significantly lower than 3 mmol/L, we would repeat this procedure.

How much K^+ do you anticipate the patient will need to bring his P_K to a safe range?

- This cannot be deduced in advance; you will have to give enough K^+ to maintain the P_K at a safe level (~3 mmol/L).

For K^+ to be retained in cells, electroneutrality must be present. Hence either K^+ must enter with an anion (usually phosphate during anabolic state such as treatment of pernicious anemia or recovery from diabetic ketoacidosis) or another cation must exit (Na^+ or H^+). There is a limited quantity of Na^+ in cells (~10 to 20 mmol/L), and not all of this Na^+ is likely to exit when K^+ enters. There are many H^+ that are bound to histidines (in proteins or in the form of carnosine, a dipeptide of alanine, and histidine in skeletal muscle cells). If entry of K^+ is accompanied by exit of H^+, the P_{HCO3} will fall and limit this process unless K^+ is given with HCO_3^- or potential HCO_3^-. In the latter instance, much more K^+ may be able to enter cells (*see margin note*).

What therapy will be needed to deal with the K^+ load that was given after K^+ started to shift out of cells?

Several strategies are needed to deal with the danger of a very large shift of K^+ from cells to the ECF compartment. First, make sure that hemodialysis is available. Second, infuse calcium to antagonize the cardiac electrical abnormalities attributable to hyperkalemia. Third, give a bolus of insulin (with enough glucose to prevent hypoglycemia). Fourth, increase the rate of excretion of K^+ in the urine with the administration of diuretics and perhaps also an exogenous mineralocorticoid (e.g., 200 μg of 9α fludrocortisone).

MAGNITUDE OF THE K^+ LOAD THAT WAS GIVEN THIS PATIENT
- The patient received ~600 mmol of K^+, which likely exceeds the total intracellular quantity of Na^+ in his cells.
- Since his P_K did not rise above 2.5 mmol/L, a large portion of this K^+ load entered cells, and it was likely accompanied by the exit of H^+.
- Perhaps the administration of K^+ with a precursor of HCO_3^- in this patient "permitted" NHE to export more H^+ and, therefore, more K^+ was needed to raise his P_K.

DIAGNOSIS

The only symptom that is attributable to hypokalemia per se is weakness, but it is not present in all patients with this electrolyte disorder. Notwithstanding, it may be more prevalent in patients with an acute and severe degree of hypokalemia.

There are no central nervous system symptoms or signs directly resulting from hypokalemia because the blood-brain barrier protects the brain from changes in the arterial P_K. Notwithstanding, patients with hypokalemia may have paresthesias and depressed deep tendon reflexes due to delayed peripheral nerve conduction. Patients with hypokalemia and magnesium deficiency usually have more severe symptoms (e.g., tetany).

An important component of the muscle weakness associated with hypokalemia is a reduction of gastrointestinal motility, with symptoms ranging from constipation to those related to paralytic ileus. The two major complications of hypokalemia in skeletal muscles are rhabdomyolysis and muscle weakness or paralysis.

Chronic hypokalemia may lead to carbohydrate intolerance and possibly overt diabetes mellitus. It has been well documented that chronic hypokalemia can predispose a patient to the development of hypertension due to the retention of NaCl.

Chronic K^+ depletion is associated with changes in renal function. Although it is said that these patients have an impaired maximum urinary concentrating ability with polydipsia and vasopressin-resistant polyuria, this is not a universal finding (discussed in more detail in Chapter 11, page 389). In the acid-base area, there is a reduced excretion of citrate and HCO_3^-, because their reabsorption in the proximal convoluted tubule is increased; this may lead to hypocitraturia and an increased precipitation of ionized calcium in the late part of the nephron. The enhanced reabsorption of HCO_3^- along with an increased rate of renal ammoniagenesis may lead to the development of metabolic alkalosis (see Chapter 7, page 199 for more discussion). Moreover, the increased formation and release of NH_4^+ into the renal vein may play a role in the pathogenesis of hepatic encephalopathy in patients with severe liver disease.

Chronic hypokalemia may be associated with tubulo-interstitial kidney disease and the formation of renal cysts. In addition, nephrocalcinosis may develop (see Chapter 4, page 103 for more discussion).

A list of the causes of hypokalemia is provided in Table 14-2.

The initial step in the diagnostic approach to patients with hypokalemia is to determine if there is an acute shift of K^+ into cells (Flow Chart 14-2).

ABBREVIATIONS
ENaC, epithelial Na^+ ion channel
EABV, effective arterial blood volume

TABLE 14-2 **CAUSES OF HYPOKALEMIA**

Decreased intake of K^+

Rarely a sole cause unless K^+ intake is very low and duration is prolonged
Can lead to a more severe degree of the hypokalemia if there is an ongoing K^+ loss

Shift of K^+ into cells

Hormones (insulin and β_2-adrenergics are most important)
Alkalemia (not a major mechanism for hypokalemia)
Anabolic state (e.g., recovery from diabetic ketoacidosis)
Other (e.g., anesthesia, hypokalemic periodic paralysis)

Increased K^+ loss

Loss of K^+ in the urine

More reabsorption of Na^+ than Cl^- in the CCD
  High aldosterone levels
  Constitutively active ENaC (e.g., Liddle's syndrome)
  Artificial ENaC (e.g., amphotericin B)
  Cortisol acts as a mineralocorticoid
    Low 11β-HSDH activity (apparent mineralocorticoid excess syndrome)
    Inhibitors of 11β-HSDH (e.g., licorice)
    Very high cortisol level (e.g., ACTH-producing tumor)
Relatively more reabsorption of Na^+ than Cl^- in the CCD
  Delivery of Na^+ with little Cl^- to the CCD and a low EABV (e.g., a Na salt of penicillin)
  Inhibition of Cl^- reabsorption in the CCD (e.g., due to bicarbonaturia)
  High delivery of Na^+ and Cl^- to the CCD and a V_{max} for Na^+ reabsorption that exceeds that for Cl^- (inhibition of NaCl reabsorption an upstream nephron segment plus a decreased EABV)

Loss of K^+ via the gastrointestinal tract

Diarrhea of any etiology (infectious, toxic, laxative abuse, villous adenoma, short bowel syndrome)

Loss of K^+ via the skin

Conditions with increased loss of K^+ in sweat (e.g., fever in a patient with cystic fibrosis)

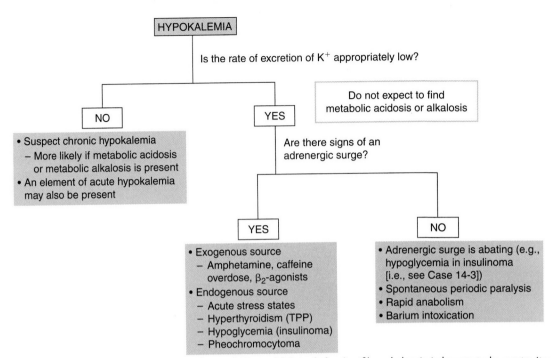

FLOW CHART 14-2 Diagnostic approach to a patient with hypokalemia. If hypokalemia is known to be acute, its basis is a recent shift of K⁺ into cells. In the absence of this evidence, the steps to follow are illustrated in the flow chart and the final diagnostic categories are in the *green shaded boxes*, preceded by a *bullet symbol*.

Steps in the clinical approach to a patient suspected of having acute hypokalemia

- Deductive reasoning is required to reach a diagnosis in most of these patients.
- The most important initial step is to establish whether the duration of illness is short.
- The following charateristics should be present if the basis is a shift of K⁺ into cells.
  - The most important etiology is an adrenergic surge that lasts for many hours.
  - There should be a minimum rate of excretion of K⁺.
  - Metabolic acidosis or metabolic alkalosis should not be present.

The only patient who will have a confirmed diagnosis of acute hypokalemia is one who has had his or her P_K measured within a short period of time prior to the development of hypokalemia. Since this is very uncommon, one must rely on deductive reasoning in most patients suspected of having hypokalemia due to an acute shift of K⁺ into cells (see Flow Chart 14-2).

Our preference is to begin by examining the rate of excretion of K⁺. The expected renal response in a patient with acute hypokalemia is the minimum rate of excretion of K⁺ in human subjects (<10 to 15 mmol/day). Since the bladder may contain an unknown volume of urine prior to beginning the timed urine collection, the measured excretion rate may be overestimation. Accordingly, we rely on the ratio of the concentrations of K^+ and creatinine in a spot urine sample to reflect the rate of excretion of K^+ because creatinine is excreted at a near constant rate throughout the day (20 mg or 200 μmol/kg body weight/min; *see margin note*). In a patient with acute hypokalemia due solely to a shift of K^+ into cells, this rate should be less than 15 mmol K^+/g creatinine or less than 1.5 mmol K^+/mmol creatinine.

There is one possible caveat in using the $U_K/U_{Creatinine}$ to determine if the basis of hypokalemia is an acute shift of K^+ into cells. This ratio may be low in a patient with chronic hypokalemia due to extrarenal loss of K^+ or a renal loss of K^+ in the recent past. In both of those settings, it is likely that a metabolic acid-base disorder will be present.

Conversely, $U_K/U_{Creatinine}$ will be higher than 15 mmol/g creatinine or higher than 1.5 mmol K^+/mmol creatinine if the diagnostic category is chronic hypokalemia. This impression is strengthened if metabolic acidosis or metabolic alkalosis is also present in that patient. Nevertheless, there could still be an element of acute hypokalemia in some of these patients.

Having established that there is an acute shift of K^+ into cells, the next step is to determine if an adrenergic surge is its cause. In these settings, tachycardia, a wide pulse pressure, and systolic hypertension are often present. It is very important to recognize this group of patients because the administration of nonspecific β-blockers can lead to a very prompt recovery (i.e., within 2 hours) without a large infusion of KCl.

These patients can be divided into two groups based on whether there is an exogenous or endogenous source of $β_2$-adrenergic agonist with a long duration of action. Be suspicious of an intake of amphetamines if the patient is obese (used to suppress appetite) or under undue stress, as in preparation for examinations (used to increase alertness while studying). Similarly, if a patient is suffering from asthma, the shift of K^+ may have been provoked by the repeated use of a large dose of $β_2$-agonists to relieve bronchospasm. Rarely, the intake of a very large quantity of caffeine (e.g., coffee, caffeinated soda pop, cocoa, or very large intake of chocolate) can provoke the attack. In the endogenous category, hypokalemia can be found in an acute and prolonged stress states (e.g., head trauma, subarachnoid hemorrhage, myocardial infarction, acute pancreatitis, alcohol withdrawal). Another example of a prolonged high adrenergic state is hyperthyroidism, especially in young Asian males (thyrotoxic periodic paralysis). In this setting, there may be an acute provocative factor to induce a shift of K^+ into cells (common ones mentioned are recovery from a bout of vigorous exercise and possibly a high intake of carbohydrates). There are other disorders with a long-acting endogenous adrenergic surge that can induce an acute shift of K^+ into cells such as hypoglycemia due to the release of insulin from an insulinoma or a pheochromocytoma.

In the absence of a high adrenergic state, suspect familial-type periodic paralysis, especially in Caucasians or the presence of a rapid anabolic state (*see margin note*).

Clinical approach to patients with chronic hypokalemia

If the patient has chronic hypokalemia, the first step is to examine the acid-base status in plasma (a list of causes of hypokalemia and metabolic acidosis or metabolic alkalosis is provided in Table 14-3).

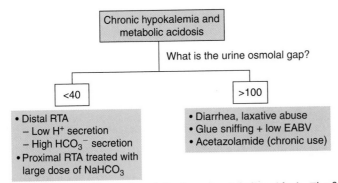

USE OF URINE OSMOLAL GAP TO ESTIMATE EXCRETION OF NH_4^+
- The advantage of using the urine osmolal gap over the urine anion gap to estimate the rate of excretion of NH_4^+ is that it does require that Cl^- be the anion excreted with NH_4^+.
- While the anion excreted with NH_4^+ is Cl^- when there is a loss of $NaHCO_3$ via the GI tract, the anion excreted with NH_4^+ is hippurate in the glue sniffer (overproduction of hippuric acid).

FLOW CHART 14-3 Chronic hypokalemia and metabolic acidosis. The first step in these patients is to estimate the concentration of NH_4^+ in the urine using the osmolal gap.

Subgroup with metabolic acidosis

The group of patients with metabolic acidosis can be divided into two categories by examining the rate of excretion of NH_4^+ (Flow Chart 14-3). To perform this task, estimate the concentration of NH_4^+ in the urine (U_{NH4}) using the urine osmolal gap (see Chapter 2, page 50; *see margin note*). To convert this concentration term into an excretion rate, divide the U_{NH4} by the $U_{Creatinine}$ and multiply by an estimate of the daily rate of excretion of creatinine.

U_{NH4} AND THE URINE OSMOLAL GAP
The U_{NH4} is the urine osmolal gap divided by 2.

Subgroup with metabolic alkolosis

Patients with chronic hypokalemia and metabolic alkalosis can be divided into two major categories based on their current rate of renal excretion of K^+ using the ratio of the concentrations of K^+ and creatinine in the urine: those with a current low rate of excretion of K^+ and those with a high current renal excretion of K^+ (Flow Chart 14-4). Those with a low value for this ratio (i.e., <30 mmol K^+ per g creatinine or per 10 mmol creatinine) will have conditions with a loss of K^+ in the past (i.e., prior but not current use of diuretics) or high rates of

TABLE 14-3 PLASMA ACID-BASE STATUS AND HYPOKALEMIA

Patients with hyperchloremic metabolic acidosis

- Gastrointestinal loss of $NaHCO_3$ (e.g., diarrhea, laxative abuse, fistula, ileus, ureteral diversion)
- Overproduction of hippuric acid (e.g., toluene abuse)
- Reduced reabsorption of $NaHCO_3$ in the proximal convoluted tubule (e.g., proximal renal tubular acidosis treated with large amounts of $NaHCO_3$, chronic use of acetazolamide)
- Distal renal tubular acidosis
  - Low distal H^+ secretion subtype
  - High distal secretion of HCO_3^- (e.g., Southeast Asian ovalocytosis with second mutation involving the Cl^-/HCO_3^- anion exchanger)

Patients with metabolic alkalosis

- Vomiting, nasogastric suction, some types of diarrhea
- Diuretic use or abuse
- Other disorders: can be classified based on blood pressure and/or P_{Renin}
  - Patients with a low effective arterial blood volume, the absence of hypertension, and a high P_{Renin} (e.g., Bartter's syndrome, Gitelman's syndrome, ligand binding to Ca-SR in thick ascending limb of the loop of Henle)
  - Patients with a high effective arterial blood volume and hypertension (e.g., renal artery stenosis, malignant hypertension, primary hyperaldosteronism, glucocorticoid remedial aldosteronism, Liddle's syndrome, apparent mineralocorticoid excess syndrome, Cushing's syndrome).

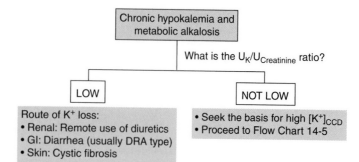

FLOW CHART 14-4 Chronic hypokalemia and metabolic alkalosis. In a patient with chronic hypokalemia and metabolic alkalosis, the first step is to determine the $U_K/U_{Creatinine}$. If this estimate of the rate of excretion of K^+ is definitely low, look for a nonrenal or a prior renal loss of K^+. Conversely, if the $U_K/U_{Creatinine}$ is *not* low, determine why the $[K^+]_{CCD}$ is higher than expected. $[K^+]_{CCD}$, concentration of K^+ in the lumen of terminal CCD.

loss of K^+ by nonrenal routes such as in sweat (e.g., cystic fibrosis) or via the GI tract (e.g., in diarrhea fluid, ileus, or drainage fluids). This latter group is considered in more detail in Flow Chart 14-5.

- The most common explanation for a high $[K^+]_{CCD}$ is a more negative voltage in the lumen of the CCD due to a higher rate of electrogenic reabsorption of Na^+ (i.e., more Na^+ is reabsorbed than Cl^-).
- There are two major categories for this high lumen-negative voltage: reabsorption of more Na^+ than Cl^- in the CCD.

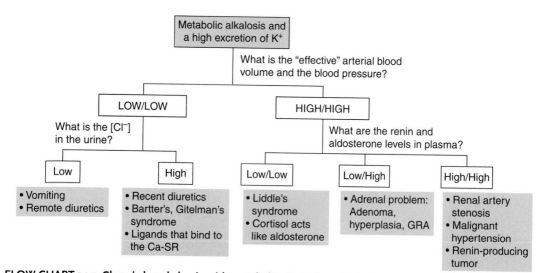

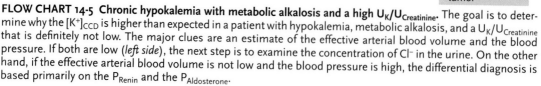

FLOW CHART 14-5 Chronic hypokalemia with metabolic alkalosis and a high $U_K/U_{Creatinine}$. The goal is to determine why the $[K^+]_{CCD}$ is higher than expected in a patient with hypokalemia, metabolic alkalosis, and a $U_K/U_{Creatinine}$ that is definitely not low. The major clues are an estimate of the effective arterial blood volume and the blood pressure. If both are low (*left side*), the next step is to examine the concentration of Cl^- in the urine. On the other hand, if the effective arterial blood volume is not low and the blood pressure is high, the differential diagnosis is based primarily on the P_{Renin} and the $P_{Aldosterone}$.

In the patients who have chronic hypokalemia and metabolic alkalosis, and a large, renal excretion of K^+, the steps to take are provided in Flow Chart 14-4. In essence, we are trying to divide these patients on the basis of a high $[K^+]_{CCD}$: those with more reabsorption of Na^+ and those with less reabsorption of Cl^- in the CCD. The clinical indices that help in the differential diagnosis are an assessment of the effective arterial blood volume, the blood pressure, and the ability to conserve Na^+ and Cl^- in response to a contracted effective arterial blood volume.

More reabsorption of Na^+ than Cl^- in the CCD

These patients are expected to have hypertension, an effective arterial blood volume that is not low, and an ability to conserve Na^+ and Cl^- in response to low effective arterial blood volume. This pathophysiology can be caused by two groups of disorders (Fig. 14-1) based on the $P_{Aldosterone}$. One group consists of conditions with high $P_{Aldosterone}$, whereas the other includes the conditions where the actions of aldosterone are mimicked, and as a result, the $P_{Aldosterone}$ is low. A list of the conditions can be found in Table 14-3 as well as in Figure 14-1. In the patient with more reabsorption of Na^+ than Cl^- in the

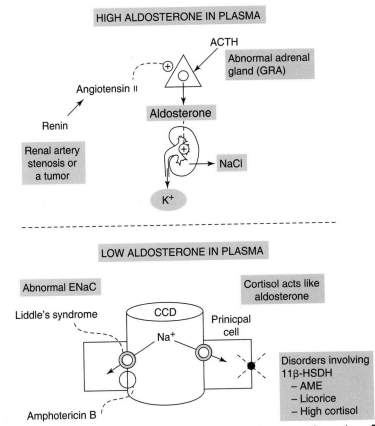

FIGURE 14-1 **Conditions causing hypokalemia with more reabsorption of Na^+ than Cl^- in the CCD.** Conditions in which there is both hypokalemia and an abnormally high $P_{Aldosterone}$ are illustrated in the *upper portion*. In contrast, conditions with hypokalemia but low $P_{Aldosterone}$ are illustrated in the *lower portion*. ACE, angiotensin-converting enzyme; ACTH, adrenocorticotropic hormone; AME, apparent mineralocorticoid excess syndrome; ENaC, epithelial Na^+ channel; GRA, glucocorticoid remediable aldosteronism; 11β-HSDH, 11β-hydroxysteroid dehydrogenase.

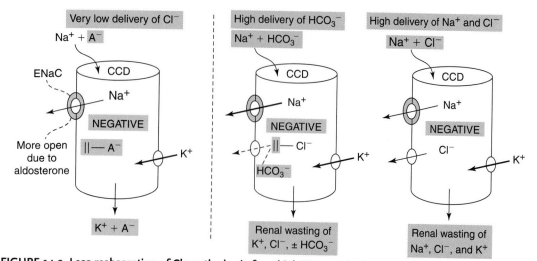

FIGURE 14-2 Less reabsorption of Cl⁻ as the basis for a high [K⁺]$_{CCD}$. The *barrel-shaped structures* represent the CCD. In all three settings, there is electrogenic reabsorption of Na⁺ because of a lower rate of Cl⁻ reabsorption in these nephron segments. As shown to the *left of the vertical dashed line*, a low distal delivery of Cl⁻ is the reason for reabsorbing more Na⁺ than Cl⁻ in the CCD (the urine contains very little Cl⁻). As shown to the *right of the vertical dashed line*, while the urine contains abundant Cl⁻, the reason for reabsorbing more Na⁺ than Cl⁻ in the CCD is either that HCO₃⁻ and/or an alkaline luminal pH decreases the "permeability" for Cl⁻ in the CCD (*middle portion*) or that there is a large delivery of Na⁺ and Cl⁻ to the CCD due to inhibition of their reabsorption in an upstream nephron segment and that aldosterone is present to open the epithelial Na⁺ channel (ENaC) units, which permits reabsorption of more Na⁺ than Cl⁻ in the CCD (*far right portion*).

CCD and a high-P$_{Aldosterone}$ type of disorder, measurement of the activity of renin in plasma (P$_{Renin}$) is helpful in determining the cause (see Table 14-2).

Less reabsorption of Cl⁻ than Na⁺ in the CCD

These patients are expected to have a low effective arterial blood volume, the absence of hypertension, and an inability to conserve Na⁺ and Cl⁻ in response to low effective arterial blood volume. The pathophysiology that leads to a lower rate of reabsorption of Cl⁻ in the CCD is illustrated in Figure 14-2. The most common causes are protracted vomiting or the use of diuretic agents (see Chapter 7, pages 211 and 212 for more discussion of this topic). The use of urine electrolytes in the differential diagnosis of hypokalemia in a patient with a contracted effective arterial blood volume is summarized in Table 14-4.

TABLE 14-4 **URINE ELECTROLYTES IN THE DIFFERENTIAL DIAGNOSIS OF HYPOKALEMIA IN A PATIENT WITH A CONTRACTED EFFECTIVE ARTERIAL BLOOD VOLUME**

Adjust values of the urine electrolyte concentration when polyuria is present.

CONDITION	URINE ELECTROLYTE	
	Na⁺	*Cl⁻*
Vomiting		
Recent	High	Low
Remote	Low	Low
Diuretics		
Recent	High	High
Remote	Low	Low
Diarrhea or laxative abuse	Low	High
Bartter's or Gitelman's syndrome	High	High

High, urine concentration > 15 mmol/L; Low, urine concentration < 15 mmol/L.

PART C
SPECIFIC CAUSES
OF HYPOKALEMIA

A list of the causes of hypokalemia is provided in Table 14-2. We begin with the disorders where there is a shift of K^+ into cells and then discuss the disorders of chronic hypokalemia in the order in Flow Charts 14-4 and 14-5.

HYPOKALEMIC PERIODIC PARALYSIS

Patients with hypokalemic periodic paralysis are divided into two categories. The first group is heterogeneous and its common feature is an absence of a hereditary basis (*see margin note*). The second group includes two entities characterized by hypokalemia and paralysis: thyrotoxic periodic paralysis and familial hypokalemia and paralysis.

The thyrotoxic subgroup is more common in Asian and Hispanic males with an age range of 20 to 50 for their first attack, whereas the familial periodic paralysis is more common in Caucasian males under the age of 20. While it is stated that attacks can be provoked by a large carbohydrate meal (release of insulin) or during the period of rest after strenuous exercise (β_2-adrenergic surge) in both of these subgroups, this correlations is not impressive when large groups of patients are studied. Moreover, it is difficult to understand how these stimuli can result in an effect that lasts for many hours.

Pathophysiology

In thyrotoxic periodic paralysis, the hyperthyroidism may be evident before the first attack, or it may be occult. At times, hyperthyroidism may become clinically evident at a much later time. The actions of thyroid hormone lead to more Na-K-ATPase in the cell membrane of skeletal muscle cells, which can contribute to a greater shift of K^+ into cells with a strong stimulus that would not cause acute hypokalemia in normal subjects. Moreover, once the acute attack is over, the patients remain normokalemic for prolonged periods of time.

Molecular basis

Genetic analyses in patients with familial periodic paralysis have suggested that the abnormality in many of these patients is linked to the gene that encodes for the α subunit of the dihydropyridine-sensitive calcium ion channel in skeletal muscles; it is not clear how this leads to the effects on resting membrane potential and P_K. The familial variety is inherited as an autosomal dominant disorder.

Clinical picture

The dominant finding is recurrent, transient episodes of muscle weakness that may progress to paralysis in association with a severe degree of hypokalemia (often <2.0 mmol/L). In Asian and Hispanic

SECONDARY CAUSES OF HYPOKALEMIA AND PARALYSIS
These conditions provoke a prolonged adrenergic surge:
- *Exogenous causes*: Ingestion of amphetamines, excessive intake of caffeine, use of β_2-adrenergics to treat asthma.
- *Endogenous causes*: Conditions with extreme stress (e.g., myocardial infection, trauma, subarachnoid hemorrhage), insulin release from an insulinoma, pheochromocytoma

populations, the disorder occurs almost exclusively in young males, and it is commonly associated with thyrotoxicosis. In Caucasian populations, the familial, nonthyrotoxic variety usually manifests in the teenage years.

Diagnosis

The diagnosis hinges on finding the characteristic clinical picture, but laboratory findings are very helpful in differentiating this form of acute hypokalemia from an acute presentation in patients with chronic hypokalemia. First, there is an absence of acid-base disorders. Second, one should anticipate a low rate of excretion of K^+ as manifested by a low $U_K/U_{Creatinine}$ ratio in the urine. If an adrenergic surge or hyperthyroidism is the basis of an acute shift of K^+ into cells, expect to find tachycardia and a wide pulse pressure on physical examination and a precipitating event. The signs of overt hyperthyroidism may be present in patients with thyrotoxic periodic paralysis and they are absent in patients with familial periodic paralysis. Plasma phosphate levels are usually somewhat low in both entities.

Differential diagnosis

The clinical and laboratory findings help to differentiate hypokalemic periodic paralysis from a chronic potassium wasting disease together with an acute shift of K^+ into cells. One other point helps in the differential diagnosis. Patients with hypokalemic periodic paralysis usually need far less KCl to bring their P_K to a safe level (~3 mmol/L) than do patients who have a chronic K^+ wasting disease together with a reason to shift K^+ acutely into cells (~1 vs. >3 mmol KCl/kg body weight).

Therapy

In an acute attack, patients are treated with KCl; its rate of administration should not exceed about 10 mmol/hr unless there is a cardiac arrhythmia. There is, however, the risk of post-treatment hyperkalemia as K^+ move back into the ECF compartment.

Patients with the thyrotoxic variety of hypokalemic periodic paralysis have been successfully treated with a nonselective β-blocker (propranolol) and a much smaller dose of KCl. In retrospective case-controlled studies, rebound hyperkalemia (>5.0 mmol/L) was observed in 30% to 70% of patients with thyrotoxic hypokalemic periodic paralysis if more than 90 mmol of KCl were given within 24 hours or at a rate of more than 10 mmol/hr. Hence, we prefer to give less than this amount unless the P_K fails to rise to a safe level of about 3 mmol/L. Propanolol may also be useful to treat hypokalemia accompanied by a high adrenergic activity, caffeine, or an excessive dose of amphetamines. Hyperthyroidism, if present, is treated in the usual fashion. Patients are advised to avoid carbohydrate-rich meals and vigorous exercise. In the longer term, nonselective β-blockers may reduce the number of the attacks of paralysis with little effect on the degree of fall in the P_K during the attack.

Acetazolamide (250–750 mg/day) has been used successfully in patients with the familial form of hypokalemic periodic paralysis, although the basis of its beneficial effect is unclear.

DISTAL RENAL TUBULAR ACIDOSIS

Pathophysiology

Hypokalemia, which can be severe at times, is commonly seen in patients with distal renal tubular acidosis that is due to a low net rate of secretion of H^+ (e.g., an inherited disorder, an acquired defect in a number of autoimmune disorders, or disorders with dysproteinemias) affecting the H^+-ATPase in the CCD or an accelerated secretion of HCO_3^- in the CCD, as in patients with Southeast Asian ovalocytosis and a second mutation affecting the Cl^-/HCO_3^- anion exchanger (see Chapter 4, page 96 for more discussion of this topic). The accelerated secretion of K^+ could be due to an effect of HCO_3^- in the lumen of the CCD and/or the alkaline luminal pH to decrease the rate of reabsorption of Cl^-, or perhaps to cause an increase the number of open ROMK channels in the luminal membrane of principal cells in the CCD.

Diagnosis

The clinical features include the presence of hypokalemia, metabolic acidosis with a normal $P_{Anion\,gap}$, a low rate of excretion of NH_4^+, and a high urine pH (~ 7). A number of these patients, however, are first diagnosed after presentation with recurrent calcium phosphate stones and possibly, nephrocalcinosis.

Therapy

- If the patient presents with a significant degree of hypokalemia, K^+ must be given as KCl.
- $NaHCO_3$ to raise the P_{HCO3} must not be administered until the P_K is increased to a safe level (>3 mmol/L).

The administration of K^+ with a precursor of HCO_3^- (e.g., citrate) seems rational to correct both the hypokalemia and metabolic acidosis. Although this therapy may lead to a further increase in urine pH and hence the fraction of divalent phosphate relative to the total amount of phosphate in the urine, the risk of this small incremental increase in the concentration of divalent phosphate must be compared with the possible benefit resulting from a lower concentration of ionized calcium in the urine, as there is an increased rate of excretion of citrate when any form of alkali is given.

GLUE SNIFFING

Pathophysiology

Metabolism of toluene leads to the production of hippuric acid (see Fig. 3-2, page 73). The excretion of hippurate anions in the urine at a rate that exceeds that of NH_4^+ leads to sodium wasting and contraction of the effective arterial blood volume. Accordingly, there is an excessive excretion of K^+ due to the electrogenic reabsorption of Na^+ in the CCD caused by more open ENaC units in the luminal membrane of principal cells in the CCD due to actions of aldosterone and the delivery of Na^+ to the CCD without Cl^- (i.e., with hippurate, an anion that cannot be reabsorbed in the CCD; see Fig. 14-2).

Diagnosis

This is based on the presence of hypokalemia, metabolic acidosis with a normal $P_{Anion\ gap}$, or a high rate of excretion of NH_4^+ in the urine with an anion other than Cl^- that has a high fractional excretion (hippurate anions are filtered and secreted in the proximal tubule). There may also be a low P_{Urea} (see Chapter 3, page 72 for more details).

Therapy

If the patient presents with a significant degree of hypokalemia, K^+ must be given as KCl; the administration of $NaHCO_3$ should be avoided until P_K has reached to a safe level (~3 mmol/L).

DIARRHEA

> • There are two groups of patients who have diarrhea and a very low P_K (Table 14-5).

The first group of patients with diarrhea has a secretory type of diarrhea, a very low effective arterial blood volume, and a large deficit of K^+. Hypokalemia, however, is usually only present in these patients *after* therapy begins. This is because severe intravascular volume depletion leads to an α-adrenergic surge and thereby inhibition of the release of insulin, which causes a shift of K^+ out of cells. This pathophysiology is reversed with reexpansion of the intravascular volume.

The second group of patients with diarrhea does not have a large delivery of Na^+ and Cl^- to the colon; rather, they have a major defect in the reabsorption of Na^+ and Cl^- in the colon. They present to the

TABLE 14-5 **HYPOKALEMIA IN A PATIENT WITH DIARRHEA**

For details, see text. The patient with secretory diarrhea has a large deficit of K^+, but only develops a low P_K after therapy with intravenous NaCl. In contrast, the patient with a diminished reabsorption of Na^+ and Cl^- in the colon will present with a low P_K but may have only a relatively small deficit of K^+ in total body terms.

FEATURES	SECRETORY DIARRHEA (e.g., CHOLERA)	LESS REABSORPTION OF Na⁺ AND Cl⁻ IN THE COLON (e.g., DRA)
Clinical	• "Explosive" onset • Hemodynamic urgency • Anticipate low P_K and pulmonary edema during therapy	• Slow onset • Mild low EABV • Danger: Possibly from a low P_K
Electrolyte issues		
• K^+	• α-adrenergic = K^+ exits cells • K^+ loss: Mainly GI, and it is large • P_K: ~4.5 mmol/L	• β₂-adrenergic = K^+ enters cells • K^+ deficit small ± renal K^+ loss • P_K: Often low
• NaCl	• Very large deficit • Extremely contracted EABV • HCO_3^- deficit visible after NaCl is given	• Deficit if low NaCl intake • Mildly contracted EABV • Causes small ↑ P_{HCO_3}
• HCO_3^-	• Very large loss in diarrhea • Deficit HCO_3^- is large • Net: P_{HCO_3} ~ 20 mmol/L	• Virtually no HCO_3^- loss in diarrhea • Mild contraction alkalosis

EABV, effective arterial blood volume.

hospital with a low P_K but only a modest deficit of K^+ unless there is *also* a cause for an increased delivery of Na^+ and Cl^- to the colon (e.g., some forms of laxative use). Accordingly, the major basis for the low P_K in this subgroup of patients is a shift of K^+ into cells secondary to a modest β-adrenergic response owing to the milder degree of contraction of the effective arterial blood volume.

Secretory diarrhea type

- This has an explosive onset and huge loss of Na^+, Cl^-, K^+, and HCO_3^- in the diarrhea fluid (e.g., the patient with cholera).
- Since the Cl^-/HCO_3^- anion exchanger has a higher maximum velocity than the Na^+/H^+ exchanger in the colonic cell luminal membrane, the diarrhea fluid typically contains 40 to 45 mmol HCO_3^-/L.
- The major issues with respect to K^+ include a large loss of K^+ via the GI tract, but hypokalemia may not be present due to a shift of K^+ out of cells.

Pathophysiology

The prototype of this type of disorder is the patient with cholera. The major feature is the delivery of more Na^+ and Cl^- to the colon than can be absorbed per unit time in this segment of the bowel. The reason for this large delivery of electrolytes is the insertion of the CFTR Cl^- channels in the luminal membrane of the early small intestine (see Chapter 4, page 107 for more discussion). If contraction of the effective arterial blood volume can be overcome by infusing isotonic saline at a very rapid rate, the quantity of Na^+ and Cl^- excreted daily in the diarrhea fluid can be twofold larger than the content of these ions in the ECF compartment (daily volume of diarrhea can exceed 20 L/day in an adult). In cholera, for example, activation of CFTR persists for the entire small intestinal crypt cell life (~7 days), as binding of the cholera toxin to these crypt cells is irreversible. Hence, the disease persists for up to 1 week, with diminished severity 3 to 4 days after the bacteria are washed away in the very large volume of diarrhea fluid.

Since the Cl^-/HCO_3^- anion exchanger has a higher maximum velocity than the Na^+/H^+ exchanger in the colonic cell luminal membrane, the diarrhea fluid typically contains 40 to 45 mmol HCO_3^-/L (*see margin note*).

Electrolyte disorders

The major effect is a very large deficit of Na^+ and Cl^- that is often close to half of their content in the ECF compartment. This large loss of ECF volume increases the P_{HCO3} markedly, but recall that there is a large deficit of $NaHCO_3$; thus, the P_{HCO3} can be close to the normal range.

The large loss of K^+ in diarrhea fluid (~15 mmol/L) leads to a major deficit of K^+. The α-adrenergic response to the very severe degree of contraction of the effective arterial blood volume leads to inhibition of the release of insulin. As a result, there is a shift of K^+ out of cells. Hence, the P_K is commonly in the higher end of the normal range.

Once the patient receives a large infusion of saline, the α-adrenergic effects are no longer present. If the $β_2$-adrenergic response persists,

EFFECT OF LARGE INFUSIONS OF NaCl ON THE P_{HCO3}
There will be a progressive fall in the P_{HCO3} for three reasons:
- Dilution due to retained $NaHCO_3$
- Increased loss of $NaHCO_3$ in the diarrhea fluid because of enhanced secretion of NaCl in the small intestine leading to large delivery of Na^+ and Cl^- to the colon
- Removal of HCO_3^- from plasma following the release of H^+ bound to histidines in skeletal muscle. This is the result of a fall in the P_{CO2} in capillaries in muscle (see Fig. 3-1, page 66).

the P_K may fall to dangerously low values. Hypokalemia may cause low GI motility, and if ileus develops, a large volume of fluid may be retained in the lumen of the GI tract (this is called *cholera sicca*).

Therapy

In the secretory diarrhea group, a very large infusion of saline is needed to partially reexpand the ECF volume. Nevertheless, this improvement in hemodynamics leads to additional problems. First, once the ECF volume is expanded sufficiently to remove the α-adrenergic response, hypokalemia will develop. Second, with the presence of a continuing stimulus to release β_2-adrenergics, there will be a large shift of K^+ into cells; a severe degree of hypokalemia may develop, especially if there is a large loss of K^+ in diarrhea fluid. Therefore, these patients will need a large quantity of KCl after the first few liters of intravenous saline are given, and one must monitor the P_K closely to plan further therapy with K^+. These patients also have a very large deficit of HCO_3^- in the ECF compartment due the loss of $NaHCO_3$ in prior diarrhea fluid. Notwithstanding, the P_{HCO3} may be close to the normal range because the ECF volume may be reduced by more than 50%; see Chapter 2, page 57 for more details on how to calculate the deficit of HCO_3^- in the ECF compartment). Hence, a severe degree of acidemia will develop and if $NaHCO_3$ is not given; in fact, some of these patients will develop pulmonary edema when there is a large infusion of saline without $NaHCO_3$ (see Chapter 3, page 70 for explanation of the mechanism). These patients should be given enough $NaHCO_3$ to prevent the development of a severe degree of acidemia. Recall that the diarrhea fluid has a high fluid concentration of HCO_3^- (~40 to 45 mmol/L). This is an exception to the rule that patients with metabolic acidosis and hypokalemia should not be treated with $NaHCO_3$ because this alkali load is being given to replace ongoing losses and to prevent a more severe degree of acidemia (i.e., it should be safe as long as the P_{HCO3} does not rise significantly). Accordingly the concentration of $NaHCO_3$ in the infusate should be equal to the P_{HCO3} when the goal is to reexpand the ECF volume, whereas the concentration of $NaHCO_3$ in the infusate should be equal to the concentration of HCO_3^- in diarrhea fluid (~40 to 45 mmol/L) when the goal is to replace ongoing losses.

Diminished reabsorption of Na⁺ and Cl⁻ in the colon

Pathophysiology

The major difference in this subtype of diarrhea is that these patients do not have a large increase in the delivery of Na⁺ and Cl⁻ to the colon—hence the volume of diarrhea fluid and the electrolyte deficits are much smaller than in the secretory subtype of diarrhea.

Electrolyte disorders

The unique problem is a decline in the activity of the Cl^-/HCO_3^- anion exchanger (AE) in the luminal membrane of colonic cells of varying severity. When this AE has a diminished catalytic activity, but still *more* than NHE, the diarrhea fluid will still contain HCO_3^-, but appreciably less than 40 mmol/L. On the other hand, if the AE has a *lower* catalytic activity than NHE, the diarrhea fluid will not contain HCO_3^- (overt downregulated in adenoma [DRA]). As a result, the P_{HCO3} will rise due to the loss of NaCl in diarrhea fluid (contraction alkalosis) and there is little if any deficit in HCO_3^- in the ECF compartment (*see margin note*).

If the subject consumes little NaCl, the deficits of Na^+ and Cl^- are somewhat larger and become manifest relatively earlier in the course of the illness. As a result of the smaller deficits of Na^+ and Cl^-, the patients have a β_2-adrenergic response, which causes a shift of K^+ into cells and hypokalemia. There is also K^+ loss in diarrhea fluid plus minor urinary K^+ loss.

Diagnosis

A history of diarrhea may be obtained; abuse of laxatives, however, may be denied. If suspected, measurement of the urine electrolytes may provide helpful clues (see Table 14-4). The U_{Na} is low if the effective arterial blood volume is contracted, but the U_{Cl} may be high if metabolic acidosis and acidemia are present, as they provide the stimulus for a high rate of excretion of NH_4^+ in the urine (*see margin note*). At times, one may have to rely on measurements of stool electrolytes and other evidence for the presence of laxatives in the stool to confirm the diagnosis (*see margin note*).

There are specific findings in individual cases. For example, in congenital chloridorrhea, there is a much earlier age of onset and persistence of the disease throughout the life of the patient. In these patients, there may be benefit from blocking the secretion of HCl in the stomach because this decreases the delivery of Cl^- (and Na^+) to the colon. When stool electrolytes are measured, the predominant electrolytes are Na^+, K^+, and Cl^-. Another group of patients may have DRA secondary to chronic inflammatory bowel disease or to an adenoma or adenocarcinoma of the colon. This topic is discussed in more detail in Chapter 4, page 82.

Therapy

In patients with diarrhea due to a reabsorptive defect in the colon, intravenous saline is also required to reexpand ECF volume, but the rate of infusion should be much slower than in the patient with secretory diarrhea, as the degree of contraction of the ECF volume is usually much less severe. One must add KCl to the first intravenous solution if the patient has an appreciable degree of hypokalemia. Glucose should not be added to the infusate because there is a shift of K^+ into cells due to the release of insulin. $NaHCO_3$ should not be infused in the patient with hypokalemia; in fact, it is not usually needed, as a large deficit of HCO_3^- is rarely observed in these patients.

If the patient has chronic hyponatremia, one should bear in mind that hypokalemia increases the incidence of osmotic demyelination with a rapid rise in the P_{Na}; hence, steps should be taken to limit the rise in the P_{Na} to less than 4 mmol/L/day (see Chapter 10, page 331 for more discussion).

DIURETICS

Pathophysiology

The increased secretion of K^+ in the CCD in these patients is due to an enhanced delivery of Na^+ and Cl^- to the CCD together with a larger capacity to reabsorb Na^+ via ENaC (because of the effects

ACID-BASED DISORDERS IN PATIENTS WHO ABUSE LAXATIVES

- In patients who abuse laxatives, there is rarely enough loss of NaCl in the stool to cause contraction alkalosis.
- There is rarely a sufficient loss of $NaHCO_3$ to cause metabolic acidosis unless there is another cause for a low rate of excretion of NH_4^+.

LOSS OF HCl IN DIARRHEA FLUID

- In the absence of luminal acceptors of H^+, the Na^+/H^+ exchanger cannot raise the luminal concentration of H^+ by appreciably more than an order of magnitude higher than the $[H^+]$ in cells of the colon; hence, this $[H^+]$ is always much less than 1 mmol/L in luminal fluid in patients with DRA or congenital chlorideorrhea. Hence, there is little direct loss of HCl.
- On the other hand, since the luminal fluid in the colon contain an appreciable amount of bacterial protein, when the luminal fluid pH is ~6, there can be appreciable binding of secreted H^+ to histidine residues in these proteins.
- As a result of reabsorption of Na^+ via the NHE, and as many of these secreted H^+ can be bound to H^+ acceptors of bacterial origin, the net effect is the addition of HCO_3^- in the body along with a deficit of Cl^-, without the presence of even 1 mmol of HCl in a liter of feces. In this setting, the feces will have a higher concentration of Cl^- as compared to the sum of the concentrations of Na^+ and K^+.

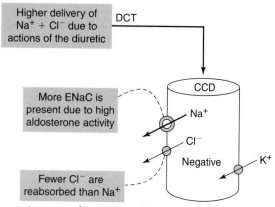

FIGURE 14-3 Augmented secretion of K$^+$ in the CCD. The *horizontal line* represents the distal convoluted tubule (DCT) and the *barrel-shaped structure* represents the CCD. A negative voltage is created in the lumen of the CCD by reabsorbing more Na$^+$ than Cl$^-$ because more open epithelial Na$^+$ channel (ENaC) are present in the luminal membranes of principal cells owing to the high $P_{Aldosterone}$.

of aldosterone released in response to a contracted effective arterial blood volume) than to reabsorb Cl$^-$ (Fig. 14-3).

Clinical picture

The hypokalemia is usually modest in degree if there is a reasonable intake of K$^+$. A P_K that is less than 3 mmol/L is observed in less than 10% of patients taking thiazide diuretics for treatment of hypertension, and it is usually present within the first 2 weeks of therapy.

Diagnosis

This diagnosis is usually evident. At times, abuse of diuretics may be denied.

Differential diagnosis

- Diuretic abuse should be suspected in a patient with hypokalemia and metabolic alkalosis if even one spot urine sample has little Na$^+$ and Cl$^-$, reflecting the normal renal response to a low effective arterial blood volume.

Screening the urine for diuretics is often helpful when diuretic abuse is suspected. The assay should be performed on urine samples that contain an appreciable amount of Na$^+$ and Cl$^-$ because this is when the diuretic would be present. Bartter's syndrome and Gitelman's syndrome are rare disorders, but they should be suspected if the patient denies the use of diuretics and every urine sample contains abundant Na$^+$ and Cl$^-$ while the effective arterial blood volume is contracted. Other diagnoses to rule out include hypercalcemia and other ligands that may bind to the calcium-sensing receptor (e.g., cationic drugs such as gentamicin, cationic proteins). Examining the concentrations of Cl$^-$ and Na$^+$ in the urine can provide clues to distinguish between patients with hypokalemia caused by diuretic abuse from those with hypokalemia caused by "occult" vomiting or the abuse of laxatives (see Table 14-4, page 476).

Therapy

Because patients with ischemic heart disease or left ventricular hypertrophy and those receiving digitalis may be at increased risk for cardiac arrhythmias in the presence of hypokalemia, even a modest degree of hypokalemia should be avoided. Of note, in patients with hypertension treated with thiazides, K^+ depletion may cause a mean rise in blood pressure by 5 to 7 mm Hg, thus diminishing the antihypertensive effect of the diuretic. One possible mechanism of this rise in blood pressure seems to be an effect of K^+ depletion to cause intracellular acidosis in proximal convoluted tubule cells. This stimulates the reabsorption of Na^+ and HCO_3^- directly and Na^+ plus Cl^- indirectly in the proximal convoluted tubule. It also diminishes the delivery of HCO_3^- to the CCD, which may permit more Cl^- to be reabsorbed with Na^+ in these nephron segments. Hence, the net effect of the actions of aldosterone is to cause retention of Na^+ and Cl^-.

Other effects of K^+ depletion include the development of nephropathy with interstitial fibrosis. In addition, there is an enhanced reabsorption of citrate in the proximal convoluted tubule; accordingly, the rate of excretion of citrate is low. The latter may be of concern in patients who are given a thiazide diuretic to prevent calcium oxalate stones.

There are several ways to minimize the degree of diuretic-induced hypokalemia. First, give the lowest effective dose of diuretic, because the risk of hypokalemia is dose dependent. In most patients with essential hypertension, a dose of 12.5 to 25 mg of hydrochlorothiazide produces as great a fall in blood pressure as higher doses of the drug. Second, the intake of K^+ should not be low. Salt substitutes such as Co-Salt (14 mmol K^+/g) are an inexpensive way to provide K^+ while decreasing the intake of Na^+. Third, lowering the rate of K^+ excretion can minimize the degree of hypokalemia. This may be achieved in part by limiting the intake and thereby the excretion of NaCl to less than 100 mmol/day. The renal loss of K^+ can be reduced with the use of potassium-sparing diuretics. We do not favor the use of tablets that combine a thiazide or a loop diuretic plus a diuretic that blocks ENaC (e.g., amiloride) because a higher distal flow rate due to the actions of a thiazide or loop diuretic lowers the luminal concentration of the blockers of ENaC; hence, they become less effective in blocking ENaC.

HYPOMAGNESEMIA

There is a clinically important relationship between hypomagnesemia and hypokalemia. Nevertheless, it is far from clear if magnesium depletion per se leads to renal potassium wasting and hypokalemia or that both the hypomagnesemia and the hypokalemia are caused by the same underlying disorder (e.g., use of diuretics). The most important fact to bear in mind is that patients who have a cardiac arrhythmia associated with hypokalemia may not have the expected response to replacement therapy with KCl until the deficit of magnesium is replaced.

VOMITING

Pathophysiology

Balance data during the drainage period from experimental studies in human volunteers have revealed that the initial deficit is primarily

ANIONS IN THE URINE AND K+ SECRETION
- Cl^-: When the urine has little Cl^-, the reabsorption of Na^+ via ENaC is electrogenic.
- *Organic anions*: A higher excretion of organic anions increases the distal delivery of Na^+ with little Cl^- (e.g., in the later phase of vomiting).

HCl, but also of KCl (see Chapter 7, page 194 for more discussion). In the postdrainage period, however, the deficits become equimolar quantities of K^+ and Cl^-. Because the K^+ concentration in gastric fluid is less than 15 mmol/L, hypokalemia in patients with vomiting or nasogastric suction results primarily from a large loss of K^+ in the urine. The renal mechanism begins with the release of aldosterone in response to angiotensin II that is produced because the effective arterial blood volume is contracted; this hormone leads to an enhanced reabsorption of Na^+ via ENaC in the CCD (see Fig. 14-3). A higher net secretion of K^+ occurs early on, and it may be due in part to the distal delivery of SO_4^{2-} with Na^+, which is the result of the ongoing production of H_2SO_4 from the oxidation of sulfur-containing amino acids, and the normal P_K at this time (see Fig. 7-4, page 200). Once the degree of hypokalemia becomes more severe, SO_4^{2-} is excreted with NH_4^+ and the rate of excretion of K^+ declines, but not to the very low rates in otherwise normal subjects consuming a low-potassium diet (*see margin note*). To a lesser extent, hypokalemia may be the result of a shift of K^+ into the ICF compartment because of the alkalemia.

Clinical picture

The patient may deny vomiting. Be suspicious in patients who are overly concerned about their body weight or body image.

Diagnosis

Key elements are a history of vomiting, a significant degree of hypokalemia, metabolic alkalosis, and a *very low* U_{Cl} (see Table 14-4, page 476). In patients with recent vomiting, the urine may contain abundant Na^+ despite contraction of the effective arterial blood volume because excretion of organic anions and possibly HCO_3^- obligates the excretion of Na^+.

Differential diagnosis

If the patient denies vomiting, other causes of hypokalemia with a low effective arterial blood volume must be considered (see Table 14-2, page 470).

Therapy

Therapy is directed toward the underlying cause of vomiting and the administration of K^+. Because these patients also have a deficit of Cl^-, KCl should be administered. If the patient also has a deficit of NaCl, this salt must be administered if the diet contains little NaCl.

BARTTER'S SYNDROME

Pathophysiology

- Bartter's syndrome can be thought of as a disorder that resembles the constant action of a loop diuretic.

Patients with Bartter's syndrome have a higher than expected rate of excretion of Na^+ and Cl^- in the urine despite a contracted effective arterial blood volume. Renal K^+ wasting results primarily from a high $[K^+]_{CCD}$. This occurs because of an enhanced distal delivery of Na^+ and Cl^- to the CCD together with more reabsorption of Na^+ than Cl^- in this nephron site because of an increased number of open ENaC in the CCD due to the effects of aldosterone, which is released in response to the low effective arterial blood volume (see Fig. 14-3).

Two other functions of the loop of Henle are compromised in patients with Bartter's syndrome. First, because this nephron segment is responsible for concentrating the urine, these patients are unable to have a high U_{Osm} when vasopressin acts. Second, because there is a large amount of calcium reabsorbed in the loop of Henle, if this reabsorption is diminished, the distal delivery of calcium can readily exceed the capacity for its reabsorption in downstream nephron segments. Accordingly, hypercalciuria is a common finding in this setting, and the index used is the urine calcium-to-creatinine ratio. In contrast, although a considerable amount of magnesium is reabsorbed in the loop of Henle, hypomagnesemia is not a common finding in patients with Bartter's syndrome because magnesium reabsorption in the distal convoluted tubule may be up-regulated in these patients; this may prevent the development of hypomagnesemia.

Molecular basis

Mutations that cause Bartter's syndrome have been identified in five separate genes (Fig. 14-4). The first two abnormalities lead to antenatal Bartter's syndrome and include mutations in the gene encoding Na^+, K^+, 2 Cl^- cotransporter (NKCC-2) and the gene

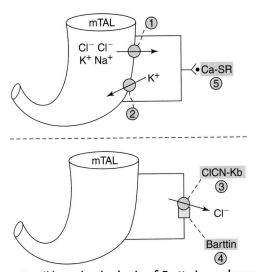

FIGURE 14-4 Possible molecular basis of Bartter's syndrome. Although the figure is shown in two parts to make the lesions less cluttered, the lesions all occur in a single cell type. The *stylized structure* is the thick ascending limb (TAL) of the loop of Henle. The defects that can lead to a diminished reabsorption of Na^+ and Cl^- and thereby Bartter's syndrome are illustrated. Those in the *upper portion* involve the luminal Na^+, K^+, 2 Cl^- cotransporter (NKCC-2; *site 1*); the ROMK channel (*site 2*); or the calcium-sensing receptor (Ca-SR; *site 5*). In the *lower portion*, lesions affecting the basolateral ClCN-Kb (*site 3*) or its β-subunit protein, Barttin (*site 4*), are shown.

encoding the luminal K^+ (rat outer medullary K^+ [ROMK]) channel. A third lesion involves the basolateral Cl^- channel (ClCN-Kb); this may also affect the functions of the distal convoluted tubule. Mutations in the gene that encodes for an essential β-subunit of this Cl^- channel, called *Barttin*, have been reported in patients with Bartter's syndrome and sensory-neural deafness. Patients with Bartter's syndrome and hypocalcemia have been reported; the basis of this disorder is an activating mutation in the gene encoding the calcium-sensing receptor.

Clinical picture

- The initial diagnosis is made early in life in most patients.
- There is often a positive family history and/or consanguinity.

The clinical picture is dominated by contraction of the effective arterial blood volume; hypokalemia; renal wasting of Na^+, Cl^-, and K^+; and metabolic alkalosis. Patients with Bartter's syndrome have an inability to excrete maximally concentrated urine when vasopressin acts. Hypercalciuria is common, but hypomagnesemia is not.

Patients with Bartter's syndrome due to a defective Cl^- channel (ClCN-Kb) may have a more severe clinical disorder, as there are also findings resulting from depressed functions of the distal convoluted tubule (e.g., hypocalciuria, hypomagnesemia) as ClCN-Kb is also expressed in this nephron segment.

Diagnosis

The clinical findings described previously leave little doubt as to the diagnosis. We discuss the acquired forms of this constellation of findings on page 493.

Differential diagnosis

The key element is to establish that the patient has a low effective arterial blood volume; a high P_{Renin} confirms this clinical impression (see Table 14-3). When present, this rules out conditions with hypokalemia in which there is an excess mineralocorticoid activity and Liddle's syndrome. Patients with these disorders are also likely to be hypertensive (see Table 14-2). Considering hypokalemia with a low effective arterial blood volume, the differential diagnosis includes abuse of diuretics or laxatives and "occult" vomiting. The use of urine electrolytes is very helpful in this differential diagnosis; sometimes measurements may need to be done in many spot urine samples to identify diuretic abuse (see Table 14-4).

There are also acquired disorders that lead to a loop diuretic–like effects and hence a Bartter's-like clinical picture. Examples include hypercalcemia and cationic drugs that bind to the calcium-sensing receptor (e.g., gentamicin). It is also possible that cationic proteins may bind to the calcium-sensing receptor and lead to a Bartter's-like clinical picture, as may be the case in a patient with multiple myeloma or in some autoimmune disorders.

Therapy

This is discussed in the section on Gitelman's syndrome.

Antenatal Bartter's syndrome

- Antenatal Bartter's syndrome results from a loss-of-function mutation in the gene encoding for either the NKCC-2 or ROMK; this is a very serious illness because the newborn has a very large degree of renal wasting of NaCl.
- The pregnancy is usually complicated by polyhydramnios and premature delivery.

Features of a defect in NKCC-2 or ROMK subtypes

The loop of Henle is an important site for the reabsorption of Na^+ and Cl^-. The following calculation uses values obtained from micropuncture studies in fed rats and applies them to adult humans for illustrative purposes even though the patient is a newborn, as data are not available in newborn rats. Human adults have about 2100 mmol of Na^+ in their ECF compartment (140 mmol Na^+/L ECF × 15 L ECF = 2100 mmol). The calculation illustrated in the *margin note* reveals that close to 3000 mmol of Na^+ are reabsorbed daily in the loop of Henle, which is appreciably greater than the content of Na^+ in their entire ECF compartment. Therefore, a complete defect in the reabsorption of Na^+ and Cl^- in the loop of Henle (i.e., in its medullary and cortical thick ascending limbs) can cause a very serious deficiency of Na^+ and Cl^-. Because patients with antenatal Bartter's syndrome survive, there must be mechanisms that will decrease the excretion of Na^+ and Cl^-.

Mechanisms that permit these patients to survive

1. *Decrease the delivery of Na^+ and Cl^- to the loop of Henle*: There is an initial large loss of Na^+ and Cl^-, which results in a marked degree of contraction of the effective arterial blood volume. As a result, there is both a large reduction in the GFR and a marked increase in the reabsorption of Na^+ and Cl^- in the proximal convoluted tubule.

2. *Up-regulation of Na^+ and Cl^- reabsorption in nephron sites downstream to the loop of Henle*: Part of this response is limited by actions of prostaglandins. Hence, inhibiting prostaglandin synthesis with cyclooxygenase inhibitors leads to an enhanced reabsorption of Na^+ and Cl^- in the late distal nephron, which makes these drugs effective to treat these patients to limit the degree of contraction of the effective arterial blood volume (see Discussion of Case 14-4, page 508 for more information). Nevertheless, there may be long-term consequences of this therapy as this class of drugs may lead to progressive renal damage.

3. *Much of the Na^+ and Cl^- reabsorbed daily in the medullary thick ascending limb of the loop of Henle is not derived from filtered Na^+ and Cl^-*: Only half of Na^+ and Cl^- reabsorbed daily in this nephron segment represents filtered Na^+ and Cl^- because a large quantity of these ions undergo recycling (enter the descending thin limbs of the loop of Henle from the interstitial compartment) by diffusion (see Chapter 9, page 264 for more discussion). Hence, there is a smaller need for reabsorption of Na^+ and Cl^- once this recycling process stops.

QUANTITATIVE ANALYSIS OF Na^+ REABSORPTION IN THE LOOP OF HENLE IN AN ADULT

- With a GFR of 180 L/day and a P_{Na} of 150 mmol Na^+ per liter of water, 27,000 mmol of Na^+ are filtered per day.
- Since five sixths of filtered Na^+ is reabsorbed proximally, one sixth of 27,000 mmol Na^+ (i.e., 4500 mmol/day) is delivered daily to the loop of Henle.
- The Na^+ concentration in fluid delivered to the early distal convoluted tubule is ~50 mmol/L, and the volume delivered is ~27 L/day; hence, 1350 mmol of Na^+ exit the loop of Henle.
- Comparing the 3000 mmol of Na^+ reabsorbed in the loop of Henle to the 2100 mmol of Na^+ in the entire ECF compartments reveals that these patients should have a life-threatening acute loss of Na^+.

Special features of the ROMK subtype

- Patients with the ROMK subtype of antenatal Bartter's syndrome present initially with hyperkalemia rather than hypokalemia.

Pathophysiology. An inactivating mutation of ROMK channels can lead to diametrically opposite effects on K^+ excretion, depending on whether transport of K^+ is limited in the CCD. In the first weeks of life, maxi-K^+ channels have not been expressed in the CCD. Hence, these patients have hyperkalemia, marked renal NaCl wasting, a very contracted effective arterial blood volume, and high aldosterone levels (an effect of both the defect in the reabsorption of Na^+ and Cl^- in the loop of Henle and a limited Na^+ reabsorption in the CCD due to the increased negative luminal voltage). One month later, maxi-K^+ channels appear to be present in the luminal membrane of the CCD. As a result, there is abundant K^+ secretion and less restriction on Na^+ reabsorption in the CCD. Accordingly, the clinical findings simply reflect events in the loop of Henle (the clinical picture of Bartter's syndrome), but with a relatively smaller degree of intravascular volume depletion.

Therapy. Nonselective cyclo-oxygenase inhibitors (e.g., indomethacin) are very effective drugs to decrease the excretion of Na^+ and Cl^- in patients with antenatal Bartter's syndrome (see the discussion of Case 14-4, page 508 for more details).

GITELMAN'S SYNDROME

Pathophysiology

- Gitelman's syndrome can be thought of as a disorder that resembles the constant action of a thiazide diuretic.
- The distinguishing findings from Bartter's syndrome include the age of clinical onset (teenage), a retained ability to have a high U_{Osm} when vasopressin acts, hypocalciuria, and hypomagnesemia.

Patients with this disorder have renal wasting of Na^+ and Cl^- and a contracted effective arterial blood volume. The combination of enhanced distal delivery of Na^+ and Cl^- to the CCD together with more reabsorption of Na^+ than Cl^- in this nephron site leads to renal potassium wasting (see Fig. 14-2).

Because the function of the loop of Henle is normal, these patients can have a high U_{Osm} when vasopressin acts. The renal handling of the divalent cations calcium and magnesium is altered when there is a lesion in the distal convoluted tubule. As discussed in the following paragraphs, there is little calcium excretion in these patients, as evidenced by a very low urine calcium-to-creatinine ratio. In contrast, hypomagnesemia and renal magnesium wasting are common in patients with a long-standing history of Gitelman's syndrome (Fig. 14-5).

Hypocalciuria

The best explanation for the hypocalciuria in patients with Gitelman's syndrome is enhanced reabsorption of calcium in the proximal convoluted tubule secondary to the contracted effective

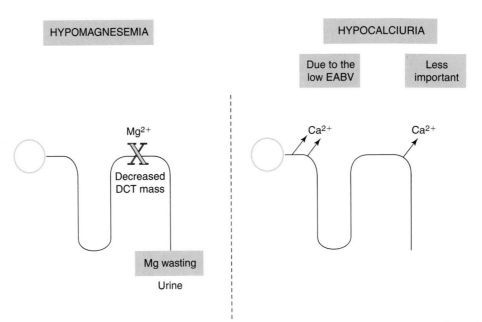

FIGURE 14-5 Hypothesis to explain the hypomagnesemia and the hypocalciuria in patients with Gitelman's syndrome. The *structure* represents a nephron. The *portion on the left* depicts the high excretion of magnesium. The most likely basis of hypomagnesemia and renal magnesium wasting is progressive atrophy or apoptosis of cells of the early distal convoluted tubule, as they constitute the last major nephron segment that reabsorbs magnesium. The *portion of the figure to the right* depicts the hypocalciuria in these patients. The major reason for the low excretion of calcium is enhanced reabsorption of calcium in the proximal convoluted tubule owing to the contracted effective arterial blood volume. Perhaps there may also be more reabsorption of calcium in the up-regulated connecting segment of the late cortical distal nephron.

arterial blood volume (*see margin note*). The reabsorption of calcium might be up-regulated in nephron segments downstream to the distal convoluted tubule. In fact, the connecting segment has all the components needed for the reabsorption of Ca^{2+}. This up-regulated calcium reabsorption might diminish the degree of hypercalciuria of Bartter's syndrome as well as cause a very low rate of excretion of calcium in patients with Gitelman's syndrome.

Hypomagnesemia

It is not clear why patients with Gitelman's syndrome have hypomagnesemia. Our preferred explanation for the renal magnesium wasting in patients with Gitelman's syndrome begins with the premise that the vast majority of distal magnesium reabsorption occurs in the distal convoluted tubule, and this nephron segment is the critical final site where reabsorption of magnesium takes place (see Fig. 14-5). A decreased reabsorption of Na^+ and Cl^- in this nephron segment for a prolonged period of time leads to apoptosis and decrease in its cell mass. Hence, renal magnesium wasting occurs, leading to hypomagnesemia.

Molecular basis

Mutations that cause Gitelman's syndrome have been identified in three separate genes (Fig. 14-6). The vast majority of patients with Gitelman's syndrome have mutations in the gene encoding the Na^+-Cl^- cotransporter in the early distal convoluted tubule. Two other molecular disorders that cause the clinical picture of Gitelman's syndrome are mutations that can lead to a defect in the γ-subunit of

CALCIUM BALANCE IN PATIENTS WITH GITELMAN'S SYNDROME

- It is not clear how patients with Gitelman's syndrome remain in balance for calcium with such a low rate of excretion of calcium.
- If the diet has not changed and it is unlikely that most of the absorbed calcium (200 mg/day) in the intestinal tract has been added to bone every day of the year for many decades, this would suggest that there is an unknown factor that influences intestinal absorption of calcium in patients with Gitelman's syndrome.

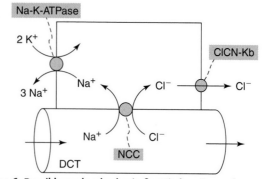

FIGURE 14-6 Possible molecular basis for Gitelman's syndrome. The most common defect causing Gitelman's syndrome is a mutation involving NCC, but mutations in genes encoding the γ-subunit of the Na-K-ATPase or the Cl^- channels (ClCN-Kb) on basolateral membranes may cause this syndrome. DCT, distal convoluted tubule; NCC, Na^+/Cl^- cotransporter.

the Na-K-ATPase in the basolateral membrane of distal convoluted tubule cells or ones that affect the gene encoding for ClCN-Kb.

Clinical picture

For the most part, this is a disease of young adults. In contrast, patients with a Cl^- channel (ClCN-Kb channel) defect often present earlier in life and the findings resemble those in a patient with Bartter's syndrome. There is often a positive family history and/or consanguinity. The main clinical symptoms are related to tetany and nonspecific findings including enuresis. The major clinical findings are secondary to the electrolyte abnormalities and/or the low effective arterial blood volume. The major laboratory abnormalities are hypokalemia, hypomagnesemia, and renal wasting of Na^+, Cl^-, K^+, and Mg^{2+}, as well as the presence of metabolic alkalosis.

Diagnosis

The typical clinical findings often leave little doubt as to the diagnosis. Nevertheless, there can be three difficulties in making this diagnosis. First, the U_{Osm} may not be as high as expected if there is renal medullary damage or if the patient has an osmotic diuresis due to the very high excretion of electrolytes (*see margin note*). Second, a low urine calcium-to-creatinine ratio may develop later in the course of the disease; early on, this may be observed only in more concentrated urines. Third, hypomagnesemia may develop later in the course of the disease.

Differential diagnosis

The differential diagnosis of hypokalemia with a low effective arterial blood volume is the same as discussed for Bartter's syndrome (page 488).

Therapy

- The following discussion applies to patients with Bartter's syndrome or Gitelman's syndrome.

EFFECT OF A HIGH RATE OF EXCRETION OF ELECTROLYTES ON THE U_{Osm}
- When these patients receive large supplements of NaCl and KCl, there is a high rate of excretion of these ions and thereby an osmotic diuresis.
- Because the same total amount of urea is excreted, but in more liters of urine, the concentration of urea is lower, and thus the maximum urine osmolality when vasopressin acts is lower, even though the nonurea osmolality is high. Therefore, examine the nonurea osmolality in the urine when vasopressin acts to evaluate the renal concentrating, process.

Correction of hypokalemia is extremely difficult in these patients, even with large supplements of K$^+$. Hypomagnesemia may be an important factor in the enhanced kaliuresis in some patients with Gitelman's syndrome. Correction of hypomagnesemia with oral magnesium is usually limited by gastrointestinal side effects. Angiotensin-converting enzyme inhibitors have been tried in some patients with variable success, but hypotension is a major concern. We have reservations about the prolonged use of nonsteroidal anti-inflammatory drugs because of the potential for chronic renal dysfunction. Potassium-sparing diuretics may help conserve K$^+$, but they may also exacerbate renal salt wasting. A common clinical observation is that even high doses of amiloride may fail to curtail the excessive kaliuresis in patients with Bartter's syndrome or Gitelman's syndrome. Part of the explanation for this diminished effect could be related to lower concentrations of these drugs in the lumen of the CCD. In more detail, lesions that inhibit the reabsorption of Na$^+$ and Cl$^-$ in the loop of Henle or the distal convoluted tubule should increase the distal delivery of osmoles and thereby the volume of fluid in the terminal CCD. This higher luminal fluid volume lowers the concentration of ENaC blockers by dilution. Therefore, to be effective, a much larger dose of amiloride must be given. Also, a potential concern of using these agents in patients with Bartter's syndrome or Gitelman's syndrome is that the sodium wasting in these patients might become a major problem, especially if dietary NaCl intake declines and/or there is a nonrenal loss of NaCl. If this were to occur, these drugs will have a higher luminal concentration and thereby become much more potent in causing an unwanted naturesis.

An interesting clinical observation in patients with Bartter's syndrome or Gitelman's syndrome is that hypokalemia persists despite large oral KCl supplements. Hence, the K$^+$ excretion rate must rise appreciably when potassium supplements are given. We offer the following speculation that focuses on modulation of the number of open ROMK channels in the luminal membranes of principal cells in the CCD. When the degree of hypokalemia becomes more severe, the number of open luminal ROMK channels in the CCD may be down-regulated; this could diminish the rate of net secretion of K$^+$ in the CCD. When the P_K rises with KCl supplementation, the number of open ROMK channels in the luminal membranes of the CCD may increase. Accordingly, the usual negative lumen voltage in the CCD could now augment the rate of secretion of K$^+$ as long as the P_K remains in this somewhat higher range.

CATIONIC DRUGS THAT BIND TO THE Ca-SR

Pathophysiology

Gentamicin and tobramycin are cationic antibiotics that bind to the calcium-sensing receptor on the basolateral aspect of cells of the thick ascending limb of the loop of Henle (Fig. 14-7). This leads to inhibition of ROMK and thus to a "Lasix-like" effect. Hence, the pathophysiology of gentamicin-induced hypokalemia can be thought of as resembling the constant weak action of a loop diuretic as gentamicin forms a covalent bond with the calcium-sensing receptor. A similar story might apply for other cationic drugs that might bind to the calcium-sensing receptor, such as cisplatin.

ABBREVIATION
Ca-SR, calcium-sensing receptor

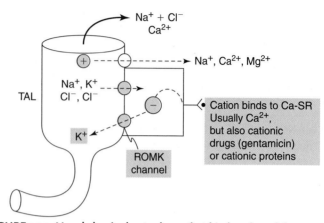

FIGURE 14-7 Hypokalemia due to drugs that bind to the calcium-sensing receptor. When ionized calcium or cationic drugs such as gentamicin bind to the calcium-sensing receptor in the basolateral membrane of cells of the medullary thick ascending limb (TAL) of the loop of Henle, ROMK channels are inhibited. Because K^+ does not enter the lumen as quickly, the flux through the Na^+, K^+, 2 Cl^- cotransporter is decreased and the lumen positive voltage is diminished. As a result, there is less reabsorption of Na^+, Cl^-, and ionized calcium in the loop of Henle. This could lead to findings akin to actions of a loop diuretic with wasting of Na^+, Cl^-, K^+, and Ca^{2+} in the urine, and the subsequent development of metabolic alkalosis.

Clinical picture

This disorder is often accompanied by the presence of a low effective arterial blood volume due to renal salt wasting, hypokalemia, hypomagnesemia, hypercalciuria, and metabolic alkalosis.

Diagnosis

This is based on the clinical picture described above in a patient who received gentamicin or other cationic drugs, which bind to the calcium-sensing receptor.

Therapy

After discontinuing the drug, there is a considerable lag time before its effects disappear because covalent binding of gentamicin to the calcium-sensing receptor may persist for a long period of time. Supportive therapy with sodium, potassium, and magnesium should be given as needed.

PRIMARY HYPERALDOSTERONISM

Pathophysiology

There is a high rate of secretion of aldosterone due to the presence of an adrenal adenoma or bilateral adrenal hyperplasia (see Fig. 14-1).

Clinical picture

This diagnosis should be suspected in patients with hypertension and unexplained hypokalemia with renal potassium wasting. Nevertheless, a large proportion of these patients do not have hypokalemia (*see margin note*).

HYPOKALEMIA IN PATIENTS WITH PRIMARY HYPERALDOSTERONISM

- A significant number of patients with primary hyperaldosteronism do not have hypokalemia, but the reason is not clear.
- Primary hyperaldosteronism should also be suspected even if the P_K is toward the lower end of the normal range but not quite in the hypokalemic range in patients who are taking drugs that may decrease the rate of excretion of K^+ (e.g., angiotensin-converting enzyme inhibitors or angiotensin II receptor blockers).

Diagnosis

The diagnosis hinges on the finding of an elevated $P_{Aldosterone}$ and a very low P_{Renin} (see Table 14-1). A high $P_{Aldosterone}$: P_{Renin} ratio in a random blood sample is usually a sufficient screening test. Primary hyperaldosteronism must be confirmed by finding a nonsuppressible high $P_{Aldosterone}$ or urinary aldosterone excretion during salt loading. A CAT scan is the best imaging test to detect an adrenal adenoma versus bilateral adrenal hyperplasia. If surgery is an option, perform adrenal vein sampling to determine if the leison detected on the CT scan is a functioning adenoma.

Differential diagnosis

The finding of very low P_{Renin} with high $P_{Aldosterone}$ separates patients with primary hyperaldosteronism from those with other causes of hypertension and hypokalemia (see Table 14-1). Patients with glucocorticoid remediable aldosteronism also have elevated $P_{Aldosterone}$ with suppressed P_{Renin} (see later discussion). In these patients, however, the $P_{Aldosterone}$ is suppressed by the administration of glucocorticoids.

Therapy

Laparoscopic unilateral adrenalectomy is generally the preferred treatment in a patient with an adrenal adenoma. If successful, it should induce a marked reduction in aldosterone secretion, a fall in blood pressure, and correction of the hypokalemia. Notwithstanding, hypertension persists in a large number of patients after unilateral adrenalectomy, especially in those with a family history of hypertension and those who were taking two or more antihypertensive medications prior to surgery.

In patients with bilateral adrenal hyperplasia, or in those with an adrenal adenoma who are not candidates for surgery, medical therapy is the preferred treatment. The goals of therapy, however, are not only to control blood pressure and to correct the hypokalemia but also to reverse the unwanted effects of hyperaldosteronism on the heart. Hence, the administration of a mineralocorticoid receptor antagonist (spironolactone or eplerenone) is preferred. Amiloride is an alternative in patients who are intolerant of these drugs. The issue about the need for a low intake of NaCl to decrease the flow rate in CCD that was discussed earlier in the Therapy section under Gitelman's Syndrome applies in this setting.

GLUCOCORTICOID-REMEDIABLE ALDOSTERONISM

Pathophysiology

This condition is a rare form of bilateral adrenal hyperplasia in which ACTH is the exclusive regulator of the secretion of aldosterone. There is also marked overproduction of C-18 oxidation products of cortisol, 18-hydroxycortisol, and 18-oxocortisol.

Molecular basis

The genetic basis for this disorder is a chimeric gene in which the regulatory region of the gene encoding for the enzyme required for the synthesis of cortisol in the zona fasciculata is linked to the coding sequence of the gene for the enzyme, aldosterone synthase that is required for the synthesis of aldosterone. Hence, ACTH regulates the secretion of aldosterone. Also, because of an apparent expression of this enzyme in the zona fasciculata, cortisol (a C-17 hydroxylated steroid) becomes hydroxylated at the C-18 position, leading to the production of cortisol-aldosterone hybrid compounds.

Clinical picture

This disease is an autosomal dominant disorder. The onset of severe hypertension usually occurs in early adulthood. There is often a strong family history of hypertension and early onset of cardiovascular and cerebrovascular diseases. Interestingly, hypokalemia is not present in a significant number of these patients.

Diagnosis

The diagnosis hinges on demonstrating suppression of aldosterone with the administration of glucocorticoids (dexamethasone or prednisone), detection of very high levels of C-18 oxidation products of cortisol in the urine, and ultimately, genetic testing to detect the chimeric gene.

Differential diagnosis

Other causes of hypertension and unexplained hypokalemia must be ruled out.

Therapy

Administration of glucocorticoids (dexamethasone or prednisone) corrects the hypersecretion of aldosterone by suppressing ACTH.

ADRENOCORTICOTROPIC HORMONE–PRODUCING TUMOR OR SEVERE CUSHING'S SYNDROME

Pathophysiology

The clinical picture is similar to that of primary hyperaldosteronism, but the $P_{Aldosterone}$ is low. Because of an overabundance of cortisol, the activity of 11β-HSDH is insufficient to inactivate all the cortisol that enters principal cells in the CCD (Fig. 14-8). As a result, cortisol binds to the mineralocorticoid receptor and exerts mineralocorticoid actions (*see margin note*).

OTHER EFFECT OF ACTH
Perhaps, very high levels of ACTH may lead to inhibition of 11β-HSDH.

Clinical picture

ACTH overproduction is commonly seen in patients with oat cell carcinoma of the lung. In patients with ACTH-producing tumors, overt signs of glucocorticoid excess may not be evident at the time of diagnosis. The P_K is often very low.

Diagnosis

The $P_{Aldosterone}$ and P_{Renin} are both suppressed (see Table 14-1). One must demonstrate very elevated plasma cortisol levels. Plasma ACTH levels are high if there is an ACTH-producing tumor and markedly suppressed in patients with Cushing's syndrome.

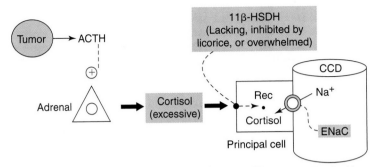

FIGURE 14-8 Conditions in which cortisol acts as aldosterone. Cortisol has a very high affinity to the aldosterone receptor. As cortisol enters principal cells of the CCD, 11β-hydroxysteroid dehydrogenase (11β-HSDH; *larger black dot inside the cell*) converts cortisol into cortisone, which cannot bind to the aldosterone receptor (Rec; *smaller black dot in the cell*). There are three circumstances in which cortisol binds to the aldosterone receptor: first, when there is a deficiency of 11β-HSDH (apparent mineralocorticoid excess syndrome); second, when an inhibitor of 11β-HSDH is present (e.g., glycyrrhetinic acid in licorice); and third, when the supply of cortisol exceeds the ability of 11β-HSDH to inactivate it (e.g., ectopic production of adrenocorticotropic hormone [ACTH] by a tumor). ENaC, epithelial Na^+ channel; PIT, pituitary gland.

Differential diagnosis

For a list of the causes of hypertension and hypokalemia, see Table 14-1, page 467.

Therapy

Therapy is directed at the primary disorder. For treatment of hypokalemia, large supplements of KCl and drugs that inhibit ENaC are often necessary.

SYNDROME OF APPARENT MINERALOCORTICOID EXCESS

Pathophysiology

The clinical picture is similar to that in patients with primary hyperaldosteronism, but the $P_{Aldosterone}$ is very low. Because of decreased activity of the enzyme 11β-HSDH, cortisol binds to the mineralocorticoid receptors and exerts mineralocorticoid actions (see Fig. 14-8).

Molecular basis

Several mutations in the gene that encodes for the kidney isoform of the enzyme 11β-HSDH-2 have been identified. These mutations result in decreased enzyme activity and therefore impaired inactivation of cortisol.

Clinical picture

This syndrome is an autosomal recessive disorder. It is characterized by juvenile onset of hypertension and hypokalemia.

OTHER POSSIBLE INHIBITORS OF 11β-HSDH
- Very large dose of flavonoids (e.g., in grapefruit juice)
- Bile acids

Diagnosis

The $P_{Aldosterone}$ and P_{Renin} are both suppressed (see Table 14-1). The diagnosis is confirmed by the finding of an elevated urinary cortisol-to-cortisone ratio.

Differential diagnosis

A similar clinical picture is seen in patients with chronic ingestion of licorice or other compounds that contain glycyrrhetinic acid, which inhibits the 11β-HSDH (*see margin note*).

Therapy

Patients respond well to blockers of the aldosterone receptor or ENaC blockers (e.g., amiloride or triamterene with the same caveat for the need for salt restriction that was noted earlier).

LIDDLE'S SYNDROME

Pathophysiology

The pathophysiology of this disorder is a constitutively active ENaC in the CCD.

Molecular basis

The key to understand this disorder is the fact that a mutation can lead to a gain of function. These mutations interfere with the process that removes ENaC units from the luminal membrane of principal cells. Several mutations in the genes encoding for the β-or γ-subunits of ENaC have been described in patients with this syndrome. Some of these mutations result in truncation of the cytoplasmic regions of the β- or γ-subunits of the ENaC complex. Others are missense mutations involving a proline-rich region (PxYY motif) of these subunits. These regions are critical in the interaction between ENaC and an intracellular protein ubiquitin ligases such as Nedd4-2 (Fig. 14-9). When Nedd4-2 binds to the β- or γ-subunit of ENaC, not only is ENaC removed from the luminal membrane but Nedd4-2 protein also ligates ubiquitin to ENaC, which results in its targeting to the proteasome for destruction. Therefore, these mutations compromise the removal of ENaC and lead to an increased number of open ENaC units in the luminal membrane of principal cells.

Clinical picture

This syndrome is an autosomal dominant inherited disorder characterized by early onset of severe hypertension and hypokalemia. Interestingly, a number of patients do not have hypokalemia.

Diagnosis

A positive family history of early-onset hypertension and hypokalemia as well as very low $P_{Aldosterone}$ and P_{Renin} are key elements in the diagnosis (see Table 14-1). There is no excess secretion of cortisol, and the urine cortisol-to-cortisone ratio is not elevated. While

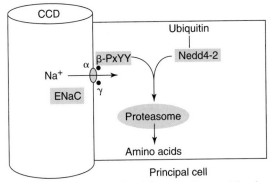

FIGURE 14-9 Molecular basis of Liddle's syndrome. The *barrel-shaped structure* represents the CCD, and the *rectangle* represents a principal cell. The *green oval* in its luminal membrane is epithelial Na^+ channel (ENaC), with its α subunit (the channel pore) and β- and γ-subunits, with their cytoplasmic tails and their PxYY motif. When the enzyme Nedd4-2 binds to the β- and γ-subunits of ENaC, ENaC is removed from the luminal membrane by endocytosis. Nedd4-2 then ligates ubiquitin to ENaC, which targets it to the proteasome for destruction. Mutations in the β- or γ-subunits of ENaC lead to defective removal of ENaC from the luminal membrane.

aldosterone receptor blockers are effective in patients with apparent mineralocorticoid excess syndrome, they are not effective in patients with Liddle's syndrome.

Differential diagnosis

Other causes of hypertension and hypokalemia must be ruled out (see Table 14-1).

Therapy

Control of hypertension and correction of hypokalemia can be achieved with the administration of large doses of ENaC blockers (amiloride and triamterene) but not with aldosterone receptor blockers (e.g., spironolactone). The effect of ENaC blockers is more evident in patients who are on a salt-restricted diet.

AMPHOTERICIN B–INDUCED HYPOKALEMIA

Pathophysiology

Amphotericin B–induced hypokalemia can be thought of as a disorder in which there are artificial ENaC-like channels that are permanently in an open configuration in the luminal membrane in the CCD. The high rate of excretion of K^+ is caused by a relatively high $[K^+]_{CCD}$, the result of reabsorbing more Na^+ than Cl^-.

Clinical picture

The clinical picture is predominantly that of the underlying illness that necessitated the administration of amphotericin B. Hypokalemia is usually associated with an expanded ECF volume.

Diagnosis

The diagnosis is suspected in a patient who develops hypokalemia while receiving amphotericin B.

Therapy

Give a sufficient quantity of KCl to raise the P_K to the normal range. Try to avoid a large intravenous infusion of saline when giving amphotericin B to avoid having a very large flow rate in the CCD when amphotericin B acts, which exacerbates the loss of K^+.

PART D
THERAPY OF HYPOKALEMIA
MEDICAL EMERGENCIES

- The major danger of a severe degree of hypokalemia is a cardiac arrhythmia.

There are two potentially life-threatening circumstances that require aggressive therapy. The most common is a cardiac arrhythmia, and the other is extreme weakness involving the respiratory muscles, especially when acidemia is present (e.g., distal renal tubular acidosis due to a low rate of secretion of H^+ or an accelerated secretion of HCO_3^- in the distal nephron, or severe diarrhea). Having decided that hypokalemia requires urgent therapy, enough K^+ must be given to raise the P_K quickly and to a high enough value (~3.0 mmol/L) to avert these dangers. The total K^+ deficit should be replaced *much* more slowly. Because large doses and high concentrations of K^+ should be infused at the outset, K^+ must be administered via a large central vein and the patient should be connected to a cardiac monitor. As a rule, the infusion should not contain glucose or HCO_3^- because this may lead to a shift of K^+ into cells, which may aggravate an already severe degree of hypokalemia. See discussion of Case 14-1 on page 468 for details of the emergency administration of K^+ via a central line.

NONMEDICAL EMERGENCIES

The specific issues in therapy of patients with hypokalemia depending on its cause were discussed previously. In this section, we provide general comments about replacing a large deficit of K^+.

General issues in treatment of the patient with hypokalemia

Magnitude of the potassium deficit

It is common practice to infer that there is a K^+ deficit of 100 to 400 mmol if the P_K is down from 4.0 to 3.0 mmol/L and that a P_K of 2 mmol/L suggests that there is a much larger deficit of K^+ (as high as 800 mmol in a 70-kg adult). In our view, there is no useful quantitative relationship between P_K and the total body K^+ deficit in an individual patient because a component of the hypokalemia often results from a shift of K^+ into cells. Hence, careful monitoring of the P_K during replacement of the K^+ deficit is mandatory.

Route of potassium administration

The oral route is preferred. Certain factors may necessitate using the intravenous route, including the urgency of therapy, the level of consciousness, and the presence of gastrointestinal problems. As a rule, the concentration of K^+ should not be greater than 40 mmol/L if infused peripherally because higher K^+ concentrations may irritate veins with a lower rate of blood flow; the rate of administration of K^+ should not exceed 60 mmol/hr in most settings.

Potassium preparations

Most preparations in tablet form release K^+ slowly. Although these are usually well tolerated, they occasionally cause ulcerative or stenotic lesions in the gastrointestinal tract owing to a high local K^+ concentration. Oral KCl can also be given in a crystalline form (e.g., salt substitutes, such as Co-Salt, which provide 14 mmol K^+ per g); this is generally well tolerated and is an inexpensive form of potassium supplementation.

For electroneutrality, a deficit of K^+ must be accompanied by the loss of Cl^- or HCO_3^-, or by a gain of Na^+. With a KCl deficit (e.g., owing to chronic vomiting or diuretic use), KCl is needed; in contrast, with a $KHCO_3$ deficit (e.g., owing to diarrhea), K^+ with HCO_3 (or a HCO_3^- equivalent; e.g., citrate) is needed. A note of caution is necessary; the administration of HCO_3^- may cause a shift of K^+ into cells in certain settings. Therefore, in a patient who is markedly hypokalemic and acidemic, KCl should be given initially; alkali in the form of $NaHCO_3$ may then be administered after the P_K approaches a safer level (~3 mmol/L). In conditions in which K^+ loss is matched by Na^+ retention (e.g., in a patient with primary hyperaldosteronism), K^+ is usually given as KCl while measures are taken to ensure that NaCl is excreted. The need for K^+ as its phosphate salt is most evident when there is rapid anabolism; examples include patients on nutritional support or those in the acute recovery phase of a catabolic disorder such as DKA. If given, phosphate should not be administered too rapidly (i.e., <50 mmol in 8 hours) because a large phosphate load has the danger of inducing metastatic calcification and hypocalcemia (see Part E, Mini-Case 14-1, page 502 for more discussion). Notwithstanding, we give K^+ as KCl in the treatment of patients with DKA and rely on the patient's diet to supply the phosphate needed for the anabolic phase of the illness, which occurs later.

Although it seems reasonable, on a superficial analysis, to increase the intake of potassium-rich foods (e.g., bananas, fruit juice), this is not an effective way to replace a K^+ deficit (*see margin note*).

Adjuncts to therapy

Administering potassium-sparing diuretics to patients with hypokalemia can diminish renal loss of K^+. Notwithstanding, this is useful only on a chronic basis and not during the treatment of acute hypokalemia, when the rate of K^+ excretion is usually less than 10 mmol/hr. Amiloride and triamterene are better tolerated than spironolactone because they lack the gastrointestinal and hormonal complications of spironolactone (amenorrhea, gynecomastia,

BANANAS TO REPLACE A DEFICIT OF K^+
- The ratio of K^+ to calories in bananas is very low. Hence, to supply a large K^+ load in this form, the excessive caloric intake can predispose to obesity.
- To provide 50 mmol K^+/day for 1 year = gain of >50 lb if there was no change in diet or activity
- Fruit provides $K^+ + HCO_3^-$, so it is not useful to replace a KCl deficit unless the patient can retain Cl^- and excrete HCO_3^-.

decreased libido). Eplerenone is a highly selective mineralocorticoid receptor antagonist that is associated with a lower incidence of these endocrine side effects, but it is also significantly more expensive than spironolactone. When using the ENaC blockers amiloride or triamterene, the patient should have a low intake of NaCl because this leads to a lower delivery of osmoles to the CCD and therefore a lower flow rate in these nephron segments. With a lower flow rate, the concentration of the drug near ENaC is higher. There is an important note of caution: Hyperkalemia may develop when K^+ is given along with potassium-sparing diuretics, especially if other conditions that may compromise potassium excretion are present.

Risks of therapy

With prolonged hypokalemia, the CCD may become hyporesponsive to the kaliuretic effect of aldosterone (probably owing to the presence of fewer luminal potassium channels in the principal cells in the CCD). This allows aldosterone to continue to be a NaCl-retaining hormone while diminishing its kaliuretic effect. Hence, it is important to monitor the P_K frequently during the treatment of hypokalemia.

Patients with renal failure and diabetes mellitus, especially if they are taking drugs that block the renin-angiotensin system, β-blockers, or nonsteroidal anti-inflammatory drugs, may be at risk for development of hyperkalemia with chronic K^+ supplementation. These patients should have their P_K monitored closely.

PART E
INTEGRATIVE PHYSIOLOGY

K^+ DEPLETION AND THE PATHOPHYSIOLOGY OF KIDNEY STONE FORMATION

- When K^+ are reabsorbed by the H^+/K^+-ATPase, K^+ *and* HCO_3^- are added to the inner medullary interstitial compartment, which becomes more alkaline.
- There are more active H^+/K^+-ATPase units in the luminal membrane of the inner medullary collecting duct when a person has a deficit of K^+ and hypokalemia.

We begin this section with a mini-case that explores the processes that may lead to precipitation of calcium salts. We use this case to illustrate the integrative physiology of the renal response to a deficit of K^+, which tends to alkalinize the renal medullary interstitial compartment and the role this may play in the initiation phase of kidney stone formation.

MINI-CASE 14-1: A SHOCKING DEVELOPMENT

A 5-year-old 20-kg male had a tonsillectomy this morning; the surgery was uneventful. As he began to recover from the anesthesia, he was restless and appeared to suffer from pain. As a result, analgesia was ordered, but he was inadvertently given an intravenous bolus of 30 mg (74 μmol) of codeine phosphate into a vein on the dorsum of his hand. Less than 10 seconds later, he collapsed and his blood pressure was not detected by palpation. He received cardiac massage and epinephrine, which led to a complete recovery. Blood drawn 18 minutes after the cardiac emergency revealed a very low ionized calcium concentration in plasma (720 μmol/L, normal value is 1200 μmol/L); in addition, he had respiratory alkalosis with a blood pH of 7.45 due to hyperventilation.

Questions

Could the 74 μmol of phosphate directly cause the very low concentration of ionized calcium in his plasma that reached the right ventricle less than 10 seconds after its administration and thus lead to his hemodynamic collapse?

What are the features that affect the diffusion of ionized calcium from the interstitial compartment of the heart to plasma in this patient?

Could the 74 μmol of phosphate cause the low concentration of ionized calcium in the blood that was drawn 18 minutes after the cardiac emergency?

What are the properties of an anion that caused the removal of ionized calcium, which persisted for 18 minutes?

What are the implications of this pathophysiology for the formation of kidney stones?

DISCUSSION OF MINI-CASE 14-1

Could the 74 μmol of phosphate directly cause the very low concentration of ionized calcium in his plasma that reached the right ventricle less than 10 seconds after its administration and thus lead to his hemodynamic collapse?

The key to answer this question is to deduce the volume of plasma that should mix with the infused codeine phosphate up to the time when it reaches the right ventricle. In fact, this volume is very small (~110 mL [*see margin note*]). The quantity of ionized calcium in plasma that reaches the right ventricle in 10 seconds is 132 μmol of ionized calcium (110 mL × 1200 μmol/L). Therefore, there was sufficient phosphate administered to cause a marked depression in the circulating ionized calcium concentration in the plasma that reached his right ventricle in 10 seconds.

What are the features that affect the diffusion of ionized calcium from the interstitial compartment of the heart to plasma in this patient?

- Diffusion is a very slow process unless there is a mechanism for rapid mixing. Hence, one needs to "stir" the interstitial compartment in the heart to accelerate diffusion.

The direction of this diffusion in this setting is from the interstitial compartment into capillaries down the concentration difference for calcium (because the concentration of ionized calcium is very low in plasma). Since the heart was beating before the arrest, there was a process to "stir" the interstitial fluid and accelerate the diffusion of ionized calcium.

VOLUME OF BLOOD THAT REACHES THE HEART IN LESS THAN 10 SECONDS
- The entire blood volume in this 20-kg boy is 1400 mL (70 mL/kg) of which ~900 mL is plasma after correcting for his hematocrit of 0.33.
- Since the volume of plasma arriving in the right ventricle is ~10% of the volume of plasma (~90 mL), in 10 seconds, and the volume in the right ventricle is 1 mL/kg or 21 mL, the volume in which the administered phosphate can distribute is ~110 mL in this patient.

On the other hand, while myocardial contractility was diminished, even if ionized calcium was administered, its diffusion from plasma to cardiac myocytes will be slow unless additional measures are taken to increase diffusion of ionized calcium at this time (administration of a stimulant of myocardial contractility).

Could the 74 μmol of phosphate cause the low concentration of ionized calcium in the blood that was drawn 18 minutes after the cardiac emergency?

There are three factors to consider. First the entire plasma volume in this patient is 0.9 L, which is about 10-fold larger than the volume that reaches the heart in 10 seconds. This plasma volume contains 1080 μmol of ionized calcium (1200 μmol/L × 0.9 L). Second, the entire interstitial volume has the same ionized calcium concentration as in plasma, and it is fourfold larger than the plasma volume. Hence, the interstitial compartment contains about 4300 μmol of ionized calcium; thus, the entire ECF compartment has almost 60-fold more calcium than the quantity of phosphate that was administered. Third, when the ionized calcium concentration falls in plasma, calcium should dissociate promptly from albumin. This pool of bound calcium is roughly equal to the quantity of ionized calcium in plasma. Therefore, it is impossible for the added phosphate (74 μmol/L) to remove enough ionized calcium to cause the observed low concentration of ionized calcium in plasma.

What are the properties of an anion that caused the removal of ionized calcium, which persisted for 18 minutes?

First, the anion that removed ionized calcium must be present in an abundant amount. Second, this anion must have a high affinity for ionized calcium and form an insoluble precipitate (e.g., carbonate) or a soluble ion complex (e.g., citrate). There is another issue: The anion that removed ionized calcium could be present in low concentrations but have a large "storage pool." In this latter regard, one must think of carbonate and its large "storage pool," HCO_3^-. Carbonate can be made from HCO_3^-; this conversion occurs when the pH rises. Hence, this will occur when there is a fall in the P_{CO_2} (hyperventilation in response to pain or anxiety) or when there is an addition of bicarbonate to the ECF compartment (e.g., due to secretion of H^+ in the stomach).

What are the implications of this pathophysiology for the formation of kidney stones?

The ion product of ionized calcium and carbonate anions in plasma indicates that this solution is supersaturated for $CaCO_3$. Therefore, the addition of calcium or of HCO_3^- will increase their ion product but not necessarily lead to precipitation of $CaCO_3$ without a nidus to cause the precipitate to form. In the renal medulla, ionized calcium is reabsorbed in the medullary thick ascending limb of the loop of Henle due its lumen-positive voltage and the permeability for calcium between its cells. This, together with the reabsorption of K^+ (and HCO_3^-) from the inner MCD via its H^+/K^+-ATPase, will increase the likelihood of $CaCO_3$ precipitation. This, however, is unlikely to be a problem because the ascending vasa recta are designed to remove small precipitates of $CaCO_3$, as there are twice as many ascending than descending vasa recta. Of greater importance, the ascending vasa recta have large fenestra (holes) through which small $CaCO_3$

precipitates can readily enter (there is a controversy as to whether these tiny precipitates are simply $CaCO_3$ or nanobacteria encased in $CaCO_3$ [for an unknown reason]). Our speculation is that $CaCO_3$ will not directly form a nidus for precipitate growth as long as luminal and interstitial fluid deep in the outer medulla have high concentrations of magnesiun (*see margin note*).

QUESTION

(*Discussed on page 510*)

14-1 *If 74 μmol of citrate were to enter the hepatic vein in a bolus form, might this cause a hemodynamic emergency?*

DISCUSSION OF CASES 14-2, 14-3, AND 14-4

CASE 14-2: HYPOKALEMIA WITH PARALYSIS

(*Case presented on page 462*)

Is there a medical emergency in this patient?

The major dangers related to hypokalemia are cardiac arrhythmias and weakness of the respiratory muscles, especially if there is a need for increased ventilation (e.g., acidemia in a patient with metabolic acidosis). There were no emergencies demanding urgent therapy; hence, the focus can shift to dangers to anticipate with therapy. The major danger to anticipate is the induction of hyperkalemia if a large dose of KCl is administered. Because the basis of the hypokalemia

MAGNESIUM AND THE PREVENTION OF KIDNEY STONES AND NEPHROCALINOSIS

- Since very little filtered magnesium is reabsorbed in the proximal convoluted tubule, whereas more than 80% of filtered calcium is absorbed in this location, fluid arriving at the bend of the loop of Henle has a much higher concentration of magnesium than calcium.

- Magnesium binds more avidly than calcium to divalent phosphate or carbonate, and this ion complex does not precipitate. Hence, luminal calcium salt precipitates should not occur.

- When the lumen-positive voltage is present in the medullary thick ascending limb of the loop of Henle, more magnesium than calcium enters the medullary interstitial compartment. This prevents the development of nephrocalcinosis. The presence of Tamm Horsfall proteins in the luminal fluid prevents the formation of calcium salts.

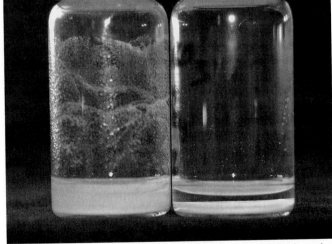

FIGURE 14-10 Conversion of CaCO3 to apatite in a phosphate buffer in vitro. Three mmol of calcium carbonate were added to 5 mL of water or to a solution that contained 5 mmol of K+ phosphate at pH 7.4 (final total concentration is 100 mmol/L to accelerate precipitation). The suspensions were left to stand for two days at room temperature. The water controls (*left*) remained as a cloudy suspension of $CaCO_3$, whereas a very firm precipitate was present in the phosphate buffer (*right*) and there was a clear solution above. The X-ray diffraction pattern of the precipitate in the phosphate buffer was composed of a mixture of $CaCO_3$ and hydroxyapatite.

CaCO3 AND KIDNEY STONE GROWTH
To test a possible role for $CaCO_3$ in kidney stone initiation, we incubated a precipitate of $CaCO_3$ in water or in a phosphate buffer at pH 7.4. Only in the latter solution was there a conversion of some of the $CaCO_3$ to apatite (Fig. 14-10). Hence, this may indicate how kidney stones are initiated as apatite in the renal inner medullary interstitial compartment.

is an acute shift of K^+ into cells due to an adrenergic surge, giving a nonselective β-blocker (e.g., propranolol) minimizes this danger, as much less K^+ will be needed to raise the P_K.

What is the basis of hypokalemia in this patient?

The short time course strongly suggests that the basis of hypokalemia in this patient was an acute shift of K^+ into cells. Moreover, he had the expected *low* rate of K^+ excretion (10 mmol K^+/g creatinine, or 1 mmol K^+/mmol creatinine) and the absence of an acid-base disorder. This conclusion is supported by the fact that his paralysis developed after exercise (β$_2$-adrenergic response) and a large glucose intake from the sugar in the soft drink (insulin actions were present). Because there was a very large intake of caffeine from the soda pop, the presumptive diagnosis is that the major basis for this shift of K^+ is an adrenergic surge (Fig. 14-11). In support of this diagnosis, he had a rapid pulse rate and a large pulse pressure. There were no abnormalities in the thyroid function tests, and he did not have a family history of paralysis or hyperthyroidism.

What effects cause a prolonged shift of K^+ into cells?

The major property is a long duration of action (several hours); the list of possible adrenergic agents includes amphetamines and stimulants such as cocaine and caffeine. As shown in Figure 14-11, a high intake of caffeine (5 L of soda pop in this case; *see margin note*) via blocking the binding of adenosine to its A_{A2} receptors can lead to a surge of catecholamines and a shift of K^+ into cells due to β$_2$-adrenergic effects. This effect of caffeine may also diminish the open probability of K^+_{ATP} channels, which may cause an even greater trapping of K^+ in cells (Fig. 14-12).

Caffeine is metabolized by one of the cytochrome P_{450} enzymes; this enzyme system was designed to protect individuals in Paleolithic times from the ingestion of toxic materials in food. Therefore, it is not surprising that this enzyme is located in cells of the intestinal tract and the liver. Although the affinity of this enzyme for caffeine is

CAFFEINE CONTENT IN BEVERAGES OR FOOD
- Coffee: ~60 mg/100 mL
- Soda: ~12 mg/100 mL
- Chocolate: 1–35 mg/oz

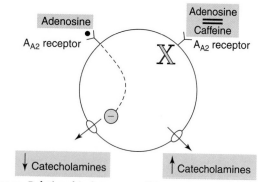

FIGURE 14-11 Relationship between caffeine and an adrenergic surge. The *circle* represents a cell membrane in the central nervous system. The receptor of interest is an adenosine A_{A2} receptor. When adenosine binds to this receptor (shown on the *left*), there is a diminished release of adrenergic hormones. In contrast, in the presence of caffeine (shown on the *right*), adenosine cannot bind to this receptor (*bold double lines*). As a result, there is no longer the inhibitory effect of adenosine and the net effect is a surge in catecholamine release.

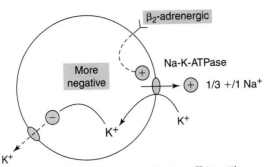

FIGURE 14-12 Cause of a K⁺ shift into cells by caffeine. The combination of activation of the Na-K-ATPase and of decreasing K⁺ exit from cells via K⁺$_{ATP}$ channels can lead to a severe degree of hypokalemia with very large intakes of caffeine.

high, its maximum velocity is *not* large. Hence, low doses of caffeine should be removed effectively but high doses would be removed *slowly* because more half-lives are needed to remove caffeine when its concentration is much greater than the substrate concentration that causes a half-maximal rate (K_m) catalyzed by the enzyme. Therefore, the very large intake of caffeine could explain its prolonged effect to cause hypokalemia.

What is the best therapy for the acute hypokalemia in this patient?

There is a danger of rebound hyperkalemia if large doses of KCl are given. Treatment of patients with an adrenergic surge with a nonselective β-blocker (e.g., propranolol) results in a disappearance of the clinical and biochemical abnormalities related to hypokalemia within 2 to 3 hours. The patient was given propranolol and a small amount of KCl. He had an impressive response to this therapy. In previous episodes when he was treated with large doses of KCl, it took close to 10 hours before there was an appreciable biochemical or clinical improvement.

He is now willing to avoid the use of drinks with a high content of caffeine to prevent recurrent attacks. There have been no further episodes since he discontinued his caffeine intake. Nevertheless, it is still possible that he has an underlying mild form of sporadic hypokalemic paralysis.

CASE 14-3: HYPOKALEMIA WITH A SWEET TOUCH

(Case presented on page 463)

Is there a medical emergency in this patient?

Although the P_K is very low, there were no changes in his electrocardiogram. Hence, there was no cardiac emergency at that moment. Despite the paralysis, he did not have a high arterial PCO_2. Therefore, emergency therapy for hypoventilation was not needed at this time.

Is there a danger to anticipate during therapy?

The major danger is overaggressive administration of KCl. Hence, the rate of administration of KCl should be faster early on but tapered as the P_K approaches about 3.0 mmol/L.

What is the basis of hypokalemia in this patient?

Shift of K^+ into cells

Based on the history and the degree of hypokalemia, there is a component of an acute shift of K^+ into his cells. Nevertheless, the major basis for hypokalemia was a chronic renal loss of K^+ because there was an acid-base disorder (metabolic alkalosis) and a high rate of excretion of K^+. In more detail, the $U_K/U_{Creatinine}$ was 50 mmol/g (5 mmol/mmol), a value that is almost five times greater than expected if the hypokalemia resulted solely from a shift of K^+ into cells or a nonrenal loss of K^+.

The basis of the shift of K^+ is likely the β_2-adrenergic released during exercise and the release of insulin following the large intake of carbohydrate. The patient may also have an underlying increased susceptibility to a shift of K^+ into cells.

Excessive excretion of K^+

This is chronic hypokalemia because his P_K was 3.3 mmol/L and he was also noted to have hypertension 1 year ago. Because the patient has metabolic alkalosis, the steps in Flow Charts 10-4 and 10-5 should be followed to seek the basis of the high ratio of K^+ to creatinine in his urine despite the presence of hypokalemia. Accordingly, the first question to ask is, "What is his effective arterial blood volume status?" Because his effective arterial blood volume was not contracted and he had hypertension, the pathophysiology is one of more reabsorption of Na^+ than reabsorption of Cl^- in the CCD. Therefore, he has an underlying disorder with increased mineralocorticoid activity (see Fig. 14-1).

Because the patient's $P_{Aldosterone}$ level was undetectable, this rules out primary or secondary hyperaldosteronism (see Table 14-1). His cortisol levels were not elevated, ruling out an ACTH-producing tumor. An inherited disorder in which ENaC is constitutively active (Liddle's syndrome) is unlikely considering the patient's age. On further detailed history, it turned out that the patient had ingested licorice in an herbal sweetener he used to add to his tea. The active ingredient in licorice (glycyrrhetinic acid) inhibits the enzyme 11β-HSDH, which inactivates cortisol in principal cells of the CCD. Therefore, cortisol acted like aldosterone and provided a major stimulus for the net secretion of K^+. On discontinuing this herbal sweetener, his P_K returned to the normal range and his blood pressure fell to normal values.

CASE 14-4: HYPOKALEMIA IN A NEWBORN

(Case presented on page 463)

Is there a medical emergency in this patient?

There is always a concern that the patient will develop a medical emergency as a result of excessive loss of Na^+ and Cl^- in his urine because he has a molecular defect that gives him lifelong complete absence of NKCC-2 and thereby an inability to reabsorb NaCl in his loop of Henle. Factors that may bring on this emergency are a sudden decrease in his ability to consume and/or absorb dietary NaCl and/or a large nonrenal loss of NaCl (e.g., diarrhea).

Is there a danger to anticipate during therapy?

The infusion of a large amount of saline could increase the excretion of K^+, but this is not a major concern in the short term.

What is the basis of hypokalemia in this patient?

The basis for the hypokalemia is excessive renal excretion of K^+ due to a very large delivery of Na^+ and Cl^- to the late cortical distal nephron. ENaC is open due to actions of aldosterone, which is released in response to a decreased effective arterial blood volume. In this setting, more Na^+ is reabsorbed than Cl^-, which should lead to increased secretion of K^+, providing that ROMK channels are open in the luminal membrane.

Why did the patient have nephrogenic diabetes insipidus?

The nephrogenic diabetes insipidus represents the usual physiology of the newborn (see Chapter 11, page 386 for more discussion of this topic). In the absence of actions of vasopressin, however, U_{Osm} depends primarily on the osmole excretion rate.

Why did his U_{Osm} fall after indomethacin was given?

In the absence of actions of vasopressin, U_{Osm} depends primarily on the osmole excretion rate. There was a marked decline in his rate of excretion of osmoles (i.e., mainly in the rate of excretion of electrolytes—U_{Na} declined from ~50 mmol/L to less than 10 mmol/L) when indomethacin was given. Since there was no change in his urine flow rate, his U_{Osm} should decline by a factor of five and now the urine is distinctly hypoosmolar.

This illustrates the need to examine the urine osmolality in terms of the urine flow rate and the rate of excretion of osmoles at the time urine was collected. Said another way, before he was given indomethacin, nephrogenic diabetes insipidus was present, but his U_{Osm} was not very low because of a high rate of excretion of electrolytes.

In what nephron segment might indomethacin have acted to curtail the natriuresis?

To decrease the excretion of Na^+ without a decrease in the urine flow rate, the site of action of indomethacin must be after the water-permeable proximal convoluted tubule. Because there is a molecular defect in the medullary thick ascending limb of the loop of Henle, which leads to a near-complete absence of this transporter, it is extremely unlikely that indomethacin has caused an increase of reabsorption of Na^+ in the loop of Henle. Therefore, the most likely site is the distal nephron, including its cortical and medullary segments.

Why is antenatal Bartter's syndrome not a lethal abnormality?

One must appreciate two facts that affect the quantity of Na^+ and Cl^- delivered to the loop of Henle in patients with antenatal Bartter's syndrome:
1. The delivery of Na^+ and Cl^- to the loop of Henle is much lower than in normal subjects because patients with antenatal Bartter's syndrome have a contracted effective arterial blood volume. As a result, they have a much lower glomerular filtration rate (the $P_{Creatinine}$ was at least three times higher than expected in this patient) and an enhanced proximal tubular reabsorption of Na^+ and Cl^-.

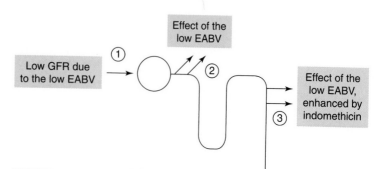

FIGURE 14-13 Reasons for having lower rates of excretion of Na$^+$ and Cl$^-$ in patients with antenatal Bartter's syndrome. The *stylized structure* represents a nephron, and the *circle* represents its glomerulus. In patients with antenatal Bartter's syndrome, there is a very contracted effective arterial blood volume. Hence, there are three major effects that lead to a reduced rate of excretion of Na$^+$. As shown in *site 1*, there is a marked reduction in the GFR and thereby in the filtered load of Na$^+$. As shown in *site 2*, the marked reduction in the effective arterial blood volume markedly augments Na$^+$ and Cl$^-$ reabsorption in the proximal convoluted tubule. As shown in *site 3*, there is up-regulation of the reabsorption of Na$^+$ and Cl$^-$ in the late distal convoluted tubule and the collecting ducts. It appears that indomethacin enhances the reabsorption of Na$^+$ and Cl$^-$ in site 3.

2. To place the numbers to be described below in perspective, we have used values in an adult. The quantity of Na$^+$ delivered daily to the loop of Henle is more than twofold larger than its content in the ECF compartment (4500 mmol Na$^+$/day versus ~2100 mmol Na$^+$ in the ECF compartment). Moreover, close to 3000 mmol of Na$^+$ are reabsorbed in the entire loop of Henle. Hence, if the delivery of Na$^+$ to the loop of Henle is reduced to one third of the normal delivery by a combination of more avid reabsorption of Na$^+$ in the proximal convoluted tubule and a lower GFR secondary to a lower effective arterial blood volume, these patients can survive. Moreover, when they are given a cyclooxygenase inhibitor to stimulate downstream reabsorption of Na$^+$ and Cl$^-$, they can survive with a smaller degree of contraction of their effective arterial blood volume.

Overall, the delivery of Na$^+$ and Cl$^-$ out the medullary thick ascending limb of the loop of Henle is much less than half of that in the normal subjects (Fig. 14-13).

DISCUSSION OF QUESTION 14-1

14-1 *If 74 μmol of citrate were to enter the hepatic vein in a bolus form, might this cause a hemodynamic emergency?*

As discussed in Mini-Case 14-1, the same quantity of phosphate did cause a cardiac arrest, so the simple, but incorrect, answer is yes. There is one major difference, however: There is not a nidus to drive the precipitation of CaCO$_3$ when citrate is added. Hence, there will only be the removal of a maximum of 74 μmol of ionized calcium from plasma. Nevertheless, our defense mechanism is the release of calcium from its bound form on albumin. Without knowing the affinity of calcium for each binding site on albumin, we cannot deduce how much ionized calcium will be released for each degree of fall in the ionized calcium concentration in plasma. Moreover, since it is very likely that this much citrate could escape removal by the liver in a single pass after drinking 1 L of orange juice (*see margin note*), this is not a threat.

CITRATE IN ORANGE JUICE
- Each liter contains 50 mmol K^+ and 50 mEq of citrate (~17 mmol; 17 μmol/mL).
- Plasma contains 1200 μmol ionized calcium/L.
- To remove half the calcium in plasma (~600 μmol), it would require the absorption of ⅓ L of orange juice, and this is extremely unlikely.
- Unlike in Mini Case 14-1, page 503, since there is no nidus when ionized calcium is chelated, there is not a progressive removal of ionized calcium in this setting. Thus, when plasma in the hepatic vein mixes with plasma in the great veins, there will be a much smaller net fall in the ionized calcium concentration; this scenario is akin to blood transfusion.

Hyperkalemia

Introduction

Hyperkalemia, usually defined as P_K greater than 5 mmol/L, is a common electrolyte disorder that is present in a number of disease states. Hyperkalemia may have detrimental effects, the most serious of which is a cardiac arrhythmia; this threat and the degree of rise in the P_K, however, are not tightly correlated.

When faced with a patient with hyperkalemia, the first step is to recognize whether an emergency is present (e.g., changes in the EKG due to hyperkalemia). If so, therapy must begin without delay.

If the time course for the development of hyperkalemia is short and/or if there has been little intake of K^+, suspect that the basis for the hyperkalemia is a shift of K^+ out of cells or pseudohypokalemia. Conversely, chronic hyperkalemia implies that there is a defect in the regulation of the excretion of K^+ by the kidney if pseudohypokalemia is not present. Notwithstanding, there may also be a component of a K^+ shift in patients with chronic hyperkalemia. Once a low rate of excretion of K^+ relative to the presence of hyperkalemia is confirmed, steps should be taken to identify why the net secretion of K^+ in the late cortical distal nephron may be low. One also should examine whether a low rate of flow in these nephron segments is a contributing factor to the low rate of excretion of K^+. Based on this analysis, one can determine where leverage can be exerted during therapy in the individual patient with hyperkalemia.

OBJECTIVES

- To point out that hyperkalemia is not a diagnostic category but a disorder that may be present in a number of disease states; its basis must be defined in each patient.
- To emphasize that hyperkalemia is a common electrolyte abnormality that may pose a major threat to survival (e.g., due to a cardiac arrhythmia).
- To provide a clinical approach to the patient with hyperkalemia based on an understanding of the physiology of shift of K^+ into cells and the renal regulation of the excretion of K^+.
- To provide an approach to the therapy of the patient with hyperkalemia.

CASE 15-1: MIGHT THIS PATIENT HAVE PSEUDOHYPERKALEMIA?

(Case discussed on page 538)

A 5-year-old male had neurosurgery to remove a vascular tumor in the frontal lobe of his brain. There were no complications during surgery, and his course in the intensive care unit was uneventful. Therefore, he was transferred to the ward for continuing care. At the time of transfer, his P_K was 4.0 mmol/L, but it was 6.0 mmol/L by the next morning. There was no hemolysis or any reason to suspect a laboratory problem. In addition, hyperkalemia was present in repeated blood testing. There was no intake of medications that would cause a shift of K^+ out of cells, and his intake of K^+ was low. He did not have a family history of hyperkalemia. The EKG did not have signs of hyperkalemia, his U_K was 10 mmol/L, and he was not polyuric. His $P_{Aldosterone}$ was very low when the results were reported at a later date. A clinical decision was made to treat him with mineralocorticoids, and several days later, his P_K returned to the normal range.

Questions

Why did hyperkalemia develop so soon after he left the intensive care unit?

What could be the basis for the high P_K, but only while the patient was on the ward?

Case 15-2: Is There an Error in the EKG?

(Case discussed on page 538)

A patient with chronic renal failure had changes in her EKG that were consistent with hyperkalemia, but her P_K was not elevated.

Question

How can this discrepancy be reconciled?

Case 15-3: Hyperkalemia with the Aid of Trimethoprim

(Case discussed on page 539)

A 23-year-old man had a long history of human immunodeficiency virus/acquired immunodeficiency syndrome (HIV/AIDS), which is now complicated by *Pneumocystis carinii* pneumonia. His dietary intake has been poor recently, and he is now malnourished. On admission, he was febrile, but his effective arterial blood volume was not contracted and plasma electrolyte values were all in the normal range. Three days after receiving treatment with sulfamethoxazole and trimethoprim, his blood pressure was low, his pulse rate was high, and his jugular venous pressure was low. Of note, his P_K was 6.8 mmol/L. Tall peaked T waves were seen on his EKG. His laboratory data on that day are summarized in the following table:

		PLASMA	URINE
Na+	mmol/L	130	60
K+	mmol/L	6.8	14
Cl−	mmol/L	105	43
BUN (Urea)	mg/dL (mmol/L)	14 (5)	100 mmol/L
Creatinine	mg/dL (μmol/L)	0.9 (100)	7 mmol/L
Osmolality	mOsm/kg H_2O	272	280
Volume	L/day	—	0.8

Questions

Why is hyperkalemia present?

What are the major issues for therapy?

If trimethoprim must be continued, what measures can be taken to minimize its ability to block ENaC?

ABBREVIATION
ENaC, epithelial Na+ channel

PART A
BACKGROUND

SYNOPSIS OF THE PHYSIOLOGY

A detailed discussion of the physiology of K+ is presented in Chapter 13. In this chapter, we provide a brief synopsis of this physiology.

Movement of K⁺ across cell membranes

- K⁺ move across cell membranes in response to an electro-chemical driving force providing that there are open K⁺ channels.
- A disorder of K⁺ distribution across cell membranes should be suspected if the time course over which hyperkalemia developed is short and/or if the input of K⁺ was low.

Negative voltage inside cells

K⁺ shift into cells when the intracellular voltage is more negative. This is present when there is more ion flux through the Na-K-ATPase, because it is an electrogenic pump (it exports 3 Na^+ and imports only 2 K^+). Flux through the Na-K-ATPase is influenced by the concentration of Na^+ in cells (this concentration of Na^+ rises when there is a spike of insulin), activation of existing Na-K-ATPase units (occurs with high levels of β_2-adrenergic hormones), and an increased number of Na-K-ATPase pump units (occurs with high levels of thyroid hormone and/or insulin). The impact of this increase in Na^+ pumping on the net cell voltage, however, depends on whether the Na^+ entry step into cells is electroneutral or electrogenic.

Electroneutral entry of Na⁺ into cells. If Na^+ enters the cell in an electroneutral fashion, its subsequent electrogenic exit via the Na-K-ATPase results in a more negative cell interior voltage, and hence there is less net exit of K^+ from these cells. This occurs when Na^+ enter cells in exchange for H^+ on the Na^+/H^+ exchanger (NHE). Although the NHE is normally *inactive* in cell membranes, it can become active if there is a spike of insulin or a higher concentration of H^+ in the intracellular fluid (ICF) compartment. The former provides the rationale for administering insulin in the emergency treatment of patients with a dangerous degree of hyperkalemia. It can also help explain why lack of actions of insulin results in a shift of K^+ out of cells and the development of hyperkalemia (e.g., in patients with diabetic ketoacidosis).

Electrogenic entry of Na⁺ in cells. The Na^+ channel in cell membranes is normally gated by voltage. When open, one cationic charge enters the cell per Na^+; its subsequent electrogenic exit via the Na-K-ATPase results in the net export of one third of a positive charge and hence the magnitude of the intracellular negative voltage diminishes. As a result, there is a net *exit* of K^+. One must recognize that depolarization is followed quickly by repolarization, during which these Na^+ are pumped out of cells by the Na-K-ATPase. This forces K^+ released during depolarization to return to the ICF compartment. To make this process efficient in skeletal muscle, the K^+ released during depolarization is trapped in a local area (T-tubular region), which prevents the development of an appreciable degree of hyperkalemia when muscles contract (*see margin note*).

K⁺ channels in cell membranes

The most important K^+ channel with respect to regulation of P_K is the K^+_{ATP} channel, which is regulated by the concentration of ADP in cells (*see margin note*).

ABBREVIATIONS

P_K and U_K, concentration of K^+ in plasma and urine, respectively

P_{Na} and U_{Na}, concentration of Na^+ in plasma and urine, respectively

P_{Cl} and U_{Cl}, concentration of Cl^- in plasma and urine, respectively

P_{Osm} and U_{Osm}, osmolality in plasma and urine, respectively

P_{HCO_3}, concentration of HCO_3 in plasma

$P_{Aldosterone}$, concentration of aldosterone in plasma

CCD, late cortical distal nephron, which includes the late distal convoluted tubule, the connecting segment, and the cortical collecting ducts

$[K^+]_{CCD}$, concentration of K^+ in the lumen of the CCD

NHE, Na^+/H^+ cation exchanger

AE, Cl^-/HCO_3^- anion exchanger

CLINICAL PEARL
Patients who are cachectic do not have this efficient trapping of K^+. Hence, they may have pseudo-hyperkalemia during repeated fist clenching in preparation for brachial venipuncture.

$[K^+]_{ATP}$ CHANNELS
- These K^+ channels are maintained in a closed configuration by the prevailing concentration of ATP in cells.
- These channels are opened when ADP binds to a regulatory site on these channels. Opening of $[K^+]_{ATP}$ in β-cells of the pancreas is involved in the secretion of insulin. Similarly, opening of these $[K^+]_{ATP}$ channels in vascular smooth muscle cells is important for the control of blood flow (see Chapter 13, page 459).

Rise in the P_K in patients with metabolic acidosis

> • Hyperkalemia occurs when the added acid is not a substrate for the monocarboxylic acid transporter (e.g., HCl, citric acid).

Transport of monocarboxylic acids (e.g., ketoacids or L-lactic acid) into cells on the monocarboxylic acid transporter does not result in a change in cell voltage and hence it does not have a direct effect on a transcellular shift of K^+. On the other hand, entry of organic acids into cells does have an important *indirect* action that promotes the entry of K^+ into cells. In more detail, as soon as L-lactic acid produced during vigorous exercise, for example, enters nonexercising cells (e.g., hepatocytes) on the monocarboxylic acid cotransporter, H^+ are released, and this creates a high local H^+ at the inner aspect of the cell membrane, which activates NHE and catalyzes the electroneutral entry of Na^+. The export of this Na^+ by the Na-K-ATPase causes a more negative voltage in cells and thereby the entry of K^+. If hyperkalemia is present in a patient with metabolic acidosis due to ketoacidosis or L-lactic acidosis, causes for hyperkalemia other than this acidemia should be sought (e.g., lack of insulin in patients with diabetic ketoacidosis, tissue injury, or a lack of ATP to drive the Na-K-ATPase in patients with L-lactic acidosis due to hypoxia).

Conversely, acids that cannot enter cells via the monocarboxylic acid transporter (e.g., HCl, citric acid) cause a shift of K^+ out of cells. Nevertheless, patients with chronic hyperchloremic metabolic acidosis may have a low P_K because of excessive loss of K^+ in diarrhea fluid in patients with chronic diarrhea or in the urine (e.g., patients with distal renal tubular acidosis due to a defect in net H^+ secretion in distal nephron).

Hyperkalemia in patients with tissue catabolism

In patients with diabetic ketoacidosis, there is a deficit of K^+ because of the catabolic state where both K^+ and phosphate anions are released from cells; then these ions are excreted in the urine. Despite this deficit of K^+, hyperkalemia is present as a result of a shift of K^+ from cells, secondary to lack of actions of insulin. The corollary is that during therapy for diabetic ketoacidosis, complete replacement of the deficit of K^+ must await the provision of cellular constituents (e.g., phosphate, amino acids, Mg^{2+}) and the presence of anabolic signals.

Hyperkalemia may be seen in patients with crush injury or tumor lysis syndrome. In these patients, factors that compromise the renal excretion of K^+ are usually present as well.

Regulation of the renal excretion of K^+

Control of the renal excretion of K^+ maintains overall daily K^+ balance. This occurs primarily in the late cortical distal nephron. Most of the secretion of K^+ occurs in the late distal convoluted tubule and the connecting segment; nevertheless, K^+ may also be secreted in the cortical collecting duct if the K^+ load is large. To be succinct, we use the abbreviation CCD to represent all of these nephron segments.

The major factor that influences the rate of excretion of K^+ is the net secretion of K^+ by principal cells in the CCD, which raises the concentration of K^+ in its lumen ($[K^+]_{CCD}$). A low delivery of Na^+ to the CCD may pose a problem for K^+ homeostasis if there is a large K^+ intake, because there may be a limited ability to generate a lumen-negative voltage in the CCD (*see margin note*). A low flow rate in the CCD may compromise the ability to secrete K^+ in the CCD by increasing the concentration of a blocker of ENaC (e.g., trimethoprim) in the luminal fluid in the CCD (see the discussion of Case 15-3, page 539).

Secretion of K^+ in the late cortical distal nephron

The driving force for the secretion of K^+ in the CCD is a lumen-negative voltage, which is generated by the electrogenic reabsorption of Na^+ in that nephron segment (reabsorption of more Na^+ than its accompanying anion, Cl^-) via the ENaC (see Fig. 13-8, page 442). Diminished actions of aldosterone reduce the number of ENaC units in the luminal membranes of principal cells and thus may decrease renal excretion of K^+.

The major pathway for Cl^- reabsorption is paracellular, and this pathway appears to be regulated. The concentration of HCO_3^- and/or an alkaline luminal fluid pH increases the net secretion of K^+ in the CCD. The mechanism has not been fully clarified, but it may result from a decrease in the apparent permeability of Cl^- and/or an increase in the number of open rat outer medullary K^+ (ROMK) channels. If the rates of reabsorption of Na^+ and Cl^- are similar in the CCD, an appreciable lumen-negative voltage will not be generated in this nephron segment, and this lowers the rate of secretion of K^+. Two factors may cause this near-equal rate of ion transport in the CCD. First, low delivery of Na^+ and Cl^- to the CCD, which occurs when the reabsorption of Na^+ and Cl^- is augmented in the distal convoluted tubule because of increased activity of Na^+, Cl^- cotransporter (NCC). Second, expansion of the effective arterial blood volume, which suppresses the release of aldosterone and leads to fewer open ENaC units; hence, the rate of reabsorption of Cl^- in the CCD may match that of Na^+. An example of this pathophysiology is the hyperkalemia in patients with Gordon's syndrome (discussed on page 526). Alternatively, Na^+ and Cl^- can be reabsorbed at comparable rates when the delivery of Na^+ and Cl^- to the CCD is normal, providing that the reabsorption of Cl^- in the CCD is stimulated. The underlying mechanism(s) that increase the permeability for Cl^- is (are) not clear, and the term *Cl^- shunt disorder* is used to describe this pathophysiology.

In addition to control by the lumen-negative voltage, the secretory process for K^+ in principal cells is dependent on having a sufficient number of open ROMK channels in the luminal membrane of principal cells. Potassium channels are abundant and have a high open probability in individuals who consume a potassium-rich diet. Therefore, ROMK channels do not seem to limit the net secretion of K^+ unless the P_K falls to the mid–3-mmol/L range. Because there is a time lag before ROMK channels are reinserted into the luminal membrane of principal cells in the CCD following chronic hypokalemia in human subjects, hyperkalemia may develop with aggressive K^+ replacement therapy in this setting.

FLOW RATE IN THE CCD

- When vasopressin acts, the osmolality is equal in the lumen of the terminal CCD and in plasma. Hence, the flow rate in the CCD is determined by the rate of delivery of osmoles (~1 L/~300 mosmol of urea and electrolytes).

- The osmole that is most important in determining the volume in the terminal CCD is urea, which usually accounts for 75% of the osmoles delivered of the CCD.

- If the flow rate in the CCD is very low, one will need a more negative luminal voltage to have a higher $[K^+]_{CCD}$ and thereby prevent a fall in the rate of excretion of K^+. If there is a limited ability to have this more negative voltage, the rate of K^+ excretion will decrease, and hyperkalemia will develop to permit the rate of excretion of K^+ to rise sufficiently to excrete the daily intake of K^+.

- A higher flow rate in the CCD, whether due to a higher intake of NaCl or protein, is not sufficient on its own to increase the excretion of K^+ without an additional stimulus to secrete K^+ in the late cortical distal nephron.

STAGES IN THE DEVELOPMENT OF HYPERKALEMIA

- *Before the defect begins:* The subject has a constant normal P_K and is in a steady state for K^+. This means that all the K^+ that is ingested each day is excreted.
- *Stage when there is a positive balance for K^+:* In this stage, there is a low rate of excretion of K^+ before chronic hyperkalemia develops.
- *Stage with chronic hyperkalemia:* A new steady state develops in which all dietary K^+ is excreted but a higher P_K is needed to increase the rate of excretion of K^+.

There are three stages in the pathophysiology of the renal process for the excretion of K^+ in patients who develop chronic hyperkalemia. In this analysis, we assume that the patient continues to eat the same diet, and therefore the delivery of Na^+ and urea, and thus the flow rate in the CCD does not limit the excretion of K^+.

1. *Before the defect begins:* In this stage, individuals have a normal ability to excrete K^+; hence, they excrete the entire absorbed dietary K^+ load and maintain a steady state with a P_K in the normal range (Fig. 15-1). The peak rate of excretion only occurs for

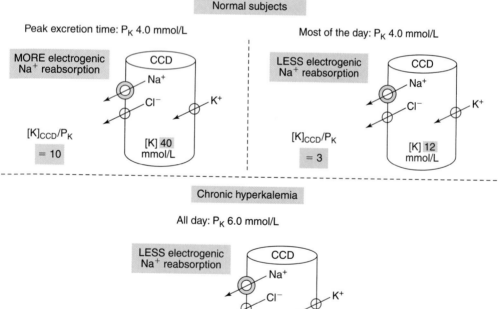

FIGURE 15-1 Excretion of K^+ in normal subjects and in patients with chronic hyperkalemia. The *barrel-shaped structures* represent the CCD. Over the 24-hour period, both the normal subject and the patient with hyperkalemia reabsorb 70 mmol more Na^+ than Cl^- and hence excrete 70 mmol of K^+, as they are in balance for K^+. The *top portion of the figure* describes normal subjects (P_K 4.0 mmol/L) and the *bottom portion* describes patients with chronic hyperkalemia. The *left section of the top part of the figure* illustrates the excretion of K^+ when it is at its usual maximum rate (close to noon) whereas the *right section* illustrates this secretory process when K^+ excretion is much lower throughout the day. In contrast, the patient with chronic hyperkalemia has a lower maximum concentration of K^+ in the lumen of the CCD. As a result, he will need to maintain peak K^+ excretion rates for all of the day, and the price to pay is chronic hyperkalemia (*lower part of the figure*).

a few hours, usually close to noon. For the majority of the day, there is a much lower rate of excretion of K^+. We emphasize that the capacity to excrete K^+ without causing the P_K to rise above the normal range is about fourfold larger (i.e., ~280 mmol/day) than the usual dietary K^+ load that must be excreted each day (~70 mmol/day) in a 70-kg adult eating a typical Western diet. Hence, one needs an enormous defect in K^+ excretion (>67%) before hyperkalemia develops (*see margin note*).

2. *The development of hyperkalemia*: The capacity to raise the $[K^+]_{CCD}$ is diminished as there is less electrogenic reabsorption of Na^+ in the CCD. As a result, the electrical gradient is diminished. Therefore, the only way to have the same $[K^+]_{CCD}$ is to have a higher P_K. Nevertheless, this patient will reach a steady state once he can excrete all the K^+ ingested each day (*see margin note*). The time needed to develop a positive balance for K^+ and thereby hyperkalemia depends on how much K^+ is ingested and how large a defect in K^+ excretion is present.

3. *The new steady state with hyperkalemia*: In this stage, the P_K is abnormally high. Nevertheless, the elevated P_K increases the capacity to secrete K^+ and the patient is now able to excrete the entire daily K^+ load by secreting K^+ at his maximal rate for the entire 24-hour period (i.e., the steady state has returned, but the price to pay is a higher P_K; see Fig. 15-1, *lower portion; see margin note*).

EFFECT OF AN ELEVATED P_K ON K^+ EXCRETION

- The events leading to a higher rate of excretion of K^+ are depicted in the following table. In this example, the flow rate in the CCD is 1 L and 40 mmol of K^+ are excreted in each subject.

SUBJECT	VOLTAGE	P_K	$[K^+]_{CCD}$
Normal	−42 mV	4	20
Hyperka-lemia	−31 mV	6	20

- Thus, when there is a lumen-negative voltage with a lower maximum value (−31 mV versus −42 mV), the same $[K^+]_{CCD}$ can be achieved as long as the P_K remains elevated (see Part E, page 535 for more discussion).

PART B
CLINICAL APPROACH

ADDRESS EMERGENCIES

It is imperative to recognize when hyperkalemia represents a medical emergency because therapy must take precedence over diagnosis (Flow Chart 15-1; see page 532 for more description). One must also anticipate the dangers associated with each mode of therapy and take steps to prevent them from occurring (see Part D, page 532 for more discussion).

DIAGNOSTIC WORKUP

Once the emergencies have been dealt with, the next step is to determine if the cause of the hyperkalemia is a shift of K^+ out of cells in vivo or in vitro (Flow Chart 15-2).

Is the time period short and/or has the intake of K^+ been low?

If the answer is yes, there are three options to consider.

1. *The high P_K could be due to a shift of K^+ out of cells in the body*. For this to occur, look for a reason to have a less negative voltage in cells. The major causes would include a lack of insulin or metabolic acidosis due to the addition of HCl or organic acids (e.g., citric acid, a tricarboxylic acid) that are not the physiologic monocarboxylic acids (e.g., L-lactic acid, ketoacids) or exhaustive exercise. A positive family history for acute hyperkalemia suggests that there may be a molecular basis for this disorder (e.g., hyperkalemic periodic paralysis).

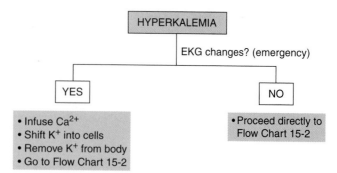

FLOW CHART 15-1 Initial treatment of the patient with hyperkalemia. If an emergency is present (usually cardiac), intravenous Ca^{2+} must be given. This treatment should act promptly. Efforts are then made to shift K^+ into cells with insulin, while preventing hypoglycemia with intravenous glucose.

2. *There is destruction of cells in the body.* In this case, the diagnosis is usually obvious (e.g., crush injury).
3. *Pseudohyperkalemia may be present.* In this setting, there will not be EKG changes associated with hyperkalemia if its only cause is pseudohyperkalemia.

Are there laboratory or technical problems?

Hemolysis, megakaryocytosis, fragile tumor cells, a K^+ channel disorder in red blood cells, and excessive fist clenching during blood sampling should be excluded. Pseudohyperkalemia can be present in cachectic patients because the normal T-tubule architecture in skeletal muscle may be disturbed. This permits more K^+ to be released into venous blood, even without excessive fist clenching during blood sampling (*see margin note*). The presence of EKG changes due to hyperkalemia means that the patient has "true" hyperkalemia, even if there are reasons for pseudohyperkalemia.

CLINICAL PEARL
Since metabolic alkalosis is not usually accompanied by hyperkalemia, suspect pseudohyperkalemia if the P_K and P_{HCO_3} are elevated.

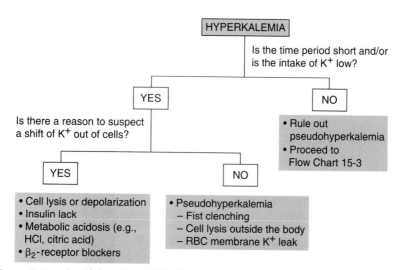

FLOW CHART 15-2 Determine if there is a shift of K^+ out of cells. The most important issue is to determine if a shift of K^+ out of cells is likely by assessing the time course for the rise in the P_K and whether there was little intake of K^+. If there is no reason to suspect a shift of K^+ out of cells, pseudohyperkalemia should be ruled out. In this latter setting, there should not be EKG changes related to hyperkalemia. The next step is to proceed to Flow Chart 15-3 and examine the rate of excretion of K^+.

Is the rate of excretion of K$^+$ high enough in a patient with hyperkalemia?

- Normal subjects in steady state excrete all the K$^+$ they ingest each day; thus, there is no normal rate of K$^+$ excretion because dietary intake of K$^+$ varies from day to day.
- Subjects with normal kidneys can excrete an enormous quantity of dietary K$^+$ per day (i.e., close to 200 mmol K$^+$) while their P$_K$ remains in the normal range.

To assess the renal response in a patient with hyperkalemia, we use the expected rate of K$^+$ excretion in normal subjects who are given a K$^+$ load; these subjects can augment the rate of excretion of K$^+$ to greater than 200 mmol/day (200 mmol/g creatinine or 20 mmol/mmol creatinine). This is achieved with only a minor increase in the P$_K$ (Flow Chart 15-3). In contrast, patients with chronic hyperkalemia will have a rate of excretion of K$^+$ that is equal to their current intake of K$^+$. Nevertheless, this can only be achieved while their P$_K$ is elevated.

It is common to rely on a 24-hour urine collection to assess the rate of excretion of K$^+$. Nevertheless, because an exact value is not needed, the ratio of the concentrations of K$^+$ and creatinine in spot urine samples (U$_K$/U$_{Creatinine}$) can be used even though there is a diurnal variation in K$^+$ excretion. This analysis is predicated on the fact that creatinine is excreted at a near-constant rate throughout the day (*see margin note*). Moreover, the U$_K$/U$_{Creatinine}$ in spot urines provides more relevant information because the stimulus to drive K$^+$ excretion (i.e., the P$_K$) is known at that time. Therefore, if fewer than 200 mmol K$^+$/g creatinine or 20 mmol K$^+$/mmol creatinine are excreted in a patient with hyperkalemia, there is a renal defect in K$^+$ excretion.

EXCRETION OF CREATININE
- The excretion of creatinine is relatively constant throughout the 24-hour period because its rate of production is constant (depends on muscle mass) and there is little variation in the glomerular filtration rate.
- The usual daily rate of excretion of creatinine is 20 mg/kg body weight (300 µmol/kg body weight).

Basis for the low [K$^+$]$_{CCD}$

- The most common explanation for a low [K$^+$]$_{CCD}$ is a less negative voltage in the lumen of the CCD due to a lower rate of electrogenic reabsorption of Na$^+$ in the CCD.

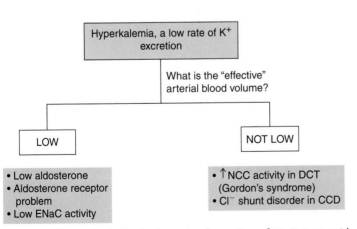

ABBREVIATION
NCC, Na$^+$, Cl$^-$ cotransporter

FLOW CHART 15-3 Basis for the low rate of excretion of K$^+$. Patients with chronic hyperkalemia can be divided into two groups based on their effective arterial blood volume (EABV). In this analysis, we have assumed that there is an adequate distal delivery of Na$^+$.

> • There are two major categories for this low lumen-negative voltage: a diminished rate of reabsorption of Na$^+$ via ENaC and conditions in which the reabsorption of Na$^+$ and Cl$^-$ occurs at near equal rates.

Diminished reabsorption of Na$^+$ via ENaC in the CCD

The first subgroup consists of patients who have a marked decrease in the effective arterial blood volume; these patients may have a sufficiently low delivery of Na$^+$ to the CCD to limit the rate of secretion of K$^+$. The hallmark for this diagnosis is the excretion of urine with a very low concentration of Na$^+$. The second subgroup consists of patients who have lesions that lead to a diminished number of open ENaCs in the luminal membrane of principal cells in the CCD. Accordingly, the reabsorption of Na$^+$ is not sufficient to generate a large lumen-negative voltage in the CCD. The basis of this slower reabsorption of Na$^+$ includes low aldosterone actions (e.g., adrenal insufficiency, blockers of the aldosterone receptor in principal cells), molecular defects that diminish the number of ENaC units in the luminal membrane of the CCD, the presence of cationic compounds in the lumen of the CCD that block ENaC (e.g., the use of potassium-sparing diuretics such as amiloride or triamterene or cationic antimicrobial agents such as trimethoprim). These patients have a low effective arterial blood volume and a higher than expected rate of excretion of Na$^+$ and Cl$^-$, and a high renin activity in plasma (P$_{Renin}$). The P$_{Aldosterone}$ is helpful to determine the reason for this diminished Na$^+$ reabsorption via ENaC in the CCD.

Reabsorption of Na$^+$ and Cl$^-$ at near-equal rates in the CCD

One subgroup seems to have an increased permeability for Cl$^-$ in the CCD (a "Cl$^-$ shunt disorder"). In another subgroup, the site of the lesion might be in the early distal convoluted tubule, where there is enhanced electroneutral reabsorption of Na$^+$ and Cl$^-$ via the NCC. Accordingly, the delivery of Na$^+$ and Cl$^-$ to the CCD is not sufficiently large to permit the rate of reabsorption of Na$^+$ to exceed the rate of reabsorption of Cl$^-$ in the CCD by an appreciable amount. In addition, there is a diminished number of open ENaC units in the luminal membranes of principal cells because of the suppression of release of aldosterone by an expanded effective arterial blood volume. Independent of the site of the lesion, these patients have an expanded effective arterial blood volume, hypertension, and a very low P$_{Renin}$. They retain the ability to excrete Na$^+$- and Cl$^-$-poor urine, however, when the effective arterial blood volume is contracted (e.g., after giving a diuretic plus a low salt diet).

PART C
SPECIFIC CAUSES
OF HYPERKALEMIA

A list of the causes of hyperkalemia based on their possible underlying pathophysiology is provided in Table 15-1. Before examining Table 15-1, pseudohyperkalemia should be ruled out. A list of drugs that may cause hyperkalemia is shown in Table 15-2.

TABLE 15-1 **CAUSES OF HYPERKALEMIA**

High intake of K⁺

- Only if combined with low excretion of K⁺

Shift of K⁺ out of cells

- Cell necrosis
- Lack of insulin
- Use of nonselective β-blockers (small effect if only factor)
- Metabolic acidosis associated with anions that are largely restricted to the extracellular fluid compartment (e.g., HCl, citric acid)
- Rare causes (e.g., hyperkalemic periodic paralysis)

Diminished K⁺ loss in the urine

- Advanced chronic renal insufficiency
- Specific lesions that may lead to a low $[K^+]_{CCD}$
  - Primary decrease in flux of Na⁺ through ENaC
    - Very low delivery of Na⁺ to the CCD
    - Low levels of aldosterone (e.g., Addison's disease)
    - Blockade of the aldosterone receptor (e.g., spironolactone)
    - Low ENaC activity (type I pseudohypoaldosteronism)
    - Blockade of ENaC (e.g., amiloride, triamterene, trimethoprim)
  - Cl⁻ reabsorbed at a similar rate as Na⁺ in the CCD
    - Increased reabsorption of Na⁺ and Cl⁻ in the distal convoluted tubule (e.g., Gordon's syndrome [WNK kinase-4 or WNK kinase -1 mutations])
    - Possible Cl⁻ shunt in the CCD (e.g., some of the causes of hyporeninemic hypoaldosteronism, diabetic nephropathy, drugs such as cyclosporin)

ENaC, epithelial Na⁺ channel; WNK, with no lysine.

TABLE 15-2 **DRUGS THAT MAY CAUSE HYPERKALEMIA**

Compounds containing K⁺ (this only increases P_K if K⁺ excretion is compromised)

- KCl, table salt substitutes that contain K⁺

Drugs that cause a shift of K⁺ from the ICF to the ECF

- Cell depolarizers such as succinylcholine
- Drugs causing cell necrosis such as chemotheraputic agents that lead to tumor lysis
- Drugs impairing insulin release from β-cells such as α-adrenergic agonists
- β₂-adrenergic receptor blockers

Drugs that interfere with K⁺ excretion in the urine

- Drugs that cause acute renal failure (acute tubular necrosis or acute interstitial nephritis)
- Drugs that lead to a low P_{Renin} (e.g., prostaglandin synthesis inhibitors [NSAID])
- Drugs that decrease the release of aldosterone (e.g., heparin, ketoconazole)
- Drugs that interfere with the renin-angiotensin II axis (e.g., angiotensin-converting enzyme inhibitors, angiotensin II receptor blockers, renin inhibitors)
- Aldosterone receptor blockers (e.g., spironolactone)
- Drugs that block ENaC in the CCD (e.g., amiloride, trimethoprim)
- Drugs that interfere with activation of ENaC via proteolytic cleavage (e.g., nafamostat mesylate)

ENaC, epithelial Na⁺ channel; NSAID, nonsteroidal anti-inflammatory drugs.

DECREASED SECRETION OF K$^+$ IN THE CCD IN PATIENTS WITH CHRONIC RENAL FAILURE

- The key issue is the low number of CCD units together with only a minimal reduction in the flow rate in the CCD (similar number of osmoles excreted, because the diet is not yet severely restricted). Hence, the flow rate through each remaining CCD is very high. This compromises the ability to reabsorb more Na$^+$ than Cl$^-$ in the CCD, and hence the lumen-negative voltage is not high enough to raise the [K$^+$]$_{CCD}$ sufficiently.
- These patients may also be taking drugs that compromise the ability to secrete K$^+$. Prominent on the list are drugs that diminish the secretion of aldosterone (angiotensin-converting enzyme [ACE] inhibitors, angiotensin II receptor blockers, or renin inhibitors) and aldosterone receptor blockers (e.g., spironolactone).

CHRONIC RENAL INSUFFICIENCY

- Hyperkalemia occurs frequently in patients with advanced chronic kidney disease, and it is due to a diminished ability to excrete K$^+$.

These patients have a limited capacity to excrete K$^+$ because they cannot generate a large enough lumen-negative voltage in their CCD (*see margin note*). The degree of hyperkalemia will be more severe when their intake of K$^+$ is large or if the rate of excretion of K$^+$ is compromised by the intake of certain drugs.

Therapy

The long-term management in patients with chronic hyperkalemia is to decrease the intake of K$^+$ and to promote K$^+$ excretion. To achieve this latter aim, one must raise the [K$^+$]$_{CCD}$ and/or increase the delivery of filtrate and/or Na$^+$ to the CCD. Specific modalities of therapy are discussed in the following disease sections and in Part E, page 537 in this chapter).

ADDISON'S DISEASE

- Adrenal crisis is a medical emergency that requires immediate therapy.
- Addison's disease is usually a chronic disorder; the symptoms are usually nonspecific.
- The major problems are caused by a lack of glucocorticoids, a low effective arterial blood volume, and hyperkalemia. Do not dismiss this diagnosis, however, if hyperkalemia is absent.

The most common cause of Addison's disease used to be bilateral adrenal destruction due to tuberculosis, but now autoimmune adrenalitis accounts for the majority of cases. Additional causes include other infectious diseases (e.g., disseminated fungal infection), adrenal replacement by metastatic carcinoma or lymphoma, adrenal hemorrhage or infarction, and drugs that impair the synthesis of aldosterone (e.g., ketoconazole and possibly fluconazole). The defect in K$^+$ excretion results from failure to generate a large enough lumen-negative voltage in the CCD because of a low number of open ENaCs in the luminal membrane of principal cells due to a lack of aldosterone.

Patients with chronic primary adrenal insufficiency may present with chronic malaise, fatigue, anorexia, generalized weakness, postural hypotension, and weight loss. Salt craving is a feature in some of these patients. On physical examination, the blood pressure is low and postural symptoms of dizziness and syncope are common. Hyperpigmentation is evident in nearly all patients.

The P$_K$ is usually close to 5.5 mmol/L. Nevertheless, hyperkalemia is not seen on presentation in approximately one third of cases. Other possible abnormal laboratory findings include hyponatremia, hyperchloremic metabolic acidosis, hypoglycemia, and eosinophilia. Some patients may present with acute adrenal crisis and shock. The diagnosis can be established by finding a low P$_{Aldosterone}$ and P$_{Cortisol}$, a high plasma renin activity, an elevated concentration of adrenocorticotropic hormone (ACTH) in plasma, and a blunted cortisol response to the administration of ACTH. A marked decrease in liver function may exacerbate the deficiency of cortisol by decreasing the conversion of cortisone to cortisol (*see margin note*).

Therapy

Adrenal crisis is an emergency that requires immediate restoration of the intravascular volume with the administration of intravenous saline and dexamethasone or hydrocortisone (*see margin note*). Avoid raising the P_{Na} too rapidly if hyponatremia is present because of the risk of osmotic demyelination in a catabolic patient. Water diuresis may ensue because of increased distal delivery of filtrate and suppression of vasopressin release with restoration of effective arterial blood volume, and because administration of glucocorticoids can lead, indirectly, to a fall in the circulating level of vasopressin. Therefore, we give desmopressin (dDAVP) at the outset of therapy to avoid a large water diuresis that could result in a sudden and excessive rise in the P_{Na}. When dDAVP is given, the patient should be water restricted for the duration of its action.

Patients with chronic adrenal insufficiency should receive chronic replacement therapy with both a glucocorticoid and a mineralocorticoid. For the former, 25 mg of hydrocortisone (15 mg in the morning and 10 mg in the afternoon) is usually given. For mineralocorticoid replacement, fludrocortisone in a single dose of 50 to 200 μg is usually used. Dose adjustments are made based on symptoms, ECF volume status, blood pressure, and P_K.

CONGENITAL ADRENAL HYPERPLASIA

These rare inherited disorders are due to deficiencies in the enzymes involved in aldosterone biosynthesis. In many of them, glucocorticoid deficiency is also present. Their common features include salt wasting, hyponatremia, hyperkalemia, and hypotension.

PSEUDOHYPOALDOSTERONISM TYPE I

- The underlying pathophysiology is a "closed" ENaC in the CCD (Fig. 15-2).
- There are two different forms of this disorder with different modes of inheritance.
- These patients fail to respond to exogenous mineralocorticoids, and their $P_{Aldosterone}$ and their P_{Renin} are markedly elevated.

Autosomal recessive form

Most mutations are frameshift or premature stop codon defects in the α-subunit of ENaC. Clinically, the disease is permanent and involves all aldosterone target organs. Patients usually present in the neonatal period with renal salt wasting, hyperkalemia, metabolic acidosis, failure to thrive, and weight loss. ENaC activity is also impaired in the lung, and this leads to excessive airway fluid accumulation and recurrent lower respiratory tract infections.

Autosomal dominant form

This form of the disorder is caused by mutations involving the mineralocorticoid receptor. It is usually mild and may remit with time. Treatment includes supplementation with NaCl and inducing

CONVERSION OF CORTISONE TO CORTISOL
- In contrast to cortisol, cortisone does not bind to the mineralocorticoid receptor, so it is biologically inactive.
- Some of the circulating pool of cortisol is continuously destroyed by 11β-HSDH in principal cells in the kidney.
- The liver can rescue this "potential cortisol" by converting cortisone back to cortisol via its 11β-HSDH. This is particularly important when the adrenal reserve is low.

ABBREVIATION
dDAVP, desamino, D-arginine vasopressin, a long-acting form of vasopressin

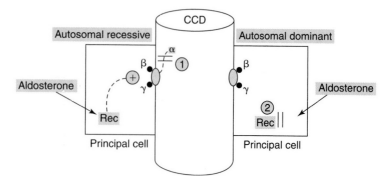

FIGURE 15-2 Molecular basis of pseudohypoaldosteronism type I. For details, see the text. The site of the lesion is the α-subunit (*green oval*) of the ENaC in the autosomal recessive form of the disorder (shown as *site 1*). This leads to an absence of the Na^+ channel per se. In contrast, the molecular defect is in the aldosterone receptor (Rec) in the autosomal dominant defect (*site 2 in the right cell*).

the loss of K^+ through the gastrointestinal tract. Dialysis may be required for treatment of life-threatening hyperkalemia.

PSEUDOHYPOALDOSTERONISM TYPE II (GORDON'S SYNDROME)

- The term *pseudohypoaldosteronism* is misleading from a physiologic perspective because patients with this syndrome have salt retention and hypertension, findings associated with higher rather than lower activity of aldosterone.
- Major deletions in the genes encoding for "with **no** lysine" (WNK) kinase-1 and WNK kinase-4 are the likely cause of this disorder (**K** is the abbreviation for lysine).

The basis for increased reabsorption of Na^+ and Cl^- in the distal convoluted tubule in this disorder has been clarified recently. Major deletions in the genes encoding for WNK kinase-1 and WNK kinase-4 have been reported in these patients (see Chapter 13, Fig. 13-15, page 452). Both of these kinases are found in the distal convoluted tubule and in the CCD. The effects of WNK kinase-4 to remove WNK-3 lead to a decrease in the number of NCC units located in the luminal membrane of the distal convoluted tubule. Therefore, if WNK kinase-4 is deleted, reabsorption of Na^+ and Cl^- by NCC in the distal convoluted tubule is augmented.

The role of WNK kinase-1 is to inactivate WNK kinase-4. As a result, there is more WNK-3, which results in an increased number of NCC units in the luminal membrane of the distal convoluted tubule. The molecular defect in WNK kinase-1 is a removal of intron bases that leads to its activation (gain-of-function mutation).

The higher activity of the thiazide-sensitive NCC could explain why hypertension, hyperkalemia, and suppressed P_{Renin} are common features in this disorder. Because angiotensin II levels are low, the release of aldosterone is decreased and $P_{Aldosterone}$ is inappropriately low in presence of hyperkalemia. The decreased delivery of Na^+ and Cl^- to the CCD together with diminished ENaC activity due to the low $P_{Aldosterone}$ prevents the reabsorption of Na^+ from being appreciably more than that of Cl⁻. The overall result is a low lumen-negative voltage in the CCD and the development of hyperkalemia (Fig. 15-1, page 518). A marked fall in blood pressure and correction of hyperkalemia are noted in these patients when treated with thiazide diuretics.

SYNDROME OF HYPORENINEMIC HYPOALDOSTERONISM

- Patients in this arbitrary diagnostic category represent a heterogeneous group with regard to the pathophysiology of their disorder.

Group 1: Patients with low capability of producing renin

The basis of the pathophysiology in this group of patients is destruction of, or a biosynthetic defect in, the juxtaglomerular apparatus that leads to hyporeninemia and thereby to a low $P_{Aldosterone}$. Accordingly, there is a relatively lower rate of reabsorption of Na^+ in the CCD. Hyperkalemia develops if there is a sufficiently large intake of K^+ such that a rise in the P_K must be present to permit the adrenal gland to secrete aldesterone and thereby allow the kidneys to excrete this K^+ and achieve balance for K^+ (see page 535 for more discussion). The effective arterial blood volume tends to be low. Patients with this disorder are expected to have a significant rise in their excretion of K^+ with the administration of exogenous mineralocorticoids.

Group 2: Patients with low stimulus to produce renin

- There are two subtypes of patients with this group of disorders.

The first subtype has an enhanced reabsorption of Na^+ and Cl^- in the distal convoluted tubule owing to an abnormal regulation of the signal system that affects the distribution of the NCC and hence more active units of NCC will reside in the luminal membrane. This has been discussed previously under the heading of Pseudohypoaldosteronism Type II (Gordon's syndrome). A hallmark of the pathophysiology in these patients is ECF volume expansion, which results in hyporeninemia, and thereby a lower than expected $P_{Aldosterone}$ in the presence of hyperkalemia. Accordingly, these patients do not have an appreciable rise in their excretion of K^+ following the administration of exogenous mineralocorticoids, but their rate of excretion of K^+ should rise when thiazide diuretics are given (higher Na^+ and Cl^- delivery to the CCD) providing that more ENaC units are present in the luminal membrane of principal cells.

The second subtype has similar clinical findings to those described previously, but there is no known molecular lesion. This syndrome is most commonly seen in some patients with diabetic nephropathy. The basis of the disorder remains to be established. It is possible that the reabsorption of Na^+ and Cl^- may be augmented in the distal convoluted tubule or that these patients may have a "Cl⁻ shunt disorder" in the CCD. If the delivery of HCO_3^- to the CCD can be increased (e.g., after the administration of acetazolamide), patients with a Cl⁻ shunt may have a significant increase in their $[K^+]_{CCD}$ and thereby in their rate of excretion of K^+.

Therapy

Differentiation between these two groups of patients with hyporeninemic hypoaldosteronism has implications for therapy. The use of exogenous mineralocorticoids (9α-fludrocortisone) is of benefit for the first group of patients (i.e., those with a defect in renin secretion) because it results in both a kaliuresis and reexpansion of the ECF volume owing to retention of Na^+. Diuretic therapy would pose a threat to these patients because it would cause a more severe degree of effective arterial blood volume contraction. In contrast, mineralocorticoids may aggravate the hypertension in the second group of patients, as they have excessive reabsorption of Na^+ and Cl^- in the distal convoluted tubule or the CCD. In this group, the administration of a thiazide diuretic to inhibit NCC should enhance the kaliuresis and lower the blood pressure. The administration of diuretics to patients with a Cl^- shunt might help lower their blood pressure and increase their rate of excretion of K^+ if it causes a sufficient degree of contraction of the effective arterial blood volume to cause the release of aldosterone and increase the number of open ENaCs in the luminal membrane of principal cells in CCD. Inducing bicarbonaturia by the administration of acetazolamide may increase the excretion of K^+; HCO_3^- loss may have to be replaced to avoid the development of metabolic acidosis.

HYPERKALEMIC PERIODIC PARALYSIS

- The defect in this disorder seems to be in the regulation of a specific population of Na^+ channels (tetrodotoxin sensitive) in muscle cell membranes.

This syndrome, which is inherited in an autosomal dominant pattern, is the result of a mutation in the α-subunit of the skeletal muscle Na^+ channel gene. When the muscle is stimulated to contract, Na^+ influx depolarizes the cell. As the membrane potential approaches −50 mV, normal Na^+ channels close. In patients with hyperkalemic periodic paralysis, these defective Na^+ channels fail to close, causing the cells to have less negative membrane potential. Depending on the absolute voltage, lesser changes may result in myotonia, whereas larger changes cause paralysis. Treatment of the acute attack involves measures to cause K^+ to shift into cells. Excessive excretion of K^+ should be avoided. Acetazolamide seems to be effective to prevent attacks, but its mechanism of action is not clear.

DRUGS ASSOCIATED WITH HYPERKALEMIA

- In general, drugs that cause hyperkalemia can be classified into those that affect the shift of K^+ into cells and those that impair its renal excretion.

Drugs that affect cellular redistribution of K^+

Nonselective $β_2$-adrenergic blockers may diminish the $β_2$-adrenergic–mediated shift of K^+ into cells. In general, only a minor rise in the P_K is observed in patients taking this class of drugs. Nevertheless, a more significant degree of hyperkalemia may develop after vigorous exercise or if there is an underlying kidney disease or the intake of drugs that may impair the excretion of K^+ by the kidney.

Digitalis overdose may be accompanied by hyperkalemia as a result of the inhibition of the Na-K-ATPase in the cell membrane of skeletal muscles. The use of depolarizing agents such as succinylcholine during anesthesia may cause a shift of K^+ from cells and cause hyperkalemia. Arginine hydrochloride (used in the treatment of hepatic coma, severe metabolic alkalosis, or upper GI bleeding) and epsilon-aminocaproic acid, a synthetic amino acid structurally similar to lysine, may cause an efflux of K^+ from cells, resulting at times in life-threatening hyperkalemia.

Impaired K^+ redistribution via the activation of K^+ channels by fluoride poisoning leads to life-threatening hyperkalemia, which may be ameliorated by the administration of quinidine and amiodarone. Drugs that have α-adrenergic agonist effects may cause hyperkalemia by inhibiting the release of insulin.

Drugs that interfere with renal K^+ excretion

With respect to many of the drugs that are associated with hyperkalemia, the mechanisms for the defect in K^+ excretion have not been studied in sufficient detail to draw unequivocal conclusions about how each drug causes hyperkalemia. This assessment requires measurement of the rate of excretion of K^+ and an evaluation of the cause of a low $[K^+]_{CCD}$ in those patients in whom hyperkalemia is caused by a low rate of excretion of K^+. The latter can be done with an assessment of the effective arterial blood volume, measurement of the P_{Renin} and the $P_{Aldosterone}$, the response to physiologic doses of exogenous mineralocorticoids (expect a rise in the rate of excretion of K^+ if the defect is a low $P_{Aldosterone}$), the administration of a thiazide diuretic (expect a rise in K^+ excretion if the basis of the defect is increased activity of NCC), and the induction of bicarbonaturia (expect a rise in the K^+ excretion if the defect is one of a "Cl^- shunt disorder"). It is possible that this information could lead to more specific modes of therapy in individual patients.

Drugs that inhibit the release of renin—nonsteroidal anti-inflammatory drugs and cyclo-oxygenase-2 inhibitors

Secretion of renin by cells in the juxtaglomerular arterioles and by cells of the macula densa in the early distal tubule appears to be mediated in part by locally produced prostaglandins. As a result, inhibition of prostaglandin synthesis will cause both the P_{Renin} and the $P_{Aldosterone}$ to be low. Nevertheless, the rise in the P_K is very small in normal subjects, but a significant degree of hyperkalemia may develop in the presence of significant kidney diseases or with the intake of other drugs that may also impair the renal excretion of K^+.

Drugs that interfere with the renin-angiotensin-aldosterone axis

The first class of these drugs includes angiotensin-converting enzyme (ACE) inhibitors, angiotensin II receptor blockers, and renin inhibitors. In more detail, the two major stimuli for the release of aldosterone are angiotensin II and a high P_K. Hyperkalemia acts in concert with angiotensin II that is generated locally within the zona glomerulosa of the adrenal gland to stimulate the release of aldosterone. Therefore, ACE inhibitors are expected to reduce aldosterone secretion and thereby impair the renal excretion of K^+. Of note, however, the $P_{Aldosterone}$ is not fully suppressed in patients on chronic therapy with ACE inhibitors. Furthermore, there are no reported studies that examined the effect of exogenous mineralocorticoids on the renal excretion of K^+ in patients who develop hyperkalemia while taking ACE inhibitors. Although it is estimated that the overall incidence of hyperkalemia is approximately 10% in patients taking this class of drugs, the rise in the P_K is less than 0.5 mEq/L in patients with relatively normal renal function. In contrast, a more severe degree of hyperkalemia may be seen in patients with renal insufficiency or the concurrent use of a drug that impairs renal K^+ excretion such as a potassium-sparing diuretic or a nonsteroidal anti-inflammatory drug.

Limited evidence suggests that the increase in the P_K may be less pronounced with use of an angiotensin II receptor blocker than with the use of an ACE inhibitor in patients with a reduced glomerular filtration rate. There are no data, however, to suggest that patients who develop a significant degree of hyperkalemia on an ACE inhibitor can be safely managed with an angiotensin II receptor blocker.

The second class of drugs that interfere with the renin-angiotensin-aldosterone axis are drugs that inhibit the synthesis of aldosterone. Aldosterone synthesis is selectively reduced in patients who are treated with heparin. This seems to be due to an effect of heparin that leads to a reduction in the number and affinity of angiotensin II receptors in the adrenal zona glomerulosa cells. Even low-dose heparin (5000 units three times daily) can lead to a reduction in the $P_{Aldosterone}$. Nevertheless, the degree of decrease in the $P_{Aldosterone}$ may not be of sufficient magnitude to affect the renal excretion of K^+ in many patients who receive this drug. It has been estimated that a greater than normal P_K occurs in 7% of patients; severe hyperkalemia occurs only if some other cause of impairment in K^+ excretion is present such as renal insufficiency or the intake of an ACE inhibitor or a potassium-sparing diuretic. Hyperkalemia has also been noted in patients receiving low-molecular-weight heparin.

The third class of drugs in this group is those that compete with aldosterone for binding to its receptor. Hyperkalemia is a potential problem in patients taking the nonspecific mineralocorticoid receptor antagonist spironolactone or the selective mineralocorticoid receptor antagonist eplenernone. The incidence of hyperkalemia is dose dependent with detectable effects even at doses of 25 mg spironolactone per day. At higher doses, the risk of severe hyperkalemia increases. Of special concern is the rise in the use of these drugs after the demonstrated improved survival with the use of aldosterone antagonists in patients with congestive heart failure. A population-based study in Canada showed that the frequency with which spironolactone was prescribed for patients with heart failure who were also taking an ACE inhibitor rose significantly. There were significant increases among these patients in the rates of hospital admissions for hyperkalemia and of in-hospital death from hyperkalemia.

The fourth class of drugs that interfere with the renin-angiotensin-aldosterone axis are those that block ENaC in the luminal membrane of principal cells in the CCD (e.g., amiloride, trimethoprim, and pentamidine). The cationic form of these drugs causes hyperkalemia and salt wasting (Fig. 15-3).

Patients with HIV and *Pneumocystis carinii* pneumonia treated with trimethoprim may develop hyperkalemia. Although this has been attributed to the use of high doses of trimethoprim in these patients, trimethoprim may cause a rise in the P_K even when used

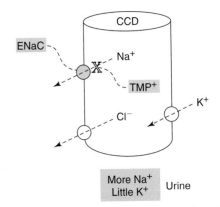

FIGURE 15-3 Mechanism of impaired excretion of K⁺ in patients on trimethoprim (TMP). The *barrel-shaped structure* represents the CCD. When TMP is in its cationic form in the lumen of the CCD, it blocks the ability of the epithelial Na⁺ channel (ENaC) to reabsorb Na⁺ (*X symbol*). As a result, there is a diminished negative voltage in the lumen of the CCD, and this leads to the wasting of Na⁺ and Cl⁻ with a decreased rate of excretion of K⁺ in the urine.

in conventional doses. Another factor that may explain the high incidence of hyperkalemia in these patients is the low flow rate in the CCD. Because the dietary intake in these patients may be very poor, the rate of delivery of osmoles (urea and NaCl) to the CCD is low and hence the flow rate in the CCD is low. This in turn increases the concentration of trimethoprim in the lumen of the CCD for a given rate of excretion of this drug (i.e., the same quantity of trimethoprim is now in a smaller volume [Fig. 15-4]). Hence, the ability of trimethoprim to block ENaC in principal cells in the CCD is enhanced.

Blockade of ENaC can cause hyperkalemia by an indirect effect that leads to a shift of K⁺ out of cells. This results from suppression of insulin release by α-adrenergics released in response to a major degree of effective arterial blood volume contraction due to salt wasting.

With regard to therapy, loop diuretics may help by increasing the flow rate in the CCD and hence lowering the concentration of

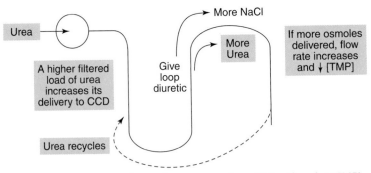

- On a mmol/mmol basis, urea is threefold more important than Na⁺ plus Cl⁻ with respect to the flow rate in the CCD.
- Ingestion of protein (rather than capsules containing urea) is much less effective in patients with AIDS because of anorexia and the usual slow rate of conversion of protein to urea.

FIGURE 15-4 Methods to lower the concentration of trimethoprim (TMP) in the CCD. The concentration of TMP falls in the lumen of the CCD when the number of osmoles delivered to this nephron segment rises. To achieve this aim, one could increase the excretion of urea (*green shading; see margin note*), or inhibit the reabsorption of Na⁺ and Cl⁻ in the loop of Henle. To avoid further contraction of the effective arterial blood volume, the patient must receive more NaCl than is excreted in the urine.

trimethoprim in the luminal fluid in the CCD. Enough NaCl must be given to defend the effective arterial blood volume. Because only the protonated form of trimethoprim blocks ENaC, increasing the pH of luminal fluid in the CCD should cause less trimethoprim to be in its cationic form, and hence its antikaliuretic effect should be minimized. Inducing bicarbonaturia with acetazolamide is a rational therapeutic option when continuation of trimethoprim is necessary and blockade of ENaC is likely. Enough alkali must be given to avoid the development of metabolic acidosis.

The fifth class of drugs in this group may cause a Cl^- shunt–type disorder. Hyperkalemia develops in some patients receiving the calcineurin inhibitors cyclosporin and FK506 following organ transplantation. The clinical signs in these patients (presence of hypertension, an effective arterial blood volume that is not low, suppressed P_{Renin}) and the finding that bicarbonaturia leads to an increase in the rate of excretion of K^+ suggest that the defect is an increased permeability for Cl^- in the CCD (Cl^- shunt disorder).

The sixth class of drugs are those that interfere with activation of ENaC via inhibiting its proteolytic cleavage. Nafamostat mesylate is a potent serine protease inhibitor that has been used in Japan for the treatment of acute pancreatitis and disseminated intravascular coagulation. It can cause hyperkalemia primarily by decreasing the urinary excretion of K^+. The mechanism is related to the metabolites of nafamostat that inhibit the aldosterone-inducible, membrane-associated channel activating proteases (*see margin note*).

CHANNEL ACTIVATING PROTEASES
- Another mechanism by which aldosterone activates ENaC involves proteolytic cleavage of the channel by serine proteases.
- These proteases activate ENaC by increasing the open probability of the channel rather than by increasing expression in the luminal membrane.

PART D
THERAPY OF HYPERKALEMIA
EMERGENCY SETTING

- The major danger of a severe degree of hyperkalemia is a life-threatening cardiac arrhythmia.

Because mild EKG changes may progress rapidly to a dangerous arrhythmia, any patient with an EKG abnormality related to hyperkalemia should be treated as a medical emergency. We would treat patients with a P_K greater than 7.0 mmol/L aggressively, even in the absence of EKG changes. Exceptions include those who develop hyperkalemia after extreme exercise (the supermarathon).

Antagonize the cardiac effects of hyperkalemia

- Calcium is the best agent; its effects should be evident within minutes, and it usually lasts 30 to 60 minutes.

Calcium is usually given as 20 to 30 mL of a 10% calcium gluconate solution (two to three ampules) or 10 mL of 10% calcium chloride (one ampule). Both solutions are equally effective, but the former is safer should the solution extravasate during the intravenous infusion because calcium gluconate is mostly nondissociated, whereas calcium chloride is nearly completely dissociated. The dose can be repeated in 5 minutes if the EKG changes persist. Extreme caution should be exerted using Ca^{2+} in patients on digitalis because hypercalcemia may precipitate digitalis toxicity.

Induce a shift of K^+ into the intracellular fluid

Insulin

- Insulin should be used as the initial therapy to induce a shift of K^+ into cells in patients with emergency hyperkalemia.
- Give enough glucose to prevent hypoglycemia; monitor the $P_{Glucose}$.

Many studies support the use of insulin in the treatment of emergency hyperkalemia. Large doses of rapidly acting insulin (e.g., 20 units of regular insulin) given as a bolus are needed for a maximal shift of K^+ into cells. Although some suggest treating nondiabetic, hyperkalemic patients with a bolus of glucose without exogenous insulin, we would not do this because high levels of insulin are required to induce an adequate shift of K^+ into cells and this may not be achieved without an infusion of insulin. Moreover, hypertonic glucose may cause K^+ to shift out of cells in patients with inadequate insulin reserves, leading to an unwanted rise in the P_K.

β_2-Adrenergic agonists

- We do not use these agents as the preferred emergency treatment for hyperkalemia.
- It remains uncertain whether β_2-agonists have a P_K-lowering effect that is additive to that of insulin.

Although a number of studies suggest that β_2-agonists (e.g., 20 mg of nebulized albuterol) are effective to lower the P_K rapidly, we do not use these agents as first-line treatment of emergency hyperkalemia for two reasons. First, they are not effective in a significant proportion of patients. In a number of studies, 20% to 40% of patients who received these agents had a decline in P_K of less than 0.5 mmol/L. It is unclear why certain patients do not exhibit a fall in P_K following the administration of β_2-agonists, and it is not possible to predict which patients will respond. Second, we are concerned about safety of the doses of these drugs that are needed to treat patients with hyperkalemia, which are four to eight times those prescribed for the treatment of acute asthma. Although no severe adverse events were reported in studies examining the use of these agents in patients with hyperkalemia, most of these studies have been performed in stable patients with a mild degree of hyperkalemia prior to their regular hemodialysis session. Moreover, a number of these studies excluded patients taking β-blockers and selected those with no significant history of coronary heart disease or unstable heart rhythms. Therefore, the safety of these agents was determined in a group of patients that may not resemble the general population with end-stage renal disease that has a high prevalence of cardiac disease.

NaHCO₃

> - NaHCO$_3$ therapy did not lower the P$_K$ acutely in a number of studies. Thus, the potential value of NaHCO$_3$ for therapy of patients with emergency hyperkalemia is not clear.
> - We would use NaHCO$_3$ in patients with significant acidemia, but we would not use it as the only emergency therapy.
> - Studies examining the combined use of NaHCO$_3$ with insulin produced conflicting results.

The first step in the action of NaHCO$_3$ is to decrease the concentration of H$^+$ in the ECF compartment and thereby to promote the electroneutral exit of H$^+$ and entry of Na$^+$ into cells via NHE. Notwithstanding, only if the NHE is active would the administration of NaHCO$_3$ have the potential to lower the P$_K$. One major activator of NHE is intracellular acidosis, because not only are H$^+$ a substrate for NHE but they also bind to a modifier site that activates it.

Of note, many of the studies that evaluated the potential role of NaHCO$_3$ to lower the P$_K$ were carried out in stable hemodialysis patients who did not have a significant degree of acidemia. In other words, these studies examined the effect of NaHCO$_3$ when the NHE was presumably in an inactive mode. The question remains as to whether NaHCO$_3$ would be effective in patients with a more significant degree of acidemia, when the NHE may become activated.

We use NaHCO$_3$ in patients with significant acidemia but not as the only emergency therapy. On the other hand, excessive administration of NaHCO$_3$ should be avoided because of the risk of inducing hypernatremia, ECF volume expansion, carbon dioxide retention, and also a fall in the concentration of ionized calcium in plasma, which may aggravate the cardiac effects of hyperkalemia.

NO MEDICAL EMERGENCIES

Removal of K$^+$ from the body

It is important to appreciate that very much less K$^+$ loss is needed to lower the P$_K$ from 7.0 to 6.0 mmol/L than to lower it from 6.0 to 5.0 mmol/L. Hence, creating a small K$^+$ loss can be very important when there is a severe degree of hyperkalemia (Fig. 15-5).

Enhancing the excretion of K$^+$ in the urine

This topic is discussed in more detail in Part E, page 537 of this chapter.

Cation exchange resins

> - Kayexalate contains 4 mmol of Na$^+$ per gram but only a small exchange of Na$^+$ for K$^+$ occurs in the gastrointestinal tract.
> - There is no benefit in using resins for the treatment of acute hyperkalemia and little if any benefit of adding resins to cathartics in the setting of chronic hyperkalemia.

The only favorable location for the exchange of Na$^+$ for K$^+$ is in the lumen of the colon. Based on data obtained from patients with an ileostomy, the amount of K$^+$ delivered to the colon that would be available for this exchange is close to only 5 mEq/day.

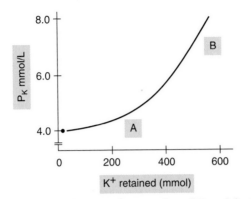

FIGURE 15-5 Relationship between the retention of K⁺ and the P$_K$. The retention of a modest quantity of K⁺ results in only a modest rise in the P$_K$ (to close to 5.0 mmol/L) because cells still have enough intracellular Na⁺ (*part A of the curve; see margin note*). Once the concentration of intracellular Na⁺ is diminished appreciably, a small additional K⁺ load causes a larger rise in the P$_K$. The corollary in therapy of hyperkalemia is that even a small K⁺ loss can cause a relatively large fall in P$_K$ in a patient with a severe degree of hyperkalemia (*part B of the curve*).

Furthermore, cations other than K⁺ such as NH_4^+, Ca^{2+}, and Mg^{2+} may exchange for resin-bound Na⁺.

One possible theoretical benefit when using cation exchange resins is if they were to lower the concentration of K⁺ in luminal water, thereby enhancing the net secretion of K⁺ by the rectosigmoid colon. But even if more K⁺ were secreted into the lumen, the low stool volume would limit the total K⁺ loss (*see margin note*). It has been shown that using resins does not result in acute lowering of P$_K$. Furthermore, the addition of resin does not result in a significant loss of K⁺ in the stool over and above that achieved with the use of cathartics alone.

Dialysis

- Hemodialysis is more effective than peritoneal dialysis for removing K⁺.

In the first hour of dialysis, approximately 35 mmol of K⁺ can be removed with a concentration of K⁺ in the bath of 1 to 2 mmol/L. As the P$_K$ is lower in subsequent periods of dialysis, less K⁺ is removed per hour (*see margin note*).

PART E
INTEGRATIVE PHYSIOLOGY
IN-DEPTH ANALYSIS OF K⁺ EXCRETION DURING CHRONIC HYPERKALEMIA

- To understand what sets the limit on the rate of excretion of K⁺ in a patient with hyperkalemia, one must apply the principles of physiology for the excretion of K⁺ and perform a quantitative analysis.

PROGRESSIVE K⁺ LOAD
The major way to shift K⁺ into cells is to have a shift of one of the following cations from the ICF.
- *Na⁺*: There is less than 20 mmol Na⁺ per liter of ICF, so this "exchange" is limited to a maximum of ~300 mmol in an adult, as some Na⁺ must remain in cells.
- *H⁺*: To make new H⁺ in the ICF, the source is $CO_2 + H_2O$. The resulting high [HCO_3^-] and pH in cells limit this "exchange" of H⁺ for K⁺.

QUANTITATIVE ANALYSIS
- If the lumen-negative transepithelial voltage in the colon is as high as −90 mV and the P$_K$ is 5 mmol/L, the concentration of K⁺ in stool water would be ~100 mmol/L.
- With a usual stool volume of 125 mL, of which 75% is water, only 10 mmol of K⁺ would be lost by this route.

K⁺ REMOVAL DURING DIALYSIS
- Removal of K⁺ from plasma is rapid.
- Removing K⁺ from most of the ECF compartment is slower, as it depends on the rate of diffusion of K⁺, which is slow.
- Removal of K⁺ from cells is even slower, as this depends on an additional step: the exit of K⁺ from cells.
- The diffusion of K⁺ into capillaries of skeletal muscle can occur at a faster rate if the patient is able to do enough exercise to increase the blood flow to skeletal muscle, as this accelerates the slow diffusion step.
- A glucose-free dialysate is preferable to avoid the glucose-induced release of insulin and thereby the subsequent shift of K⁺ into cells, which decreases the removal of K⁺. Notwithstanding, there is danger of inducing hypoglycemia if the patient received a bolus of insulin during emergency therapy for hyperkalemia.

Patients who will develop chronic hyperkalemia have a renal defect characterized by an inability to create a lumen voltage in the CCD that is sufficiently negative to excrete all of their current daily intake of K^+. Nevertheless, ultimately a steady state will develop in which they can excrete their K^+ intake, but they need a high P_K to do this (see Fig. 15-1, page 518). To illustrate the implications of this pathophysiology, we shall begin our analysis with the "big picture" (external K^+ balance), and proceed stepwise to the next logical issues, ending with a clinical application in which we examine the development of hyperkalemia in patients taking inhibitors of the renin-anigiotensin-aldosterone axis and suggest options for therapy that may permit a steady state to be achieved with a lesser degree of hyperkalemia in this setting.

1. *External balance*: The basic premise is that a steady state will be achieved in a chronic condition. Therefore, all the K^+ that is consumed each day will be excreted in the 24-hour urine if there is no loss of K^+ via nonrenal routes. *Thus, if a patient with chronic hyperkalemia and a normal subject each has an intake of 70 mmol of K^+ per day and no nonrenal K^+ loss for simplicity, each will excrete 70 mmol of K^+ in the urine daily.*

2. *Driving force to excrete K^+*: This driving force to secrete K^+ in the CCD is electrical (*see margin note*). Hence, 1 mmol of Na^+ must be reabsorbed via ENaC without Cl^- for each mmol of net secretion of K^+ into the lumen of these nephron segments. In our example, each subject will excrete 70 mmol of K^+ per day in steady state. *Therefore, both the normal subject and the patient with chronic hyperkalemia will reabsorb 70 mmol more Na^+ than Cl^- in the CCD. Notwithstanding, the patient with hyperkalemia has a defect that leads to a diminished ability to generate the required lumen-negative voltage in his CCD.*

3. *Compared to the K^+ load they ingest, normal subjects have a much larger capacity to secrete K^+ in the CCD*: In fact, they excrete most of their daily K^+ load in short time period close to noon (Fig. 15-1, page 518). Conversely, K^+ is also excreted throughout the day in normal subjects consuming a typical Western diet, but at a much lower rate. While we do not know the mechanism for stimulating the secretion of K^+ in the CCD close to noon, it is likely due to a greater lumen-negative voltage in this nephron segment, as there is little diurnal variation in the P_K and in the flow rate traversing the CCD (the osmole excretion rate undergoes only modest changes). Notwithstanding, the mechanism should lead to reabsorption of more Na^+ than Cl^- in the CCD; for example, it should cause more open ENaC in the luminal membrane of principal cells (e.g., actions of aldosterone) or cause less reabsorption of Cl^- in the CCD (e.g., the presence of HCO_3^- or a more alkaline pH in the lumen of the CCD). Since consuming $NaHCO_3$ or acetazolamide (which inhibits proximal HCO_3^- reabsorption) results in a prompt and large kaliuresis, an effect that is not observed with the ingestion of a "physiologic" amount of the synthetic mineralocorticoid fludrocortisone later in the day, we suspect that a larger delivery of HCO_3^- may be part of the physiologic control system for the net secretion of K^+ in the CCD.

4. *Excretion of 70 mmol of K^+ in a patient with chronic hyperkalemia*: Bearing in mind that patients with chronic hyperkalemia have a less negative luminal votage in the CCD and that they will have the same flow rate traversing the CCD (same rate of excretion of osmoles, as they consume the same diet as the normal subjects in this hypothetical example), they must have a lower luminal

DELIVERY OF K^+ TO THE CCD

- The concentration of K^+ in the lumen of the terminal cortical thick ascending limb of the loop of Henle is ~1.5 mmol/L (in a fed rat).
- Extrapolating from micropuncture data in the fed rat, there appears to be ~27 L of filtrate delivered to the early distal convoluted tubule each day in a human adult. Hence, close to 40 mmol of K^+ are delivered daily to the CCD (27 L/day × 1.5 mmol K^+/L).
- For simplicity, we shall ignore the quantity of K^+ delivered to the CCD in our calculations, as this is unlikely to be very different in the normal subjects and in patients with chronic hyperkalemia. In addition, a lumen-negative voltage is required to retain this K^+ in the luminal fluid in the CCD.

K^+ concentration relative to their P_K. Nevertheless, they can excrete the same K^+ load as normal subjects for two reasons:

    A. *A higher P_K*: A less negative lumen voltage in the CCD will tend to decrease the luminal K^+ concentration in this nephron segment, but this will tend to be offset when the P_K is in a higher range (*see margin note*).

    B. *A longer duration for maximal rate of K^+ secretion*: In the normal subject, there are only several hours during the day when the K^+ secretion process is maximally stimulated, whereas much less K^+ is excreted per hour for the rest of the 24-hour period (*see margin note*). In contrast, if the lumen-negative voltage is reduced, the maximal possible rate of K^+ secretion will need to be sustained for many more hours during the day to achieve the desired rate of K^+ excretion. To maintain this maximal rate of K^+ secretion, a higher P_K is required.

Implications for the patient with chronic hyperkalemia

1. Since the lumen-negative voltage in the CCD is low, this patient will have to maintain a degree of hyperkalemia throughout the 24-hour period (*see margin note*). Moreover, the P_K will rise when K^+ is absorbed from the intestinal tract, and this higher P_K will need to be maintained for the time period during which maximal K^+ excretion is required to achieve K^+ balance.

2. The use of diuretics to increase the excretion of K^+ depends on their effect to increase the delivery of Na^+ and Cl^- to the CCD and thereby the flow rate in the CCD, as the net secretion of K^+ is rarely limited by the luminal Na^+ concentration. Nevertheless, when the effective arterial blood volume declines, more Na^+ and Cl^- will be reabsorbed in the proximal convoluted tubule and less Na^+ and Cl^- are delivered distally. The net effect is new steady state with a rate of excretion of Na^+ and Cl^- that is equal to their dietary intake of NaCl. Nevertheless, since their effective arterial blood volume is lower, more Na^+ and Cl^- are reabsorbed proximally, while less Na^+ and Cl^- are reabsorbed distally owing to the actions of the natriuretic agent (in steady state, these two effects have the same magnitude). Thus, there is only a transient period (less than 7 days) when a diuretic augments K^+ excretion (i.e., while the negative balance of Na^+ and Cl^- is being induced). Therefore, for diuretics to be effective in lowering P_K, the patient must ingest more NaCl to diminish the degree of contraction of his or her effective arterial blood volume to maintain the increase in the delivery of Na^+ and Cl^- to the CCD.

3. A low-NaCl diet or enhanced nonrenal loss of NaCl will lower the delivery of Na^+ and Cl^- and thereby the flow rate in the CCD. Hence, the entire K^+ load can be excreted only if there is a greater degree of hyperkalemia.

Application of these principles to the management of chronic hyperkalemia in patients taking ACE inhibitors, angiotensin II receptor blockers, or direct renin inhibitors

The ingestion of these drugs (± the underlying disorder) may lead to a less negative luminal voltage in the CCD and thereby a lower $[K^+]_{CCD}$. As long as these patients eat enough protein and salt to maintain their flow rate in the CCD, they will be able to excrete all their dietary K^+ without an appreciable rise in their P_K. Should they

---

RELATIONSHIP BETWEEN THE P_K AND THE LUMEN-NEGATIVE VOLTAGE ON THE LUMINAL K^+ CONCENTRATION

- *Normal subject:* A more negative lumen voltage is the mechanism that raises the $[K^+]_{CCD}$ (top line of table below).
- *Hyperkalemic patient:* The less negative voltage in this patient tends to lower the $[K^+]_{CCD}$, but hyperkalemia allows a similar $[K^+]_{CCD}$ to be achieved.

P_K (mmol/L)	FOLD RISE IN $[K^+]_{CCD}$	$[K^+]_{CCD}$ (mmol/L)
4.0	3	12
6.0	2	12

MAXIMAL K^+ EXCRETION RATE

- The volume traversing the CCD is 6 L/day because 1800 mosmol traverse the lumen of the CCD each day.
- The are only 75 mOsm/L of electrolytes in luminal fluid in the CCD, as its osmolality is 300 mOsm/L and three fourths of these luminal osmoles are urea. Hence, the maximal Na^+ concentration in the lumen is 37.5 (half of 75 mmol/L). In addition, the total amount of Na^+ delivered daily to the CCD is 225 mmol (37.5 mmol/L × 6 L/day).
- Therefore, the 70 mmol of K^+ can be excreted in 2 L, which is one third of 6 L.
- Obviously, some K^+ is excreted in the other 4 L of fluid traversing the CCD. Thus, the duration of peak kaliuresis and/or the maximal K^+ concentration will be less in normal subjects.
- Since 1 mmol Na^+ must be reabsorbed to secrete 1 mmol of K^+, the maximal $[K^+]_{CCD}$ is ~35 mmol/L. Moreover, since not all the Na^+ delivered to the CCD will be reabsorbed in this nephron segment, the maximal luminal concentration of K^+ will be less than 35 mmol/L.

K^+ EXCRETION IN A PATIENT WITH HYPERKALEMIA
This patient has a lower magnitude for the lumen-negative voltage in the CCD. Hence, there is a reduced maximal $[K^+]_{CCD}$ (i.e., ~12 mmol/L in this example). Therefore his maximal rate of K^+ secretion must be sustained throughout the 24-hour period to excrete 70 mmol of K^+ (i.e., 6 L/day exiting the CCD x ~12 mmol K^+/L).

THERAPY WITH DIURETICS

- A common clinical practice is to place patients on diuretics while they are also on angiotensin-converting enzyme inhibitors or angiotensin II receptor blockers to enhance their antihypertensive effect or if the patient develops hyperkalemia. From the analysis in this section of the chapter, one can understand why hyperkalemia may develop or become worse if the patient becomes intravascular volume depleted (more reabsorption of Na^+ and Cl^- in the proximal convoluted tubule).

- Although diuretics increase the excretion of Na^+ and Cl^- temporarily, they do not do this in steady state. Rather, they permit the same quantity of Na^+ and Cl^- to be excreted as is ingested, but in a setting with a lower effective arterial blood volume. Hence, this is not a good sole form of therapy for a patient with chronic hyperkalemia.

be advised to eat less protein and/or less NaCl, however, or become intravascular volume depleted with the administration of diuretics (*see margin note*), their flow rate in the CCD could fall enough in steady state to compromise their ability to excrete their entire dietary K^+ load with the development of a much higher P_K. If this occurs, therapy should include measures to increase protein intake if it was significantly reduced or to increase the intake of NaCl if effective circulating volume appears to be low and hypertension is not an important constraint.

In summary, the interaction of electrogenic reabsorption of Na^+ (equal to K^+ intake), the ability to generate a given lumen-negative voltage (e.g., availability of enough aldosterone), and the rate of excretion of osmoles must be integrated to understand how a patient with chronic hyperkalemia could remain in K^+ balance without a large increase in P_K. This analysis places in perspective the options for management of a patient with hyperkalemia. Hence, one can decrease K^+ intake, increase the number of osmoles of urea and NaCl delivered to the terminal CCD, and/or increase the lumen-negative voltage in the CCD (e.g., give acetazolamide to decrease the reabsorption of $NaHCO_3$ in the proximal convoluted tubule) to increase the rate of secretion of K^+ in the CCD.

DISCUSSION OF CASES

CASE 15-1: MIGHT THIS PATIENT HAVE PSEUDOHYPERKALEMIA?

(Case presented on page 513)

Why did hyperkalemia develop so soon after he left the intensive care unit?

To develop hyperkalemia without an intake of K^+ implies that the basis for the high P_K is a shift of K^+ out of cells. The question is, "Did this shift of K^+ occur from cells in the body or from red blood cells while they were sitting in the test tube?" Moreover, the very low $P_{Aldosterone}$ suggests that there was an adrenal problem as well or that the shift of K^+ into plasma occurred outside the body. If the latter were true, the patient may really have hypokalemia and this would explain the low rate of excretion of K^+ and the low $P_{Aldosterone}$.

The next step was to test whether there was a leak of K^+ from red blood cells while they were stored on ice. One blood sample from the patient and one from his physician were drawn. To be certain to control for time before analysis, the blood sample was assayed after 2 hours and 6 hours later. One portion of the blood was left to stand at room temperature and another was stored on ice.

There was no change in the P_K at 2 hours and 6 hours in both subjects, whereas the P_K rose to 6.0 mmol/L in both subjects when blood was stored on ice. Hence, inhibition of the Na-K-ATPase in red blood cells by cold could cause the P_K to rise. Nevertheless, there was no defect in blood cells to explain the hyperkalemia. Therefore one should ask, "What could be the basis for the high P_K that occurred only while the patient was on the ward?"

What could be the basis for the high P_K, but only while the patient was on the ward?

A likely explanation is that K^+ shifted out of cells locally into capillaries drained by the site of venipuncture. In fact, blood was drawn *slowly* from a T-tube connector in a vein on the dorsum of his wrist in the ICU—thus, there was no pain and the drainage bed had few muscle cells. On the ward, however, the child struggled vigorously and had to be restrained to draw blood from his brachial vein (venous drainage from a large muscle mass). Accordingly, he had pseudo-hyperkalemia. When blood was drawn using the same technique as in the intensive care unit, his P_K was 3.4 mmol/L, and this is a likely explanation for the low $P_{Aldosterone}$. Therefore, one must rule out pseudohyperkalemia before accepting a blood value when there is an unusual setting for hyperkalemia.

CASE 15-2: IS THERE AN ERROR IN THE EKG?

(Case presented on page 514)

How can this discrepancy be reconciled?

The reasoning in this case was as follows. The EKG changes suggested that the patient did have hyperkalemia. Therefore, a reason for *pseudohypokalemia* was suspected (e.g., the uptake of K^+ in vitro by circulating tumor cells). Another speculation was that the P_K was lowered by dilution of plasma in the test tube containing the blood sample. In fact, the test tubes used contained 0.3 mL of anticoagulant. Since the volume of blood sampled was quite small, this could now explain how a much lower than expected P_K could be found in plasma—an artifact due to dilution by the volume of the anticoagulant. If this is the correct mechanism, the P_{Na} should also be low.

CASE 15-3: HYPERKALEMIA WITH THE AID OF TRIMETHOPRIM

(Case presented on page 514)

Why is hyperkalemia present?

Although an element of pseudohyperkalemia is suspected in this cachectic patient, it is not the only or the major cause of hyperkalemia because his EKG shows signs of hyperkalemia (tall peaked T waves). Hence emergency treatment of hyperkalemia is needed.

The next step is to examine the rate of excretion of K^+ as outlined in Flow Chart 15-2. The facts that the time course is short and especially that there was little ingestion of K^+ provided strong evidence that a major basis for the hyperkalemia is a shift of K^+ out of cells. The fact that he had a very low intake of NaCl, which implies a lower ECF volume prior to taking trimethoprim and a natriuresis due to renal actions of this drug, means that there could have been enough contraction of his effective arterial blood volume to induce an α-adrenergic response. This latter setting could inhibit the release of insulin from β-cells of the pancreas and thereby induce a shift of K^+ out of skeletal muscle cells.

The degree of hyperkalemia will depend on how readily the kidneys will excrete this K^+. Accordingly, the next step is to look at the rate of excretion of K^+. This rate of excretion is very low because the U_K is 14 mmol/L and the 24-hour urine volume is 0.8 L (K^+ excretion is 11 mmol/day vs. an expected rate of more than 200 mmol/day). Similarly, the $U_K/U_{Creatinine}$ ratio is only 2 (14/7 mmol/L), which is much less than the expected rate of 15 mmol K^+/mmol creatinine in spot urines. Accordingly, the next step is to determine why the patient has such a low $[K^+]_{CCD}$ (see Flow Chart 15-3).

The low $[K^+]_{CCD}$ results from less electrogenic reabsorption of Na^+ in the CCD. As he has a low effective arterial blood volume and a U_{Na}

and U_{Cl} that are inappropriately high in the presence of a contracted effective arterial blood volume, his low $[K^+]_{CCD}$ is probably caused by inhibition of ENaC by trimethoprim. Both his P_{Renin} and $P_{Aldosterone}$ (which become available later) were high; this suggests that the actions of aldosterone are deficient.

This patient also has a low flow rate traversing his CCD because his osmole excretion rate is low (0.8 L/day × 270 mOsm/L = 216 mOsm/day). The low protein intake causes a low rate of delivery of urea to the CCD (*see margin note*), and the low salt intake with the low effective arterial blood volume cause a low rate of delivery of Na^+ and Cl^-. This reduced flow rate in the CCD increases the concentration of trimethoprim in its lumen for a given amount of this drug. Hence, trimethoprim becomes a more effective blocker of ENaC.

UREA
Urea is normally responsible for 75% of this flow owing to recycling of urea in the renal outer medulla (see Chapter 9, page 291 for more discussion).

What are the major issues for therapy?

This cachectic patient is very unlikely to have a high intake of food containing K^+; in support of this presumption, his osmole excretion rate is very low. Hence, it is unlikely that he has a large positive balance for K^+. Therefore, although the rise in P_K occurred over several days, a shift of K^+ from cells rather than a large positive external balance for K^+ is the major cause of hyperkalemia. This is important to recognize because one should not induce a large loss of K^+ and cause an overall total body K^+ deficit during therapy, because this may lead to a severe degree of hypokalemia when K^+ shift back into cells.

If trimethoprim must be continued, what measures can be taken to minimize its ability to block ENaC?

Trimethoprim is needed to treat the pneumonia; hence, it should be continued. To avoid developing a life-threatening degree of hyperkalemia and a very contracted effective arterial blood volume, it is essential to remove trimethoprim's ability to block ENaC in the CCD. Therefore, the objective is to lower the concentration of trimethoprim in the lumen of the CCD. To achieve this aim, the flow rate in the CCD must be higher by increasing the delivery of osmoles to the CCD. To raise the delivery of urea to the CCD in a cachectic patient who is unlikely to eat much more protein, one may administer urea in capsular form. One may also increase the delivery of NaCl with the administration of a loop diuretic. To avoid a further contraction of his effective arterial blood volume, enough NaCl must be infused to create a positive balance for Na^+ and Cl^- to reexpand his ECF volume if a loop diuretic is given. Inducing bicarbonaturia could also be considered to lower the concentration of H^+ in the luminal fluid in the CCD and thereby the concentration of the cationic form of the drug that blocks ENaC (see equation).

$$Trimethoprim^0 + H^+ \rightleftharpoons Trimethoprim^+ \ (active\ form)$$

section four
Integrative Physiology

Hyperglycemia

Introduction

This chapter has been placed at the end of the book because hyperglycemia is associated with many electrolyte and acid-base disorders and hence requires an integrative analysis. In addition, the approach outlined and the rationale for our decision making during therapy are recapitulations of those used in the previous chapters. Moreover, because diabetes mellitus in poor control represents a common disorder, we believe that it is useful to have a separate chapter on this topic. In particular, it is a strong supplement to Chapter 5, on ketoacidosis, because both ketoacidosis and hyperglycemia are components of the picture of diabetic ketoacidosis (DKA) and possibly the hyperglycemic hyperosmolar syndrome.

We begin this chapter with a section on metabolic regulation to explain the biochemical basis of hyperglycemia. This is followed by a section in which the emphasis is on the physiology of osmotic diuresis and the influence of hyperglycemia on cell size in different organs. In the clinical section, we discuss the problem of the hyperglycemic hyperosmolar state and analyze the findings in this setting with an emphasis on the importance of a quantitative analysis of the extracellular fluid (ECF) volume. This is followed by an outline of therapy for patients with hyperglycemia; this emphasizes how to minimize the risk of developing cerebral edema, a complication that may arise during therapy, particularly in children with DKA.

ABBREVIATIONS

$P_{Glucose}$, concentration of glucose in plasma

P_{Na}, concentration of Na^+ in plasma

P_K, concentration of K^+ in plasma

$P_{Creatinine}$, concentration of creatinine in plasma

P_{Urea}, concentration of urea in plasma

$P_{Effective\ osm}$, effective osmolality in plasma

GFR, glomerular filtration rate

DKA, diabetic ketoacidosis

HHS, hyperglycemic hyperosmolar state

OBJECTIVES

- To emphasize that when there is a relative lack of insulin, a severe degree of hyperglycemia develops if there is a marked reduction in glomerular filtration rate (GFR) and/or a large intake of glucose.
- To illustrate the importance of a quantitative analysis in the clinical management of patients with DKA and hyperglycemic hyperosmolar syndrome.
- To illustrate that the type of fluid intake, which is usually large due to polydipsia, influences the electrolyte and acid-base parameters in these patients and the implications this has for therapy.
- To outline the principles of therapy in patients with hyperglycemia with an emphasis on measures to minimize the risk of developing cerebral edema, especially in children with DKA.

CASE 16-1: AND I THOUGHT WATER WAS GOOD FOR ME!

(Case discussed on page 569)

A 14-year-old, 50-kg girl has a long history of poorly controlled type 1 diabetes mellitus because she does not take insulin regularly. In the past 48 hours, she was thirsty and drank large volumes of fruit juice. She noted that her urine volume was very high. While in the emergency department, she did not have fruit juice, so she drank tap water (*see margin note*). On physical examination, her blood pressure was 105/66 mm Hg, her heart rate was 80 beats per minute, there were no significant postural changes in blood pressure and heart rate, and her jugular venous pressure was not

"OCCULT" DANGER OF CEREBRAL EDEMA

- Beware, there is a danger that this patient will develop cerebral edema!
- To prevent this dreaded complication, the approach to therapy must often be different from the current guidelines.

low. Her urine flow rate was 10 mL/min over two consecutive 100-minute periods. Her laboratory data are presented in the following table:

		ADMISSION		AT 100 MIN		AT 200 MIN	
		PLASMA	URINE	PLASMA	URINE	PLASMA	URINE
Glucose	mg/dL	1260	6300	1260	6300	630	6300
Glucose	mmol/L	70	350	70	350	35	350
Na$^+$	mmol/L	125	50	125	50	123	50
Osmolality	mOsm/L	320	500	320	500	281	500
Hematocrit		0.45	—	0.45	—	0.45	—

Other plasma laboratory data on admission: pH 7.33, P_{HCO3} 28 mmol/L, $P_{Anion\ gap}$ 16 mEq/L, BUN 22 mg/dL (P_{Urea} 8 mmol/L), $P_{Creatinine}$ 1.0 mg/dL (88 μmol/L; her usual $P_{Creatinine}$ is 0.7 mg/dL [60 μmol/L]).

Questions

What is the basis of the polyuria?

How can the effective arterial blood volume and $P_{Effective\ osm}$ be defended during therapy?

Why did her $P_{Glucose}$ fail to fall in the first 100 minutes?

Why did the $P_{Glucose}$ and the $P_{Effective\ osm}$ fall in the second 100 minutes?

In what way did a severe degree of hyperglycemia "help" this patient?

CASE 16-2: I AM NOT "JUICED UP"

(Case discussed on page 571)

An 8-year-old, 27-kg girl with no prior history of diabetes mellitus complained of intense "air hunger," cough, and difficulty breathing without an obvious cause. On more detailed questioning, she also had polyuria, polydipsia, fatigue, and a weight loss of 5 lb (2.3 kg) over the past 2 weeks. Of note, to quench her thirst, she drank a large volume of water, but little fruit juice. Physical examination revealed a blood pressure of 113/73 mm Hg, a heart rate of 123 beats per minute, a respiratory rate of 34 breaths per minute, and a temperature of 36.6° C. The laboratory data are:

Glucose	mg/dL	350	Glucose	mmol/L	19.5
Na$^+$	mmol/L	133	K$^+$	mmol/L	3.3
Cl$^-$	mmol/L	112	HCO$_3^-$	mmol/L	<3
pH (arterial)		6.81	pH (venous)		6.88
Pco$_2$ (arterial)	mm Hg	8	Pco$_2$ (venous)	mm Hg	11
Anion gap	mEq/L	19	Hematocrit		0.48
Creatinine	mg/dL	0.6	Creatinine	μmol/L	56
BUN	mg/dL	11	Urea	mmol/L	4.0

Question

Why did she have such a severe degree of acidemia, a $P_{Glucose}$ that was not very high, a modest degree of contraction of the effective arterial blood volume, and a lower than expected P_K?

PART A
BACKGROUND

REVIEW OF GLUCOSE METABOLISM

A more comprehensive discussion of principles of metabolic control is provided at the beginning of Chapter 5. The following points highlight pertinent aspects with regard to normal control of metabolism of glucose.

NET INSULIN ACTIONS
Low "net insulin actions" refers to low levels of insulin and high levels of hormones with actions that oppose those of insulin, including glucagon. The converse is also true.

Brain fuels

• When the $P_{Glucose}$ is low, a fat-derived fuel (ketoacids) must be provided for the brain.

Glucose is the principal fuel oxidized by the brain in the fed state (Fig. 16-1). A lack of insulin or a resistance to its actions (*see margin note*) makes fatty acids almost the only fuel available for oxidation in this setting. Notwithstanding, fatty acids cannot cross the blood-brain barrier at a rapid enough rate—hence, they are not an important fuel for the

PHOSPHOFRUCTOKINASE
This is the enzymatic step in the glycolytic pathway where control is exerted by the concentration of ATP (it is not shown in the schematic representation of glycolysis).

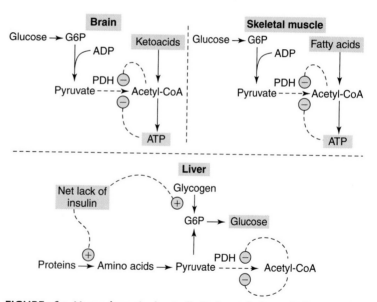

ABBREVIATION
PDH, pyruvate dehydrogenase
ATP, adenosinetriphosphate
ADP, adenosinediphosphate
NAD, nicotineadeninediphosphate

FIGURE 16-1 Hyperglycemia due to limited metabolism of glucose. The metabolic control that allows for reduced oxidation of glucose in the brain and skeletal muscle when there is a relative lack of insulin is illustrated in the *upper portion of the figure*. The critical fact is that oxidation of glucose must have a continuing regeneration of ADP, as it is the other substrate for glycolysis (*see margin note*). Because pyruvate may also be produced during amino acid oxidation, having the products of fat oxidation, acetyl-CoA, NADH (not shown), and ATP lead to a lower activity of pyruvate dehydrogenase (PDH) ensures that these precursors of pyruvate cannot be oxidized in states with a relative lack of insulin. The metabolic events in the liver are illustrated in the *lower portion of the figure*. Glucagon activates the enzymatic pathways for the breakdown of glycogen in the liver to produce glucose as well as those involved in the conversion of amino acids to glucose (gluconeogenesis). Inhibition of PDH ensures that the flux of carbon proceeds toward the synthesis of glucose.

brain. To provide a fat-derived fuel for the brain, fatty acids must be converted into water-soluble compounds—ketoacids—in the liver.

Steady-state hyperglycemia

- In a steady state, the rates of input and output of glucose must be equal. Therefore, hyperglycemia develops if there is a diminished output of glucose (mainly via oxidation and/or renal excretion) and/or a large input of glucose.

The brain oxidizes ketoacids in preference to glucose if both are present, even if the $P_{Glucose}$ is high. The basis for this statement is that the products of the oxidation of fat-derived fuels (e.g., ketoacids) inhibit the enzyme PDH and hence the complete oxidation of glucose. Although a mild degree of hyperglycemia develops as a result of a lack of insulin (see Fig. 16-1), a severe degree of hyperglycemia requires an additional factor, either an extraordinary large intake of glucose or, much more commonly, a low rate of excretion of glucose because of a very low GFR (Fig. 16-2).

Hierarchy of fuel oxidation

- To conserve glucose for the brain, fatty acids and/or ketoacids must be oxidized.
- Organs other than the brain will oxidize glucose at appreciable rates only when fatty acids and ketoacids are no longer available.

The basis for this hierarchy of fuel oxidation is that fuels compete for the availability of ADP for their oxidation. Furthermore, the activity of PDH, the highly regulated enzyme that controls the complete oxidation of glucose, is reduced by the products of the oxidation of fatty acids or ketoacids (acetyl-CoA, NADH, and, indirectly, ATP; see Fig. 16-1 and *margin note*).

CONTROL OF THE RATE OF FUEL OXIDATION BY ATP AND ADP

- ATP, but not ADP, exerts feedback control on the glycolytic enzyme phosphofructokinase-1.
- Absolute control of glucose oxidation, however, is mediated by the *availability* of NAD+ and/or ADP because ADP is an obligatory substrate in glucose oxidation (see Chapter 6, page 155). Therefore, the rate of glucose oxidation is diminished when there is insufficient work to regenerate ADP.
- Oxidation of glucose is diminished when ketoacids in the brain or fatty acids in skeletal muscle are oxidized because their oxidation "steals NAD+ and/or ADP," making them become unavailable for the oxidation of glucose.

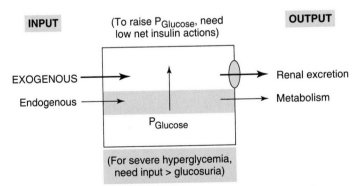

FIGURE 16-2 Development of a severe degree of hyperglycemia. The $P_{Glucose}$ rises when there is a low net insulin action (called *hormonal permission* for simplicity). When the rise in $P_{Glucose}$ does not exceed the renal threshold (i.e., $P_{Glucose}$ 10 mmol of glucose per liter GFR; *green shaded area*), the output of glucose depends solely on its removal via metabolism (*smaller arrows*). If the GFR is very low, very little glucose is excreted and a severe degree of hyperglycemia develops even in the absence of a very large intake of glucose, because the pool size for glucose is small. In the absence of a marked reduction in GFR, a severe degree of hyperglycemia develops only if there is a very large input of glucose.

QUANTITATIVE ANALYSIS OF GLUCOSE METABOLISM

- The quantity of glucose in the body is very small relative to the amount of glucose consumed and oxidized each day.
- In steady state, the output of glucose by metabolism (i.e., oxidation, conversion to storage fuels) equals its input (i.e., from diet, liver glycogen breakdown, gluconeogenesis [i.e., conversion of protein to glucose]).
- Because of the low caloric density in glycogen (has bound water), the stores of glycogen are small.

To understand why the concentration of a metabolite is abnormal (glucose in this case), one requires a quantitative analysis of its rates of input and output. The daily rate of input and output of glucose typically exceeds its pool size by close to 20-fold (Fig. 16-3). Extremely sensitive controls maintain a tiny pool of glucose in the body despite a high flux of glucose through this pool. If these controls do not operate properly, hyperglycemia develops; at times, this can occur rapidly.

Pool size for glucose

- The pool size for glucose is only ~100 mmol or 18 g in a 70-kg adult.

Most of the glucose in the body is in the ECF compartment. There is some glucose in cells of organs that do *not* require insulin to transport glucose across their cell membranes (i.e., most organs other than skeletal muscle and adipose tissue; the intracellular fluid [ICF] volume of these organs is ~5 L). If the $P_{Glucose}$ is 5 mmol/L (100 mg/dL), and the volume of distribution of glucose is 20 L in a 70-kg adult (15 L ECF + 5 L ICF), there is close to 100 mmol (18 g) of glucose in the body.

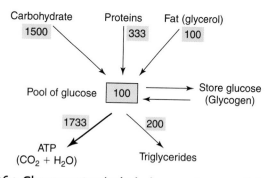

FIGURE 16-3 **Glucose content in the body versus turnover of glucose on a typical Western diet.** The pool of glucose in the body (*green shaded rectangle*) is very small (~100 mmol, or 18 g) relative to the turnover of glucose each day (~1933 mmol, or 312 g). Conversion of proteins to glucose is small compared with input of glucose from dietary sources, and it does not occur at a rapid rate. All the numbers are in mmol of glucose; multiply by 0.18 to convert to grams.

Input of glucose

From the diet

Adults on a typical Western diet consume close to 270 g (1500 mmol) of carbohydrate each day (see Fig. 16-3). Some glucose is also synthesized during the metabolism of ingested proteins (60 g, 333 mmol/day) and from the glycerol portion of dietary triglycerides (18 g, 100 mmol/day). The daily input of glucose (i.e., 350 g) is close to 20 times larger than the entire pool of free glucose in the body.

From stores of glycogen

Glycogen is stored primarily in the liver and skeletal muscle.

Glycogen in the liver

• The major function of glycogen in the liver is to supply the brain with glucose when the $P_{Glucose}$ declines (e.g., between meals). The main activator of glycogenolysis in the liver is the hormone, glucagon.

The size of the pool of glycogen in the liver is only 100 g (600 mmol). This stored glycogen can provide glucose on a "one time only" basis. This store of glycogen becomes depleted under the catabolic signals of a lack of insulin and high levels of glucagon.

Glycogen in skeletal muscle

• The major function of glycogen in skeletal muscle is to enable the regeneration of ATP at the fastest possible rate during vigorous exercise.
• Adrenergic hormones are released when the $P_{Glucose}$ is low, and this causes the breakdown of glycogen in skeletal muscle. The final carbon product in muscles is L-lactic acid, however, and not glucose. L-Lactic acid can be converted into glucose in the liver and in the cortex of the kidney.

Large amounts of glucose (450 g, 2500 mmol) are stored as glycogen in skeletal muscle cells. Because muscles lack the enzyme glucose-6-phosphatase, breakdown of glycogen does not result in the release of glucose from muscle. The major setting for a high rate of breakdown of glycogen in muscle is exercise, and this process is stimulated by a high adrenergic activity. During a sprint, when glycogenolysis is very rapid, ATP is regenerated very quickly. To complete the picture, L-lactic acid is released, and it is converted into glucose in the liver and in the cortex of the kidney—hence, the net result is the conversion of glycogen in muscle to glucose in these organs. During hypoglycemia, adrenergic hormones are released and glycogen in muscle is converted to L-lactic acid, which is then converted to glucose in the liver and in the cortex of the kidney. This process can be viewed as an emergent but temporary supply of glucose for the brain (*see margin note*).

RELEASE OF L-LACTIC ACID FROM SKELETAL MUSCLE IN RESPONSE TO HYPOGLYCEMIA

• The brain consumes 0.5 mmol of glucose per liter of blood flow to regenerate all the ATP it needs to perform its biologic work.
• The liver can convert 4 mmol of L-lactic acid into 2 mmol of glucose per minute (or per liter of blood flow) and hence the liver regenerates an appropriate amount of glucose on a temporary basis.

METABOLISM OF DIETARY PROTEIN
• The liver is virtually the only organ where this pathway occurs because it contains all the enzymes required for the metabolism of the 20 amino acids in proteins.
• If 100 g of protein are fully oxidized in the liver, this would yield 400 kcal (4 kcal/g), whereas the liver needs only close to 300 kcal/day. Therefore, conversion of protein to glucose is an obligatory pathway for protein metabolism in the fed state in the liver; the major carbon end product is glycogen rather than glucose.

FUELS COMPETE FOR AVAILABLE ADP IN THE LIVER DURING STARVATION AND DKA
The conversion of protein to glucose (gluconeogenesis, GNG) consumes ADP. This means that the higher the rate of GNG, the lower the rate of ketoacid formation if hepatic consumption of O_2 is to remain constant (ADP is available from work or if there is uncoupling of oxidative phosphorylation; see Chapter 5, page 145).

Conversion of protein to glucose

> • Gluconeogenesis (GNG) is obligatorily linked to ureagenesis when the substrate is proteins.

The quantity of glucose formed from dietary proteins is not large when compared with dietary carbohydrate intake (333 mmol/day vs. 1500 mmol/day; *see margin note.*)

Approximately 60% of the weight of proteins can be converted to glucose because some of the amino acids cannot be metabolized in this pathway (ketogenic amino acids) and others must be partially oxidized in the tricarboxylic acid cycle (e.g., only three carbons of the five-carbon skeleton in glutamine, the most abundant amino acid in proteins, are converted to the three-carbon gluconeogenic intermediate, pyruvate). It is important to recognize when protein is being converted to glucose at an appreciable rate, because this indicates a catabolic state or the breakdown of proteins in blood in the lumen of the gastrointestinal (GI) tract.

This process of conversion of the carbon skeleton in amino acids to pyruvate is obligatorily linked to the conversion of the nitrogen in amino acids to urea (Fig. 16-4). The stoichiometry of this is the production of 60 g (333 mmol) of glucose and 16 g N (equivalent to almost 600 mmol of urea) from the metabolism of 100 g of protein.

Output of glucose

> • Metabolic removal of glucose is via its oxidation or its conversion to storage compounds.
> • Under conditions of low net insulin actions, renal excretion is the only major pathway for removal of glucose.

Removal of glucose via metabolism

There are two major metabolic means of removing glucose from the circulation: oxidation to regenerate ATP and conversion to its storage forms—glycogen or neutral fat (triglycerides).

Oxidation of glucose. Oxidation of glucose can occur only when the availability of fat-derived fuels (fatty acids or ketoacids) is low because their oxidation decreases the availability of ADP and the products of fat oxidation inhibit the complete oxidation of glucose at

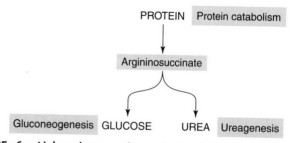

FIGURE 16-4 Linkage between the synthesis of glucose and urea during protein catabolism. It is inaccurate to describe gluconeogenesis and ureagenesis as two separate metabolic pathways, because both pathways are linked in the process of protein oxidation; in fact, they share a common intermediate, argininosuccinate, near the end of this pathway.

pyruvate dehydrogenase (see Fig. 16-1). The brain oxidizes close to 5 g (28 mmol) of glucose per hour if the concentration of ketoacids in plasma is not elevated. In contrast, if the concentration of ketoacids in plasma is elevated, oxidation of glucose is markedly diminished (*see margin note*). In this setting, the only major option for removal of glucose is glucosuria (see Fig. 16-2).

Conversion of glucose to storage forms. High net insulin actions lead to the synthesis (induction) of important enzymes and provide the signals required for the conversion of glucose to glycogen. In addition, there must be a high $P_{Glucose}$ to drive the conversion of glucose to glucose-6-phosphate, the substrate for glycogen synthesis. Nevertheless, a high $P_{Glucose}$ is not sufficient on its own to stimulate glycogen synthesis. To synthesize a large quantity of glycogen in muscle, there must be prior depletion of this pool by exercise.

In the liver, glucose is also converted to triglycerides, which are then stored in adipose tissue, but this pathway proceeds at a slow rate and only when there is more acetyl-CoA available than is needed to regenerate ATP (i.e., when there is limited availability of ADP). The rate-limiting enzyme in this pathway of fat synthesis, acetyl-CoA carboxylase, is stimulated by insulin and is inhibited by adrenergic hormones (see Fig. 5-5, page 118).

Excretion of glucose in the urine

Glucose is not excreted in the urine in normal physiology—this prevents the loss of a precious fuel for the brain. Glucose is excreted in the urine when the $P_{Glucose}$ exceeds the renal threshold for its reabsorption (~10 mmol [~1.8 g] of glucose/L GFR). When glucose is excreted, it "drags" valuable ions (e.g., Na^+ and K^+) and water into the urine. In addition, if the source of urinary glucose is endogenous proteins, the cost in terms of loss of lean body mass is large (*see margin note*).

PART B
RENAL ASPECTS OF HYPERGLYCEMIA

RENAL HANDLING OF GLUCOSE

- The maximum amount of glucose that can be reabsorbed is close to 10 mmol (1.8 g)/L GFR or 1800 mmol (325 g)/day with a GFR of 180 L/day in a 70-kg adult.

Reabsorption of glucose occurs in the proximal convoluted tubule via a Na^+-linked glucose transporter in the luminal membrane (SLGT2); this transporter is different from the one in the intestinal lumen (SLGT1) because its stoichiometry is 1 Na^+/glucose instead of 2 Na^+/glucose (*see margin note*; Fig. 16-5). The exit of glucose from proximal convoluted tubular cells is via a glucose transporter on the basolateral membrane that is independent of Na^+ (GLUT2). The renal handling of glucose is discussed in more detail in Part D of this chapter.

CLINICAL PEARL
When insulin is given to a diabetic in poor control, the rate of glucose oxidation is low until the circulating levels of fatty acids and ketoacids decline markedly.

GLUCOSURIA AND LOSS OF LEAN BODY MASS
- One liter of urine usually contains close to 300 mmol of glucose during a glucose-induced osmotic diuresis.
- If the source of this glucose is from catabolism of proteins, close to 300 mmol of glucose can be formed during the breakdown of 100 g of protein.
- One hundred grams of protein is derived from 0.5 kg (about 1 lb) of muscle (80% of weight of muscle is water).

INHIBITION OF SLGT2 IN THE KIDNEY
- The reabsorption of glucose in the kidney is inhibited by phloridzin derivatives.
- This may become a new strategy to minimize the degree of hyperglycemia in patients with diabetes mellitus.

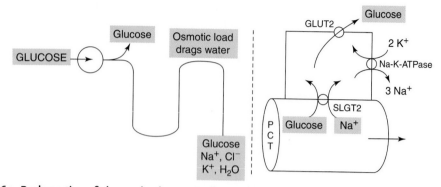

FIGURE 16-5 Reabsorption of glucose by the proximal convoluted tubule. As shown on the *left*, reabsorption of glucose occurs in the proximal convoluted tubule (PCT). Limits are usually set by the GFR (10 mmol glucose re-absorbed/L GFR). When too much glucose is filtered (>10 mmol/L GFR), the extra glucose is delivered distally, where it cannot be absorbed. As a result, an osmotic diuresis occurs. As shown on the *right*, the Na$^+$-linked glucose transporter that carries out the bulk of the glucose reabsorption in the luminal membrane, SLGT2, is located in the early portion of the PCT and transports 1 Na$^+$/glucose. The Na$^+$ absorbed is pumped out of cells by the Na-K-ATPase, which lowers the concentration of Na$^+$ in cells; this provides the driving force to absorb Na$^+$ and glucose from the lumen. The exit of glucose from cells of the PCT is via a glucose transporter on the basolateral membrane that is independent of Na$^+$ (GLUT2).

GLUCOSE-INDUCED OSMOTIC DIURESIS

There are two factors that cause a high volume of urine during an osmotic diuresis: an increased number of effective osmoles in the urine and a lower osmolality in the fluid of the interstitial compartment of the renal medulla (Fig. 16-6). The major effective osmole in the urine in a patient with hyperglycemia is glucose

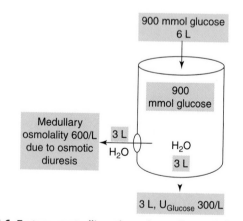

FIGURE 16-6 Factors controlling the urine volume during a glucose-induced osmotic diuresis. The *cylindrical structure* represents the medullary collecting duct (MCD). When vasopressin acts, the MCD is permeable to water. For simplicity, in this example, glucose is the only effective luminal osmole that will be excreted in the urine. Because the osmolality at the end of the cortical collecting duct is similar to the P$_{Osm}$ (300 mOsm/L for easy calculation), 900 mmol of glucose are delivered to the MCD in 6 L of filtrate along with 900 mosmol of other solutes (not shown). If the medullary interstitial osmolality is 600 mOsm/kg H$_2$O, 3 L of water would be absorbed and 3 L would be excreted with the 900 mmol of glucose because the concentration of glucose in the final urine is 300 mmol/L.

TABLE 16-1 **COMPOSITION OF ONE LITER OF GLUCOSE-INDUCED OSMOTIC DIURESIS***

GLUCOSE (mmol/L)	UREA (mmol/L)	Na⁺ (mmol/L)	K⁺ (mmol/L)
300–350	100–200	40	20

*These values serve as reasonable approximations.

(~300 to 350 mmol/L). During an osmotic diuresis, the urine also contains a much lower concentration of other effective osmoles (Na⁺ 40 mmol/L, K⁺ 20 mmol/L, and NH_4^+ plus their anions; Table 16-1).

Effect of a fall in the glomerular filtration rate on the $P_{Glucose}$

As shown in Table 16-2, a large amount of glucose is excreted in the urine when there is both a significant degree of hyperglycemia and a near-normal GFR. A very large intake of glucose is needed to maintain a steady state with a significant degree of hyperglycemia in this setting.

As the GFR falls progressively because of the deficit of Na⁺ created by the glucose-induced osmotic diuresis, the effective arterial blood volume becomes more contracted, and there is a diminished filtered load of glucose. As shown in Table 16-2, much less glucose is excreted for a given $P_{Glucose}$ when the GFR is lower.

In quantitative terms, adults typically consume close to 270 g of glucose per day, of which close to 100 g is metabolized in organs that do not require insulin for the transport of glucose (e.g., the brain). Therefore, with this usual daily intake of glucose, a steady-state $P_{Glucose}$ of 1000 mg/dL can be maintained only if the GFR is less than 25 L/day (see Table 16-2). A steady state with a $P_{Glucose}$ of 500 mg/dL can be achieved only with the usual intake of glucose if the GFR is 50 L/day (*see margin note*). Conversely, if the GFR is 180 L/day, a steady state with a $P_{Glucose}$ of 500 mg/dL would require the daily intake of 575 g of glucose.

Fall in the $P_{Glucose}$ during therapy of hyperglycemia

The $P_{Glucose}$ falls during therapy because of dilution with the administered intravenous isotonic saline because this expands the ECF volume. In addition, reexpansion of the effective arterial blood volume raises the GFR, which leads to more glucosuria. Table 16-2 indicates how much glucose will be excreted with a given GFR at a certain $P_{Glucose}$.

STEADY-STATE HYPERGLYCEMIA

- These calculations are provided to illustrate the effect of a fall of GFR and the intake of glucose on the degree of hyperglycemia.
- It is not likely that a steady state will be maintained, because the GFR will fall further as the effective arterial blood volume becomes more contracted due to the loss of Na⁺ in the urine during the glucose-induced osmotic diuresis.

TABLE 16-2 **EFFECT OF HYPERGLYCEMIA AND THE GFR ON THE EXCRETION OF GLUCOSE**

Excretion of glucose (g/day) = (GFR [L/day] × $P_{Glucose}$ [g/L] – 1.8 g glucose × GFR [L/day]). With the usual daily intake of glucose (260 g or ~1500 mmol) minus the amount that can be oxidized in the brain (~100 g/day), there is a net input of 160 g/day in a patient with a lack of actions of insulin. Thus, the only setting in which a steady state will develop with a $P_{Glucose}$ of 500 mg/dL is if the GFR falls to 50 L/day (shown in bold type).

	GFR (L/day)			
	180	100	50	25
$P_{Glucose}$ *(mg/dL)*	GLUCOSE EXCRETED *(g/day)*			
250	125	70	35	0
500	575	320	**160**	0
1000	1475	820	410	205

IMPACT OF HYPERGLYCEMIA ON BODY COMPARTMENT VOLUMES

Hyperglycemia has two major influences on the ECF and ICF volumes. First, if glucose is added without water, there is a severe degree of hyperglycemia and a high $P_{Effective\ osm}$, which leads to a shift of water from the ICF compartment to the ECF compartment. Second, water and electrolytes are lost in the urine as a result of a hyperglycemia-induced osmotic diuresis. Therefore, the ECF volume will decrease.

Shift of water across cell membranes

- During severe hyperglycemia accompanied by a rise in the $P_{Effective\ osm}$, muscle cells shrink, and hepatocytes swell if hyponatremia is present.
- The size of individual cells in the brain depends on whether glucose can enter these cells rapidly enough for them to have a glucose concentration close to that in plasma.

To understand the impact of hyperglycemia on a shift of water across cell membranes, one must recognize that there are two classes of particles to consider in this analysis.

Particles that do not cause a shift of water

Particles that can achieve equal concentrations in the ECF and ICF compartments raise the P_{Osm} but do not cause a water shift—examples include urea and ethanol.

Particles that do cause a shift of water

Particles that are restricted to one or the other compartment (e.g., Na^+ in the ECF, K^+ in the ICF) cause water to shift out of or into that compartment when their concentrations fall or rise, in a given compartment (*see margin note*).

Glucose and the intracellular fluid volume

Skeletal muscle cells. The concentration of glucose is always much higher outside skeletal muscle cells because they depend on insulin for the transport of glucose, and thus glucose behaves like Na^+ in effective osmole terms. Hence, if hyperglycemia is associated with a rise in the $P_{Effective\ osm}$, water will shift out of skeletal muscle cells (Fig. 16-7).

Hepatocytes. Glucose is not an effective osmole for hepatocytes because its transport in these cells is independent of insulin. As a result, its concentration is equal in both the ECF and the ICF compartments in the liver. Hence, hyperglycemia per se does not cause a shift of water out of liver cells. If hyponatremia is present, however, water will shift from the ECF compartment into hepatocytes, and hence they swell.

Cells in the brain. It is difficult to make a definitive statement about brain cell volume in patients with DKA who present with hyperglycemia, a low ECF volume, and a high $P_{Effective\ osm}$. There are two issues to consider. On one hand, it appears that some brain cells (e.g., neuronal cells of the hypothalamus, which are responsible for sensing the P_{Na}) behave as if glucose is *not* an effective osmole. On the other hand, glucose seems to be an effective osmole for some of the other cells in the brain. In fact, radiologic studies prior to therapy in pediatric patients with DKA suggest that the brain is swollen. There is reason to believe

---

K+ AND THE ICF VOLUME
- If K^+ were to exit from cells and H^+ were to enter, there will be a loss of particles in cells, as the H^+ will bind to proteins and/or remove HCO_3^-; therefore, the cell volume will decline.
- If K^+ were to exit and Na^+ were to enter in a 1:1 stoichiometry, there will be no change in ICF particles and therefore no change in cell volume.
- In the catabolic phase of diabetes mellitus in poor control, there is a decreased content of the major form of organic phosphate (RNA) in cells. As a result, K^+ and inorganic phosphate enter the ECF compartment. When examined, this accounts for almost half of the loss of K^+ from cells (primarily in hepatocytes).

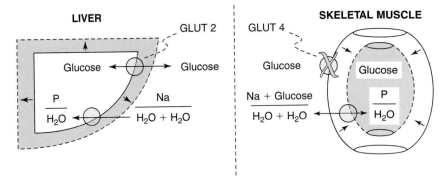

FIGURE 16-7 Hyperglycemia and a shift of water across cell membranes. The *solid outlines* represent the normal size of the organs, whereas the *dashed outlines* represent their size during hyperglycemia. The *X* represents the low ability to transport glucose into skeletal muscle cells in the absence of insulin, which makes the concentration of glucose in these cells always very low in comparison to the $P_{Glucose}$ (represented by a smaller font). Hence, if the $P_{Effective\ osm}$ is elevated during hyperglycemia, water shifts into the extracellular fluid (ECF) compartment. As a result, muscle cells shrink, and the concentration of Na^+ in the ECF falls. In contrast, the concentration of glucose in hepatocytes is equal to the $P_{Glucose}$. Hence, hyperglycemia per se does not cause a shift of water out of liver cells. Hyponatremia, however, causes water to enter hepatocytes, and they swell. GLUT is a glucose transporter.

that the extra water is in both the ICF and ECF compartments. Of note, it is very important to prevent a fall in the $P_{Effective\ osm}$ during therapy to minimize the risk of swelling of brain cells and the development of cerebral edema, especially in children with DKA.

Quantitative relationship between the rise in the $P_{Glucose}$ and the fall in the P_{Na}

- There is *no reliable quantitative relationship* between the rise in the $P_{Glucose}$ and the fall in the P_{Na} in an individual patient with hyperglycemia.

The calculations that adjust the P_{Na} for the rise in $P_{Glucose}$ are based on the assumption that glucose was added *without* water. One cannot know, however, whether glucose was added with or without water in an individual patient and also what the balances for water and Na^+ were prior to therapy (*see margin note*). To illustrate this point, the $P_{Glucose}$ is raised using two different settings in the following sample calculations. For simplicity, we consider the ECF compartment and the ICF compartment of only skeletal muscle in each example.

DATA FROM CLINICAL STUDIES
The data reported in the literature about the ratio of the fall in P_{Na} and the rise in $P_{Glucose}$ from studies in a large number of patients are not helpful in an individual patient with hyperglycemia because these data apply to an "average" patient who may or may not be similar to your patient.

Sample calculation

A 50-kg patient has an ECF volume of 10 L and a skeletal muscle ICF volume of 15 L. The ECF compartment contains 1400 mmol of Na^+ (P_{Na} 140 mmol/L × 10 L) and 50 mmol of glucose ($P_{Glucose}$ 5 mmol/L × 10 L) before hyperglycemia developed.

Add an iso-osmotic solution of glucose

In this example, 2 L of 285 mmol of glucose/L (an iso-osmotic solution) are added and all of the glucose and water are retained in the ECF compartment. Because there is no change in the $P_{Effective\ osm}$, water does not move across cell membranes in skeletal muscle. Hence, the $P_{Glucose}$ rises and the P_{Na} falls because Na^+-free water is retained in the ECF compartment. Thus, the ECF volume increases from 10 to 12 L (*see margin note*; see Table 16-3).

CHANGE IN P_{Na} FROM ADDING 2 L OF ISO-OSMOLAL GLUCOSE SOLUTION
- The ECF volume is now 12 L (10 + 2 L) and the $P_{Glucose}$ rises by 47.5 mmol/L ([285 mmol/L × 2 L] ÷ 12 L).
- The new P_{Na} decreases to 117 mmol/L (1400 mmol Na^+ ÷ 12 L). Thus, the fall in the P_{Na} is 23 mmol/L and the rise in $P_{Glucose}$ is 47.5 mmol/L—the ratio of the fall in P_{Na} to the rise in $P_{Glucose}$ is 0.5 in mmol/L terms.

TABLE 16-3 **FALL IN THE P$_{Na}$ WHEN THERE IS A RISE IN THE P$_{Glucose}$** *

WATER AND GLUCOSE ADDED	NEW ECFV (L)	FALL IN P$_{Na}$ (mmol/L)	RISE IN P$_{Glucose}$ (mmol/L)	RATIO ↓P$_{Na}$/ ↑P$_{Glucose}$
2 L, 570 mmol	12.0	23	47.5	~0.50
0 L, 570 mmol	11.1	14	51.4	~0.27

*These values serve as reasonable approximations.
ECFV, extracellular fluid volume.

Add glucose but no water

In this example, 570 mmol of glucose without water are added to and retained in the ECF compartment. Because there is a rise in the P$_{Effective osm}$, water shifts from muscle cells to the ECF compartment; the volume of water that is shifted depends on the rise in the P$_{Effective osm}$ (*see margin note*).

As evident from the calculations in the margin notes, which are summarized in Table 16-3, there is *not* an expected fall in the P$_{Na}$ for a given rise in the P$_{Glucose}$ because one cannot know how much glucose versus water was retained or how much Na$^+$ and water were excreted in a given patient. Said in stronger terms *do not calculate this ratio*. You know that water has shifted from muscle cells only if there was a rise in the P$_{Effective osm}$. In addition, this calculation should not be used to predict a rise in P$_{Na}$ for a given fall in the P$_{Glucose}$. It is important to prevent a fall in the P$_{Effective osm}$ for at least the first 10 to 15 hours of therapy, because this may help diminish the risk of developing cerebral edema (this is discussed later in this chapter).

Impact of an osmotic diuresis on body fluid composition

- The major losses in a glucose-induced osmotic diuresis are glucose, Na$^+$, K$^+$, Cl$^-$, and water.
- In quantitative terms, the concentrations of glucose (300 to 350 mmol/L), Na$^+$ (40 mmol/L), and K$^+$ (20 mmol/L) in the urine usually do not vary appreciably.
- To calculate the deficit of Na$^+$ in the ECF compartment, one needs a quantitative estimate of the ECF volume.

The total deficits of Na$^+$, K$^+$, and water have been estimated in balance studies in patients with diabetes mellitus who had insulin therapy withheld or from retrospective studies using the average amounts of Na$^+$, K$^+$, and water that were retained during therapy of patients with DKA. These estimates, however, are not accurate because when more Na$^+$ is infused than needed, patients with prior effective arterial blood volume contraction retain a quantity of Na$^+$ that overexpands their ECF volume; some of them retained enough Na$^+$ to develop edema. Moreover, these approximations are not really helpful to determine the deficits for an *individual* patient who presents with severe hyperglycemia. Hence, we describe how to estimate the deficit of Na$^+$ and HCO$_3^-$ in an individual patient with a severe degree of hyperglycemia prior to instituting therapy.

While one knows the P$_{Na}$, one needs a *quantitative* estimate of the ECF volume to calculate the deficit of Na$^+$. This can be obtained using the hematocrit (or hemoglobin level) on presentation (in the absence of prior anemia or polycythemia), but not from the physical examination (see Chapter 2, page 57 for more discussion).

CHANGE IN THE P$_{Na}$ WHEN 570 mmol OF GLUCOSE ARE ADDED WITHOUT WATER

- The initial total number of mosmol in the ECF compartment plus in the ICF of skeletal muscles is 7125 ([10 L + 15 L] × 285 mOsm/L); after the addition of 570 mmol glucose, the total number of mosmol is now 7695. Hence, the osmolality rises to 308 mOsm/L (7695 ÷ 25 L).
- Dividing the number of mosmol in skeletal muscle (15 L × 285 mOsm/L = 4275 mOsm) by the new P$_{Effective osm}$ (308 mOsm/L) yields a new ICF volume in skeletal muscle of 13.9 L. Hence, 1.1 L of water has shifted into the ECF compartment.
- The new ECF volume is 11.1 L (10 + 1.1 L).
- The P$_{Glucose}$ has risen by 51.4 mmol/L (570 mmol ÷ 11.1 L) and with no change in the content of Na$^+$ in the ECF compartment, the P$_{Na}$ falls to 126 mmol/L (1400 mmol ÷ 11.1 L).
- Hence, the ratio of the fall in P$_{Na}$ (14 mmol/L) to the rise in P$_{Glucose}$ (51.4 mmol/L) is 0.27, a value that is almost half that obtained after the addition of the same amount of glucose as an iso-osmotic solution described previously!

Sample calculation

A 50-kg patient presented to hospital with DKA; the $P_{Glucose}$ was 900 mg/dL (50 mmol/L), the P_{Na} was 120 mmol/L, and the hematocrit was 0.50. Prior to the illness, this patient had a P_{Na} of 140 mmol/L and an ECF volume of 10 L, and hence the ECF volume contained 1400 mmol of Na^+.

A hematocrit of 0.40 represents a red blood cell volume of 2 L and a blood volume of 5 L (2 L red blood cells + 3 L plasma). When the hematocrit is 0.50, the red blood cell volume and plasma volumes are equal; hence, the plasma volume is now only 2 L (two thirds of normal). Accordingly, the ECF volume is two thirds of normal (~6.7 L). Multiplying the ECF volume by the P_{Na} (120 mmol/L) yields the present content of Na^+ in the ECF compartment (~800 mmol). Therefore, the deficit of Na^+ in this patient is close to 600 mmol (1400 − 800); this provides an estimate of the total negative balance for Na^+ in the ECF compartment. This calculation, however, overestimates the loss of Na^+ from the body because approximately half the loss of K^+ in the urine was accompanied by a gain of Na^+ in the ICF compartment.

IMPACT OF THE INGESTION OF FRUIT JUICE

- The composition of fruit juice represents the ICF of fruit; it contains sugar (~750 mmol/L), K^+ (~50 mEq/L), and potential HCO_3^- (~50 mEq/L), but little Na^+ and Cl^-. Hence, look for clues related to each of these constituents in a patient with diabetes mellitus in poor control who consumed a large quantity of fruit juice.

Sugar

When a patient develops DKA, the hyperglycemia induces an osmotic diuresis, and the urine contains Na^+ (~40 to 50 mmol/L) and K^+ (~20 mmol/L). Because dietary Na^+ is usually low, a deficit of Na^+ develops, and there is a fall in the ECF and the effective arterial blood volumes. The latter triggers thirst, which causes patients to increase their fluid intake. When they drink fruit juice, the degree of hyperglycemia becomes more severe. For example, 1 L of apple juice contains 750 mmol of glucose. Nevertheless, the amount of ingested glucose that enters the ECF compartment may be less than the quantity ingested, because hyperglycemia causes a delay in gastric emptying; this topic is discussed in more detail on page 562. Notwithstanding, a vicious cycle is created; when the effective arterial blood volume becomes more contracted, thirst becomes more intense, and, as a result, more fruit juice is ingested, which increases the degree of hyperglycemia. The ingestion of a large volume of fruit juice usually produces a large volume of osmotic diuresis until the GFR falls appreciably as the result of the fall in the effective arterial blood volume and possibly also because of a high $P_{Albumin}$ (*see margin note*).

Na^+ and Cl^-

The presence of a large osmotic diuresis causes an appreciable loss of Na^+ in the urine (*see margin note*). The ingestion of more fruit juice usually produces a large volume of osmotic diuresis and thus increases the deficit of Na^+. The magnitude of the deficit of Na^+ is also influenced by the quantity of Na^+ that is ingested.

$P_{Albumin}$ **AND THE GFR**
- The higher the $P_{Albumin}$, the greater the colloid osmotic pressure.
- In the capillaries of the glomerulus, this colloid osmotic pressure decreases the net driving force for filtration.

LOSS OF Na^+ WHEN 1 L OF FRUIT JUICE IS INGESTED AND ITS SUGAR IS EXCRETED IN THE URINE
- One liter of urine contains close to 350 mmol of glucose and 50 mmol of Na^+ in this setting.
- One liter of fruit juice contains ~750 mmol of sugar and no Na^+.
- If all this ingested sugar is excreted at a concentration of 350 mmol of glucose per liter, the urine volume will be 2 L.
- Thus, there is a negative balance of ~100 mmol of Na^+, which is equivalent to the quantity of Na^+ in two thirds of a liter of ECF.

Potassium

- Patients who consume fruit juice should have a higher P_K than patients who consume little fruit juice during the course of their illness.

The magnitude of the deficit of K^+ depends on how many K^+ are excreted (which depends on the exogenous glucose load because this induces an osmotic diuresis) and how much K^+ is ingested. The major source of dietary K^+ in this setting is from fruit juice; the principal cation in fruit juice is K^+, and its concentration is close to 50 mmol/L.

Potential HCO_3^-

- The major anions in fruit juice are a family of organic anions (e.g., citrate), which provides close to 50 mEq/L of potential HCO_3^- per liter of fruit juice.

The magnitude of the deficit of HCO_3^- depends on how much potential HCO_3^- is ingested. If a patient with DKA does not ingest much fruit juice, there is a much smaller input of potential HCO_3^- and, as a result, a more severe degree of acidemia.

PART C
CLINICAL APPROACH
CLASSIFICATION OF HYPERGLYCEMIA

- A very high $P_{Glucose}$ indicates a marked reduction in GFR and/or a very large input of glucose if the GFR is not markedly reduced.
- When there is a net lack of insulin actions, a large change in the $P_{Glucose}$ can occur quickly because the pool size of glucose in the body is small.

Low net insulin actions are required to develop chronic hyperglycemia. A marked reduction in GFR and/or a very large intake of glucose causes the degree of hyperglycemia to become very severe. The natural history of this hyperglycemic state begins with a polyuric phase during which the ECF volume and the GFR have not yet declined appreciably. The major cause of the hyperglycemia at this stage is a large intake of glucose in a setting where the metabolic removal of glucose is very low. After excreting a large volume of urine during an osmotic diuresis, the result is a large deficit of Na^+. Accordingly, there is a decline in the effective arterial blood volume, and thereby the GFR falls. Hence, at this stage, the urine flow rate declines and a greater degree of hyperglycemia develops if there is a continuing input of glucose that exceeds its rate of excretion. Based on these principles, we call the polyuric phase the "*drinker*" stage and the oliguric phase the "*prune*" stage of hyperglycemia. The best initial way to deduce the major cause of the hyperglycemia is to examine the

TABLE 16-4 **ISSUES IN DIAGNOSIS AND THERAPY OF PATIENTS WITH HYPERGLYCEMIA**

	DIAGNOSTIC FEATURE	SPECIAL FINDINGS	THERAPEUTIC EMPHASIS
Polyuric group (urine flow rate > 3 mL/min)			
The "drinker"	• Large ingestion of glucose	• Rate of gastric emptying influences the rise in $P_{Glucose}$	• Not likely the sole cause of a severe degree of hyperglycemia
Catabolic state*	• High rate of appearance of urea	• Breakdown of endogenous proteins	• Address the cause of the protein catabolism or gastrointestinal bleeding
Oliguric group			
The "prune"	• Very low EABV	• Hemodynamic instability	• Reexpand EABV volume rapidly at first to restore blood pressure • Prevent a fall in $P_{Effective\ osm}$
Chronic renal insufficiency	• Expanded extracellular fluid volume	• Congestive heart failure • Hyperkalemia	• After giving insulin, the fall in $P_{Glucose}$ may take hours to occur

EABV, effective arterial blood volume.
*A catabolic state causes an appreciable rise in the $P_{Glucose}$ only in patients who are already hyperglycemic.

urine flow rate (Table 16-4), the plasma creatinine, and the effective arterial blood volume (Flow Chart 16-1).

Polyuric group

High sugar–intake type (the "drinker")

> • A very large glucose intake and rapid stomach emptying are required to maintain a severe degree of hyperglycemia.

An extraordinarily large input of glucose can overwhelm the normal kidney's ability to excrete it for a period of time; this may lead to a severe degree of hyperglycemia. Most commonly, the source of glucose is an excessive intake of fruit juice or sweetened soft drinks (~750 mmol of glucose per liter) that are consumed in response to thirst.

Stomach emptying is usually slow in the patient with a high $P_{Glucose}$. Nevertheless, an abrupt increase in $P_{Glucose}$ and/or in the urine flow rate may occur because of a sudden increase in stomach emptying and absorption of glucose in the small intestine. This may also be suspected if the fall in $P_{Glucose}$ during therapy is less than expected from the degree of reexpansion of the ECF volume (dilution) and the degree of osmotic diuresis (see the discussion of Case 16-1 and page 562).

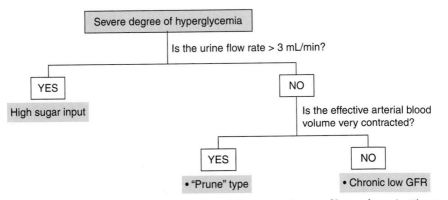

FLOW CHART 16-1 Diagnostic approach to the patient with a severe degree of hyperglycemia. The steps to follow are outlined in the flow chart. The final diagnostic categories appear after the *bullets* at the bottom of each column. We have selected a urine flow rate of 3 mL/min, but this is admittedly an arbitrary value.

High protein catabolism

> • Look for an increased rate of appearance of urea (the amount of urea excreted in the urine plus the change in the content of urea in the body).

This alone cannot be the sole cause of a sustained and severe degree of hyperglycemia because breakdown of 100 g of protein provides the carbon skeleton for the synthesis of only close to 333 mmol of glucose (equal to the content of glucose in 1 L of osmotic diuresis; see Table 16-1). Nevertheless, an increased endogenous input of glucose can result *transiently* from the breakdown of a large quantity of protein (e.g., increased amino acid absorption after major GI bleeding). This may be suspected if the fall in the $P_{Glucose}$ is less than expected during therapy and if the P_{Urea} is higher than expected as compared to the $P_{Creatinine}$ (breakdown of 100 g of protein provides the nitrogen for the synthesis of ~600 mmol of urea).

Oliguric group

Patients with prerenal failure

As shown in Table 16-2, the excretion of glucose may be small during severe hyperglycemia if the GFR is very low because the filtered load of glucose can now be almost completely reabsorbed. Most commonly, this reduction in the GFR is secondary to the low effective arterial blood volume due to the large negative balance for Na^+, as a result of the prior osmotic diuresis.

Patients with chronic renal failure

The excretion of glucose should be very low in patients with advanced, chronic renal disease because they cannot have an osmotic diuresis owing to their very low GFR. In this setting, the ECF volume is expanded. Water will be drawn into the ECF compartment from cells that require insulin for the transport of glucose (primarily skeletal muscles, which represent almost half of total body water) if the $P_{Effective\ osm}$ is high. These patients are not in negative balance for Na^+ because their hyperglycemia could not cause an osmotic diuresis.

THERAPY FOR THE PATIENT WITH HYPERGLYCEMIA

> • The major issue is to prevent a fall in the $P_{Effective\ osm}$ in the first 10 to 15 hours after therapy begins to minimize the risk of brain cell swelling.

Administration of Na^+ and water

> • Infuse saline rapidly only if there is hemodynamic instability (Table 16-5).

TABLE 16-5 **INTRAVENOUS THERAPY IN A PATIENT WITH A SEVERE DEGREE OF HYPERGLYCEMIA**

COMPARTMENT	SPEED	IV FLUID TONICITY	COMMENTS
ECF			
Replace deficit of Na+	• Fast only in an emergency	• Isotonic to the ECF, or to the urine if polyuric	• Bolus of saline increases risk of cerebral edema
Loss of glucose in the urine may be from the ECF or from the stomach	• Replace the glucose lost from the ECF with NaCl • Do not replace glucose from the stomach	• Prevent a fall in the $P_{Effective\ osm}$	• Fast in "drinker" • Retained glucose helps to defend the ECF volume
ICF			
Keep a constant ICF volume	—	• Same as urine if polyuria is present	• Important to prevent cerebral edema, especially in children

ECF, extracellular fluid; GFR, glomerular filtration rate; ICF, intracellular fluid.

- To minimize the risk of cerebral edema during therapy of DKA, avoid an excessive administration of saline (use the brachial venous P_{CO_2} and the hematocrit to guide the rate of infusion of saline), do *not* administer a bolus of insulin, and do not permit the $P_{Effective\ osm}$ to fall in the first 10 to 15 hours of therapy.
- Beware of abrupt stomach emptying, which may cause a fall in the $P_{Effective\ osm}$ early on if there was a recent large intake of water or later on if glucose and water were ingested and the glucose is removed rapidly by metabolism (i.e., due to insulin actions).

The major cause of morbidity and mortality in children with DKA is cerebral edema; this does not seem to be a risk in most adult patients with a severe degree of hyperglycemia. Nevertheless, since subtle changes in brain function could occur, our major goal during therapy is to prevent brain swelling in all patients with severe chronic hyperglycemia. The risk factors for development of cerebral edema during therapy of DKA in children are discussed in detail in Chapter 5, page 127. Therefore, we provide only a brief summary of important issues in therapy in this chapter.

Treat a hemodynamic emergency only if it is present

- A bolus of saline should be given *only* if there is a hemodynamic emergency.
- Consider other causes for hemodynamic instability if the patient remains hemodynamically unstable after the infusion of an appreciable volume of isotonic saline.

Although a true hemodynamic emergency is *not* common in children with DKA, this could be a problem in adults with a severe degree of contraction of their effective arterial blood volume due to a large deficit of Na+ and/or an underlying disorder (e.g., prior therapy with diuretics). It is important to recognize that a bolus of intravenous saline can be a risk factor for the development of cerebral edema because it increases the hydrostatic pressure and diminishes the colloid osmotic pressure in capillaries in the blood-brain barrier.

In the absence of a hemodynamic emergency, we use the brachial venous P_{CO_2} as a guide to the initial rate of infusion of saline. Enough saline should be administered to lower this venous P_{CO_2} to a value that is not more than 10 mm Hg higher than the arterial P_{CO_2}. This ensures that the bicarbonate buffer system in skeletal muscle is effective in

EXPRESSING THE AMOUNT OF SALINE PER kg BODY WEIGHT
Because patients with DKA differ in size, one cannot talk about absolute volumes to infuse. Therefore, one must express these volumes per kg body weight as illustrated in the following example:
• in a 50-kg person, the ECF volume is 10 L.
• Note that 3 mmol Na^+/kg = 150 mmol Na^+ = 1 L of isotonic saline; this is equal to 10% of the normal ECF volume.

ISSUES IN THERAPY
1. Avoid a large fall in the $P_{Effective\ osm}$.
2. Anticipate the composition of stomach contents by taking a careful history.
3. Cerebral edema may develop anytime due to the provision of water. In contrast, cerebral edema may develop later in time when insulin acts if glucose plus water are absorbed in the intestinal tract and insulin actions cause the rapid metabolism of glucose.

Na^+ DEFICIT
• The calculated deficit represents Na^+ that was lost from the ECF compartment (see sample calculation on page 557).
• Not all of that Na^+ loss from the ECF compartment was excreted; some Na^+ shifted into cells in response to the exit of K^+ from these cells.
• When balance studies were performed in patients with DKA, close to half of the loss of K^+ from cells represented a shift of K^+ for Na^+ (also some for H^+), and the other half represented a loss of K^+ and inorganic phosphate (Fig. 16-8).

buffering an added H^+ load and hence binding of H^+ to intracellular proteins in vital organs (e.g., brain cells) is diminished. One must consider other causes for hemodynamic instability if it persists after the infusion of an appreciable volume of saline (*see margin note*).

Avoid a large fall in the $P_{Effective\ osm}$

> • An important objective during therapy is to prevent brain cell swelling, which may occur if the $P_{Effective\ osm}$ falls.

The most common cause of a large fall in the $P_{Effective\ osm}$ is a large decrease in the $P_{Glucose}$ early during therapy. Therefore, the P_{Na} must rise by half of the fall in the $P_{Glucose}$ to prevent a fall in the $P_{Effective\ osm}$ (see Chapter 5, page 130 for more discussion of this topic). To achieve this, the effective osmolality of the infusate should be equal to that of the urine in a polyuric patient. Therefore, infuse isotonic saline with 40 mmol KCl added per liter when K^+ is needed—this results in an effective osmolality of close to 380 mOsm/L, a value that is reasonably close to the effective osmolality of the urine in a glucose-induced osmotic diuresis (see Table 16-1). Although one may be tempted to switch to hypotonic saline to treat the hyperosmolar state, it is our view that this is especially *dangerous* in children because it increases the risk of developing cerebral edema. As discussed previously, one should not adjust the P_{Na} for the degree of hyperglycemia.

"Occult" stomach emptying. When subjects drink beverages that contain sugar to quench their thirst, some of this glucose remains in the stomach because hyperglycemia slows stomach emptying. The following observations are clues that stomach emptying and absorption of ingested fluid that contains glucose has occurred in a patient with hyperglycemia (*see margin note*):
1. A rise in $P_{Glucose}$ in the absence of an infusion of solutions containing glucose or L-lactate. A much better clue is a rise in the $P_{Glucose}$ in arterial blood, as this rise may not be seen in brachial venous blood owing to dilution with the large interstitial fluid volume.
2. A sudden large rise in the urine output due to glucose-induced osmotic diuresis
3. Absence of a sufficient fall in $P_{Glucose}$ despite glucose being excreted in the urine
4. An unexpected rise in the in the $P_{Effective\ osm}$

If a patient drank water recently, stomach emptying results in an intravenous infusion of water via the portal vein. The key finding is a fall in the $P_{Effective\ osm}$; this will be more evident in arterial blood, as mentioned above.

Longer-term consideration: Reexpand the extracellular fluid volume

Having defined the safe rate and tonicity of the fluid to infuse, the issue now is to define what is a reasonable total volume to infuse to avoid overexpansion of the ECF volume, especially in children, because this may be a risk factor for cerebral edema. To assess the deficit of Na^+ in the ECF compartment, one needs a quantitative estimate of the ECF volume. This can be obtained using the hematocrit or the total plasma protein concentration. Nevertheless, not all of this Na^+ deficit in the ECF compartment represents a loss of Na^+ from the body (*see margin note*).

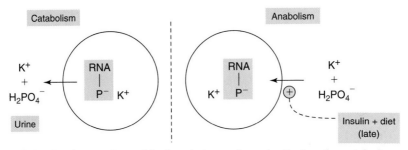

FIGURE 16-8 Deficit of K⁺ in a patient with chronic hyperglycemia. During the catabolism phase of DKA (*left of the vertical dashed line*). RNA breakdown leads to the release of inorganic phosphate and K⁺ from the intracellular fluid compartment. A major site for this catabolism is in the liver. These changes are reversed after a significant delay, when insulin is administered (*right of the vertical dashed line*). Therefore, this portion of the K⁺ deficit cannot be replaced early in therapy. Rather, it requires dietary intake of phosphate and K⁺. The administration of KCl early in therapy is to replace a deficit of K⁺ in cells that occurred when there was a gain of H⁺ (due to the gain of ketoacids) and a shift of some Na⁺ into cells (not shown in the figure).

Replace the urine volume early in therapy with a saline solution that is isotonic to the urine. To maintain the desired ECF volume early in therapy, ongoing losses of Na⁺ in the urine need to be replaced. Because the hyperglycemia helped maintain the ECF volume early on, loss of glucose that was in the ECF compartment and excreted in the urine should be replaced by giving different effective osmoles for the ECF compartment (i.e., Na⁺ and Cl⁻; *see margin note*). The loss of glucose in the urine in excess of this amount should *not* be replaced because the source of this glucose is likely to be glucose absorbed from the upper GI tract during therapy.

Potassium therapy

- The portion of intracellular K⁺ loss that was associated with a net entry of Na⁺ or H⁺ into cells can be replaced with KCl.
- The portion of intracellular K⁺ loss that was associated with a loss of phosphate in the urine will be replaced days later, when the anabolic effects of insulin are present and phosphate is supplied in the diet.

The total loss of K⁺ is said to be close to 5 mmol/kg of body weight. Approximately half of these K⁺ were lost from the ICF compartment in conjunction with phosphate anions. Because the net charge on intracellular phosphate diesters is −1, an equal amount of K⁺ should leave the cells with phosphate. Replacement of this K⁺ deficit occurs over days with the intake of phosphate in the diet and requires the presence of anabolic signals (i.e., actions of insulin).

The remaining half of the ICF K⁺ loss largely represents K⁺ that shifted in exchange for Na⁺ and were excreted in the urine with Cl⁻ or potential HCO_3^- (ketoacid anions). Therefore, this represents, at most, a loss of 1.5 L of ECF volume in a 50-kg person. This portion of the K⁺ deficit is replaced early in therapy by the administration of KCl (see Fig. 16-8; *see margin note*).

CALCULATION OF EXTRA GLUCOSE IN THE BODY IN A 50-kg PATIENT
- This patient has a normal ECF volume of 10 L. Because the normal $P_{Glucose}$ is 5 mmol/L and glucose distributes in the ECF compartment (10 L) as well as in 5 L of the ICF compartment in this patient, the content of glucose is 75 mmol before the development of hyperglycemia.
- Assume that the patient has a hematocrit of 0.50 (ECF volume is two thirds of its normal value [i.e., 6.7 L]) and a $P_{Glucose}$ of 900 mg/dL (50 mmol/L). Hence, the content of glucose in this patient is currently 585 mmol; the ECF volume (6.7 L) + 5 L of ICF = 11.7 L × 50 mmol/L.
- Accordingly, we must replace close to 500 mmol of glucose with a positive balance of 250 mmol of NaCl (2 mosmol in 1 mmol of NaCl).

SHIFT OF Na⁺ INTO CELLS
It is not clear why the extra Na⁺ are retained in cells (i.e., they are not exported by the Na-K-ATPase).

(Discussion on page 573)

16-1 *If a patient with diabetes mellitus in poor control has GI bleeding and digests and absorbs all the protein in 1 L of blood, how much extra glucose and urea are produced?*

16-2 *A patient presented to the hospital with DKA; the initial $P_{Glucose}$ was 60 mmol/L (1080 mg/dL) and the P_{Na} was 140 mmol/L ($P_{Effective\ osm}$ 340 mOsm/L). After 48 hours of therapy, the $P_{Glucose}$ was 15 mmol/L (270 mg/dL) and the P_{Na} was 160 mmol/L ($P_{Effective\ osm}$ 335 mOsm/L). Over the next 6 hours, the $P_{Glucose}$ fell to 10 mmol/L (180 mg/dL) and his P_{Na} declined to 140 mmol/L. Of note, the patient did not drink or receive hypotonic fluids. Why did his P_{Na} decline over this time period and what are the implications for therapy?*

PART D
INTEGRATIVE PHYSIOLOGY

EFFECTS OF INSULIN ON Na⁺ AND K⁺ HOMEOSTASIS: AN INTEGRATIVE PERSPECTIVE

- Think of control mechanisms in the context of providing an advantage for survival in Paleolithic times.
- Actions of insulin to cause the excretion of K^+ and retention of Na^+ were required in Paleolithic times, when the diet was rich in K^+ and poor in NaCl. It made sense to endow insulin with these actions because the diet (fruit and berries), which provided K^+, was also high in sugars.

MINI-CASE 16-1: A PATIENT WITH ANOREXIA NERVOSA

A 16-year-old girl has lost 25 kg (55 lb) in the past 8 months as a result of diminished intake of food, high level of exercise, and an unknown number of episodes of self-induced vomiting. She was admitted to the hospital for nutritional therapy. The values for her electrolytes, albumin, and glucose in plasma were all in the normal range, and her serum creatinine were in the expected range considering her markedly reduced muscle mass. She gained 9 lb (4 kg) in the first week of feeding.

Questions

What are the major dangers to anticipate with feeding, and how can they be minimized?

What may be responsible for an excessive gain of weight in this patient during refeeding?

Discussion of Mini-Case 16-1

What are the major dangers to anticipate with feeding, and how can they be minimized?

Hypoglycemia

- The Paleolithic diet contained large amount of sugar, which raises the $P_{Glucose}$ and thereby causes the release of insulin.

When food is ingested, the $P_{Glucose}$ rises and insulin is released. Accordingly, hypoglycemia could develop when the dietary intake is started and then is stopped. Hence, it is prudent to provide a hypocaloric diet with small frequent meals and keep a close watch on the $P_{Glucose}$ during this initial phase of refeeding. It is interesting to note, however, that patients with this disorder would have likely had intermittent periods when food was ingested prior to admission to hospital without developing a serious degree of hypoglycemia.

Hypophosphatemia

- A major action of insulin is to increase the synthesis of proteins; this requires the production of ribosomes that are composed principally of RNA, which contains phosphate. Hence, there is an immediate demand for inorganic phosphate in cells to synthesize this RNA during feeding.

Because most diets do not contain enough inorganic phosphate for the burst of RNA synthesis in the short-term, there is a major shift of phosphate into cells, and this may result in a serious degree of hypophosphatemia. To minimize this complication, begin feeding with very small and frequent meals and add supplements of phosphate.

Hypokalemia

- Insulin causes a rapid shift of K^+ into skeletal muscle cells.
- In Paleolithic times, actions of insulin were likely required to cause a rapid and large kaliuresis, and to prevent a natriuresis because the diet contained a large amount of K^+ (with organic anions) but a small quantity of NaCl.

Shift of K^+. Insulin causes a shift of K^+ into cells because it activates the Na^+/H^+ exchanger and the Na-K-ATPase in cell membranes of skeletal muscle cells. In addition, there is a burst of synthesis of organic phosphates (e.g., RNA) early during feeding. As a result, these cells retain K^+. These patients are often profoundly K^+ depleted because of previous vomiting with renal K^+ loss. In this setting, insulin may provoke a hypokalemic emergency.

Excretion of K^+. Insulin may promote a rapid excretion of K^+, which is best understood in terms of the Paleolithic diet with its high content of K^+ and organic anions (potential HCO_3^-).

The actions of insulin resemble (and are addictive to) those of aldosterone in the late cortical distal nephron (i.e., it causes the generation of a lumen-negative voltage, and it may also have an effect to insert rat outer medullary K^+ channels [ROMK] into the luminal membrane of principal cells). In support of this speculation, the late cortical distal nephron has a very high density of insulin receptors. Actions of insulin may lead to an increase in the conductance of ENaC for Na^+, as well as increase the number of ENaC units in the luminal membranes of principal cells in the late cortical distal nephron.

Clinical implications for the effect of insulin to cause Na^+ retention. Mechanisms were required in Paleolithic times, when the diet contained little NaCl, to prevent the natriuresis; this may have clinical implications in modern times. For example, patients with DKA usually have a large deficit of Na^+, and physicians usually administer much more NaCl than needed to replace the deficit of Na^+ in these patients (see Chapter 5, page 131 for more discussion). Hence, it is not surprising that insulin may play a role in the retention of this extra NaCl, and if the quantity is large enough, the patient may develop obvious edema (*see margin note*). The same phenomenon may provide an explanation for the development of edema in patients who have consumed too few calories for a protracted period of time (e.g., patients with kwashiorkor, marasmus, or anorexia nervosa when the intake of calories and salt is increased [called *refeeding edema*]).

What may be responsible for an excessive gain of weight in this patient during refeeding?

- Because water is the most abundant mass in the body, it is likely that a sudden and large gain in weight resulted from a gain of water.

There are two locations where there is a gain of water: in cells and in the ECF compartment.

Gain of water in cells

- There can be a gain of water in cells if there is a gain of effective osmoles in cells and/or a fall in the P_{Na}.

Although the normal value for the P_{Na} suggests that there is no gain of water in cells, this is a superficial analysis because there is a gain of effective osmoles in cells, which leads to a gain of water. Although the gain of phosphate does not lead directly to more osmoles because RNA is a macromolecule, the gain of a cation (principally K^+) in cells for electroneutrality is the cause for a gain in effective osmoles and therefore leads to a gain of water and expansion of the ICF volume.

When sugar is ingested and insulin acts, glycogen is synthesized. Two to three grams of water are bound in each gram of glycogen that accumulates. Hence, if this glycogen-depleted patient accumulates 500 g of glycogen, an extra 1000 to 1500 g (1 to 1.5 L) of water is retained.

Gain of water in the extracellular fluid compartment

- A low $P_{Albumin}$ has been suggested as a likely mechanism to cause the edema; however, edema cannot merely result from a shift of saline from plasma into the interstitial compartment because there is not enough plasma volume for edema to develop (i.e., there must be a positive balance for Na^+).

A large quantity of Na^+ must be ingested or infused and retained for edema to develop, because the ECF volume must be expanded by many liters. A low $P_{Albumin}$ may provide the signal to retain this dietary Na^+ because it leads to a low plasma oncotic pressure and thereby to a fall in the effective arterial blood volume. As discussed previously, the release of insulin in response to feeding may cause the retention of Na^+ in these subjects with a prior very low intake of NaCl. Since the P_{Na} did not change appreciably in this patient, there was retention of water and of Na^+.

FACTORS THAT LEAD TO THE RETENTION OF NaCl AND WATER
In addition to the potential role for insulin, the following factors may contribute to avid retention of dietary or infused NaCl:
- Prior K^+ depletion
- Prior contraction of the effective arterial blood volume
- Prior high angiotension II levels

Patients with anorexia nervosa are very concerned about their body weight. Therefore, the feeding strategy should include a low intake of NaCl while the Na^+-retaining actions of insulin are still very prominent.

Implications for patients eating a typical Western diet

- Insulin does not cause Na^+ retention in normal subjects eating NaCl-rich Western diets.

Actions of insulin to cause the excretion of K^+ and retention of Na^+ were required in Paleolithic times, when the diet was rich in K^+ and poor in NaCl. This control mechanism may provide an explanation for the edema that may develop in conditions in which insulin is given or is released in subjects who have a deficit of NaCl in their body in modern times (e.g., when refeeding begins after prolonged fasting). Conversely, insulin does not lead to continuing retention of NaCl in subjects consuming a typical Western diet with its abundant quantity of NaCl. There is a parallel here to the *escape from chronic high aldosterone levels,* in which once aldosterone leads to expansion of the effective arterial blood volume, the kidneys do not continue to retain Na^+ despite the continued actions of aldosterone. Notwithstanding, retention of Na^+ does occur in a very small subgroup of patients with diabetes mellitus who eat a diet with abundant NaCl after they are treated with insulin (*see margin note*).

"INSULIN EDEMA" IN PATIENTS WITH DIABETES MELLITUS
There are a number of case reports, mainly from Japan, that have described the association between edema and administration of insulin in patients with a mitochondrial DNA mutation that results in a single amino acid substitution. Of interest, the patients seem to benefit from therapy with coenzyme Q.

RENAL GLUCOSURIA

- Failure to reabsorb all the filtered glucose will lead to a loss of more than half of the glucose that is ingested each day.
- Isolated renal glucosuria is a benign condition that is rarely a clinical problem.
- The diagnosis is often made when the urine is tested for sugar in a routine examination.

RENAL GLUCOSURIA
This topic is discussed because inhibitors of renal glucose reabsorption may be used in the future to lower the $P_{Glucose}$ in patients with diabetes mellitus.

In normal subjects, virtually all of the glucose that is filtered is reabsorbed in the proximal convoluted tubule. Two transport systems are involved in this process: one on the luminal membrane and another on the basolateral membrane.

Luminal transport of glucose

The luminal transport system for glucose in the proximal convoluted tubule consists of two different active Na^+-linked glucose transporters (SLGTs) that act in tandem. The one that carries out the bulk of the glucose reabsorption, SLGT2, is located in the early portion of the proximal convoluted tubule; it transports 1 Na^+/glucose (*see margin note*). It has a low affinity for glucose, but it has a high capacity to reabsorb glucose. The second luminal transporter, SLGT1, is located later in the proximal convoluted tubule; its function is to reabsorb the remaining luminal glucose and galactose. It has a different stoichiometry in that it requires 2 Na^+/glucose. Of interest, the important transporter for glucose absorption in the small intestine is SLGT1.

NOMENCLATURE USED FOR Na^+-LINKED GLUCOSE TRANSPORTER
Unfortunately, the numbers do *not* reflect the stoichiometry of the SLGT.

Quantities

> • The filtered load of glucose is ~180 g/day (~1000 mmol/day) in an adult with a GFR of 180 L/day.

The filtered load of glucose (180 g/day) is equivalent to close to two thirds of the daily intake of carbohydrate (270 g/day or 1500 mmol/day) in a 70-kg adult eating a typical Western diet. Nevertheless, 90 mg/dL (5 mmol/L) for the $P_{Glucose}$ is not a constant value throughout the day; it is higher after meals and lower between meals. These high values for glucose excretion were observed in patients with a mutation that completely inactivated SLGT2 (called *type 0*, a truncating mutation); somewhat lower rates of excretion of glucose were observed when the mutation simply decreased the amount of SLGT2.

Clinical features

The main complaint in these patients is nocturia due to the glucose-induced osmotic diuresis. If 150 g of glucose per day were excreted, the urine volume resulting from this osmotic load is close to 3 L because each liter of osmotic diuresis contains close to 50 g of glucose (~300 mOsm). In fact, most of these patients actually excrete considerably less than 150 g of glucose per day.

Basolateral transport of glucose

The exit step for glucose on the basolateral membrane is not linked to Na^+ (the transporter is called *GLUT2*). This transporter is passive and simply requires a higher concentration of glucose in the cell compared with the ECF compartment. This GLUT2 is also located in the liver cell membranes and in β-cells of the pancreatic islets of Langerhans. Thus, there are other problems in addition to glucosuria in patients who have defective GLUT2.

Liver

There is a slower uptake of glucose in the liver after meals, and hyperglycemia can be present in the fed state. In contrast, there can be a slower output of glucose from the liver in the fasting state, and this can lead to hypoglycemia between meals.

β-cells of the pancreas

There is an inability to recognize a high $P_{Glucose}$. Therefore, there is an impaired release of insulin after meals, leading to diabetes mellitus.

Kidneys

In cells of the proximal convoluted tubule, there is a very high concentration of glucose, and this leads to an accumulation of glycogen. Over time, these proximal convoluted tubular cells fail to carry out many of their usual functions. As a result, a clinical picture of Fanconi syndrome develops; another name for this disorder is *Fanconi-Bickel syndrome*.

DISCUSSION OF CASES

CASE 16-1: AND I THOUGHT WATER WAS GOOD FOR ME!

(Case presented on page 544)

What is the basis of the polyuria?

The U_{Osm} of 450 mOsm/kg H_2O indicates that this is an osmotic diuresis. Because her $P_{Glucose}$ was 1260 mg/dL (70 mmol/L) and her GFR was only modestly low, this is a glucose-induced osmotic diuresis. This was confirmed because the $U_{Glucose}$ was 320 mmol/L.

How can the effective arterial blood volume and the $P_{Effective\ osm}$ be defended during therapy?

Effective arterial blood volume

To avoid hemodynamic instability, ongoing losses of Na^+ in the urine must be replaced. Because the high $P_{Glucose}$ helped to maintain the ECF volume, the loss of *this portion of the glucose* in the urine should be replaced with NaCl. Hence, one needs to replace the effective osmoles (Na^+, Cl^-, and glucose) excreted in the urine in the early few hours of therapy. If her ECF volume is 8 L, the Na^+ content in her ECF compartment would be reduced by 400 mmol (1400 mmol − [8 × 125 mmol/L]). Not all of this Na^+ deficit must be replaced, however, because there may have been a shift of Na^+ into cells. Giving KCl restores this component of the deficit of Na^+ the ECF volume.

$P_{Effective\ osm}$

> • By infusing fluid with the same effective osmolality as the urine, a fall in the $P_{Effective\ osm}$ could be prevented. Nevertheless, a fall in the $P_{Effective\ osm}$ may occur if a large volume of hypotonic fluid is absorbed from the GI tract.

The goal is to prevent a fall in the $P_{Effective\ osm}$ ($P_{Glucose}$ + 2 P_{Na}) in the first 10 to 15 hours to avoid inducing ICF volume expansion and, as a result, brain cell swelling (see Fig. 5-9, page 130). If the rise in P_{Na} is half the fall in the $P_{Glucose}$, the $P_{Effective\ osm}$ will be maintained. To achieve this, the effective osmolality of the infusate should be equal to that of the urine in a polyuric state.

Why did her $P_{Glucose}$ fail to fall in the first 100 minutes?

The answer is simply a matter of balance.

Output

The major output of glucose is in the urine in a patient with a very high $P_{Glucose}$ and a reasonable GFR. Because the urine volume and the likely concentration of glucose in each liter of osmotic diuresis are known, the loss of glucose in the urine can be calculated (i.e., 350 mmol/L × 1 L of urine in the first 100 minutes). Conversion of glucose to its metabolic products, glycogen and CO_2, should be very low in this setting.

• These cases are presented to emphasize the effects of drinking fruit juice on the clinical and laboratory findings in patients with diabetes mellitus in poor control.

• Case 16-1 illustrates two main points: the importance of both stomach emptying and a recent change in the composition of ingested fluid.

INPUT OF GLUCOSE

- Although entry of glucose into its pool can be from endogenous sources, these can be dismissed in this case because of the low rate of gluconeogenesis (as deduced from the low rate of appearance of urea) and that there was a small quantity of glycogen in the liver.
- Although there is a large quantity of glycogen in skeletal muscle (~500 g in a 70-kg adult), it cannot be released as glucose because skeletal muscles lack the necessary enzyme (glucose-6-phosphatase) to do so. From a Paleolithic perspective, muscle glycogen is "reserved" because this permitted our starved ancestors to sprint and obtain food for survival.
- This patient needed a large reservoir of glucose—most likely glucose that was retained in her stomach—and a very rapid rate of gastric emptying to permit this high glucose input. This is unusual because gastric emptying is usually slow in patients with hyperglycemia.

Input

There are two sources to examine (*see margin note*). The first source of glucose is that which can be made from glycogen or from protein in the body. Because glycogen stores in the liver are very low and there was no huge increase in urea appearance, there is only a minor endogenous input of glucose. The second source of glucose is the glucose stored in the stomach of the patient, and this amount can be very large. Therefore, our best guess is that this patient had some gastric emptying and fortuitously, the amount was similar to the quantity of glucose lost in the urine. Because there was no change in the P_{Na}, there was probably an input of close to 1 L of water along with this glucose and this replaced the 1 L of water that was excreted in the urine.

Why did the $P_{Glucose}$ and the $P_{Effective\ osm}$ fall in the second 100 minutes?

The first step is to examine the balance for water. The patient was given 1 L of water with 150 mmol NaCl (isotonic saline) and excreted 1 L of urine. Thus, there appears to be external water balance. Again, we turn to the $P_{Glucose}$ for an additional clue. The fall in the $P_{Glucose}$ was consistent with the amount excreted, and this suggests that there was little glucose absorbed from the GI tract in the second 100 minutes. Notwithstanding, the P_{Na} should rise if this is a complete description of the events (positive balance of 100 mmol of Na^+ [input of 150 mmol − output of 50 mmol in the urine] and nil balance for water). Because the P_{Na} actually fell by 3 mmol/L, there must be an occult gain of water that prevented the rise in the P_{Na}. Recall that the patient changed her intake from fruit juice to water in the emergency department.

Implications for the risk of developing cerebral edema

- These observations might be important to understand how cerebral edema may occur prior to therapy in young patients with DKA.
- In fact, close to 5% of patients who develop cerebral edema do so before therapy begins.

The volume of the ICF compartment rises if the $P_{Effective\ osm}$ declines while the number of effective osmoles in the ICF compartment remains largely unchanged. In the second 100 minutes, her calculated $P_{Effective\ osm}$ fell from 320 to 281 mOsm/kg H_2O (2 × P_{Na} of 123 mmol/L + 35 mmol of glucose/L) as she changed her intake from fruit juice, which contained the effective osmole glucose, to water. Hence, brain cell swelling is now a threat to the patient, and death may result from herniation of the brain through the foramen magnum.

In what way did a severe degree of hyperglycemia "help" this patient?

- This degree of hyperglycemia helped her maintain an adequate circulating volume!
- The extra glucose in the ECF compartment is 520 mmol; this must be replaced with 260 mmol of NaCl to prevent a fall in the ECF volume.

A quantitative assessment of her ECF volume is needed to illustrate this point. Fortunately, her hematocrit was measured. Her plasma volume was 2.4 L, a decrease of close to 20% (*see margin note*). Thus, her ECF volume was likely decreased by 20% to 8 L. With an ECF volume of 8 L, she had an extra 520 mmol of glucose in her ECF compartment ($[70 - 5 \text{ mmol/L}] \times 8 \text{ L}$). With a $P_{\text{Effective osm}}$ of 320 mOsm/L, this degree of hyperglycemia would be responsible for maintaining close to 1.6 L (out of 8 L) in her ECF compartment (520 mosmol/320 mOsm/L). Beware; the loss of *this glucose* in the urine represents the loss of ECF volume. To maintain hemodynamic stability, this volume of urine needs to be replaced with a solution that contains other effective ECF osmoles (i.e., NaCl).

"Take home" messages concerning this case

> - This fall in the $P_{\text{Effective osm}}$ could have occurred without the clinician knowing about it if the patient had arrived in the emergency department *after* the first 100 minutes. The question is this: *"If all the relevant information were known in a timely fashion in this case, would the reader be persuaded to infuse enough hypertonic saline to return the $P_{Effective\ osm}$ to its original value?"* In retrospect, the authors would have raised the $P_{\text{Effective osm}}$ by giving this patient hypertonic saline based on these data.
> - This process of "occult entry of water into the body" may place the patient at risk for cerebral edema *any time* in the course of therapy for DKA. Accordingly, in our opinion, a careful history concerning oral intake prior to arrival in the hospital is mandatory (*see margin note*).

CASE 16-2: I AM NOT "JUICED UP"

(Case presented on page 545)

Why did she have such a severe degree of acidemia, a P_{Glucose} that was not very high, a modest degree of contraction of the effective arterial blood volume, and a lower than expected P_K?

The modest degree of hyperglycemia suggests a low input of glucose. This could be the result of consuming a smaller amount of glucose-containing drinks.

The major fate of ingested glucose is its excretion in the urine when the P_{Glucose} is greater than 10 mmol/L (180 mg/dL); during glucosuria, there is an obligatory loss of Na^+ and Cl^- in the urine. Thus, there should be a major loss of Na^+ when there is a large osmotic diuresis. A quantitative assessment of the ECF volume using the hematocrit (0.45) reveals that the plasma volume is reduced by close to 20% before therapy began and hence her ECF volume is probably also decreased by close to 20%. In support of a modest degree of contraction of her effective arterial blood volume, the P_{CO_2} in the brachial vein is only 3 mm Hg higher than the P_{CO_2} in the arterial blood. Because there was not a large deficit of NaCl in this child, it appears she did not have a large osmotic diuresis because there was a low intake of glucose.

In summary, the relatively small rise in the P_{Glucose} reflects a small exogenous intake of glucose. Hence, it does not imply that the metabolic lesion causing the DKA was less severe. One should consider the

QUANTITATIVE ESTIMATE OF THE EXTRACELLULAR FLUID VOLUME
The hematocrit was 0.45, and we assume that her normal blood volume is 5 L, red blood cell (RBC) volume is 2 L, and the plasma volume is 3 L.

$$0.45 = 2 \text{ L RBC volume} \div X \text{ L blood volume}$$
$$X = 4.4 \text{ L}$$
Plasma volume = (4.4 L − 2.0 L RBC) = 2.4 L

Hence, her plasma volume was reduced by close to 20%, and by inference, so was her ECF volume.

FALL IN THE $P_{\text{Effective osm}}$ WHEN FRUIT JUICE IS INGESTED
If this is absorbed when fatty acid and ketoacid anion levels are low due to actions of insulin, the glucose will be oxidized, leaving the water behind.

NOTE
- This case illustrates the effects of a low intake of fruit juice in a patient with a severe degree of acidemia during DKA.
- The features are summarized in Figure 16-9.

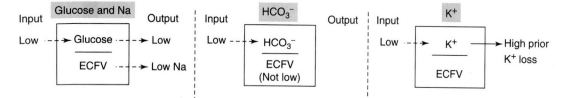

FIGURE 16-9 Balances when there is a low intake of fruit juice in a patient with diabetic ketoacidosis. One liter of fruit juice contains close to 750 mmol of glucose plus fructose after digestion, and it also contains 50 mmol of K^+ and a similar quantity of potential HCO_3^- in the form of organic anions such as citrate. Citrate is converted to HCO_3^- in a single pass through the intestinal and hepatic cells. The *dashed arrows* indicate low fluxes and the *solid arrows* indicate high fluxes. As shown on the *left*, the low intake of fruit juice could lead to a relatively lower $P_{Glucose}$, less osmotic diuresis, and a smaller deficit of Na^+ and can therefore lead to a smaller decline in the extracellular fluid volume (ECFV). As shown in the *center*, the low intake of fruit juice could lead to a low P_{HCO_3} because of both a smaller content of HCO_3^- and a smaller degree of contraction of ECFV. As shown on the *right*, the low intake of fruit juice could lead to a low P_K, primarily as a result of the smaller intake of K^+ and loss of K^+ in the urine prior to arrival in the hospital.

composition of fruit juice and think about the implications of the low intake of fruit juice, with its sugar, K^+, and potential HCO_3^-, for the findings in this patient (Fig. 16-9).

The very low P_{HCO_3} on admission

Because the arterial P_{CO_2} is in the expected range, the acidemia in this patient reflects the balance between processes that cause a disappearance of HCO_3^- and those that add HCO_3^- to the body. The rate of production of ketoacids is increased when there are low net insulin actions. To have very high rates, one needs an increased delivery of fatty acids to the liver and "permission" to have a larger availability of the cofactors ADP and NAD^+ in the liver (see Chapter 5, page 116 for more discussion). Nevertheless, unless there was an ingestion of a large quantity of an uncoupler of oxidative phosphorylation (e.g., high dose of aspirin), one would be hard pressed to find support for an unusually high rate of production of ketoacids.

In addition, because the brain and the kidneys remove ketoacids in patients with DKA, and there is no evidence for reduced function of the brain (sedation, coma) or the kidneys ($P_{Creatinine}$ is only 0.6 mg/dL), we must look for a different reason for the severe degree of acidemia. In this context, there is no evidence of an excessive loss of $NaHCO_3$ via the GI tract and no evidence of prior renal disease (renal tubular acidosis). The most likely cause of the severe degree of acidemia is a low ingestion of HCO_3^- or potential HCO_3^-. Consistent with this impression is the fact that the patient did not consume a large amount of fruit juice.

The severe degree of acidemia is surprisingly well tolerated in this patient, and this suggests that the majority of the H^+ load is buffered by HCO_3^- in skeletal muscle. Key to this interpretation is the low brachial venous P_{CO_2}, because this reflects the P_{CO_2} in capillaries draining skeletal muscle. This P_{CO_2} is in equilibrium with the bicarbonate buffer system in the ECF and ICF compartments in this organ. In addition, the modest degree of contraction of the effective arterial blood volume should permit continued autoregulated blood flow to the brain and thereby minimize H^+ binding to neuronal proteins.

The very low P_K on admission

There is a lower than expected P_K on admission in this patient (who also has a low rate of excretion of K^+ prior to therapy; see Fig. 16-9). This, too, suggests a lower intake of K^+ than in other patients with DKA. For completeness, we should also consider a possible shift of K^+ into cells. One potential mechanism is a high β_2-adrenergic surge, because this hormone activates the Na-K-ATPase in the cell membrane of skeletal muscle cells (see Chapter 13, page 432 for more discussion). It is possible that the air hunger due to the very severe acidemia has led to an unusually high adrenergic drive, and this may have increased the shift of K^+ into muscle cells. Of note, if insulin is given before K^+ replacement and if $NaHCO_3$ is administered, there may be a large fall in the P_K due to a shift of K^+ into cells, which may lead to a cardiac arrhythmia (*see margin note*).

INITIAL THERAPY IN THIS PATIENT
- The first step is to assess threats to life.
- *Acute fall in P_K:* Since there is a risk of developing a dangerous degree of hypokalemia, add KCl (40 mmol/L) to the initial IV fluid.
- *Severe acidemia:* There are two competing issues: the severe acidemia and the danger of inducing a dangerous fall in the P_K. Therefore, we would add 40 mmol of $NaHCO_3$ plus the 40 mmol KCl to the initial IV fluids.
- Because of the risk associated with this fall in P_K, we would delay administering insulin until the P_K is in a safe range (i.e., 4 mmol/L).
- Further decisions will depend on the P_K and the P_{HCO3} plus the clinical status after 1 hour of therapy.

DISCUSSION OF QUESTIONS

16-1 *If a patient with diabetes mellitus in poor control has GI bleeding and digests and absorbs all the protein in 1 L of blood, how much extra glucose and urea are produced?*

Only 60% of the weight of protein can be converted to glucose. In 1 L of blood, there is 140 g of hemoglobin in red blood cells and 70 g of protein in plasma. Thus, there are 210 g of protein, which may be converted to 126 g of glucose. Because the molecular weight of glucose is 180, 700 mmol of glucose would be formed. This can drive the excretion of 2 L of urine because of the glucose-induced osmotic diuresis.

Because one sixth of the protein is nitrogen, the 210 g of protein contains 35 g of nitrogen. Each mmol of urea has 28 mg of nitrogen. Therefore, 1250 mmol of urea will be formed.

16-2 *A patient presented to the hospital with DKA; the initial $P_{Glucose}$ was 60 mmol/L (1080 mg/dL) and the P_{Na} was 140 mmol/L ($P_{Effective\ osm}$ 340 mOsm/L). After 48 hours of therapy, the $P_{Glucose}$ was 15 mmol/L (270 mg/dL) and the P_{Na} was 160 mmol/L ($P_{Effective\ osm}$ 335 mOsm/L). Over the next 6 hours, the $P_{Glucose}$ fell to 10 mmol/L (180 mg/dL) and his P_{Na} declined to 140 mmol/L. Of note, the patient did not drink or receive hypotonic fluids. Why did his P_{Na} decline over this time period and what are the implications for therapy?*

- For the P_{Na} to fall, there must be an addition of water to the ECF compartment and/or a decrease in the content of Na^+ in this compartment.

Gain of water: If the patient has access to water or was given ice chips and/or hypotonic saline, the P_{Na} can fall because of a positive balance for water. These sources of water were not present in this patient. Hence, the focus should now be on the loss of hypertonic saline in the urine.

Negative balance for Na^+: The urine should be maximally concentrated, because the patient does not have diabetes insipidus and hypernatremia is a powerful stimulus for the secretion of vasopressin. In fact, the U_{Na} rose from 50 mmol/L to 265 mmol/L, whereas the U_{Osm} did not change appreciably. In more detail, in earlier urines during the glucose-induced osmotic diuresis, the major urine osmole was glucose; hence the concentration of Na^+ in the urine was low (typically in the 40- to 50-mmol/L range). Later on, because the patient was not very hyperglycemic, there was virtually no glucose in the urine. In addition, this patient, like almost every patient treated for DKA, has been given far too much Na^+ and Cl^-; therefore, he had a major stimulus to excrete a large quantity of Na^+ and Cl^-. In the presence of vasopressin and a normal renal medulla, he was producing large volumes of urine that had a very high concentration of Na^+. As a result, this, on its own, could have caused a major decline in his P_{Na}.

The issue to be considered at this point is whether this 20 mmol/L fall in the P_{Na} in a period of 6 hours (160 mmol/L to 140 mmol/L) will harm the brain. There are three reasons why this may be dangerous. First, the brain on presentation is swollen in other young patients with DKA, despite the fact that the ECF volume was contracted and the $P_{Effective\ osm}$ was high (340 mOsm/kg H_2O) on admission. There are no data to know how long it will take for this swelling of the brain to resolve. Second, it is possible that brain cells have adapted over the close to 30-hour exposure to a high P_{Na} and have imported new effective osmoles to reexpand their ICF volume. Third, one cannot be certain about how much fluid is still in the stomach of this patient and what its composition is. It is important to recognize that the levels of fatty acids and ketoacid anions in plasma are no longer elevated owing to actions of insulin (this is likely to occur 5 to 15 hours after insulin was administered). If the stomach were to contract and its contents entered the intestinal tract and absorption occurred in this period, the glucose could be oxidized and/or converted to glycogen and the water would be left in the body. As a result, the P_{Na} and the $P_{Effective\ osm}$ may fall and cause life-threatening cerebral edema.

Options for therapy: The authors would elect to raise his P_{Na} by 10 mmol/L to 150 mmol/L with hypertonic saline now to minimize the risk of developing brain herniation. We would keep the P_{Na} in this area for about 12 hours and then lower the P_{Na} to 140 mmol/L over the subsequent 24 hours.

Suggested Readings

ACID BASE

A broad view of integrative physiology with an emphasis on acid base

Brosnan ME, Brosnan JT: Renal arginine metabolism. J Nutrition 134:S2791–S2795, 2004.

Davids MR, Edoute Y, Jungas RL, et al: Facilitating an understanding of integrative physiology: emphasis on the composition of body fluid compartments. Can J Physiol Pharmacol 80:835–850, 2002.

Kamel KS, Lin S-H, Cheema-Dhadli S, et al: Prolonged total fasting: a feast for the integrative physiologist. Kidney Int 53:531–539, 1998.

Role of H+ in the production of ATP and uncoupling of oxidative phosphorylation

Brand MD, Esteves TC: Physiological functions of the mitochondrial uncoupling proteins UCP2 and UCP3. Cell Metab 2:85–93, 2005.

Buffering of an acid load by the bicarbonate buffer system

Gowrishankar M, Kamel KS, Halperin ML: Buffering of a H+ load: a 'brain-protein-centered' view. J Amer Soc Nephrol 18:2278–2280, 2007.

Acid balance

Halperin ML, Jungas RL: Metabolic production and renal disposal of hydrogen ions. Kidney Int 24:709–713, 1983.

Kamel KS, Cheema-Dhadli S, Shafiee MA, et al: Dogmas and conundrums for the excretion of nitrogenous wastes in human subjects. J Exp Biol 207:1985–1991, 2004.

Base balance

Cheema-Dhadli S, Lin S-H, Halperin ML: Mechanisms used to dispose of a progressively increasing alkali load in the rat. Am J Physiol 282:F1049–F1055, 2002.

Simpson D: Citrate excretion: a window on renal metabolism. Am J Physiol 244:F223–F234, 1983.

Net negative voltage on albumin

Kamel KS, Cheema-Dhadli S, Halperin FA, et al: Anion gap: do the anions restricted to the intravascular space have modifications in their valence? Nephron 73:382–389, 1996.

Synopsis of molecular advances

Fry AC, Karet FE: Inherited renal acidoses. Physiology (Bethesda) 22:202–211, 2007.

Weiner D: The Rh gene family and ammonium transport. Curr Opin Nephrol Hypertens 13:533–540, 2004.

Kidney stones

Evan AP, Lingeman JE, Coe F, et al: Randall's plaque of patients with nephrolithiasis begins in basement membranes of thin loops of Henle. J Clin Invest 111:607–616, 2003.

Kamel KS, Cheema-Dhadli S, Halperin ML: Studies on the pathophysiology of the low urine pH in patients with uric acid stones. Kidney Int 61:988–994, 2002.

Kamel KS, Cheema-Dhadli S, Shafiee MA, et al: Identifying the lesions causing an alkaline urine pH in patients with calcium hydrogen phosphate kidney stones. Nephrol Dial Transplant 21:424–431, 2007.

Clinical approach to the patient with metabolic acidosis

Kamel KS, Halperin ML: An improved approach to the patient with metabolic acidosis: a need for four amendments. Clin Nephrol 65:S76–S85, 2006.

Renal tubular acidosis

Carlisle EJF, Donnelly SM, Vasuvattakul S, et al: Glue-sniffing and distal renal tubular acidosis: sticking to the facts. J Am Soc Nephrol 1:1019–1027, 1991.

Donnelly SM, Kamel KS, Vasuvattakul S, et al: Might distal renal tubular acidosis be a proximal disorder? Am J Kidney Dis 19:272–281, 1992.

Halperin ML, Kamel KS, Ethier JH, et al: What is the underlying defect in patients with isolated, proximal renal tubular acidosis? Am J Nephrol 9:265–268, 1989.

Kaitwatcharachai C, Vasuvattakul S, Yenchitsomanus P, et al: Distal renal tubular acidosis in a patient with Southeast Asian ovalocytosis: possible interpretations of a high urine PCO_2. Am J Kidney Dis 33:1147–1152, 1999.

Kamel KS, Briceno LF, Santos M, et al: A new classification for renal defects in net acid excretion. Am J Kidney Dis 29: 126–136, 1997.

Diabetic ketoacidosis

Atchley D, Loeb R, Richards D Jr, et al: On diabetic ketoacidosis: detailed study of electrolyte balances following the withdrawal and reestablishment of insulin therapy. J Clin Invest 12: 297–326, 1933.

Carlotti A, Bohn D, Halperin M: Importance of timing of risk factors for cerebral oedema during therapy for diabetic ketoacidosis. Arch Dis Child 88:170–173, 2003.

Carlotti AP, St George-Hyslop C, Guerguerian A-M, et al: Occult risk factor for the development of cerebral edema in children with diabetic ketoacidosis: possible role for stomach emptying. Ped Diabetes 10:522–533, 2009.

Edge J, Jakes R, Roy Y: The UK case-control study of cerebral oedema complicating diabetic ketoacidosis in children. Diabetologia 49:2002–2009, 2006.

Glaser N, Barnett P, McCaslin I, et al: Risk factors for cerebral edema in children with diabetic ketoacidosis. N Engl J Med 344:264–269, 2001.

Halperin M, Bohn D, Carlotti ACP, et al: Principles of fluid and electrolyte therapy in patients with diabetes mellitus in poor control. Acta Nephrol 22:1–13, 2008.

Hoorn E, Carlotti ACP, Costa LA, et al: Preventing a drop in effective plasma osmolality to minimize the likelihood of cerebral edema during treatment of children with diabetic ketoacidosis. J Pediatr 150:467–473, 2007.

Toxins and metabolic acidosis

Barceloux DG, Krenzelok EP, Olson K, Watson W: American Academy of Clinical Toxicology Practice Guidelines on the treatment of ethylene glycol poisoning. J Toxicol Clin Toxicol 37:537–560, 1999.

Barceloux DG, Krenzelok EP, Olson K, Watson W: American Academy of Clinical Toxicology Practice Guidelines on the treatment of methanol poisoning. J Toxicol Clin Toxicol 40: 415–446, 2002.

Brent J: Current management of ethylene glycol poisoning. Drugs 61:979–988, 2001.

Oh M, Halperin ML: Toxin-induced metabolic acidosis. In Gennari FJ, Adrogue HJ, Galla JH, Madias NE (eds): Acid-Base Disorders and Their Treatment, Vol 1. Boston, Marcel Decker, 2005, pp 377–409.

Pathophysiology of cholera

Field M: Intestinal transport and the pathophysiology of diarrhea. J Clin Invest 111:931–943, 2003.

Watten RH, Morgan FM, Songkhla YN, et al: Water and electrolyte studies in cholera. J Clin Invest 38:1879–1889, 1959.

Zalunardo N, Lemaire M, Davids MR, et al: Acidosis in a patient with cholera: a need to redefine concepts. QJM 97:681–696, 2004.

Metabolic alkalosis

Kassirer JP, Schwartz WB: The response of normal man to selective depletion of hydrochloric acid. Am J Med 40:10–18, 1996.

Scheich A, Donnelly S, Cheema-Dhadli S, et al: Does saline 'correct' the abnormal mass balance in metabolic alkalosis associated with chloride-depletion in the rat? Clin Invest Med 17: 448–460, 1994.

SODIUM AND WATER

Integrative physiology

Machnik A, Neuhofer W, Titze J: Macrophages regulate salt-dependent volume and blood pressure by a vascular endothelial growth factor-C–dependent buffering mechanism. Nat Med 15, 545–552, 2009.
Schmidt-Nielsen K: Animal Physiology: Adaptation and Environment, 5th ed. Cambridge, Cambridge University Press, 1997.
Ziomber A, Machnik A, Titze J: Sodium-, potassium-, chloride-, and bicarbonate-related effects on blood pressure and electrolyte homeostasis in deoxycorticosterone acetate-treated rats. Am J Physiol Renal Physiol 295:F1752–F1763, 2008.

Classical references

Edelman I, Leibman J: Anatomy of body water and electrolytes. Am J Med 27:256–277, 1959.
Gamble JL, McKhann CF, Butler AM, et al: An economy of water in renal function referable to urea. Am J Physiol 109:139–154, 1934.
Kleinschmidt-DeMasters KB, Norenberg MD: Rapid correction of hyponatremia causes central pontine myelinolysis. Science 211:1068–1070, 1981.
McCance RA: Medical problems in mineral metabolism. III. Experimental human salt deficiency. Lancet 230:823–830, 1936.
Schwartz WB, Bennett W, Curelops S, et al: Syndrome of renal sodium loss and hyponatremia probably resulting from inappropriate secretion of antidiuretic hormone. Am J Med 23: 529–542, 1957.
Watanabe S, Kang D-H, Feng L, et al: Uric acid, hominoid evolution, and the pathogenesis of salt-sensitivity. Hypertension 40:355–360, 2002.
Welt LG, Orloss J, Kydd DM, et al: An example of cellular hyperosmolarity. J Clin Invest 29: 935–939, 1950.

Pediatric issues

Aperia A, Broberger O, Thodenius K, et al: Development of renal control of salt and fluid homeostasis during the first year of life. Acta Paediatr Scand 64:393–398, 1975.
McCance RA: Renal physiology in infancy. Am J Med 9:229–241, 1950.

Physiology

Bhalla V, Hallows KR: Mechanisms of ENaC regulation and clinical implications. J Am Soc Nephrol 19:1845–1854, 2008.
Gowrishankar M, Lenga I, Cheung RY, et al: Minimum urine flow rate during water deprivation: importance of the permeability of urea in the inner medulla. Kidney Int 53:59–66, 1998.
Halperin ML, Kamel KS, Oh MS: Mechanisms to concentrate the urine: an opinion. Curr Opin Nephrol Hypertens 17:416–422, 2008.
Halperin ML, Oh MS, Kamel KS: Integrating effects of aquaporins, vasopressin, distal delivery of filtrate and residual water permeability on the magnitude of a water diuresis. Nephron 114:11–17, 2010.
Lassiter WE, Gottschalk CW, Mylle M: Micropuncture study of net transtubular movement of water and urea in non-diuretic mammalian kidney. Am J Physiol 200:1139–1146, 1961.
Nielsen S, Frokiaer J, Marples D, et al: Aquaporins in the kidney: from molecules to medicine. Physiol Rev 82:205–244, 2002.
Nofziger C, Blazer-Yost R: PPARγ agonists, modulation of ion transporters, and fluid retention. J Am Soc Nephrol 20:2481–2483, 2009.
Robertson GL. Thirst and vasopressin. In Alpern R, Hebert SC (eds): The Kidney, 4th ed, Vol 1. New York, Raven Press, 2008, pp 1143–1123.
Sands JM, Knepper MA: Urea permeability of mammalian inner medullary collecting duct system and papillary surface epithelium. J Clin Invest 79:138–147, 1987.
Shafiee MA, Charest AF, Cheema-Dhadli S, et al: Defining conditions that lead to the retention of water: the importance of the arterial sodium concentration. Kidney Int 67:613–621, 2005.
Zhai X, Fenton R, Andreasen A, et al: Aquaporin-1 is not expressed in descending thin limbs of short-loop nephrons. J Am Soc Nephrol 18:2937–2944, 2007.

Molecular advances

Feldman BJ, Rosenthal S, Vargas GA, et al: Nephrogenic syndrome of inappropriate antidiuresis. N Engl J Med 352:1884–1890, 2005.
Hebert SC: Extracellular calcium-sensing receptor: implications for calcium and magnesium handling in the kidney. Kidney Int 50: 2129–2139, 1996.
Lifton RP: Genetic dissection of human blood pressure variation: common pathways from rare phenotypes. Harvey Lect 100:71–101, 2004–2005.
Luft FC: Mendelian forms of human hypertension and mechanism of disease. Clin Med Res 1:291–300, 2003.

Ring AM, Leng O, Reinhart J: An SGK1 site in WNK4 regulates Na$^+$ channel and K$^+$ channel activity and has implications for aldosterone signaling and K$^+$ homeostasis. Proc Nat Acad Sci U S A 104:4025–4029, 2007.

Scheinman SJ, Guay-Woodford LM, Thakker RV, et al: Genetic disorders of renal electrolyte transport. N Engl J Med 340:1177–1187, 1999.

Zhou B, Zhuang J, Gu D, et al: WNK4 enhances the degradation of NCC through a sortilin-mediated lysosomal pathway. J Am Soc Nephrol 21:82–92, 2010.

Hyponatremia: Clinical tools

Carlotti AP, Bohn D, Mallie J-P, Halperin ML: Tonicity balance and not electrolyte-free water calculations more accurately guide therapy for acute changes in natremia. Intensive Care Med 27:921–924, 2001.

Hyponatremia: Clinical assessment of the ECF volume

Chung HM, Kluge R, Schrier RW: Clinical assessment of extracellular fluid volume in hyponatremia. Am J Med 83:905–908, 1987.

Maesaka, J, Fishbane S: Regulation of renal urate excretion: a critical review. Am J Kidney Dis 32:917–933, 1998.

McGee S, Abernethy WB, Simel DL: Is this patient hypovolemic? JAMA 17:1022–1029, 1999.

Napolova O, Urbach S, Davids MR, et al: How to assess the degree of extracellular fluid volume contraction in a patient with a severe degree of hyperglycemia. Nephrol Dial Trans 18: 2674–2677, 2003.

Hyponatremia: Acute

Bohn D, Davids MR, Friedman O, et al: Acute and fatal hyponatraemia after resection of a craniopharyngioma: a preventable tragedy. QJM 98:691–704, 2005.

Cherney DZI, Davids MR, Halperin ML: Acute hyponatraemia and MDMA ("Ecstasy"): insights from a quantitative and integrative analysis. QJM 95:475–483, 2002.

Rosner M, Kirven J: Exercise-associated hyponatremia. Clin J Am Soc Nephrol 2:151–161, 2007.

Hyponatremia: Chronic

Anderson RJ: Hospital associated hyponatremia. Kidney Int 29:1237–1247, 1986.

Berl T: Treating hyponatremia: damned if we do and damned if we don't. Kidney Int 37: 1006–1018, 1990.

Decaux G, Brimioulle S, Genette F, et al: Treatment of the syndrome of inappropriate secretion of antidiuretic hormone by urea. Am J Med 69:99–106, 1980.

Ellison D, Berl T: The syndrome of inappropriate antidiuresis. N Engl J Med 356:2064–2072, 2005.

Halperin ML, Kamel KS: A new look at an old problem: therapy of chronic hyponatremia. Nat Clin Pract Nephrol 3:1–3, 2007.

Kengne FG, Soupart A, Pochet R, et al: Re-induction of hyponatraemia after rapid overcorrection of hyponatremia reduces mortality in rats. Kidney Int 76:614–621, 2009.

Lohr JW: Osmotic demyelination syndrome following correction of hyponatremia: association with hypokalemia. Am J Med 96:408–413, 1994.

Oh MS, Kim HJ, Carroll HJ: Recommendations for the treatment of chronic hyponatremia. Nephron 70:143–150, 1995.

Sterns RH: Severe symptomatic hyponatremia: treatment and outcome. A study of 64 cases. Ann Intern Med 107:656–664, 1987.

Sterns RH, Hiks JK: Overcorrection of hyponatremia is a medical emergency. Kidney Int 76: 587–589, 2009.

Verbalis J, Goldsmith S, Greenberg A, et al: Hyponatremia Treatment Guidelines 2007: Expert Panel Recommendations. Am J Med 120:S1–S21, 2007.

Cerebral salt wasting

Harrigan MR: Cerebral salt wasting: a review. Neurosurgery 38:152–160, 1996.

Singh S, Bohn D, Cusimano M, et al: Cerebral salt wasting; truths, fallicies, theories and challenges. Crit Care Med 30:2575–2579, 2002.

Edema states

Abassi ZA, Winaver J, Skorecki KL: Control of extracellular fluid volume and the pathophysiology of edema formation. In Brenner BM (ed): Brenner's & Rector's The Kidney, 7th ed, Vol 1. Philadelphia, WB Saunders, 2003, pp 777–855.

Ehrlich S, Querfeld U, Pfeiffer E: Refeeding oedema. An important complication in the treatment of anorexia nervosa. Eur Child Adolesc Psychiatry 15:241–243, 2006.

Creatinine

Carlotti APCP, Bohn D, Matsuno et al: Indicators of lean body mass catabolism: emphasis on the creatinine excretion rate. QJM 101:197–205, 2008.

Walser M: Creatinine excretion as a measure of protein nutrition in adults of varying age. J Parenter Enter Nutr 11:73S–78S, 1987.

POTASSIUM

Ellison DH: Voltage channel K subunit Kv1.1 links kidney and brain. J Clin Invest 119:763–766, 2009.

Glaudemans B, van der Wijst J, Rosana H, et al: Missense mutation in the Kv1.1 voltage-gated potassium channel-encoding gene KCNA1 is linked to human autosomal dominant hypomagnesemia. J Clin Invest 119:936–942, 2009.

Janssen AGH, Scholl U, Domeyer C, et al: Disease-causing dysfunctions of Barttin in Bartter syndrome IV. J Am Soc Nephrol 20:145–153, 2009.

Integrative physiology

Bockenhauer D, Cruwys M, Kleta R, et al: Antenatal Bartter's syndrome: why is this not a lethal condition? QJM 101:927–942, 2008.

Eaton SB, Konner M: Paleolithic nutrition. N Engl J Med 312:283–289, 1985.

Halperin ML, Kamel KS: Dynamic interactions between integrative physiology and molecular medicine: the key to understand the mechanism of action of aldosterone in the kidney. Can J Physiol Pharm 78:587–594, 2000.

K+ channels

Hebert SC, Desir G, Giebisch G, et al: Molecular diversity and regulation of renal potassium channels. Physiol Rev 85:319–371, 2005.

Landry DW, Oliver JA: The pathogenesis of vasodilatory shock. N Engl J Med 345:588–595, 2001.

WNK kinase system

Huang CL, Yang SS, Lin SH: Mechanism of regulation of renal ion transport by WNK kinases. Curr Opin Nephrol Hypertens 17:519–525, 2008.

Kahle KT, Ring AM, Lifton RP: Molecular physiology of the WNK kinases. Ann Rev Physiol 70:329–355, 2008.

Advances in physiology

Cheema-Dhadli S, Chong C-K, Lin S-H, et al: Control of potassium excretion, a Paleolithic approach. Curr Opin Nephrol Hypertens 15:430–436, 2006.

Cheema-Dhadli S, Lin S-H, Keong-Chong CK, et al: Requirements for a high rate of potassium excretion in rats consuming a low electrolyte diet. J Physiol London 572:493–501, 2006.

Garty H: Regulation of the epithelial Na+ channel by aldosterone: open questions and emerging answers. Kidney Int 57:1270–1276, 2000.

Hadchouel J, Delaloy C, Faure S, et al: Familial hyperkalemic hypertension. J Am Soc Nephrol 17:208–217, 2006.

Halperin ML, Gowrishankar M, Mallie JP, et al: Urea recycling, an aid to the excretion of potassium during antidiuresis. Nephron 72:507–511, 1996.

Diurnal variation in K+ excretion

Moore-Ede MC, Herd JA: Renal electrolyte circadian rhythms: independence from feeding and activity patterns. Am J Physiol 232:F128–F135, 1977.

Steele A, deVeber H, Quaggin SE, et al: What is responsible for the diurnal variation in potassium excretion? Am J Physiol 36:R554–R560, 1994.

Tools to assess the excretion of K+: importance of the recycling of urea

Halperin ML, Kamel KS, Oh MS: Mechanisms to concentrate the urine: an opinion. Curr Opin Nephrol Hypertens 17:416–422, 2008.

Acute shift of K+ into cells

Al-Alazami M, Lin S, Chih-Jen C, Davids M, Halperin M: Unusual causes of hypokalaemia and paralysis. QJM 99: 81–192, 2006.

Lin SH, Lin YF: Propranolol rapidly reverses paralysis, hypokalemia, and hypophosphatemia in thyrotoxic periodic paralysis. Am J Kidney Dis 37:620–624, 2001.

Lin SH, Lin YF, Halperin ML: Hypokalemia and paralysis: Clues on admission to help in the differential diagnosis. QJM 94:133–139, 2001.

Sterns RH, Cox M, Feig PU, et al: Internal potassium balance and the control of the plasma potassium concentration. Medicine 60:339–354, 1981.

Clinical approach

Groeneveld JHM, Sijpkens YWJ, Lin SH, et al: Approach to the patients with a severe degree of hypokalemia: the potassium quiz. QJM 98:305–316, 2005.

Halperin ML, Kamel KS: Potassium. Lancet 352:135–142, 1998.

Treatment of patients with hypokalemia and hyperkalemia

Kamel KS, Oh MS, Lin S-H, Halperin ML: Treatment of hypokalemia and hyperkalemia; a companion to Brenner and Rector's The Kidney. In Wilcox CS, Berl T, Himmelfarb J, et al (eds): Therapy in Nephrology and Hypertension, 3rd ed. Philadelphia, WB Saunders/Elsevier, 2008, pp 353–367.

Kamel KS, Wei C: Controversial issues in treatment of hyperkalemia. Nephrol Dial Transpl 18:2215–2218, 2003.

Schreiber MS, Chen C-B, Lessan-Pezeshki M, et al: Antikaliuretic action of trimethoprim is minimized by raising the urine pH. Kidney Int 49:82–87, 1996.

MAGNESIUM

Knoors NV: Inherited forms of renal hypomagnesemia: an update. Ped Nephrol 26:697–705, 2009.

Martin KG, Gonzalez EA, Slatopolsky E: Clinical consequences and management of hypomagnesemia. J Am Soc Nephrol 20:2291–2295, 2009.

Thebault S, Alexander RT, Woulter M, et al: EGF increases TRPM6 activity and surface expression. J Am Soc Nephrol 20:78–85, 2009.

Tiel WM, Groenestege T, Thebault S, et al: Impaired basolateral sorting of pro-EGF causes isolated recessive renal hypomagnesemia. J Clin Invest 117:2260–2267, 2007.

HYPOXIA

Gleadle J: How cells sense oxygen: lessons from and for the kidney. Nephrology 14:86–93, 2009.

HYPERGLYCEMIA

Biochemistry

Halperin ML, Rolleston FS: Clinical Detective Stories: A Problem-based Approach to Clinical Cases in Energy and Acid-Base Metabolism. London, Portland Press, 1993.

Jungas RL, Halperin ML, Brosnan JT: Lessons learnt from a quantitative analysis of amino acid oxidation and related gluconeogenesis in man. Physiol Rev 72:419–448, 1992.

Physiology

Carlotti APCP, Bohn D, Jankiewicz N, et al: Hyperglycaemic hyperosmolar state in a young child: diagnostic insights from a quantitative analysis. QJM 100:125–137, 2007.

Halperin M, Bohn D, Carlotti ACP, et al: Principles of fluid and electrolyte therapy in patients with diabetes mellitus in poor control. Acta Nephrol 22:1–13, 2008.

West ML, Marsden PA, Singer GG, et al: A quantitative analysis of glucose loss during acute therapy for the hyperglycemia hyperosmolar syndrome. Diabetes Care 9:465–471, 1986.

Acid-base issues

Gowrishankar M, Carlotti APCP, St George-Hyslop C, et al: Uncovering the basis of a severe degree of metabolic acidosis in a patient with diabetic ketoacidosis. QJM 100:721–735, 2007.

Halperin ML, Cherney DZI, Kamel KS: Ketoacidosis. In DuBose TD Jr, Hamm LL (eds): Acid-Base and Electrolyte Disorders: A Companion to Brenner and Rector's, The Kidney. Philadelphia, WB Saunders, 2002, pp 67–82.

Sodium and water issues

Halperin ML, Goguen JM, Scheich AM, et al: Clinical consequences of hyperglycemia and its correction. In Seldin DW, Giebisch G (eds): Clinical Disturbances of Water Metabolism. New York, Raven Press Ltd, 1993, pp 249–272.

Index

Note: Page numbers followed by c indicate flow charts; those followed by f indicate figures; those followed by t indicate tables.